AF581896

Antimicrobial Prescribing and Stewardship, 2nd Volume

Antimicrobial Prescribing and Stewardship, 2nd Volume

Editor

Diane Ashiru-Oredope

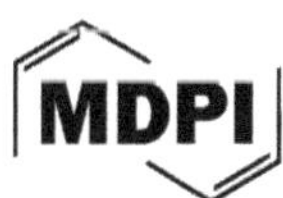

Basel • Beijing • Wuhan • Barcelona • Belgrade • Novi Sad • Cluj • Manchester

Editor
Diane Ashiru-Oredope
School of Pharmacy
University of Nottingham
Nottingham
United Kingdom

Editorial Office
MDPI
St. Alban-Anlage 66
4052 Basel, Switzerland

This is a reprint of articles from the Special Issue published online in the open access journal *Antibiotics* (ISSN 2079-6382) (available at: www.mdpi.com/journal/antibiotics/special_issues/Stewardship_2nd).

For citation purposes, cite each article independently as indicated on the article page online and as indicated below:

Lastname, A.A.; Lastname, B.B. Article Title. *Journal Name* **Year**, *Volume Number*, Page Range.

ISBN 978-3-0365-9209-1 (Hbk)
ISBN 978-3-0365-9208-4 (PDF)
doi.org/10.3390/books978-3-0365-9208-4

© 2023 by the authors. Articles in this book are Open Access and distributed under the Creative Commons Attribution (CC BY) license. The book as a whole is distributed by MDPI under the terms and conditions of the Creative Commons Attribution-NonCommercial-NoDerivs (CC BY-NC-ND) license.

Contents

About the Editor ix

Preface xi

Christopher Kiss, Declan Connoley, Kathryn Connelly, Kylie Horne, Tony Korman and Ian Woolley et al.
Long-Term Outcomes in Patients on Life-Long Antibiotics: A Five-Year Cohort Study
Reprinted from: *Antibiotics* **2022**, *11*, 62, doi:10.3390/antibiotics11010062 1

Xinjun Li, Kristina Sundquist and Filip Jansåker
Fluoroquinolones and Other Antibiotics Redeemed for Cystitis—A Swedish Nationwide Cohort Follow-Up Study (2006–2018)
Reprinted from: *Antibiotics* **2022**, *11*, 172, doi:10.3390/antibiotics11020172 9

Sana M. Mohayya, Navaneeth Narayanan, Daniel Cimilluca, Alexander Malanowski, Parth Vaidya and Tanaya Bhowmick
Effectiveness of an Electronic Automated Antibiotic Time Out Alert in the Setting of Gram-Negative Bacteremia
Reprinted from: *Antibiotics* **2021**, *10*, 1078, doi:10.3390/antibiotics10091078 18

Güzin Surat, Pascal Meyer-Sautter, Jan Rüsch, Johannes Braun-Feldweg, Christoph-Thomas Germer and Johan Friso Lock
Retrospective Cohort Analysis of the Effect of Antimicrobial Stewardship on Postoperative Antibiotic Therapy in Complicated Intra-Abdominal Infections: Short-Course Therapy Does Not Compromise Patients' Safety
Reprinted from: *Antibiotics* **2022**, *11*, 120, doi:10.3390/antibiotics11010120 27

Angel-Orión Salgado-Peralvo, Juan-Francisco Peña-Cardelles, Naresh Kewalramani, Alvaro Garcia-Sanchez, María-Victoria Mateos-Moreno and Eugenio Velasco-Ortega et al.
Is Antibiotic Prophylaxis Necessary before Dental Implant Procedures in Patients with Orthopaedic Prostheses? A Systematic Review
Reprinted from: *Antibiotics* **2022**, *11*, 93, doi:10.3390/antibiotics11010093 37

Catherine V. Hayes, Bláthnaid Mahon, Eirwen Sides, Rosie Allison, Donna M. Lecky and Cliodna A. M. McNulty
Empowering Patients to Self-Manage Common Infections: Qualitative Study Informing the Development of an Evidence-Based Patient Information Leaflet
Reprinted from: *Antibiotics* **2021**, *10*, 1113, doi:10.3390/antibiotics10091113 48

Shweta Khare, Ashish Pathak, Cecilia Stålsby Lundborg, Vishal Diwan and Salla Atkins
Understanding Internal and External Drivers Influencing the Prescribing Behaviour of Informal Healthcare Providers with Emphasis on Antibiotics in Rural India: A Qualitative Study
Reprinted from: *Antibiotics* **2022**, *11*, 459, doi:10.3390/antibiotics11040459 64

Laura M. Hamill, Julia Bonnett, Megan F. Baxter, Melina Kreutz, Kerina J. Denny and Gerben Keijzers
Antimicrobial Prescribing in the Emergency Department; Who Is Calling the Shots?
Reprinted from: *Antibiotics* **2021**, *10*, 843, doi:10.3390/antibiotics10070843 80

Ingrid Christensen, Jon Birger Haug, Dag Berild, Jørgen Vildershøj Bjørnholt, Brita Skodvin and Lars-Petter Jelsness-Jørgensen
Factors Affecting Antibiotic Prescription among Hospital Physicians in a Low-Antimicrobial-Resistance Country: A Qualitative Study
Reprinted from: *Antibiotics* **2022**, *11*, 98, doi:10.3390/antibiotics11010098 . . . . **94**

António Teixeira Rodrigues, João C. F. Nunes, Marta Estrela, Adolfo Figueiras, Fátima Roque and Maria Teresa Herdeiro
Comparing Hospital and Primary Care Physicians' Attitudes and Knowledge Regarding Antibiotic Prescribing: A Survey within the Centre Region of Portugal
Reprinted from: *Antibiotics* **2021**, *10*, 629, doi:10.3390/antibiotics10060629 . . . . **105**

Diane Ashiru-Oredope, Ella Casale, Eleanor Harvey, Eno Umoh, Sagar Vasandani and Jacqui Reilly et al.
Knowledge and Attitudes about Antibiotics and Antibiotic Resistance of 2404 UK Healthcare Workers
Reprinted from: *Antibiotics* **2022**, *11*, 1133, doi:10.3390/antibiotics11081133 . . . . **115**

Maria-Eirini Oikonomou, Despoina Gkentzi, Ageliki Karatza, Sotirios Fouzas, Aggeliki Vervenioti and Gabriel Dimitriou
Parental Knowledge, Attitude, and Practices on Antibiotic Use for Childhood Upper Respiratory Tract Infections during COVID-19 Pandemic in Greece
Reprinted from: *Antibiotics* **2021**, *10*, 802, doi:10.3390/antibiotics10070802 . . . . **129**

Essam M. Abdelfattah, Pius S. Ekong, Emmanuel Okello, Deniece R. Williams, Betsy M. Karle and Terry W. Lehenbauer et al.
Factors Associated with Antimicrobial Stewardship Practices on California Dairies: One Year Post Senate Bill 27
Reprinted from: *Antibiotics* **2022**, *11*, 165, doi:10.3390/antibiotics11020165 . . . . **140**

Nduta Kamere, Sandra Tafadzwa Garwe, Oluwatosin Olugbenga Akinwotu, Chloe Tuck, Eva M. Krockow and Sara Yadav et al.
Scoping Review of National Antimicrobial Stewardship Activities in Eight African Countries and Adaptable Recommendations
Reprinted from: *Antibiotics* **2022**, *11*, 1149, doi:10.3390/antibiotics11091149 . . . . **158**

Omotola Ogunnigbo, Maxencia Nabiryo, Moses Atteh, Eric Muringu, Olatunde James Olaitan and Victoria Rutter et al.
Exploring the Antimicrobial Stewardship Educational Needs of Healthcare Students and the Potential of an Antimicrobial Prescribing App as an Educational Tool in Selected African Countries
Reprinted from: *Antibiotics* **2022**, *11*, 691, doi:10.3390/antibiotics11050691 . . . . **175**

Mark Kizito, Rejani Lalitha, Henry Kajumbula, Ronald Ssenyonga, David Muyanja and Pauline Byakika-Kibwika
Antibiotic Prevalence Study and Factors Influencing Prescription of WHO Watch Category Antibiotic Ceftriaxone in a Tertiary Care Private Not for Profit Hospital in Uganda
Reprinted from: *Antibiotics* **2021**, *10*, 1167, doi:10.3390/antibiotics10101167 . . . . **189**

Reuben Kiggundu, Rachel Wittenauer, JP Waswa, Hilma N. Nakambale, Freddy Eric Kitutu and Marion Murungi et al.
Point Prevalence Survey of Antibiotic Use across 13 Hospitals in Uganda
Reprinted from: *Antibiotics* **2022**, *11*, 199, doi:10.3390/antibiotics11020199 . . . . **199**

Nikki D'Arcy, Diane Ashiru-Oredope, Omotayo Olaoye, Daniel Afriyie, Zainab Akello and Daniel Ankrah et al.
Antibiotic Prescribing Patterns in Ghana, Uganda, Zambia and Tanzania Hospitals: Results from the Global Point Prevalence Survey (G-PPS) on Antimicrobial Use and Stewardship Interventions Implemented
Reprinted from: *Antibiotics* **2021**, *10*, 1122, doi:10.3390/antibiotics10091122 . . . . **220**

Kittiya Jantarathaneewat, Anucha Apisarnthanarak, Wasithep Limvorapitak, David J. Weber and Preecha Montakantikul
Pharmacist-Driven Antibiotic Stewardship Program in Febrile Neutropenic Patients: A Single Site Prospective Study in Thailand
Reprinted from: *Antibiotics* **2021**, *10*, 456, doi:10.3390/antibiotics10040456 . . . . **235**

Federica Calò, Lorenzo Onorato, Margherita Macera, Giovanni Di Caprio, Caterina Monari and Antonio Russo et al.
Impact of an Education-Based Antimicrobial Stewardship Program on the Appropriateness of Antibiotic Prescribing: Results of a Multicenter Observational Study
Reprinted from: *Antibiotics* **2021**, *10*, 314, doi:10.3390/antibiotics10030314 . . . . **244**

Saleh Alghamdi, Ilhem Berrou, Eshtyag Bajnaid, Zoe Aslanpour, Abdul Haseeb and Mohamed Anwar Hammad et al.
Antimicrobial Stewardship Program Implementation in a Saudi Medical City: An Exploratory Case Study
Reprinted from: *Antibiotics* **2021**, *10*, 280, doi:10.3390/antibiotics10030280 . . . . **255**

Diane Ashiru-Oredope, Maxencia Nabiryo, Andy Yeoman, Melvin Bell, Sarah Cavanagh and Nikki D'Arcy et al.
Development of and User Feedback on a Board and Online Game to Educate on Antimicrobial Resistance and Stewardship
Reprinted from: *Antibiotics* **2022**, *11*, 611, doi:10.3390/antibiotics11050611 . . . . **270**

David F. Léger, Maureen E. C. Anderson, François D. Bédard, Theresa Burns, Carolee A. Carson and Anne E. Deckert et al.
Canadian Collaboration to Identify a Minimum Dataset for Antimicrobial Use Surveillance for Policy and Intervention Development across Food Animal Sectors
Reprinted from: *Antibiotics* **2022**, *11*, 226, doi:10.3390/antibiotics11020226 . . . . **284**

Francesca Menegon, Katia Capello, Jacopo Tarakdjian, Dario Pasqualin, Giovanni Cunial and Sara Andreatta et al.
Antibiotic Use in Alpine Dairy Farms and Its Relation to Biosecurity and Animal Welfare
Reprinted from: *Antibiotics* **2022**, *11*, 231, doi:10.3390/antibiotics11020231 . . . . **302**

Xavier Khan, Caroline Rymer, Partha Ray and Rosemary Lim
Categorisation of Antimicrobial Use in Fijian Livestock Production Systems
Reprinted from: *Antibiotics* **2022**, *11*, 294, doi:10.3390/antibiotics11030294 . . . . **311**

About the Editor

Diane Ashiru-Oredope

Professor Diane Ashiru-Oredope PhD FFRPS, FRPharmS is the Lead Pharmacist for healthcare-associated infections (HCAIs) and antimicrobial resistance (AMR) at UK Health Security Agency and is Chair of the English Surveillance Programme for Antimicrobial Utilisation and Resistance (ESPAUR). She is also Honorary Chair and Professor of Pharmaceutical Public Health at the University of Nottingham.

An antimicrobial pharmacist by background, Diane has led several projects that have shaped national and international policy in tackling antimicrobial resistance, including creating the global Antibiotic Guardian campaign in 2014. From 2016 to March 2022, she was advisor and Global AMR lead for the Commonwealth Pharmacists Association. Diane remains research active, with more than 70 peer-reviewed publications, and is one of the editors for BMC Public Health. She recently led the UK-wide evidence review on Pharmaceutical Public Health, commissioned by the four UK Chief Pharmaceutical Officers. In 2022, she was credentialed as a consultant pharmacist through the Royal Pharmaceutical Society's national credentialing and assessment processes. She has been recognised nationally, including through awards, nominations to deliver two TEDx talks, and fellowships with the Royal Pharmaceutical Society (FRPharmS and FFRPS).

Preface

Antimicrobial stewardship, as "a coherent set of actions which promote using antimicrobials in ways that ensure sustainable access to effective therapy for all who need them" (Dyar, O.J.; 2017), is critical (alongside, e.g., infection prevention and control strategies) for tackling antimicrobial resistance/drug-resistant infections. Volume 2 of Antimicrobial Prescribing and Stewardship builds on the success of volume 1 of this Special Issue. This Special Issue consists of manuscripts, including original research articles, review articles, and opinion papers on antimicrobial stewardship-related topics, including:

- Disease-based/organism-based antimicrobial stewardship;
- The influence of antimicrobial utilization changes on antimicrobial resistance;
- The impact of antimicrobial stewardship on quality performance measures and patient outcomes;
- Novel antimicrobial stewardship education and training approaches or interventions aimed toward public and/or healthcare workers;
- Behavioral change approaches to antimicrobial stewardship;
- Collaborative practice agreements in antimicrobial stewardship;
- Antimicrobial stewardship in special populations (e.g., pediatrics, geriatrics, emergency medicine, hematology/oncology);
- Tackling AMR through antimicrobial stewardship in low- and middle-income countries;
- Antimicrobial stewardship for animal health;
- Antimicrobial stewardship in alternative settings (e.g., community practice, long-term care, resource-limited settings, small and rural hospitals);
- Antimicrobial use and stewardship in the context of the COVID-19 pandemic;
- Global collaborations to tackle AMR through antimicrobial stewardship.

Diane Ashiru-Oredope
Editor

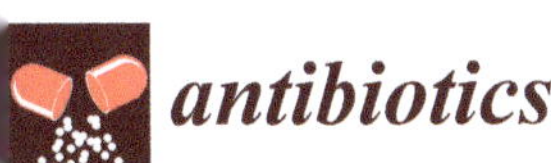
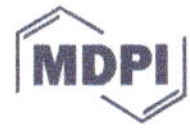
Brief Report

Long-Term Outcomes in Patients on Life-Long Antibiotics: A Five-Year Cohort Study

Christopher Kiss [1], Declan Connoley [1], Kathryn Connelly [1,2], Kylie Horne [1], Tony Korman [1], Ian Woolley [1,2] and Jillian S. Y. Lau [1,2,*]

[1] Monash Infectious Diseases, Monash Medical Centre, Monash Health, Clayton, VIC 3168, Australia; c.r.kiss89@gmail.com (C.K.); declan.connoley@gmail.com (D.C.); kathryn.connelly@monash.edu (K.C.); Kylie.Horne@monashhealth.org (K.H.); tony.korman@monash.edu (T.K.); ian.woolley@monash.edu (I.W.)
[2] Faculty of Medicine, Nursing and Health Sciences, Monash University, Clayton, VIC 3800, Australia
* Correspondence: jillian.lau@monash.edu; Tel.: +61-395944564

Abstract: Background: Little is known about the impacts at an individual level of long-term antibiotic consumption. We explored health outcomes of long-term antibiotic therapy prescribed to a cohort of patients to suppress infections deemed incurable. Methods: We conducted a 5-year longitudinal study of patients on long-term antibiotics at Monash Health, a metropolitan tertiary-level hospital network in Australia. Adults prescribed antibiotics for >12 months to suppress chronic infection or prevent recurrent infection were included. A retrospective review of medical records and a descriptive analysis was conducted. Results: Twenty-seven patients were followed up during the study period, from 29 patients originally identified in Monash Health in 2014. Seven of the 27 patients (26%) died from causes unrelated to the suppressed infection, six (22%) ceased long-term antibiotic therapy and two (7%) required treatment modification. Fifteen (56%) were colonised with multiresistant microorganisms, including vancomycin resistant Enterococci, methicillin resistant *Staphylococcus aureus*, and carbapenem resistant Enterobacteriaciae. Conclusions: This work highlights the potential pitfalls of long-term antibiotic therapy, and the frailty of this cohort, who are often ineligible for definitive curative therapy.

Keywords: antibiotics; life-long; suppression; antimicrobial resistance; multi-resistant organisms

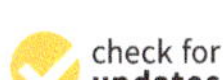

Citation: Kiss, C.; Connoley, D.; Connelly, K.; Horne, K.; Korman, T.; Woolley, I.; Lau, J.S.Y. Long-Term Outcomes in Patients on Life-Long Antibiotics: A Five-Year Cohort Study. *Antibiotics* **2022**, *11*, 62. https://doi.org/10.3390/antibiotics11010062

Academic Editor: Seok Hoon Jeong

Received: 28 November 2021
Accepted: 24 December 2021
Published: 5 January 2022

Publisher's Note: MDPI stays neutral with regard to jurisdictional claims in published maps and institutional affiliations.

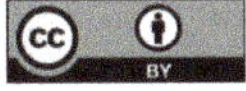

Copyright: © 2022 by the authors. Licensee MDPI, Basel, Switzerland. This article is an open access article distributed under the terms and conditions of the Creative Commons Attribution (CC BY) license (https://creativecommons.org/licenses/by/4.0/).

1. Introduction

Antibiotics were originally developed and then used as short-term therapy for bacterial infections [1]. Evaluation of their utility was thus focused on short term harm and benefits. Subsequent evidence supports specific long-term effective use of certain antibiotics for prophylaxis against infection following transplantation, splenectomy and for recurrent urinary tract infections (UTI) [2], though less evidence supports their use in other settings, such as for infected prosthetic material not amenable to removal and for nonantibacterial effects such as immunomodulation [2]. In this context, the evidence is limited, as is the measurement of the adverse consequences of long-term therapy [3].

Pitfalls associated with long-term antibiotic use include development of antimicrobial resistance (AMR) and cumulative risk of adverse events. AMR is a growing global concern with multiresistant microorganisms (MROs) responsible for greater than 35,000 deaths annually in the United States [4]. Emergence of AMR has been demonstrated after prolonged antibiotic usage in multiple conditions including post-splenectomy, rheumatic fever and UTI prophylaxis [2].

We previously reviewed antibiotic prescribing practices at Monash Health, a large tertiary-level, university-affiliated health service in Melbourne, Australia, and found that long-term antibiotic therapy made up only a small proportion (202/66,127, 0.3%) of total prescriptions, with great heterogeneity in indication for use [5]. Long-term therapy was defined as an intended treatment course of greater than 12 months. Out of the 202 patients on long-term antibiotic therapy identified in this previous study, 29 patients were prescribed this therapy for infections deemed incurable [3,5]. We looked more closely at this cohort of 29 patients and found one in five patients screened to be colonised with multiresistant microorganisms (MROs) including vancomycin resistant Enterococci (VRE) and methicillin resistant *Staphylococcus aureus* (MRSA) [3]. Furthermore, nearly half of the patients in this cohort described adverse drug reactions (ADRs) attributable to long-term antibiotic consumption [3].

Despite being a recognised treatment strategy [2], there is limited information on the outcomes in patients who are prescribed long-term antibiotics for suppression of infections deemed otherwise uncurable. The aim of this study was to describe the impact of long-term antibiotic use on health outcomes in this cohort of patients originally identified in 2015, and explore issues such as tolerance of therapy, treatment modification, adverse events and colonisation with MROs.

2. Results

2.1. Patient Demographics

Of the 29 patients originally identified in our previous study [3], two had no follow-up through our institution and were excluded from this analysis. Baseline demographics and clinical information for the 27 eligible patients are presented in Table 1. The median age was 73 (range of 47–93). Fourteen (52%) were female. Fifteen different antibiotic regimens were used, with combination rifampicin and fusidic acid (6/27, 22%), and cefalexin monotherapy (6/27, 22%) prescribed most commonly. Indications for long-term antibiotic prescriptions were diverse, the most frequent being prosthetic joint infection (PJI) (15/27, 56%), vascular graft infection (VGI) (3/27, 11%), and recurrent *Staphylococcus aureus* bacteraemia (3/27, 11%). The Charlson Comorbidity Index (CCI) increased over the study period from 5 (median, range 1–13, interquartile range 3–7) at baseline, to 7 (median, range 1–13, interquartile range of 4–9) by the end of follow-up.

2.2. Patient Outcomes

Patient outcomes are summarised in Figure 1. At the conclusion of the study period seven patients had died (26%), two of whom died from infection, (not the original suppressed infection). No deaths were attributed to treatment-related adverse drug reactions. Six patients (22%) ceased long-term antibiotic therapy: three completed their therapy, two ceased because of adverse drug reactions including acute kidney injury (AKI) and vaginal thrush, and one patient ceased therapy due to anticipated drug interactions with new medications. These six patients had previously taken prolonged antibiotics for between 2 to 10 years. They were followed up for between 3 months and 2 years following cessation of antibiotics prior to discharge from clinic. Four had prosthetic joint infections and had further surgery (two had joint revision surgery, one had washout/liner exchange, one had joint arthroscopy without washout). All six were discharged from infectious diseases (ID) outpatient follow-up and have not had any relapse of their suppressed infection.

2.3. Follow Up

Of the 14 patients who had remained on long-term antibiotic therapy (52%), eight had been discharged from ID without any plan to cease therapy, tolerating their regimen without issue. Three of these eight were discharged with no further input from our healthcare network. The other five were followed up by specialty units within the network including orthopaedics, cardiology and haematology, and are clinically stable. Of the six patients with ongoing follow-up, three are reviewed annually, two reviewed six-monthly, and one every three months. Two patients had modifications to their regimen, one because of diarrhea, and another because a new organism was identified in a subsequent surgical procedure. Four patients remained on their initial regimen and continue to attend ID outpatients.

Table 1. Patient characteristics.

Age	Sex	Antibiotic Regimen	Indication	Targeted Organism/s	Charlson Comorbidity Index Baseline	End	MRO—Isolate Site	Cause of Death	Hospital Admission Days (Total/Infection Related/ICU)	Ongoing ID Follow Up	Duration of Follow Up (Years)	Regimen Adjust-ment/Reason	Adverse Drug Reactions ^
70	M	Amoxycillin	PVI	*E. faecalis*	13	13	ESBL *E. coli*—Urine	Lung Cancer	13/7/0	N/A	5 months	N/A	
76	F	Rifampicin, Fusidic Acid, Pristi-namycin	Chronic hip osteomyelitis (OM)	MRSA	3	7	MRSA—hip tissue VRE—Screening swab	Unknown (coroner's case)	109/64/5	N/A	7	N/A	
79	M	amoxicillin/ clavulanic acid, Ciprofloxacin	PJI	*S. marcescens*	11	12	VRE—Screening swab	Heart failure	64/30/0	N/A	4	Ceased amoxi-cillin/Deemed unnecessary + ADR	Oral Thrush
56	F	Flucloxacillin	PJI	MSSA	4	6	VRE—Screening swab ESBL *E. coli*—urine	Unknown (coroner's case)	106/102/14	N/A	4	Added ciprofloxacin/ Relapsed infection	Reflux
70	M	Cephalexin	Recurrent MSSA bacteraemia	MSSA	6	7	VRE—Screening swab	Chest sepsis	17/15/15	N/A	4	N/A	
87	F	Rifampicin, Fusidic Acid, ciprofloxacin	PJI	MRSA	10	10	MRSA—joint tissue	Myocardial Infarction	7/0/0	N/A	2	N/A	
63	F	Rifampicin, Amoxy-cillin, Doxycy-cline	PJI	*C. amycolatum*, *E. faecalis*, *S. epidermidis*	2	2	ESBL *E. coli*—urine	Intra-abdominal haemor-rhage	22/22/2	N/A	2	N/A	
65	M	Cephalexin	Recurrent MSSA bacteraemia	MSSA	3	7	No	N/A	86/79/2	No	5	Ceased/deemed unnecessary	
65	M	Rifampicin, Fusidic Acid	PJI	MRSA	5	5	MRSA—joint tissue	N/A	9/8/0	No	5	Ceased/projected medication interactions	

Table 1. *Cont.*

Age	Sex	Antibiotic Regimen	Indication	Targeted Organism/s	Charlson Comorbidity Index Baseline End		MRO—Isolate Site	Cause of Death	Hospital Admission Days (Total/Infection Related/ICU)	Ongoing ID Follow Up	Duration of Follow Up (Years)	Regimen Adjust-ment/Reason	Adverse Drug Reactions ^
68	M	Pristinamycin, Cotrimoxa-zole, Ciprofloxacin, Fluconazole	VGI	*S. maltophilia*, VRE, *P. moteilii*, *C. albicans*	4	7	VRE—abdominal pus ESBL *K. pneumoniae*—screening swab	N/A	4/4/0	No	4	Ceased/ADR	Acute kidney and liver injury
70	M	Amoxycillin	PJI	*S. agalactiae*	6	8	ESBL *E. coli*—urine	N/A	7/2/0	No	1	Ceased/Deemed unnecessary	
56	F	Cephalexin	PJI	MSSA	4	7	No	N/A	0/0/0	No	3	Ceased/Deemed unnecessary	Vaginal thrush
59	F	Cephalexin	PJI	*S. agalactiae*	6	6	MRSA—wound swab	N/A	41/36/0	No	4	Ceased/Inefficacy + ADR	Vaginal thrush
65	F	Flucloxacillin, Ciprofloxacin	PJI	MSSA, *C. aurimucosum*	5	5	VRE—screening swab	N/A	360/314/8	Yes	7	Changed to doxycy-cline/Failed definitive surgery, new target organism	
69	F	Rifampicin, Fusidic Acid	PJI	MRSA	3	4	MRSA—joint tissue	N/A	25/0/0	Yes	5	N/A	
74	M	amoxicillin-clavulanic acid Pristi-namycin	VGI	*S. typhimurium*, VRE	6	10	VRE, CRE, *E. cloacae*—screening swab	N/A	3/0/0	Yes	5	Changed amoxi-cillin/clavulanic acid to amoxi-cillin/ADR	Diarrhoea
78	M	Rifampicin, Fusidic Acid	PJI	MRSA	5	13	MRSA, ESBL K. pneumoniae—Knee tissue	N/A	12/9/0	Yes	6	N/A	
45	F	Rifampicin Fusidic Acid	PJI	*S. epidermidis*, MSSA	1	2	No	N/A	30/30/0	Yes	6	N/A	

Table 1. *Cont.*

Age	Sex	Antibiotic Regimen	Indication	Targeted Organism/s	Charlson Comorbidity Index Baseline	End	MRO—Isolate Site	Cause of Death	Hospital Admission Days (Total/Infection Related/ICU)	Ongoing ID Follow Up	Duration of Follow Up (Years)	Regimen Adjust-ment/Reason	Adverse Drug Reactions ^
69	M	Rifampicin, Fusidic Acid	PJI	MRSA	2	3	MRSA—joint tissue	N/A	0/0/0	Yes	9	N/A	
77	M	Cephalexin	PJI	MSSA	4	5	No	N/A	0/0/0	No	5 months	N/A	
73	F	Amoxycillin	Infected spinal metal-ware	PSSA	9	9	No	N/A	0/0/0	No	2 months	N/A	
45	F	Penicillin	PVI	*C. acnes*	1	3	No	N/A	0/0/0	No	1	N/A	
42	F	Nitrofurantoin	Recurrent urinary tract infection	*E. faecalis*	1	1	No	N/A	29/0/0	No	1	N/A	
59	M	Clindamycin, Amoxy-cillin	VGI	*S. epidermidis*	3	4	No	N/A	0/0/0	No	1	N/A	
88	F	Cephalexin	Recurrent MSSA bacter-aemia, OM	MSSA	7	7	MRSA, VRE—screening swab	N/A	0/0/0	No	1	N/A	
86	F	Rifampicin, Fusidic Acid	PJI	MRSA	9	9	MRSA—joint tissue	N/A	34/26/0	No	4	N/A	
71	M	Ciprofloxacin	Post laminec-tomy infection	*E. cloacae, P. mirabilis*	7	7	No	N/A	2/0/0	No	1	N/A	

M—male; F—female; PJI—prosthetic joint infection; PVI—prosthetic valve infection; MSSA—methicillin susceptible *Staphylococcus aureus*; OM—osteomyelitis; VGI—vascular graft infection; MRO—multi-resistant microorganisms; MRSA—methicillin resistant *Staphylococcus aureus*; VRE—vancomycin resistant Enterococci; CRE—carbapenem resistant Enterobacteriaciae; ICU—intensive care unit; ADR—adverse drug reaction. Charlson Comorbidity Index—baseline refers to time of recruitment to study in 2015, end refers to the last available review. MRO; multi-resistant organism; ^ reported during follow-up period.

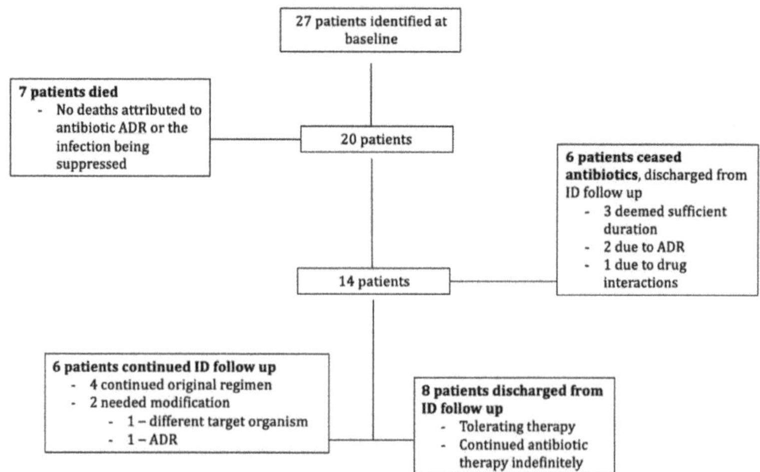

Figure 1. Patient outcomes. ADR, adverse drug reaction; ID, infectious diseases.

2.4. Adverse Events

Twenty patients required hospital admission in the follow-up period, 15 of these for an infection unrelated to the one requiring suppressive therapy. Two patients experienced adverse drug events newly identified in the follow up period. One had severe cholestatic liver function derangement (peak GGT 1562, ALP 600) and significant kidney injury (eGFR 37 from 75) with associated metabolic acidosis, which occurred two years following commencement of suppressive therapy. The other patient experienced recurrent vaginal thrush.

The rest of the reported adverse drug events were noted during our original study [5], and included gastrointestinal side effects such as nausea, vomiting, stomach discomfort, reflux and diarrhoea, itch/rash, weight gain, thrush, confusion, alopecia, fatigue, and headache).

2.5. MRO Colonisation

We found 18 patients to be colonised with MROs (18/27, 67%). Of these patients, vancomycin resistant Enterococci (VRE) was isolated in eight patients, methicillin resistant *Staphylococcus aureus* (MRSA) in nine patients, carbapenem resistant Enterobacteriaciae (CRE) in one patient, and five patients had extended-spectrum beta-lactamase organisms (ESBL) isolated (three with *Escherichia coli*, two with *Klebsiella pneumoniae*). Six patients had more than one MRO identified. Of the 24 organisms isolated across the 18 patients, 14 organisms were isolated from clinical specimens, the remaining 10 organisms were isolated from screening purposes either from admission infection control or research purposes.

Eight patients had MROs detected after the commencement of suppressive therapy (ranging between 6 months to 5 years following commencement). Eight patients had MROs detected at the time of commencement of suppressive therapy, and two had MROs detected prior to suppressive therapy (both detected 1 year prior).

3. Discussion

We observed a cohort of patients who had been prescribed long-term antibiotics over a five-year period. The key finding of our study was a high overall mortality rate of 26% over five years. Twenty-two percent of the cohort ceased their antimicrobials, with intolerable medication side effects being the reason for cessation in a third of these cases.

The mortality rate of 26% is higher than in previous studies focusing on single indications for long-term antibiotic therapy. A mortality rate of 17.4% was previously demonstrated in a cohort of 23 patients with infected prosthetic hip joints after a mean follow up of 33 months [6]. Reassuringly, no patients in our study died from the underlying infection requiring suppressive therapy, or from adverse effects of the suppressive therapy itself. Factors such as older age and comorbidities likely contributed to the observed mortality rate. This is supported by the high median CCI of five of our cohort, which has an estimated 1-year mortality of 85% [7], as well as the admission frequency for both infective and noninfective indications seen over the follow-up period, unrelated to chronic infection and suppressive antibiotics. We postulate that patients selected for suppressive antibiotic therapy are likely ineligible for definitive (and usually more aggressive) management, reflecting a frailer cohort with more comorbidities. Such patients are also at higher risk of adverse effects from long-term antibiotics, which was seen in our study with 19% needing modification or cessation of their treatment regimen most commonly due to adverse drug reactions or medication interactions. This highlights the complexities of managing these patients over time, and balancing infection suppression with the risks of long-term antibiotics in the context of comorbidities and polypharmacy.

No recurrences of infection were noted in the patients who ceased antibiotic therapy and continued to be followed up in our healthcare network. This may indicate that these patients may not have actually required long-term antibiotics for their original infective indications. Alternatively, this may reflect the small sample size of our cohort, as it does not match previous studies that have stopped long-term antibiotics following prosthetic joint infection [8].

A major strength of this study is the longitudinal design with long-term follow-up over five years. There are few similar studies [2], of which most have focused on suppressive antibiotics in the setting of a particular intervention such as debridement and implant retention for PJI [6,9], or VGI [10]. These studies did not measure outcomes such as rates of continued follow-up in ID clinic, and antibiotic discontinuation.

Our study has several limitations. First, the small cohort size from a single healthcare network, and second reliance on medical records as the sole source of data. Nevertheless, this study is important because long-term antibiotic prescribing may contribute significantly to antibiotic consumption and associated morbidity, particularly in indications where the evidence for their use is unclear. MROs were still detected in 67% of our cohort from clinical specimens and screening for infection control and previous study purposes. This suggests an association between long-term antibiotic consumption and AMR, which is likely underestimated in our study as there was no routine MRO screening. Another limitation is the heterogeneity of our cohort, including differing indications and antibiotic regimens. Although this limits our ability to draw specific conclusions, it does reflect the real-life challenges of managing these heterogeneous and often medically complex patients on long-term antibiotics.

4. Materials and Methods

We conducted a longitudinal study of patients taking long-term antibiotics at Monash Health, a large tertiary-level, university affiliated health service in Melbourne, Australia comprising five hospitals and servicing more than 1.5 million people. Patients were followed up for five years between April 2015 and May 2020. This study was approved by the Monash Health Human Research Ethics Committee: approval number 14379A.

Adult patients prescribed long-term antibiotics were identified at baseline using the hospital drug management system (Merlin Ver. 4.94, Pharmhos Software, Port Melbourne, VIC, Australia) as previously described [3,5]. Patients prescribed antibiotics for longer than 12 months to suppress chronic infection or prevent recurrent infection were included. Patients were excluded if they were aged under 18 years, unable to give informed consent, if they were prescribed prophylaxis in the context of immunocompromise and if they received antibiotic therapy outside of our hospital network.

This study reports five-year follow-up of this patient cohort. Medical records were retrospectively reviewed to determine baseline demographic characteristics and outcomes, including rates of ongoing antibiotic therapy and cessation, adverse events (including side effects attributable to antibiotic therapy and infection-related hospital admission), mortality, and isolation of MROs from clinical specimens, infection control screening and our previous study's swabs [3]. A CCI was calculated as a validated method to identify comorbidity extent in our population at baseline and the end of the follow-up period [11]. A descriptive analysis was performed.

5. Conclusions

Our study demonstrates the pitfalls of long-term antibiotic therapy. A high 5-year mortality rate reflects the older and more comorbid population of patients being prescribed this therapy. Further research is needed to elucidate which antimicrobials are associated with higher risk of adverse drug events and failure in this population, along with detailing true rates of MRO colonisation.

Author Contributions: C.K., I.W. and J.S.Y.L. devised and developed the study. C.K. and D.C. conducted the data collection and analysis of the data. C.K., K.C., T.K. and K.H. drafted the paper. All authors reviewed, edited and commented on previous versions of the manuscript. All authors have read and agreed to the published version of the manuscript.

Funding: This research received no external funding.

Institutional Review Board Statement: The study was conducted according to the guidelines of the Declaration of Helsinki, and approved by the Monash Health Human Research Ethics Committee: approval number 14379A.

Informed Consent Statement: No medical records, and no identifying information has been published. Informed consent was not obtained from the individual patients described in this study.

Data Availability Statement: The data used in this study has been presented in table format in the results section. Any further deidentified information can be made available in deidentified format upon reasonable request.

Conflicts of Interest: The authors declare no conflict or competing interest.

References

1. Chain, E.; Florey, H.W.; Adelaide, M.B.; Gardner, A.D.; Heatley, N.G.; Jennings, M.A.; Orr-Ewing, J.; Sanders, A.G. Penicillin as a chemotherapeutic agent. *Clin. Orthop. Relat. Res.* **1940**, *236*, 226–228. [CrossRef]
2. Lau, J.S.Y.; Korman, T.M.; Woolley, I. Life-long antimicrobial therapy: Where is the evidence? *J. Antimicrob. Chemother.* **2018**, *73*, 2601–2612. [CrossRef] [PubMed]
3. Lau, J.S.Y.; Bhatt, S.; Streitberg, R.; Bryant, M.; Korman, T.M.; Woolley, I. Surveillance of life-long antibiotics-A cross-sectional cohort study assessing patient attitudes and understanding of long-term antibiotic consumption. *Infect. Dis. Health* **2019**, *24*, 179–186. [CrossRef] [PubMed]
4. CDC. *Antibiotic Resistance Threats in the United States, 2019*; U.S. Department of Health and Human Services, CDC: Atlanta, GA, USA, 2019.
5. Lau, J.S.; Kiss, C.; Roberts, E.; Horne, K.; Korman, T.M.; Woolley, I. Surveillance of life-long antibiotics: A review of antibiotic prescribing practices in an Australian Healthcare Network. *Ann. Clin. Microbiol. Antimicrob.* **2017**, *16*, 3. [CrossRef] [PubMed]
6. Leijtens, B.; Weerwag, L.; Schreurs, B.W.; Kullberg, B.J.; Rijnen, W. Clinical Outcome of Antibiotic Suppressive Therapy in Patients with a Prosthetic Joint Infection after Hip Replacement. *J. Bone Jt. Infect.* **2019**, *4*, 268–276. [CrossRef] [PubMed]
7. Charlson, M.E.; Pompei, P.; Ales, K.L.; MacKenzie, C.R. A new method of classifying prognostic comorbidity in longitudinal studies: Development and validation. *J. Chronic Dis.* **1987**, *40*, 373–383. [CrossRef]
8. Byren, I.; Bejon, P.; Atkins, B.L.; Angus, B.; Masters, S.; McLardy-Smith, P.; Gundle, R.; Berendt, A. One hundred and twelve infected arthroplasties treated with 'DAIR' (debridement, antibiotics and implant retention): Antibiotic duration and outcome. *J. Antimicrob. Chemother.* **2009**, *63*, 1264–1271. [CrossRef] [PubMed]
9. Segreti, J.; Nelson, J.A.; Trenholme, G.M. Prolonged suppressive antibiotic therapy for infected orthopedic prostheses. *Clin. Infect. Dis.* **1998**, *27*, 711–713. [CrossRef] [PubMed]
10. Erb, S.; Sidler, J.A.; Elzi, L.; Gurke, L.; Battegay, M.; Widmer, A.F.; Weisser, M. Surgical and antimicrobial treatment of prosthetic vascular graft infections at different surgical sites: A retrospective study of treatment outcomes. *PLoS ONE* **2014**, *9*, e112947. [CrossRef] [PubMed]
11. Quan, H.; Li, B.; Couris, C.M.; Fushimi, K.; Graham, P.; Hider, P.; Januel, J.-M.; Sundararajan, V. Updating and validating the Charlson comorbidity index and score for risk adjustment in hospital discharge abstracts using data from 6 countries. *Am. J. Epidemiol.* **2011**, *173*, 676–682. [CrossRef] [PubMed]

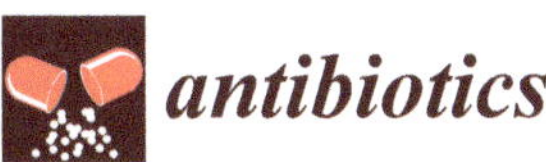

MDPI

Article

Fluoroquinolones and Other Antibiotics Redeemed for Cystitis—A Swedish Nationwide Cohort Follow-Up Study (2006–2018)

Xinjun Li [1], Kristina Sundquist [1,2,3] and Filip Jansåker [1,*]

1 Center for Primary Health Care Research, Department of Clinical Sciences Malmö, Lund University, 205 02 Malmö, Sweden; xinjun.li@med.lu.se (X.L.); kristina.sundquist@med.lu.se (K.S.)
2 Center for Community-Based Healthcare Research and Education (CoHRE), Department of Functional Pathology, School of Medicine, Shimane University, Matsue 690-0823, Japan
3 Department of Family Medicine and Community Health, Department of Population Health Science and Policy, Icahn School of Medicine at Mount Sinai, New York, NY 10029, USA
* Correspondence: filip.jansaker@med.lu.se; Tel.: +46-4039-1376

Abstract: Background: Antibiotics are commonly prescribed for outpatient management of cystitis. Previous evidence suggests that certain factors likely beyond the infection seem to influence the choice of antimicrobial treatment. However, studies on the specific antibiotic treatments for cystitis are lacking. This study aimed to explore the antibiotic treatments for cystitis using nationwide primary healthcare data and investigate if factors beyond the infection could be associated with fluoroquinolone treatment. Methods: This nationwide follow-up cohort study consisted of 352,507 women with cystitis. The primary aim was to investigate what specific classes of antibiotics were redeemed by patients within five days from the cystitis diagnosis. Each patient could only be included once. Logistic regression models were also used to examine the relationship between fluoroquinolone (FQ) treatment, parity, and sociodemographic factors. Results: In total, 192,065 antibiotic prescriptions were redeemed. Pivmecillinam (58.4%) followed by nitrofurantoin (22.2%), trimethoprim (12.0%), fluoroquinolone (5.6%), and cephalosporins (1.5%) were the most redeemed antibiotics. Sociodemographic factors were weakly associated with fluoroquinolone treatment; young age was inversely associated with fluoroquinolone treatment. Parity and cervical cancer history were not associated with fluoroquinolone treatment. The proportion of fluoroquinolone and trimethoprim treatments decreased over time, while pivmecillinam and nitrofurantoin increased. Conclusions: The treatment trends of antibiotics redeemed within five days from a cystitis diagnosis were similar to the national surveillance program of these antibiotics (not diagnosis linked). Fluoroquinolones were weakly associated with sociodemographic factors, which likely is only of historical relevance.

Keywords: antibiotics; cystitis; fluoroquinolones

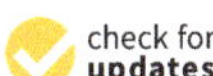

Citation: Li, X.; Sundquist, K.; Jansåker, F. Fluoroquinolones and Other Antibiotics Redeemed for Cystitis—A Swedish Nationwide Cohort Follow-Up Study (2006–2018). *Antibiotics* **2022**, *11*, 172. https://doi.org/antibiotics11020172

Academic Editor: Masafumi Seki

Received: 13 December 2021
Accepted: 25 January 2022
Published: 28 January 2022

Publisher's Note: MDPI stays neutral with regard to jurisdictional claims in published maps and institutional affiliations.

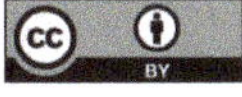

Copyright: © 2022 by the authors. Licensee MDPI, Basel, Switzerland. This article is an open access article distributed under the terms and conditions of the Creative Commons Attribution (CC BY) license (https://creativecommons.org/licenses/by/4.0/).

1. Introduction

Uncomplicated lower urinary tract infection (UTI), also known as uncomplicated cystitis, is one of the most common bacterial infections in women. About one in ten women have at least one infection each year and therefore cystitis is an important contributor to antibiotics exposure in otherwise healthy women in Sweden and worldwide [1–5].

However, over the last decades, safe and effective treatment options have decreased. This is partly due to an increase in antibiotic resistance, making certain antibiotics, such as fluoroquinolones, less suitable as empirical treatment options for cystitis. For example, fluoroquinolone resistance has passed 20% in several countries worldwide. Furthermore, certain UTI antibiotics have also been found to be more associated with collateral damage and severe adverse effects. For example, suspected cardiotoxicity and neuropsychiatric conditions have been related to fluoroquinolones [6–20].

All this considered, the treatment guidelines for cystitis (including in Sweden) have turned away from certain antibiotics—mainly fluoroquinolones, reserved for more serious infections—towards more narrow-spectrum antibiotics, such as nitrofurantoin and pivmecillinam, with lower resistance rates and more suitable safety profiles for use in the treatment of cystitis [8,19,21]. The national antibiotic surveillance program has demonstrated this shift [22], which has also been seen in smaller local but diagnosis-linked studies [23,24]. However, no study has investigated on a population-based dataset UTI treatment trends for a diagnosis of uncomplicated cystitis, nor how large of a proportion of certain antibiotics (e.g., fluroquinolones) comprise and if this could vary due to factors beyond the infection.

The gap in previous research is most likely due to the lack of nationwide population-based data from primary healthcare, where UTIs are mostly managed. We recently identified that about 54.5% of women diagnosed with uncomplicated cystitis in Sweden redeemed an antibiotic for their prescription. Furthermore, the study found that certain factors (likely beyond the infection) were associated with antibiotic treatment for cystitis [4]. In this follow-up study, by using a similar method [4], we aimed to study what specific classes of antibiotics were redeemed for cystitis in Sweden over a 13-year time period and determine if the annual trends were similar to the national surveillance program of antibiotics. We also intended to study if factors likely beyond the infection (e.g., history of cervical cancer and parity, and sociodemographic factors) could be associated with fluoroquinolone treatment.

2. Results

Table 1 includes the annual proportional distribution of each of the investigated antibiotic groups amongst the 192,065 antibiotic treatments for uncomplicated cystitis during the study period. The table shows that penicillins with extended spectrum (pivmecillinam) were used in 58.4% of all cases, followed by nitrofurantoin (22.2%), trimethoprim (12.0%), fluoroquinolones (5.6%), cephalosporins (1.5%), sulphonamides/trimethoprim combinations (0.4%), and beta-lactam/beta-lactamase inhibitors (<0.1%). During the first couple of years, treatment with fluoroquinolones, cephalosporins, and especially trimethoprim was more common but declined prominently in the following years. Nitrofurantoin was not widely used in our population during the first years, but as fluoroquinolones and trimethoprim use decreased, nitrofurantoin treatment increased. From 2011–2018, nitrofurantoin was used in about one-third of all cases. Pivmecillinam was used in about 60% of all cases annually (except for the first two years). Supplementary Table S1 includes data on when seven-level ATC codes from 2006 to 2013 were available. Pivmecillinam (J01CA08) accounted for about 57.4% of all these, followed by nitrofurantoin (20.1%), trimethoprim (13.6%), and fluoroquinolones (5.9%). Pivmecillinam also accounted for 99.4% of the penicillin with extended spectrum (amoxicillin, J01CA04, accounted for the other 0.6%). The proportion of nitrofurantoin and pivmecillinam treatments also seemed to increase in parallel to the decline of trimethoprim and fluoroquinolone treatments.

Table 2 presents a fully adjusted model of the associations between the individual sociodemographic variables and fluoroquinolone treatment within five days after the uncomplicated cystitis event. Age and education level were weakly associated with fluoroquinolone treatment. For example, middle followed by low education level had higher odds compared to high education level. Low income was associated with an increased odds of fluoroquinolone treatment. For example, the lowest income quartile had an OR of 1.30 (95% CI 1.23–1.38) compared to the highest income quartile. Living outside larger cities was strongly associated with lower odds of fluoroquinolone treatment. Country of origin did not seem to have a strong association with fluoroquinolone treatment in general. However, women from Western countries, Asia (excluding the Middle East) and Oceania, and Latin America and the Caribbean seemed to have significantly increased odds of fluoroquinolone treatment compared to Swedish women. History of cervical cancer and parity were associated with a decreased odds of fluoroquinolone treatment, however, only to a statistically significant extent for the latter. Year of infection (continuously increasing) was significantly associated with a decrease in fluoroquinolone treatment.

Table 1. Treatment trends of the 192,065 antibiotics redeemed for uncomplicated cystitis (2006–2018).

Antibiotic Groups in Order of Total Proportion (%)	Year													
	2006	**2007**	**2008**	**2009**	**2010**	**2011**	**2012**	**2013**	**2014**	**2015**	**2016**	**2017**	**2018**	**All**
Penicillins with extended spectrum (J01CA)	46.6	51.8	62.6	62.3	60.6	61.6	61.5	63.5	62.6	64.5	62.1	59.2	59.2	58.4
Nitrofuran derivatives (J01XE)	10.6	14.2	13.2	21.7	26.8	29.0	30.9	29.5	31.8	29.5	33.0	35.3	35.1	22.2
Trimethoprim and derivatives (J01EA)	28.0	22.1	16.2	10.5	7.7	5.2	3.5	2.7	1.7	1.6	0.9	0.8	0.5	12.0
Fluoroquinolones (J01MA)	11.4	9.0	5.6	4.1	3.7	3.1	2.9	3.3	3.0	3.5	2.9	3.7	4.1	5.6
Cephalosporins (J01DB-E,I)	3.0	2.5	2.0	1.2	0.9	0.8	0.9	0.8	0.7	0.7	1.0	0.5	0.7	1.5
Sulphonamides/Trimethoprim combinations (J01EE)	0.5	0.4	0.5	0.3	0.4	0.4	0.3	0.2	0.2	0.2	0.1	0.4	0.4	0.4
	100.0	100.0	100.0	100.0	100.0	100.0	100.0	100.0	100.0	100.0	100.0	100.0	100.0	100.0

No sulphonamide antibiotics (J01EB, J01EC, J01ED) were identified. Less than 0.1% of the antibiotic treatments were a beta-lactam/b-lactam inhibitor combination (J01CR, i.e., amoxicillin/clavulanic acid), hence why it is not part of the table. During 2006–2013, when seven-level ATC coding was available, in regard to J01CA, >99% was pivmecillinam and the remaining was amoxicillin; J01XE was nitrofurantoin; J01EA was trimethoprim; J01MA was ciprofloxacin (62%) and norfloxacin (38%). No sulphonamide antibiotics (J01EB, J01EC, J01ED) or fosfomycin (J01XX01) were identified. Each patient could only be included once during the study period. Data is from the Swedish Prescribed Drug Register.

Table 2. The association between history of cervical cancer, parity, and individual sociodemographic factors and fluoroquinolone treatment (10,684 cases) for uncomplicated cystitis.

Covariates	* OR	95% CI		*p*-Value
Gynecological history (ref. no history)				
Parity	0.92	0.87	0.96	<0.001
Cervical cancer	0.92	0.83	1.02	0.126
Age (ref. age 45–50 years)				
15–24	1.02	0.95	1.09	0.674
25–34	0.88	0.83	0.94	<0.001
35–44	0.95	0.90	1.01	0.082
Educational level (ref. ≥ 12 years)				
≤9	1.06	1.00	1.12	0.060
10–11	1.12	1.06	1.18	<0.001
Family income (ref. high)				
Low	1.30	1.23	1.38	<0.001
Middle-low	1.19	1.13	1.26	<0.001
Middle-high	1.07	1.01	1.13	0.019
Region of residence (ref. large cities)				
Southern Sweden	0.88	0.83	0.92	<0.001
Northern Sweden	0.84	0.78	0.91	<0.001
Country of origin (ref. Sweden)				
Eastern Europe	1.05	0.97	1.14	0.246
Western countries	1.21	1.10	1.33	<0.001
Middle East/North Africa	0.94	0.86	1.02	0.112
Africa (excluding North Africa)	1.05	0.92	1.19	0.502
Asia (excluding Middle East) and Oceania	1.25	1.13	1.37	<0.001
Latin America and the Caribbean	1.19	1.04	1.36	0.013
Year of infection (increasing)	0.93	0.92	0.93	<0.001

CI: confidence interval. OR: odds ratio. * Fully adjusted for all covariates. Time period: 2006–2018.

3. Discussion

This study presents diagnosis-linked antibiotic treatment trends for uncomplicated cystitis on a nationwide level. As expected, pivmecillinam and nitrofurantoin were the two most used antibiotics. The annual proportion of these antibiotics increased over time, as the proportion of trimethoprim and fluoroquinolones decreased. Year of infection (continuously increasing) was also inversely associated with fluoroquinolone treatment rates. These trends were in accordance with the national guidelines [21] and the general trend of UTI antibiotics (not linked to diagnoses) in women in the national surveillance program over the same time period [25]. Furthermore, annual treatment trends were comparable to that of smaller local studies [23,24]. The consistencies support our findings, and altogether this indicates that the national surveillance program of antibiotics [25] seems to be representative and valid for cystitis. These findings could represent important information for healthcare planners working on national antibiotic surveillance and for the clinical implications of these programs for this very common bacterial infection.

Less than six percent of all the antibiotic treatments linked to uncomplicated cystitis were fluoroquinolones (mainly ciprofloxacin). Factors likely beyond the infection—such as sociodemographic factors and history of cervical cancer and parity—did not seem to be associated with fluoroquinolone treatment for uncomplicated cystitis to a high extent. Women from low family income backgrounds seemed to have received more fluoroquinolone treatments than women of higher socioeconomic status. For country of origin, only MENA women had lower odds of fluoroquinolone compared to Swedish-born women (although statistically non-significant), while women from Asia (excluding Middle East) and Oceania, Western countries, and Latin America and the Caribbean had weak but significantly higher odds of fluoroquinolone treatment compared to Swedish-born women. The mechanisms behind these sociodemographic differences in fluoroquinolone treatment of uncomplicated cystitis, which were similar to the odds for antibiotic treatment in general [4], could, inter alia, be attributed to uncertainty in diagnostic testing [18]. During the last decade, it has not been recommended to prescribe fluoroquinolones as a first-line prescription for uncomplicated cystitis [19], as these antibiotics ought to be limited to serious infections and not uncomplicated cystitis due to concern of worrisome collateral damage and adverse effects associated with these antibiotics [15–20]. If the sociodemographic differences associated with fluoroquinolones still exist, it would be of particular concern. However, fluoroquinolones were not included in the recent Swedish guidelines for cystitis [21], and the prescription of these drugs has in general been drastically declining over the recent years [25], which was also seen in our study with diagnosis-linked data. Hence, it is possible that these findings are of more historic relevance in Sweden.

Limitations of this study were that we did not have access to data on the symptoms or clinical presentation in the patients, nor did we have data on adherence rates. Therefore, no firm conclusion can be made on whether the differences in fluoroquinolone treatment could have been due to unequal healthcare (differences in prescription rates) or differences in adherence (differences in pick-up rates). Further studies could examine possible mechanisms behind the found associations of factors likely beyond the infection and antibiotic treatments [4]. The main strengths of this study include that this study involved several highly validated nationwide patient and population data registries including nationwide primary healthcare data. Previous population-based studies on antibiotic treatments of primary healthcare infections have, to the best of our knowledge, not included data of diagnoses linked to antibiotic prescriptions.

Antibiotics are important drugs for patients worldwide [26] and should be given when needed. However, due to the growing threat of antimicrobial resistance [10,13,14] and potential severe adverse reactions [15–20], certain drugs, such as fluoroquinolones, ought to be saved for more serious infections. This study demonstrates that the shift in treatment recommendations for uncomplicated cystitis seems to have been followed. In addition to this, the findings support that the national surveillance program of antibiotics, although lacking the diagnoses linked to the antibiotics, likely is representative, at least for UTI antibiotics in women. Further population-based diagnosis-linked studies using primary healthcare data are needed to validate these findings on other infections before a general conclusion can be made.

4. Materials and Methods

4.1. Study Design

This was a population-based cohort register study and follow-up to a recent nationwide study of ours [4]. The time period was from 1 January 2006 to 31 December 2018. The study used several national registers together with nationwide primary healthcare data.

4.2. Setting

This research was conducted at the Center for Primary Health Care Research at Lund University and Region Skåne, Malmö, Sweden. The STROBE statement for cohort studies was considered when conducting this study and in the writing process [27].

4.3. Study Population

The study population consisted of 352,507 women [4] between the age of 15 and 50 years at the time of being diagnosed with a first event of uncomplicated cystitis during the study period. The 10th revision of the International Classification of Diseases (ICD-10) was used to identify the code N30 for acute infective cystitis [5]. Cases with diagnoses not considered to be in accordance with uncomplicated cystitis were not included in the study: i.e., ICD-10 codes of N301-304, and N308, or co-morbidities (ICD-10: B20-24, C64-68, D41, D80-89, E10-11, M623, N03, N07, N11, N13-23, N25-29, N32, Q60-64) diagnosed within two years prior to the cystitis episode. Women with ongoing pregnancy or treatment with immunomodulating agents were also not considered [4]. Each woman could only be included once.

4.4. Outcome Variable

The outcome variable (redeemed antibiotic prescription) was defined as the first UTI antibiotic redeemed (measured as prescription from a physician dispensed at a pharmacy) within five days after a diagnosis of uncomplicated cystitis. The outcome is generally referred to as "antibiotic treatment" in the manuscript. The following antibiotic groups were assessed based on their ATC code: penicillins with extended spectrum (J01CA), for example, pivmecillinam; beta-lactam/b-lactam inhibitor combinations (J01CR); cephalosporins (J01DB-E,I); trimethoprim derivatives (J01EA), i.e., trimethoprim; sulphonamides/trimethoprim combinations (J01EE), i.e., trimethoprim/sulphamethoxazole; fluoroquinolones (J01MA), for example ciprofloxacin; and nitrofuran derivatives, i.e., nitrofurantoin (J01XE). Seven-level ATC codes were available during the first eight years (2006–2013) of the study. Oral drugs were exclusively assessed. Monosulphonamide antibiotics and fosfomycin were not considered, as these antibiotics were not widely available in Sweden at the time of the study. We did not consider either antibiotics that were not recommended [19,21] to be used or generally prescribed for patients with cystitis (e.g., tetracyclines, macrolides).

4.5. Predictor Variables for Fluoroquinolone Treatment

The predictors investigated were measured at baseline (i.e., time of the cystitis diagnosis). Age groups were defined as being between 15–24, 25–34, 35–44, or 45–50 years of age. Country of origin was categorized as originating from any of the following countries/regions: Sweden; Eastern European countries; Western countries; Middle East/North Africa (MENA); Africa (excluding North Africa); Asia (excluding Middle East) and Oceania; or Latin America/the Caribbean. Countries with geographical proximity and/or cultural and economic similarities were categorized together. Both first- and second-generation immigrants were included in country groups other than Sweden. The categories for this study were based on the definition used in a previous study of ours [5]. Educational level was classified into three different categories based on the duration of school years attended: compulsory schooling or less ($\leq$9 years); short or partially completed high school education (10–11 years); or completed high school education or more, such as university or college education ($\geq$12 years). For those aged 15–17 years in the youngest age group, the highest educational level of the parents was used. Family income was categorized into four groups based on a weighted average income in each family: low (lowest income quartile of the study population), middle low/middle high (second/third quartiles), and high (highest quartile). Region of residence was grouped as large cities, Southern Sweden, and Northern Sweden. Parity was defined from the Swedish Medical Birth Register and categorized as no child (nullipara) or at least one child. Cervical cancer (Yes/No) was defined from the Swedish Cancer Register according to ICD-7 code 171. As the prescription rate of fluoroquinolone decreased in Sweden [25] during the time period, the year of infection was included as a continuous (increasing) variable in the analysis.

4.6. Data Sources

This cohort study population was identified through population-based primary healthcare data (1997–2018) accessed from 21 out of 22 administrative regions in Sweden during the study period. The coverage of these data varied by time and region based on when the patient records were digitalized. The database included around 72% of the population in Sweden in 2015 and around 90% of the population at the end of the study. The following nationwide registers, managed by the National Board of Health and Welfare (in Swedish: *Socialstyrelsen*), were used to identify the outcome, parity, cervical cancer, as well as comorbidities or other complicating factors not aligned with uncomplicated cystitis: [1,28] the Swedish Prescribed Drug Register (2005–2018), which contains the specific ATC codes on redeemed drug prescriptions from all pharmacies in Sweden; the Medical Birth Register (1973–2018); the National Patient Register (including inpatient (1964–2018) and outpatient data (2001–2018)); the Cause of Death Register (1961–2018); and the Swedish Cancer Register (1958–2018). The Total Population Register (1968–2018) was used to collect data on age, country of origin, education, income, and region of residence. All linkages between the individual-level data in the databases were performed using a pseudonymized (encrypted) version of the unique 10-digit personal identification number (assigned to each person residing in Sweden during their lifetime).

4.7. Statistical Analysis

Descriptive statistics on the annual treatment trends (redeemed antibiotic prescription five days after a diagnosis of uncomplicated cystitis) were calculated for each antibiotic based on the five-level-ATC-code antibiotic group for the whole study period (Table 1). During the years when seven-level-ATC-code were available, a sub-analysis of specific antibiotic treatment proportions was conducted (Supplementary Material Table S1). To test for the association between the predictor variables and fluoroquinolone treatment, adjusted logistic regression models (Table 2) were used to estimate odds ratios (ORs) and 95% confidence intervals (CIs). The study period started on 1 January 2006 and proceeded until redeemed antibiotic prescription (within five days), death, emigration, or the end of the study period on 31 December 2018. Missing values (range 0.0–1.3%) were not excluded. A two-tailed p-value of <0.05 was used to define statistical significance. SAS version 9.4 (SAS Institute Inc.; Cary, NC, USA) was used for all statistical analyses.

4.8. Ethical Consideration

The present study was a non-intervention nationwide register study of pseudonymized secondary data obtained from Swedish authorities and was approved by the Ethical Review Board in Lund. All methods were performed in accordance with the relevant guidelines and regulations.

4.9. Role of Funding Source

The funding sources of this study were all non-commercial and had no role in the study design; the collection, analysis, and interpretation of data; the writing of the report; or the decision to submit the paper for publication.

5. Conclusions

The treatment trends of antibiotics (for urinary tract infections) redeemed within five days from a cystitis diagnosis were similar to the national surveillance program of these antibiotics (not diagnosis linked). The decreasing treatment rate of fluroquinolones over time was also in accordance with the national surveillance program. This indicates that the national surveillance program is likely representative and valid in identifying antibiotics treatments for urinary tract infections. Fluoroquinolone treatment was weakly associated with some sociodemographic factors and parity, which likely are beyond the infection but only of historical relevance, as these antibiotics seem to be used less for this infection in Sweden, in accordance with national guidelines. These findings represent important new information, particularly for healthcare planners involved with the national antibiotic surveillance of this very common bacterial infection in women.

Supplementary Materials: The following are available online at https://www.mdpi.com/article/10.3390/antibiotics11020172/s1, Table S1: Number of specific UTI antibiotics in the four most common antibiotic treatment groups for uncomplicated cystitis (2006–2013).

Author Contributions: Concept and visualization: F.J. Development of idea and design: F.J., K.S. and X.L. Access, acquisition, and analysis of data: K.S. Statistical analysis and tables: X.L. Interpretation of data: all authors. Literature search and drafting of manuscript: F.J. Critical revision of the manuscript for intellectual content: all authors. The authors attest that all listed authors meet authorship criteria and that no others meeting the criteria have been omitted. All authors have read and agreed to the published version of the manuscript.

Funding: This work was supported by non-commercial research grants, i.e., funding granted to F.J. from the Primary Healthcare Management, and by governmental funding (Alf funding) of clinical research within the NHS (National Health Services), both Region Skåne (Sweden) and the Swedish Society of Medicine. It was also funded by grants provided to K.S. from the Swedish Research Council.

Institutional Review Board Statement: This study was conducted according to the guidelines of the Declaration of Helsinki and approved by the Ethical Review Board in Lund (2008/471, 2012/795 and later approved amendments).

Informed Consent Statement: Due to pseudonymized secondary register data, the need for individual consent was waived by the ethical review board.

Data Availability Statement: This study made use of several national registers and, owing to legal concerns, data cannot be made openly available. Further information regarding the health registries is available from the Swedish National Board of Health and Welfare: https://www.socialstyrelsen.se/en/statistics-and-data/registers/ (accessed on 26 October 2021), and Kristina Sundquist.

Acknowledgments: We thank Patrick Reilly for helping with language edits.

Conflicts of Interest: The authors declare no conflict of interest.

Abbreviations

ATC	Anatomic Therapeutic Chemical classification system
CI	Confidence interval
ICD	International Classification of Diseases
MENA	Middle East/North Africa
OR	Odds ratio
UTI	Urinary tract infection

References

1. Nicolle, L.E. Uncomplicated urinary tract infection in adults including uncomplicated pyelonephritis. *Urol. Clin. N. Am.* **2008**, *35*, 1–12. [CrossRef] [PubMed]
2. Foxman, B.; Barlow, R.; D'Arcy, H.; Gillespie, B.; Sobel, J.D. Urinary tract infection: Self-reported incidence and associated costs. *Ann. Epidemiol.* **2000**, *10*, 509–515. [CrossRef]

3. Butler, C.C.; Hawking, M.K.; Quigley, A.; McNulty, C.A. Incidence, severity, help seeking, and management of uncomplicated urinary tract infection: A population-based survey. *Br. J. Gen. Pract.* **2015**, *65*, e702–e707. [CrossRef]
4. Jansåker, F.; Li, X.; Knudsen, J.D.; Milos Nymberg, V.; Sundquist, K. The Effect of Sociodemographic Factors, Parity and Cervical Cancer on Antibiotic Treatment for Uncomplicated Cystitis in Women: A Nationwide Cohort Study. *Antibiotics* **2021**, *10*, 1389. [CrossRef] [PubMed]
5. Jansåker, F.; Li, X.; Sundquist, K. Sociodemographic factors and uncomplicated cystitis in women aged 15–50 years: A nationwide Swedish cohort registry study (1997–2018). *Lancet Reg. Health-Eur.* **2021**, *4*, 100108. [CrossRef] [PubMed]
6. Schito, G.C.; Naber, K.G.; Botto, H.; Palou, J.; Mazzei, T.; Gualco, L.; Marchese, A. The ARESC study: An international survey on the antimicrobial resistance of pathogens involved in uncomplicated urinary tract infections. *Int. J. Antimicrob. Agents* **2009**, *34*, 407–413. [CrossRef] [PubMed]
7. Kahlmeter, G.; Poulsen, H.O. Antimicrobial susceptibility of Escherichia coli from community-acquired urinary tract infections in Europe: The ECO.SENS study revisited. *Int. J. Antimicrob. Agents* **2012**, *39*, 45–51. [CrossRef]
8. Poulsen, H.O.; Johansson, A.; Granholm, S.; Kahlmeter, G.; Sundqvist, M. High genetic diversity of nitrofurantoin- or mecillinam-resistant Escherichia coli indicates low propensity for clonal spread. *J. Antimicrob. Chemother.* **2013**, *68*, 1974–1977. [CrossRef]
9. Kahlmeter, G.; Ahman, J.; Matuschek, E. Antimicrobial Resistance of Escherichia coli Causing Uncomplicated Urinary Tract Infections: A European Update for 2014 and Comparison with 2000 and 2008. *Infect. Dis. Ther.* **2015**, *4*, 417–423. [CrossRef]
10. Holmes, A.H.; Moore, L.S.; Sundsfjord, A.; Steinbakk, M.; Regmi, S.; Karkey, A.; Guerin, P.J.; Piddock, L.J. Understanding the mechanisms and drivers of antimicrobial resistance. *Lancet* **2016**, *387*, 176–187. [CrossRef]
11. Abdelrady, A.M.; Zaitone, S.A.; Farag, N.E.; Fawzy, M.S.; Moustafa, Y.M. Cardiotoxic effect of levofloxacin and ciprofloxacin in rats with/without acute myocardial infarction: Impact on cardiac rhythm and cardiac expression of Kv4.3, Kv1.2 and Nav1.5 channels. *Biomed. Pharmacother.* **2017**, *92*, 196–206. [CrossRef] [PubMed]
12. Sellick, J.; Mergenhagen, K.; Morris, L.; Feuz, L.; Horey, A.; Risbood, V.; Wojciechowski, A.; Ruh, C.; Bednarczyk, E.; Conway, E.; et al. Fluoroquinolone-Related Neuropsychiatric Events in Hospitalized Veterans. *Psychosomatics* **2018**, *59*, 259–266. [CrossRef] [PubMed]
13. Laxminarayan, R.; Van Boeckel, T.; Frost, I.; Kariuki, S.; Khan, E.A.; Limmathurotsakul, D.; Larsson, D.G.J.; Levy-Hara, G.; Mendelson, M.; Outterson, K.; et al. The Lancet Infectious Diseases Commission on antimicrobial resistance: 6 years later. *Lancet Infect. Dis.* **2020**, *20*, e51–e60. [CrossRef]
14. Roberts, S.C.; Zembower, T.R. Global increases in antibiotic consumption: A concerning trend for WHO targets. *Lancet Infect. Dis.* **2021**, *21*, 10–11. [CrossRef]
15. Kalghatgi, S.; Spina, C.S.; Costello, J.C.; Liesa, M.; Morones-Ramirez, J.R.; Slomovic, S.; Molina, A.; Shirihai, O.S.; Collins, J.J. Bactericidal antibiotics induce mitochondrial dysfunction and oxidative damage in Mammalian cells. *Sci. Transl. Med.* **2013**, *5*, 192ra185. [CrossRef] [PubMed]
16. Kaur, K.; Fayad, R.; Saxena, A.; Frizzell, N.; Chanda, A.; Das, S.; Chatterjee, S.; Hegde, S.; Baliga, M.S.; Ponemone, V.; et al. Fluoroquinolone-related neuropsychiatric and mitochondrial toxicity: A collaborative investigation by scientists and members of a social network. *J. Community Support. Oncol.* **2016**, *14*, 54–65. [CrossRef]
17. Kuula, L.S.M.; Viljemaa, K.M.; Backman, J.T.; Blom, M. Fluoroquinolone-related adverse events resulting in health service use and costs: A systematic review. *PLoS ONE* **2019**, *14*, e0216029. [CrossRef]
18. Redgrave, L.S.; Sutton, S.B.; Webber, M.A.; Piddock, L.J. Fluoroquinolone resistance: Mechanisms, impact on bacteria, and role in evolutionary success. *Trends Microbiol.* **2014**, *22*, 438–445. [CrossRef]
19. Gupta, K.; Hooton, T.M.; Naber, K.G.; Wullt, B.; Colgan, R.; Miller, L.G.; Moran, G.J.; Nicolle, L.E.; Raz, R.; Schaeffer, A.J.; et al. International clinical practice guidelines for the treatment of acute uncomplicated cystitis and pyelonephritis in women: A 2010 update by the Infectious Diseases Society of America and the European Society for Microbiology and Infectious Diseases. *Clin. Infect. Dis.* **2011**, *52*, e103–e120. [CrossRef]
20. Mathews, B.; Thalody, A.A.; Miraj, S.S.; Kunhikatta, V.; Rao, M.; Saravu, K. Adverse Effects of Fluoroquinolones: A Retrospective Cohort Study in a South Indian Tertiary Healthcare Facility. *Antibiotics* **2019**, *8*, 104. [CrossRef]
21. *Drug Treatment of Urinary Tract Infections in Outpatient Care—Treatment Recommendation: Information from the Swedish Medical Products Agency. [Läkemedelsbehandling av Urinvägsinfektioner i Öppenvård—Behandlingsrekommendation: Information från Läkemedelsverket]*; Swedish Medical Products Agency: Uppsala, Sweden, 2017; Volume 5, pp. 21–36. Available online: https://www.lakemedelsverket.se/uvi (accessed on 26 October 2021). (In Swedish)
22. Ternhag, A.; Grunewald, M.; Naucler, P.; Wisell, K.T. Antibiotic consumption in relation to socio-demographic factors, co-morbidity, and accessibility of primary health care. *Scand. J. Infect. Dis.* **2014**, *46*, 888–896. [CrossRef] [PubMed]
23. Lindback, H.; Lindback, J.; Melhus, A. Inadequate adherence to Swedish guidelines for uncomplicated lower urinary tract infections among adults in general practice. *APMIS* **2017**, *125*, 816–821. [CrossRef] [PubMed]
24. Kornfalt Isberg, H.; Melander, E.; Hedin, K.; Molstad, S.; Beckman, A. Uncomplicated urinary tract infections in Swedish primary care; etiology, resistance and treatment. *BMC Infect. Dis.* **2019**, *19*, 155. [CrossRef] [PubMed]
25. *SWEDRES-SVARM 2019. Consumption of Antibiotics and Occurrence of Resistance in Sweden*; Public Health Agency of Sweden: Solna, Sweden, 2019; ISSN 1650-6332.
26. Adedeji, W.A. The Treasure Called Antibiotics. *Ann. Ib. Postgrad. Med.* **2016**, *14*, 56–57.

27. Von Elm, E.; Altman, D.G.; Egger, M.; Pocock, S.J.; Gotzsche, P.C.; Vandenbroucke, J.P.; Initiative, S. The Strengthening the Reporting of Observational Studies in Epidemiology (STROBE) statement: Guidelines for reporting observational studies. *Lancet* **2007**, *370*, 1453–1457. [CrossRef]
28. Sabih, A.; Leslie, S.W. Complicated Urinary Tract Infections. In *StatPearls*; StatPearls Publishing: Treasure Island, FL, USA, 2020.

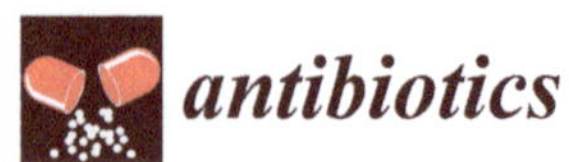

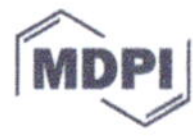

Article

Effectiveness of an Electronic Automated Antibiotic Time Out Alert in the Setting of Gram-Negative Bacteremia

Sana M. Mohayya [1,*], Navaneeth Narayanan [1,2,3], Daniel Cimilluca [4], Alexander Malanowski [3], Parth Vaidya [2] and Tanaya Bhowmick [3]

1 Department of Pharmacy, Robert Wood Johnson University Hospital, New Brunswick, NJ 08901, USA; navan12@pharmacy.rutgers.edu
2 Department of Pharmacy Practice and Administration, Ernest Mario School of Pharmacy, Rutgers University, Piscataway, NJ 08854, USA; parthv18@gmail.com
3 Department of Medicine, Division of Allergy, Immunology, Infectious Diseases, Rutgers Robert Wood Johnson Medical School, New Brunswick, NJ 08903, USA; ajm421@rwjms.rutgers.edu (A.M.); bhowmita@rwjms.rutgers.edu (T.B.)
4 Department of Pathology and Laboratory Medicine, Robert Wood Johnson University Hospital, New Brunswick, NJ 08901, USA; dc1251@rwjms.rutgers.edu
* Correspondence: sanamohayya@gmail.com

Abstract: To minimize complications associated with over-utilization of antibiotics, many antimicrobial stewardship programs have incorporated an antibiotic time out (ATO); however, limited data are available to support its effectiveness. This was a single-center retrospective cohort study assessing the impact of the automated electronic ATO in the setting of Gram-negative bacteremia. The primary outcome was the proportion of patients who received a modification of therapy within 24 h of final culture results. Secondary outcomes included modification at any point in therapy, time to modification of therapy, time to de-escalation, and days of therapy of broad-spectrum antibiotics. There was a total of 222 patients who met inclusion criteria, 97 patients pre-ATO and 125 patients post-ATO. The primary outcome of modification of therapy within 24 h of final culture results was not significantly different (24% vs. 30%, $p = 0.33$). The secondary outcome of modification of therapy at any point in therapy was not significantly different between the two groups (65% vs. 67%, $p = 0.73$). All other secondary outcomes were not significantly different. The ATO alert was not associated with a higher rate of antibiotic modification within 24 h of culture results in patients with GNB. Further efforts are needed to optimize the ATO strategy and antibiotic prescribing practices.

Keywords: antimicrobial stewardship; antibiotics; antimicrobial prescribing; behavior change

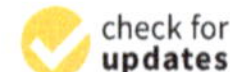

Citation: Mohayya, S.M.; Narayanan, N.; Cimilluca, D.; Malanowski, A.; Vaidya, P.; Bhowmick, T. Effectiveness of an Electronic Automated Antibiotic Time Out Alert in the Setting of Gram-Negative Bacteremia. *Antibiotics* **2021**, *10*, 1078. https://doi.org/10.3390/antibiotics10091078

Academic Editor: Seok Hoon Jeong

Received: 30 July 2021
Accepted: 3 September 2021
Published: 6 September 2021

Publisher's Note: MDPI stays neutral with regard to jurisdictional claims in published maps and institutional affiliations.

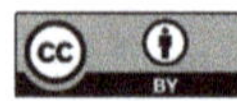

Copyright: © 2021 by the authors. Licensee MDPI, Basel, Switzerland. This article is an open access article distributed under the terms and conditions of the Creative Commons Attribution (CC BY) license (https://creativecommons.org/licenses/by/4.0/).

1. Introduction

While broad-spectrum antibiotics may be effective to treat a variety of infections, their over-utilization may lead to superinfections and contribute to the development of antimicrobial resistance. In an effort to minimize these complications, antimicrobial stewardship programs have been developed with the goal of optimizing antibiotic therapy by using the most targeted regimen whenever possible. Stewardship programs include a variety of effective strategies to optimize antimicrobial therapy, including an antibiotic time out (ATO). An ATO is a strategy endorsed by the Centers for Disease Control and Prevention (CDC) and the Joint Commission (TJC), which encourages a re-evaluation of antibiotic therapy at a pre-specified time point during empiric treatment after clinical results have been reported [1,2]. Despite the increasing adoption of an ATO, the optimal strategy and timing have not yet been established.

Previous studies [3–5] have assessed the efficacy of an ATO strategy involving prospective audit and feedback (PAF) in which an infectious diseases (ID) physician or pharmacist reviews individual patient cases and intervenes when a change in therapy is deemed appropriate. These studies suggested that this type of intervention may be effective as an adjunct to other stewardship interventions, but the impact of a self-driven ATO was uncertain. A more recent study [6] evaluated the concept of self-stewardship, which prompts the primary care provider to re-evaluate therapy when more data was available and found that providers were more likely to de-escalate antibiotics. The results of these studies have been inconsistent as some have shown utility while others have not [3–6] and the optimal method of delivery of this alert has not yet been demonstrated. This study aimed to address these inconsistencies by analyzing an automated ATO in patients who have a true infection and who received at least 72 h of antibiotic treatment. We chose to focus on Gram-negative bloodstream infections (GNB) because it is classified as a definitive disease state without concern for the possibility of colonization or misclassification. GNB is a high yield stewardship research opportunity for modification of therapy, as it is common practice to de-escalate or escalate and, therefore, may have a better yield in terms of clinical impact [7].

ATOs have been adopted broadly as an antimicrobial stewardship tool, despite limited evidence supporting their effectiveness. This study was designed to analyze an automated tool built into the electronic medical record (EMR). The objective of the study was to assess the impact of an automated EMR-integrated ATO on the proportion of antibiotic modification for patients with Gram-negative bacteremia (GNB).

2. Results

Of the 570 adult inpatients with GNB between September 2016 and December 2018, 222 patients were eligible to be included in the study (Figure 1). A total of 97 patients were included in the pre-ATO cohort and 125 patients in post-ATO cohort. Patient demographics and other covariates were assessed (Table 1). Overall, there were no statistically significant differences in baseline characteristics between the two cohorts. The predominant source of bacteremia was urinary (95/222 (43%)) and the most common isolated taxon was *E. coli* (127/222 (57%)). All other encounter characteristics, including Pitt bacteremia score and ICU admission, were similar between the two groups. All positive cultures resulted by time of decision making.

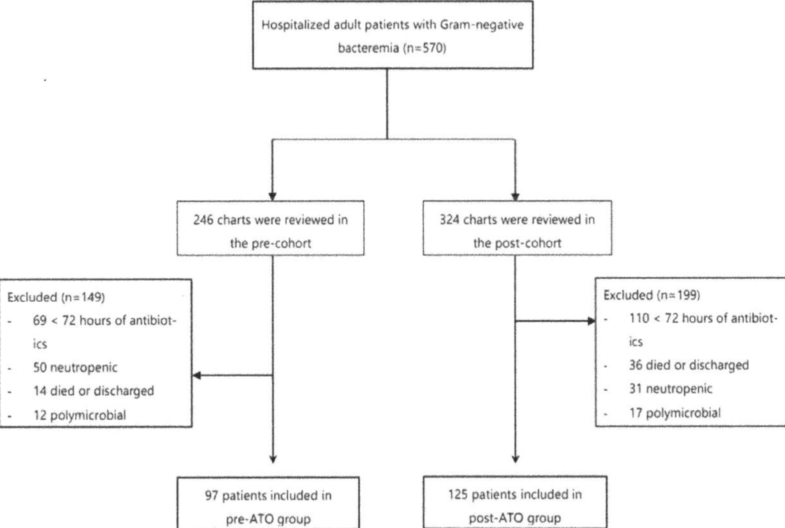

Figure 1. Study flowchart.

Table 1. Baseline demographics and clinical characteristics of patients included in the study.

Characteristic	Pre-Intervention (*n* = 97)	Post-Intervention (*n* = 125)	*p*-Value
Patient demographics			
Age, y, mean (SD)	66 (50–82)	69 (55–83)	0.62
Female sex	43 (44)	63 (50)	0.42
CKD	25 (26)	40 (32)	0.37
Encounter characteristics			
Pitt Bacteremia Score, mean (SD)	2 (0–5)	2.2 (0–5)	0.76
ICU admission while on antibiotic	38 (39)	44 (35)	0.58
Vasopressor use	20 (21)	31 (25)	0.52
Isolated taxon			0.63
Escherichia coli	55 (57)	72 (58)	
Klebsiella spp.	19 (20)	28 (22)	
Proteus mirabilis	5 (5)	10 (8)	
Enterobacter spp.	6 (6)	9 (7)	
Serratia marcescens	5 (5)	4 (3)	
Pseudomonas aeruginosa	2 (2)	0 (0)	
Stenotrophomonas maltophilia	2 (2)	1 (0.8)	
Acinetobacter baumannii	1 (1)	1 (0.8)	
Citrobacter freundii	2 (2)	0 (0)	
Antibiotic resistance [a]			0.25
Carbapenem-resistant	6 (6)	2 (2)	
Ceftriaxone-resistant	18 (19)	23 (18)	
Fluoroquinolone-resistant	28 (29)	29 (23)	
Allergies [b]	22 (23)	32 (26)	0.64
Beta-lactam allergy	18 (19)	20 (16)	
Antibiotic allergy in addition to beta-lactam	6 (6)	5 (4)	
Other antibiotic allergy(non-beta-lactam)	4 (4)	12 (10)	
Anaphylaxis reported	5 (5)	5 (4)	
Likely source of bacteremia			0.65
Urinary only	38 (39)	57 (46)	
Abdominal only	25 (26)	27 (22)	
Respiratory only	8 (8)	6 (5)	
Other site	12 (12)	16 (13)	
Multisite	7 (7)	13 (10)	
Unknown	5 (5)	2 (2)	
Skin and soft tissue only	1 (1)	3 (2)	
Other positive culture [c]			
Same pathogen as index blood culture	26 (27)	48 (38)	0.70
Same sensitivity profile as index blood culture [d]	22 (85)	40 (83)	
Focus of infection [e]	29 (30)	45 (36)	0.42
Removed	20 (69)	36 (80)	
Not removed	9 (31)	9 (20)	
Antibiotic at time of final culture results			
Piperacillin-tazobactam	61 (63)	75 (60)	0.82
Ceftriaxone	10 (10)	16 (13)	
Meropenem	9 (9)	15 (12)	
Other [f]	17 (18)	19 (15)	
Modified antibiotic [g]			0.93
Ceftriaxone	18 (28)	25 (30)	
Levofloxacin	12 (19)	18 (21)	
Cefazolin	8 (13)	10 (12)	
Meropenem	8 (13)	7 (8)	
Other [h]	17 (27)	24 (29)	
Primary hospital service at time of culture results			0.62
Internal medicine	47 (48)	77 (62)	
Pulmonary	22 (23)	26 (21)	
Surgical	13 (13)	14 (11)	
Cardiovascular	4 (4)	4 (3)	

Table 1. *Cont.*

Characteristic	Pre-Intervention (n = 97)	Post-Intervention (n = 125)	p-Value
Other [i]	11 (11)	4 (3)	
Discharge status			0.38
Home	52 (54)	56 (45)	
Institution [j]	32 (33)	52 (42)	
Death [k]	13 (13)	17 (14)	

Data are presented as no. (%), unless otherwise indicated. Abbreviations: CKD, chronic kidney disease; ICU, intensive care unit; ID, infectious disease. [a] Category of resistance is mutually exclusive and only highest level of resistance was recorded. Intermediate resistance patterns were considered resistant. [b] Of the patients who reported a beta-lactam allergy, 33% of the pre-cohort and 4% of the post-cohort had additional antibiotic allergies. Anaphylaxis included patients with allergy to any antibiotic with documentation of serious anaphylactic reactions, including symptoms of shortness of breath and swelling. [c] A positive culture from another source (i.e., urine, tissue, body fluid) that had final results prior to or within 24 h of final blood culture results. [d] Proportion of other cultures with same sensitivities are reported on the basis of the frequencies of cultures with same pathogen as blood culture. [e] Removed focus of infection includes patients who had a source of infection that may require removal to achieve source control. The percentages reported are based on the total number of patients who had a removable source of infection. [f] Other antibiotics include aztreonam, levofloxacin, ertapenem, ceftazidime, cefazolin, cefepime, ampicillin-sulbactam, ciprofloxacin, ceftazidime-avibactam, and ceftolozane-tazobactam. [g] If antibiotic was modified. Percentages are calculated based on the total number of patients who modified therapy. [h] Other antibiotics after modification included amoxicillin, amoxicillin-clavulanate, ampicillin-sulbactam, sulfamethoxazole-trimethoprim, ceftazidime, ceftazidime-avibactam, ceftolozane-tazobactam, cephalexin, ciprofloxacin, and ertapenem. In cases when escalation of therapy was indicated, piperacillin-tazobactam and meropenem were initiated. [i] Other services include hematology/oncology, gynecology/oncology, neurology, heart transplant, infectious disease, and nephrology. [j] Institution is defined as discharged to another institution, including another hospital, rehabilitation center, long-term care facility, or skilled nursing facility. [k] Death includes patients who were discharged to hospice.

The primary outcome of modification of therapy within 24 h of final culture results was not significantly different for patients in the pre-ATO and post-ATO groups (24% vs. 30% (p = 0.33)), as shown in Table 2. The secondary outcome of modification of therapy at any point in therapy after final culture results was not significantly different between the two groups (65% vs. 67%, p = 0.73). Of the 147 patients who received a modification of therapy, the mean time to modification from time of final culture results was not significantly different between the two cohorts (27.2 h vs. 25.4 h, p = 0.09). All other secondary outcomes were not significantly different between study groups including days of broad-spectrum antibiotic therapy.

Table 2. Primary and secondary outcomes.

	Pre-Intervention (n = 97)	Post-Intervention (n = 125)	p-Value
Primary outcome			
Modification within 24 h of culture results [a]	23 (24)	37 (30)	0.33
Secondary outcomes			
Modification at any point in therapy	63 (65)	84 (67)	0.73
Time to modification (hours)–median (±IQR) [b]	27.2 (21–52)	25.4 (10–48)	0.09
14-day in-hospital mortality	8 (8)	12 (10)	0.73
DOT [c] of broad-spectrum antibiotic–median (±IQR)	6 (2–10)	5 (2–8)	0.08
C. difficile infection	2 (2)	9 (7)	0.08

Data are presented as no. (%), unless otherwise indicated. Abbreviations: AKI, acute kidney injury; DOT, days of therapy. [a] Therapy modification is defined as the action of de-escalating to targeted regimen or escalating to broader coverage based on culture results. One patient in the pre-cohort was classified as a discontinuation of antibiotics due to allergic reaction to the empiric therapy and subsequent modification of therapy to an inactive agent. [b] Time to modification among patients who modified at any point in therapy. [c] Days of therapy was calculated from day of therapy initiation through day of discontinuation. Broad-spectrum antibiotic includes piperacillin-tazobactam, ceftriaxone, meropenem, aztreonam, levofloxacin, ertapenem, ceftazidime, cefazolin, cefepime, ciprofloxacin, ceftazidime-avibactam, and ceftolozane-tazobactam.

An exploratory subgroup analysis of patients who did not achieve the primary outcome was performed to assess for differences among these patients (Table 3). A total of 75 patients were included (34 patients from the pre-cohort and 41 patients from the post-cohort). There were no significant differences in the characteristics, including ICU admission (29% vs. 29%, $p = 0.99$) and vasopressor use (21% vs. 17%, $p = 0.93$) during therapy. Resistance patterns were also similar ($p = 0.57$). Within this subgroup, we also assessed if the infectious diseases team was consulted (59% vs. 66%, $p = 0.70$), as well as if the consult occurred prior to culture results (44% vs. 39%, $p = 0.42$).

Table 3. Subgroup analysis of patients who did not achieve primary outcome.

Characteristics	Pre-Intervention ($n = 34$)	Post-Intervention ($n = 41$)	p-Value
ICU admission while on antibiotic	10 (29)	12 (29)	0.82
Vasopressor use	7 (21)	7 (17)	0.99
Antibiotic resistance			0.57
Carbapenem resistant	1 (3)	1 (2)	
Ceftriaxone resistant	5 (15)	11 (27)	
Fluoroquinolone resistant	7 (21)	3 (7)	
ID consult	20 (59)	27 (66)	0.70
ID consult before culture results	15 (44)	16 (39)	0.42

A separate analysis of the ATO data was performed for the intervention cohort (supplementary material: Table S1). Among the 125 patients included in the intervention cohort, 109 patients (87.2%) triggered the automated ATO within the EMR. Of those, 36 patients (28.8%) achieved the primary outcome of modification within 24 h of final culture results. A total of 88 patients (70.4%) had a modification of therapy at any point in the hospitalization.

3. Discussion

In this observational study evaluating the effect of an automated ATO alert in patients with GNB, we did not find a significant difference in the primary outcome. While more patients in the post-implementation cohort had a modification of antibiotic therapy within 24 h of final culture results, this difference was not statistically significant. In addition, the secondary outcome of modification at any point in therapy was not statistically significant between the two cohorts. The time to modification was shorter in the post-cohort, however this difference was not significant. The other secondary outcomes of 14-day in-hospital mortality, days of therapy, and incidence of *C. difficile* infections were also not found to be significant.

Our results may be comparable to Gruber et al. [3] who implemented an electronic antimicrobial dashboard that required physicians to complete an electronic form and a documented note within the EMR. The authors measured discontinuations of vancomycin and piperacillin-tazobactam, two of the most commonly used broad-spectrum agents. The authors found a higher rate of discontinuation of vancomycin, but, similar to our study, also found no difference for piperacillin-tazobactam. Our study included other broad-spectrum antibiotics and focused primarily on GNB, but the results were comparable.

Similar to other studies, we found that an automated ATO alert may not be as effective as the sole stewardship intervention. A passive automated alert in addition to an active intervention may be most effective. Thom et al. [5] evaluated the effect of a provider-driven paper ATO tool that consisted of a structured conversation during clinical rounds, prompted by the provider without direction from the stewardship team, and subsequent completion of a form which included current antibiotic data. The authors found a significant difference in the proportion of modification or discontinuation of antibiotics, which was analyzed as a secondary outcome. The contrasting results may indicate that an active provider-led intervention may be more effective than a more passive, automated alert as we analyzed in our study. Similarly, other studies which have assessed an active in-person ATO have reported comparable results [3,8].

Wolfe et al. [6] conducted a retrospective study evaluating all positive blood cultures including both Gram-positive and Gram-negative organisms and found that there was a significant increase in antibiotic de-escalation after the implementation of the automated ATO. The results of our study may differ largely be due to the patient population included, as Wolfe et al. included patients with all types of infections. Our study only included

Gram-negative infections, which are generally more severe infections and may be a reason for prescribers to be less inclined to de-escalate antibiotics.

The timing of the alert may have been a factor affecting our results. The ATO was designed to trigger after 72 h of antibiotic initiation to allow ample time for final cultures and sensitivities to be reported. At this point, teams would be able to make an informed and confident decision to de-escalate, escalate, or appropriately continue antibiotics. A study conducted by Van Schooneveld et al. [9] evaluated an ATO led by a pharmacist which was performed 72 h after antibiotic initiation and after ≤5 days of initiation. The authors did not find a significant difference in antibiotic use, which suggests that timing of the intervention may not be a significant factor.

Paulson et al. [10] also evaluated a pharmacist-led ATO intervention at 48 h after antibiotic initiation and evaluated antibiotic use after 72 h. The authors evaluated antibiotic use by documentation of an antibiotic plan in the EMR, which was significantly improved in the ATO group. This suggests that the 72 h timepoint may be appropriate. This study also further suggests our earlier point that an active intervention as part of an ATO may be more effective.

We hypothesized that the implementation of a physician-driven ATO would change physician practice in favor of antimicrobial stewardship measures. However, this was not observed. We speculate that this may be due to alert fatigue, as prescribers at our institution also encounter other alerts during order entry. In addition, despite widespread education of providers prior to and during implementation, further interventions may have been required, especially amongst newer prescribers.

Limitations of this study include the retrospective design of the study, which would make it difficult to control for confounding factors. Another limitation is that the ATO was designed to alert if an order was active for 72 h. Therefore, it would not account for initial one-time orders, which was true for most patients who initiated therapy in the emergency department. Our study did include one-time orders when calculating the duration of an antibiotic, and therefore the timing may not have correlated accurately with the timing of the alert for the provider in real-time. Moreover, the automated ATO allowed physicians to defer the alert, which may also have had an effect on the time when antibiotic modification was performed. However, the alert was intended to act as a reminder so even if action was not taken at that time, it may have prompted a discussion or reassessment which could lead to discontinuation at a later point. Furthermore, the EMR triggered an alert if one particular antibiotic order was active for 72 h so it would be less likely to alert for patients whose antibiotics had been reordered. For example, a dose modification resulting in the discontinuation and re-entry of the antibiotic would postpone the alert. In addition, the ATO was designed to alert only during daytime hours, so any patient eligible for the alert during evening or overnight hours may not have received the alert. It is also important to note that not all in the post-intervention cohort was eligible to receive the ATO. The authors designed the study to analyze real-world impact of the alert, rather than only eligible patients. Moreover, as mentioned earlier, the ATO implemented at our institution was a passive intervention. To build upon our results, it may be beneficial to incorporate other active stewardship tools. For example, our institution recently initiated an antimicrobial stewardship response team. This team, consisting of infectious diseases physicians, faculty members, and pharmacists, contacts providers when culture results are reported so they may provide guidance on treatment. Further studies may look into the effect of this program, or a similar intervention, in addition to an ATO. Another limitation was that there is not a well-established sample size in the literature to calculate sample size. Also, the sample is constrained by the implementation study period so our study was a convenience sampling. It is possible that our study is underpowered but because many of the referred studies also had similar results, this may not be the case.

There are also several strengths of our study. This is the first study assessing the effect of an ATO in a focused population of GNB. By including only GNB, we mitigate the risk of confounding factors due to the type of infection and inappropriate discontinuation of therapy. Another strength was that all patient-related factors, other than the intervention, were similar between the two groups, indicating minimal seasonal or secular trends that could introduce confounding factors.

An effective ATO would optimize antimicrobial usage by encouraging providers to perform timely modification of therapy. This may lead to a reduction in the duration of broad-spectrum antibiotics and, as a result, decrease the possible induction of drug resistance and other associated adverse effects. In addition, with increasing antibiotic resistance, an ATO would alert providers to escalate therapy in the case of bacteria that are resistant to the empiric antibiotic chosen. Due to its considerable potential, the ATO is being increasingly adopted across a variety of platforms and methods. This study was designed to evaluate a passive provider-driven EMR delivered ATO in patients with GNB.

While this data may not support the use of an ATO as the sole stewardship intervention, it may provide further insight into the future of antimicrobial stewardship. As clinicians continue to discover the optimal stewardship strategy, the role of the ATO may be become more pronounced. Other forms of stewardship tools, such as active in-person interventions, may be an important component of an ATO. Further studies investigating the role of an automated time out in combination with other active interventions are needed.

4. Materials and Methods

4.1. Study Design

This was a single-center, retrospective, observational, before-and-after cohort study conducted at a 625-bed academic medical center (Robert Wood Johnson University Hospital, New Brunswick, NJ, USA). The data was collected via EMR chart reviews of inpatient encounters from January 2018 to December 2018 (intervention cohort) and September 2016 to September 2017 (historical cohort). The sampling was conducted using convenience sampling of first episode per patient during the specified study period.

The EMR used at the institution is Sunrise Clinical Manager (Allscripts, Chicago, IL, USA). The study was approved by the local Institutional Review Board at Rutgers University in New Brunswick, NJ, USA.

4.2. Participants

We included hospitalized adults ($\geq$18 years) with GNB, as indicated by a positive blood culture with a Gram-negative pathogen, who received at least 72 h of empiric antibiotics at any point in hospitalization. Only Gram-negative isolates were included as these were likely indicative of true infections. Patients who received less than 72 h of empiric antibiotics would not have triggered the alert. Patients were excluded if they had neutropenia, or absolute neutrophil count (ANC) below 500 cells/m^3 at time of antibiotic initiation and during empiric therapy. These neutropenic patients would be more likely to continue broad-spectrum antibiotics for longer duration, independent of clinical response or culture results. Patients were also excluded if antibiotics were initiated prior to the patient's admission on the basis of the outside hospital's culture results since therapy would already be targeted to recovered pathogen, or if more than one pathogen was identified in the set of blood cultures as other culture results may impact the provider's decision to continue or modify antimicrobial therapy.

4.3. Routine Work-Up and Reporting from the Microbiology Laboratory

The microbiology laboratory is located on-site at Robert Wood Johnson University Hospital. All positive blood culture Gram stain results are called to the nurse caring for the patient who then informs the patient's physician. Final culture results with identification of organism and susceptibility to antimicrobials are available in the EMR. During both the historical and intervention cohort time periods, there were no changes to laboratory processes or reporting of positive blood cultures as positive. No rapid diagnostic testing strategies were employed for identification of Gram-negative organisms from blood culture isolates. In addition, the antimicrobial stewardship program was not directly involved with routine review, reporting, or guidance of Gram-negative blood culture isolates during the entire study period.

4.4. Intervention

The ATO was an automated dashboard built into the EMR displayed to ordering providers. This was implemented in October 2017. The alert was triggered after a patient received at least 72 h of any antibiotic and after a provider entered any new order for that patient in an effort to avoid interruption of workflow. The dashboard displayed the patient's relevant data, including culture results (if any), temperature curve, laboratory trends, and current antibiotics (supplementary material: Figure S1). The user had the option to either continue or discontinue each antibiotic within that screen. The user was also given the option to defer, in the event that the user cannot make a decision on the basis of the results at that time. Deferring the alert would cause the alert to trigger again after 12 h for that individual provider. In addition, the alert did not fire overnight when the on-call providers were less likely to make decisions on patients for whom they were not the primary care provider. The ATO was designed to alert providers when there may be a potential to optimize antimicrobial therapy in a timely and convenient manner. Educational efforts were provided to all ordering providers prior to the implementation via in-person sessions and electronic distribution through the medical staff newsletter.

4.5. Outcomes

The primary outcome was the proportion of patients who received a modification of therapy for GNB within 24 h of final culture results. Modification of therapy was defined as either a de-escalation to a targeted agent or escalation of therapy to broader coverage based on susceptibilities of blood cultures. De-escalation was defined as a change in antibiotic from a broad-spectrum agent to a more targeted agent on the basis of the results of the culture. Escalation was a change in antibiotic to an agent with a broader spectrum on the basis of the results of the culture. Secondary outcomes included modification at any point in therapy and time to modification among those patients. All outcomes measuring time were measured from the time of final culture susceptibilities reported ("time zero"). Other outcomes included 14-day in-hospital mortality, *C. difficile infection* incidence, and days of therapy of empiric antibiotics.

4.6. Statistical Analysis

Continuous data were reported as means with standard deviations or medians with interquartile ranges (IQR), as appropriate. All categorical data were reported as percentages. Continuous data were analyzed with using Student's *t*-test or Wilcoxon rank sum test for nonparametric distribution. Categorical data were analyzed using the chi-squared test or Fisher's exact test, as appropriate. The significance level was determined as a *p*-value of <0.05 (two-sided). A subgroup analysis of baseline characteristics was performed for patients who did not achieve the primary outcome. Data were analyzed using R software (version 1.0.136).

5. Conclusions

In conclusion, the results of our study indicate that a provider-driven automated ATO did not have a significant effect on modifying antibiotic therapy following culture results. However, future studies are required to determine the optimal timing of the alert, especially in the setting of rapid diagnostics. By optimizing the ATO, we can improve antimicrobial stewardship on a global scale and ultimately lessen the risk of antimicrobial resistance.

Supplementary Materials: The following are available online at https://www.mdpi.com/article/10.3390/antibiotics10091078/s1, Table S1: Antibiotic time out data for intervention cohort. Figure S1: Example of time out alert.

Author Contributions: D.C., A.M. and T.B. contributed to the conceptualization. D.C., P.V. and S.M.M. contributed to the data curation. S.M.M., N.N. and T.B. contributed to writing and revision of the work. All authors have read and agreed to the published version of the manuscript.

Funding: This research received no external funding.

Institutional Review Board Statement: Ethical approval for this study was obtained from the Rutgers Institutional Review Board and Research Utilization Group (Pro20170000887, 26 November 2018). The study was conducted according to the guidelines of the Declaration of Helsinki.

Informed Consent Statement: Patient consent was waived due to retrospective nature of study which had little to no risk to subjects.

Data Availability Statement: The datasets generated during and/or analyzed during the current study are available from the corresponding author upon reasonable request.

Conflicts of Interest: The authors declare no conflict of interest.

References

1. Centers for Disease Control and Prevention. *Core Elements of Hospital Antibiotic Stewardship Programs*; US Department of Health and Human Services, CDC: Atlanta, GA, USA, 2019. Available online: https://www.cdc.gov/antibiotic-use/core-elements/hospital.html (accessed on 29 July 2019).
2. The Joint Commission. *New Antimicrobial Stewardship Standard*; Joint Commission Perspectives: Oak Brook, IL, USA, 2016; Volume 36, Available online: https://www.jointcommission.org/-/media/enterprise/tjc/imported-resource-assets/documents/new_antimicrobial_stewardship_standardpdf.pdf?db=web&hash=69307456CCE435B134854392C7FA7D76&hash=69307456CCE435B134854392C7FA7D76 (accessed on 29 July 2019).
3. Graber, C.J.; Jones, M.M.; Glassman, P.A.; Weir, C.; Butler, J.; Nechodom, K.; Kay, C.L.; Furman, A.E.; Tran, T.T.; Foltz, C.; et al. Taking an Antibiotic Time-out: Utilization and Usability of a Self-Stewardship Time-out Program for Renewal of Vancomycin and Piperacillin-Tazobactam. *Hosp. Pharm.* **2015**, *50*, 1011–1024. [CrossRef] [PubMed]
4. Lee, T.C.; Frenette, C.; Jayaraman, D.; Green, L.; Pilote, L. Antibiotic Self-stewardship: Trainee-Led Structured Antibiotic Time-outs to Improve Antimicrobial Use. *Ann. Intern. Med.* **2014**, *161*, S53–S58. [CrossRef] [PubMed]
5. Thom, K.A.; Tamma, P.D.; Harris, A.D.; Dzintars, K.; Morgan, D.J.; Li, S.; Pineles, L.; Srinivasan, A.; Avdic, E.; Cosgrove, S.E. Impact of a Prescriber-driven Antibiotic Time-out on Antibiotic Use in Hospitalized Patients. *Clin. Infect. Dis.* **2018**, *68*, 1581–1584. [CrossRef] [PubMed]
6. Wolfe, J.R.; Bryant, A.M.; Khoury, J.A. Impact of an automated antibiotic time-out alert on the de-escalation of broad-spectrum antibiotics at a large community teaching hospital. *Infect. Control Hosp. Epidemiol.* **2019**, *40*, 1287–1289. [CrossRef] [PubMed]
7. Bhowmick, T.; Kirn, T.J.; Hetherington, F.; Takavarasha, S.; Sandhu, S.S.; Gandhi, S.; Narayanan, N.; Weinstein, M.P. Collaboration between an antimicrobial stewardship team and the microbiology laboratory can shorten time to directed antibiotic therapy for methicillin-susceptible staphylococcal bacteremia and to discontinuation of antibiotics for coagulase-negative staphylococcal contaminants. *Diagn. Microbiol. Infect. Dis.* **2018**, *92*, 214–219. [CrossRef] [PubMed]
8. Senn, L.; Burnand, B.; Francioli, P.; Zanetti, G. Improving appropriateness of antibiotic therapy: Randomized trial of an inter-vention to foster reassessment of prescription after 3 days. *J. Antimicrob. Chemother.* **2004**, *53*, 1062–1067. [CrossRef] [PubMed]
9. Van Schooneveld, T.C.; Rupp, M.E.; Cavaleiri, R.J.; Lyden, E.; Rolek, K. Cluster randomized trial of an antibiotic time-out led by a team-based pharmacist. *Infect. Control Hosp. Epidemiol.* **2020**, *41*, 1266–1271. [CrossRef] [PubMed]
10. Paulson, C.M.; Handley, J.F.; Dilworth, T.J.; Persells, D.; Prusi, R.Y.; Brummitt, C.F.; Torres, K.M.; Skrupky, L.P. Impact of a Systematic Pharmacist-Initiated Antibiotic Time-Out Intervention for Hospitalized Adults. *J. Pharm. Pract.* **2020**, *2020*. [CrossRef]

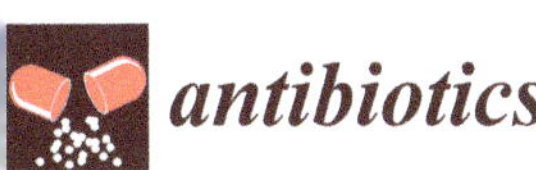

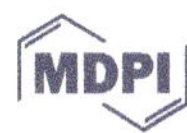

Article

Retrospective Cohort Analysis of the Effect of Antimicrobial Stewardship on Postoperative Antibiotic Therapy in Complicated Intra-Abdominal Infections: Short-Course Therapy Does Not Compromise Patients' Safety

Güzin Surat [1,*], Pascal Meyer-Sautter [2], Jan Rüsch [2], Johannes Braun-Feldweg [2], Christoph-Thomas Germer [2] and Johan Friso Lock [2]

1 Unit for Infection Control and Antimicrobial Stewardship, University Hospital of Würzburg, 97080 Würzburg, Germany

2 Department of General-, Visceral-, Transplant-, Vascular- and Pediatric Surgery, University Hospital of Würzburg, 97080 Würzburg, Germany; meyer-sautter.p@gmx.de (P.M.-S.); jan-ruesch@t-online.de (J.R.); johannes.braun-feldweg@gmx.de (J.B.-F.); germer_c@ukw.de (C.-T.G.); lock_j@ukw.de (J.F.L.)

* Correspondence: surat_g@ukw.de

Abstract: Background: Recent evidence suggests that short-course postoperative antibiotic therapy (PAT) of intra-abdominal infections is non-inferior considering clinical outcomes. The aim of this study was to compare the outcome of short vs. long PAT in complicated intra-abdominal infections (cIAIs) without sepsis. Methods: We performed a single center-quality improvement study at a 1500 bed sized university hospital in Bavaria, Germany, with evaluation of the length of antibiotic therapy after emergency surgery on cIAIs with adequate source control during 2016 to 2018. We reviewed a total of 260 cases (160 short duration vs. 100 long duration). The antibiotic prescribing quality was assessed by our in-house antimicrobial stewardship team (AMS). Results: No significant differences of patient characteristics were observed between short and long PAT. The frequency of long PAT declined during the observation period from 48.1% to 26.3%. Prolongation of PAT was not linked with any clinical benefits, on the contrary clinical outcome of patients receiving longer regimes were associated with higher postoperative morbidity. AMS identified additional educational targets to improve antibiotic prescribing quality on general wards like unnecessary postoperative switches of antibiotic regimes, e.g., unrequired switches to oral antibiotics as well as prolongation of PAT due to elevated CRP. Conclusion: Short-course antibiotic therapy after successful surgical source control in cIAIs is safe, and long-duration PAT has no beneficial effects.

Keywords: antimicrobial stewardship; antibiotic prescribing quality; low-risk intra-abdominal infections; post-operative antibiotic treatment

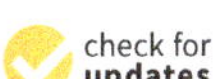

Citation: Surat, G.; Meyer-Sautter, P.; Rüsch, J.; Braun-Feldweg, J.; Germer, C.-T.; Lock, J.F. Retrospective Cohort Analysis of the Effect of Antimicrobial Stewardship on Postoperative Antibiotic Therapy in Complicated Intra-Abdominal Infections: Short-Course Therapy Does Not Compromise Patients' Safety. *Antibiotics* **2022**, *11*, 120. https://doi.org/10.3390/antibiotics11010120

Academic Editors: Diane Ashiru-Oredope and Marc Maresca

Received: 22 December 2021
Accepted: 15 January 2022
Published: 17 January 2022

Publisher's Note: MDPI stays neutral with regard to jurisdictional claims in published maps and institutional affiliations.

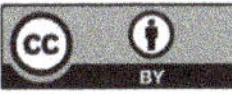

Copyright: © 2022 by the authors. Licensee MDPI, Basel, Switzerland. This article is an open access article distributed under the terms and conditions of the Creative Commons Attribution (CC BY) license (https://creativecommons.org/licenses/by/4.0/).

1. Introduction

Antimicrobial stewardship programs (ASPs) are gaining, globally, increasing in merited recognition and acceptance and were primarily launched to stop antimicrobial resistance (AMR) [1,2]. As antibiotic consumption is considered the main driver for AMR—natural factors, such as intrinsic or acquired genetic resistance patterns, environmental sources and missing hygiene measures are contributing effects too—one of the starting-points includes improving the social and prescribing attitude towards the use of antimicrobial agents [3–6]. Indication, choice of antimicrobial agent, way of application, de-escalation efforts and duration are amongst the markers to be evaluated each time antibiotics are prescribed [7–9]. Incorporating multimodal concepts by engaging the responsible physicians without neglecting nurse staff and undergraduate trainees embedded in a multidisciplinary team, including infectious diseases specialists, microbiologists, pharmacists and infection control physicians in charge, is by far the most worthwhile strategy in order to assure sustainable success for AMR to be antagonized [10–13]. Postantibiotic duration for complicated surgical intra-abdominal infections (cIAIs) attracts focus and motivates progressively more data suggesting that a short regimen may suffice for an optimal clinical recovery applying for both, complicated mild/moderate IAIs and severe postoperative IAIs in critically ill patients, provided source control has been achieved [14–16]. Maximizing the clinical benefit by minimizing collateral damage remains the curative principle especially given the high rates of mortality and morbidity in patients with (uncontrolled) cIAIs [17–19]. Uncomplicated IAIs are managed either only surgically or conservatively with antibiotics alone. For cIAIs the approach encloses timely performed surgical source control with appropriate antimicrobial treatment; community or hospital acquired IAIs may be uncomplicated or complicated by definition as well [17,20–22].

This study is to be understood as a sequel to previously published data by Surat et al. on the impact of antimicrobial stewardship on antibiotic consumption for non-elective surgical IAIs [12]. However, this sub-analysis opens the chapter to postantibiotic therapy (PAT) in complicated mild/moderate community-acquired IAIs in non-septic patients with achieved source control, also encompassing de-escalation manners e.g., switching to oral therapy conducted on general wards and aim at confirming the trend that a short duration of PAT is again not afflicted with higher rates of postoperative infectious complications or worse clinical outcomes.

2. Methods

This quality improvement study entails a period of 3 years (2016–2018) and was conducted retrospectively in a 1500 bed tertiary hospital in Germany, with an in-hospital ASP officially launched in 2015, gradually reaching out to all departments including the department of general surgery by 2018. The backbone of the in-house AMS team consists of infection control physicians, microbiologists, pharmacists and infectious diseases (ID) consultants with an ID physician responsible for the leadership. The prequel of this project included 776 patients and focused on the impact of antimicrobial stewardship interventions on surgical antibiotic prescription behavior of surgical IAIs, especially postoperative antibiotic use and the appropriateness of indication. The previous analysis revealed a significant reduction of total days of antibiotic therapy and fewer patients receiving PAT altogether [12]. The intention of this subsequent analysis was to assess the impact of antimicrobial stewardship implementations on patients actually receiving PAT due to cIAIs but were non-septic or had life-threatening conditions.

2.1. Study Design

The effects of different durations of antibiotic therapy in IAIs were examined by a retrospective cohort analysis. All data were retrieved from the hospital information system and transferred in a pseudonymous database with multiple variables containing baseline patient characteristics, pre-, peri- and postoperative antibiotic therapy (ABT), surgical therapy, and postoperative 30-day outcome. We defined two groups based of the duration of PAT. The short duration group was limited to a maximum of 4 days post-surgery, leant on the STOP-IT trial by Sawyer et al. (sPAT group) [14]. Patients with longer PAT were included in the lPAT group. Any extension beyond this had to be discussed with the in-hospital AMS-team. Reasons for allowed extensions of therapy were immune suppression or other present infections such as pneumonia or urinary tract infection. The follow-up was limited to 30 days.

2.2. Patients

All patients ≥18 years undergoing emergency abdominal surgery with IAI and PAT during 01.01.2016 and 31.12.2018 were included with the following selection criteria: Diagnosis of peritonitis (ICD-10 K65.0–K65.9), acute cholecystitis (ICD-10 K80.0-K80.01, K81.0), acute appendicitis (ICD-10 K35.2–K35.8), acute diverticulitis (ICD-10 K57.2–K57.22), or intestinal perforation (K25.1–K25.2, K26.1–K26.2, K63.0–K63.2). Patients with the following criteria were excluded from analysis: Acute pancreatitis, acute mesenteric ischemia, acute leukemia, end-stage malignant disease in palliative care, ASA score > IV, extra-abdominal infectious focus requiring antimicrobial therapy before and after surgery. For this subgroup analysis, we included only non-septic patients with complicated IAIs with successfully achieved surgical source control. Patients with postoperative anastomotic insufficiency were excluded in this analysis.

2.3. Outcome Assessment

Postoperative outcome assessment up to 30 days postoperative. Postoperative complications were graded according to Clavien-Dindo [23]. Clavien-Dindo grade I-II complications were appraised as no severe complications, whereas Clavien-Dindo grade IIIa-V complications were appraised as severe complications. Surgical site infections (SSI) were defined according to the Centers for Disease Control and Prevention (CDC) criteria [24].

2.4. Statistical Analysis

All statistical analyses were performed using IBM SPSS Statistics, version 26 (International Business Machines Corporation, Armonk, NY, USA). Descriptive data were reported as means with standard deviation, unless otherwise noted. Groups were compared using the Chi-square, Fisher's exact Test or Mann–Whitney U test according to the data scale and distribution. The level of statistical significance was 0.05 (two-sided).

3. Results

Patients' Baseline Characteristics and Indications for Emergency Surgery

There were no significant disparities in the preoperative risk-stratification between the two groups. Shorter therapies were significantly more common in 2018 than in the previous two years. The collected risk scores (Charlson comorbidity index and ASA score) did not either differ significantly between both groups. Severe previous liver or kidney disease or immunosuppression at the time of surgery were generally rare in the observed cohort and similarly distributed between both groups. Preoperative risk factors such as prolonged hospitalizations or pre-operations were also not present in greater numbers in either group. Intraoperative findings revealed a higher prevalence of peritonitis in the sPAT group (Table 1). There were slightly more cases of cholecystitis in the sPAT, and slightly more cases of appendicitis and colonic perforations in the lPAT group.

Insignificantly more patients (sPAT 50% vs. lPAT 38%) were admitted directly to the normal ward compared to patients who required intensive care support (sPAT 33.8% vs. lPAT 48%). Accordingly, these patients were more often postoperatively ventilated (sPAT 21.3% vs. lPAT 31%) and received vasopressors (sPAT 17.5% vs. lPAT 26%). However, these differences were again not statistically significant. There were almost twice as many surgical side infections in the lPAT group (sPAT 6.9% vs. lPAT 12%), almost as many as non-intra-abdominal infections (lPAT 11.9% vs. lPAT 10%), but this effect was also not statistically significant. Importantly the groups differed significantly regarding postoperative complications. The rate of necessary re-interventions was almost twice as high in long-treated patients (sPAT 15% vs. lPAT 27%). Of these re-interventions many had to be performed as re-operations (sPAT 8.8% vs. lPAT 23%). Accordingly, the postoperative complications classified as per Clavien–Dindo were found to be to the disadvantage of the lPAT group (sPAT 11.9% vs. lPAT 23%) (a complication-free course was significantly more frequent in the short treated group (sPAT 36.3% vs. lPAT 16%). Length-of-stay (LOS) differed significantly in the sPAT group (median 7 days) compared to the lPAT group (median 11 days). In contrast, there was no difference in LOIS (Table 2). While the total duration of PAT in the short-treated group was 4 days on average and median, patients in the lPAT group were treated for more than twice as long (median 8; Table 2).

Table 1. Preoperative patient characteristics and intraoperative findings.

Characteristic	Patients, No. (%)		p Value [b]
	Postoperative Antibiotic Therapy		
	Short (n = 160)	Long (n = 100)	
2016	42 (51.9)	39 (48.1)	0.015
2017	59 (59.6)	40 (40.4)	
2018	59 (73.8)	21 (26.3)	
age, mean (median)	58.00 (61.50)	58.40 (62.00)	0.910
ASA classification			
1	15 (9.4)	8 (8.0)	0.281
2	77 (48.1)	43 (43.0)	
3	58 (36.3)	36 (36.0)	
4	9 (5.6)	13 (13.0)	
BMI, mean (median)	27.30 (27.00)	27.00 (27.0)	0.832
CCI			
none (0)	41 (25.6)	27 (27.0)	0.264
low (1–2)	33 (20.6)	17 (17.0)	
moderate (3–4)	52 (32.5)	25 (25.0)	
severe (>4)	34 (21.3)	31 (31.0)	
liver cirrhosis	1 (0.6)	1 (1.0)	0.736
chronic kidney disease	15 (9.4)	17 (17.0)	0.069
current immunosuppressive drugs	9 (5.6)	8 (8.0)	0.451
community-acquired IAI	133 (83.1)	83 (83.0)	0.979
hospital-aquired IAI	27 (16.9)	17 (17.0)	
high-risk of MDR	28 (17.5)	17 (17.0)	0.917
preoperative [a] LOS, mean (median), d	14.00 (0.00)	13.00 (0.00)	0.724
surgery	15 (9.4)	8 (8.0)	0.704
MDR	5 (3.1)	5 (5.0)	0.444
MRSA	1 (0.6)	0 (0.0)	0.737
VRE	2 (1.3)	2 (2.0)	
3MRGN	1 (0.6)	2 (2.0)	
intraoperative peritonitis	90 (56.3)	49 (49.0)	0.254
gastric perforation	10 (6.3)	4 (4.0)	0.612
small intestine perforation	10 (6.3)	9 (9.0)	
colonic perforation	20 (12.5)	17 (17.0)	
appendicitis	55 (34.4)	39 (39.0)	
cholecystitis	57 (35.6)	28 (28.0)	
intestinal obstruction	7 (4.4)	3 (3.0)	

[a] Within 30 days prior index surgery; [b] p values were derived from Chi-square, Fisher's exact or Mann-Whitney U tests, depeding upon data scale. Abbreviations: ASA, American Society of Anesthesiologists; BMI, body mass index; CCI, Charlson comorbidity index; IAI, intra-abdominal infection; LOS, length of hospital stay; ABT, antibiotic therapy; MDR, multidrug-resistant bacteria, GI: gastrointestinal.

Table 2. Postoperative outcome.

Characteristic [a]	Patients, No. (%)		p Value [d]
	Postoperative Antibiotic Therapy		
	Short (n = 160)	Long (n = 100)	
postoperative transfer to			
general ward	80 (50.0)	38 (38.0)	0.069
IMC	26 (16.3)	14 (14.0)	
ICU	54 (33.8)	48 (48.0)	
postoperative organ support			
ventilation	34 (21.3)	31 (31.0)	0.077
vasopressors	28 (17.5)	26 (26.0)	0.100
SSI	11 (6.9)	12 (12.0)	0.157
other postoperative infections [b]	19 (11.9)	10 (10.0)	0.640
re-intervention necessary	24 (15.0)	27 (27.0)	0.018
re-operation necessary	14 (8.8)	23 (23.0)	0.001
postoperative findings			
MDR	4 (2.5)	3 (3.0)	0.809
postoperative complications [c]			
none	58 (36.3)	16 (16.0)	0.001
no severe complications	83 (51.9)	61 (61.0)	
severe complications	19 (11.9)	23 (23.0)	
postoperative mortality	2 (1.3)	0 (0)	0.262
LOS mean (median)	10.00 (7.00)	14.00 (11.00)	<0.001
LOIS mean (median)	2.00 (1.00)	3.00 (1.00)	0.138
duration of PAT mean (median) in days	4 (4)	9 (8.5)	<0.001

[a] Within 30 days after the index surgery; [b] non-intraabdominal infection such as urinary tract infection, pneumonia, etc; [c] according to the Clavien–Dindo classification; [d] p values were derived from Chi-square, Fisher's exact or Mann-Whitney U tests, depeding upon data scale. Abbreviations: IMC, intermediate care unit; ICU, intensive care unit; SSI, surgical site infection; MDR, multi-drug-resistance bacteria discovered postoperative; PAT, postoperative antibiotic therapy; AMS, antimicrobial stewardship; LOS, length of stay; LOIS, length of stay on ICU.

The initial empiric antibiotic regimens between both groups were quite similar. Patients on long therapy were more frequently subject to switches (sPAT 19.4% vs. lPAT 56%). Switches were rarely due to AMS recommendations in either group (sPAT 9.7% vs. lPAT 1.8%), nor to keeping with the actual resistograms. Undocumented indications for the use of antibiotics were still high (sPAT 77.4% vs. lPAT 72.7%; Table 3). Nevertheless, most indications were deemed appropriate by our in-house AMS-team (sPAT 75.6% vs. lPAT 77%). Inappropriate indications were mostly due to prolongations of the perioperative prophylaxis (PAP). There were large differences in the management of switches, for example 32% of those treated long were incorrectly escalated (mostly from a 1st/2nd generation cephalosporin to an oral 3rd generation cephalosporin, in comparison to 9.4% in the short-treated group (Table 3). As per general definition a switch form intravenous to oral antibiotic therapy is considered de-escalation, we defined this step as 'escalation' when the selected oral antibiotic belonged to 3rd generation cephalosporins such as cefpodoxime [7].

Table 3. Postoperative antibiotic therapy.

Characteristic	Patients, No. (%)		*p* Value [a]
	Postoperative Antibiotic Therapy		
	Short (n = 160)	Long (n = 100)	
Initial Regimen:			
cephalosporins	76 (72.4)	52 (67.5)	0.641
broad-spectrum penicillin	26 (24.8)	21 (27.3)	
carbapenems	3 (2.9)	4 (5.2)	
switch of antibiotic agent	31 (19.4)	56 (56.0)	<0.001
postoperative day of switch, mean (median), d	3.00 (2.00)	4.00 (3.00)	0.004
Reason for Switch of Antibiotic Agent			
not documented	24 (77.4)	40 (72.7)	0.123
resistogram	4 (12.9)	14 (25.5)	
AMS council	3 (9.7)	1 (1.8)	
switch in ICU or IMC	7 (22.6)	9 (16.4)	0.567
switch on general ward	24 (77.4)	46 (83.6)	
Assessment Based on AMS-Guidelines			
PAT necessary	121 (75.6)	77 (77.0)	0.800
de-escalation or discontinuation correct	154 (96.3)	79 (79.0)	<0.001
missing de-escalation	4 (2.5)	20 (20.0)	
missing escalation	2 (1.3)	1 (1.0)	
Switch of Empirical Antibiotic Therapy			
not required or correctly performed	143 (89.4)	65 (65.0)	<0.001
wrong de-escalation	2 (1.3)	3 (3.0)	
wrong escalation	15 (9.4)	32 (32.0)	
efficacy			
not effective against strains	96 (60.0)	57 (57.0)	0.632
effective against detected strains	64 (40.0)	43 (43.0)	
Biochemical Values After PAT			
leukocytes. mean (median)	9.60 (8.60)	10.20 (9.90)	0.076
CRP mean (median)	10.30 (8.00)	6.10 (4.00)	<0.001
PCT mean (median)	6.90 (0.80)	0.50 (0.50)	0.643

[a] *p* values were derived from Chi-square, Fisher's exact or Mann-Whitney U tests, depeding upon data scale. Abbreviations: AMS, antimicrobial-stewardship as defined by current AMS-standards; ICU, intensive care unit; IMC, intermediate care unit; PAT, postoperative antibiotic therapy; CRP, C-reactive protein; PCT, procalcitonin.

4. Discussion

In this retrospective single-center study we analyzed patients requiring emergency surgery for complicated IAIs over 2016–2018 with attention on the length of PAT. Yet, unlike to the prequel published by Surat et al. these findings included only non-septic patients with adequate source control [12,25]. This time the prescribing attitudes of surgeons on general wards were the focus of our observations, within the wider ambition of discerning the influence of biochemical inflammation markers such as C-reactive protein (CRP) or procalcitonin (PCT) on the duration of PAT.

In accordance with the data released on postsurgical antimicrobial management in complicated community acquired (or healthcare associated IAIs) so far, our results support that shortened PAT is not associated with worse clinical outcomes. The surgical and clinical conditions that warranted interventions in this study were similar to the general published data (e.g., peritonitis, appendicitis, cholecystitis) [14,15,26–28]. Here, both groups did not differ in the risk-profile and yet the long-duration arm became evident with a significantly higher rate of infectious complications and, in consequence necessitated more re-operations. Continuing misuse of antibiotics has been linked with avoidable adverse events, emergence of antibiotic resistance and unnecessary monetary burden for the health system and demands a change in the prescribing culture of antibiotics [9,29]. The debate about the duration of PAT is still ongoing and remains an important key factor for ASPs to target on for it is deemed to being the main reason for inappropriate use of antibiotics in managing IAIs [20,30]. Fortunately, our results re-emphasize the role of ASPs on antibiotics for the postsurgical therapy of complicated IAIs: over the observed three years (2016–2018) the duration of PAT successively shortened, which is mainly attributed to the roll-out of our in-hospital ASP involving general wards in the already regularly happening antibiotic ward rounds and discussions in intensive care units. Although this finding was not statistically significant, long-duration PAT, on the other hand, did not prevent the significant need for re-interventions, even given the fact that PAT was administered twice as long within the long-duration group. These results are in line with data from Tellado et al. that showed that inappropriate indication for the empiric use of antibiotics was associated with unsuccessful outcomes and a higher rate of e.g., re-operations [31].

Looking further into the quality of antibiotic utilization, the long-duration group happened to have not only a higher rate of switches of the empirically selected antibiotic agents, but these switches mainly took place on the general surgical wards resulting in 'escalations' to oral antibiotics–reasonable, one might think given patients surgical and clinical status and the fact that AMS consultations for general wards were missing at the time. Although intravenous to oral antibiotic switch is a main tool in ASPs, in our study these actions were considered inappropriate by our in-hospital AMS team for it prolonged unnecessarily the duration wherein treatment could have been stopped. Importantly, the choices of oral antibiotics were not in keeping with the in-house AMS de-escalation standards (2nd- and 3rd-generation cephalosporin with poor oral bioavailability lacking efficacy; data not available in the result part) [7,9,28].

Guiding antibiotic therapy by inflammatory markers (e.g., leukocyte count, CRP, PCT or interleukin 6), has been numerously investigated in hospitalized patients including those critically ill. PCT carries more specificity and sensitivity in the detection of truly bacterial infections and the guidance of antibiotic duration by PCT may result in significant reduction of antibiotic consumption and mortality [32–36]. Data on the prescribing behavior in cIAIs directed by named markers remain sparse and yet the results, so far, attest PCT a useful tool for both the diagnosis of bacterial infections and discontinuation of antibiotics; yet, it must be stressed that biomarkers should not be read outside the clinical setting [35,37,38]. The power and the nature of this study does not allow to draw a conclusion regarding the role of PCT in terms of ceasing PAT or the safeness of such a course, yet following the decrease of the CRP level was associated with longer PAT.

Discussing the results of this study on the whole, the point of its research nature as in the meaning of monocentric and retrospective limits their interpretation. Furthermore, the power of the study cannot be used to reason that shortened duration of PAT is associated with improved outcomes, but it clearly suggests that a longer duration of antibiotic therapy is tied with more complications and does do more harm than good. The subject of the influence of laboratory markers on the duration of PAT and the detailed appropriateness and quantification of switches from intravenous to oral antibiotics will be outlined in future investigations. In conclusion, our results confirm that short-course antibiotic therapy after successful surgical source control in cIAIs is safe.

Author Contributions: All authors significantly contributed to the design of the study, the acquisition or interpretation of data. G.S. and J.F.L. wrote the manuscript. P.M.-S., J.R. and J.B.-F. collected and analyzed the data. C.-T.G. contributed to the design of the study and revised the manuscript. All authors have read and agreed to the published version of the manuscript.

Funding: There was no funding for this study.

Institutional Review Board Statement: The analysis was approved by the ethics committee of the Julius-Maximilians University of Würzburg (Ref. 20210505 03).

Informed Consent Statement: Not applicable.

Data Availability Statement: The data presented in this study are available on request from the corresponding author. The data are not publicly available due to European General Data Protection Regulation (GDPR).

Acknowledgments: We all consent to thank Ulrich Vogel for the assistance during design and conduct of the study.

Conflicts of Interest: The authors declare no conflict of interest.

References

1. Sartelli, M.; Labricciosa, F.M.; Barbadoro, P.; Pagani, L.; Ansaloni, L.; Brink, A.J.; Carlet, J.; Khanna, A.; Chichom-Mefire, A.; Coccolini, F.; et al. The Global Alliance for Infections in Surgery: Defining a model for antimicrobial stewardship-results from an international cross-sectional survey. *World J. Emerg. Surg.* **2017**, *12*, 34. [CrossRef]
2. Owens, R.C., Jr. Antimicrobial stewardship: Concepts and strategies in the 21st century. *Diagn. Microbiol. Infect. Dis.* **2008**, *61*, 110–128. [CrossRef]
3. Davey, P.; Marwick, C.A.; Scott, C.L.; Charani, E.; McNeil, K.; Brown, E.; Gould, I.M.; Ramsay, C.R.; Michie, S. Interventions to improve antibiotic prescribing practices for hospital inpatients. *Cochrane Database Syst. Rev.* **2017**, *2*, CD003543. [CrossRef] [PubMed]
4. Charani, E.; Castro-Sanchez, E.; Sevdalis, N.; Kyratsis, Y.; Drumright, L.; Shah, N.; Holmes, A. Understanding the determinants of antimicrobial prescribing within hospitals: The role of "prescribing etiquette". *Clin. Infect. Dis.* **2013**, *57*, 188–196. [CrossRef] [PubMed]
5. Vikesland, P.; Garner, E.; Gupta, S.; Kang, S.; Maile-Moskowitz, A.; Zhu, N. Differential Drivers of Antimicrobial Resistance across the World. *Acc. Chem. Res.* **2019**, *52*, 916–924. [CrossRef] [PubMed]
6. Holmes, A.H.; Moore, L.S.P.; Sundsfjord, A.; Steinbakk, M.; Regmi, S.; Karkey, A.; Guerin, P.J.; Piddock, L.J.V. Understanding the mechanisms and drivers of antimicrobial resistance. *Lancet* **2016**, *387*, 176–187. [CrossRef]
7. de With, K.; Wilke, K.; Kern, W.V.; Strauß4, R.; Kramme, E.; Friedrichs, A.; Holzmann, T.; Geiss, H.K.; Isner, C.; Fellhauer, M.; et al. AWMF-S3-Leitlinie Strategien zur Sicherung Rationaler Antibiotika-Anwendung im Krankenhaus. Available online: https://www.awmf.org/leitlinien/detail/ll/092-001.html (accessed on 5 March 2019).
8. Tarchini, G.; Liau, K.H.; Solomkin, J.S. Antimicrobial Stewardship in Surgery: Challenges and Opportunities. *Clin. Infect. Dis.* **2017**, *64*, S112–S114. [CrossRef]
9. Barlam, T.F.; Cosgrove, S.E.; Abbo, L.M.; MacDougall, C.; Schuetz, A.N.; Septimus, E.J.; Srinivasan, A.; Dellit, T.H.; Falck-Ytter, Y.T.; Fishman, N.O.; et al. Implementing an Antibiotic Stewardship Program: Guidelines by the Infectious Diseases Society of America and the Society for Healthcare Epidemiology of America. *Clin. Infect. Dis.* **2016**, *62*, e51–e77. [CrossRef]
10. Majumder, M.A.A.; Rahman, S.; Cohall, D.; Bharatha, A.; Singh, K.; Haque, M.; Gittens-St Hilaire, M. Antimicrobial Stewardship: Fighting Antimicrobial Resistance and Protecting Global Public Health. *Infect. Drug Resist.* **2020**, *13*, 4713–4738. [CrossRef] [PubMed]
11. Majumder, M.A.A.; Singh, K.; Hilaire, M.G.; Rahman, S.; Sa, B.; Haque, M. Tackling Antimicrobial Resistance by promoting Antimicrobial stewardship in Medical and Allied Health Professional Curricula. *Expert Rev. Anti-Infect. Ther.* **2020**, *18*, 1245–1258. [CrossRef]
12. Surat, G.; Vogel, U.; Wiegering, A.; Germer, C.T.; Lock, J.F. Defining the Scope of Antimicrobial Stewardship Interventions on the Prescription Quality of Antibiotics for Surgical Intra-Abdominal Infections. *Antibiotics* **2021**, *10*, 73. [CrossRef]
13. Wang, R.; Degnan, K.O.; Luther, V.P.; Szymczak, J.E.; Goren, E.N.; Logan, A.; Shnekendorf, R.; Hamilton, K.W. Development of a Multifaceted Antimicrobial Stewardship Curriculum for Undergraduate Medical Education: The Antibiotic Stewardship, Safety, Utilization, Resistance, and Evaluation (ASSURE) Elective. Elective. *Open Forum Infect. Dis.* **2021**, *8*, ofab231. [CrossRef]
14. Sawyer, R.G.; Claridge, J.A.; Nathens, A.B.; Rotstein, O.D.; Duane, T.M.; Evans, H.L.; Cook, C.H.; O'Neill, P.J.; Mazuski, J.E.; Askari, R.; et al. Trial of short-course antimicrobial therapy for intraabdominal infection. *N. Engl. J. Med.* **2015**, *372*, 1996–2005. [CrossRef]
15. Schein, M.; Assalia, A.; Bachus, H. Minimal antibiotic therapy after emergency abdominal surgery: A prospective study. *Br. J. Surg.* **1994**, *81*, 989–991. [CrossRef]

16. Montravers, P.; Tubach, F.; Lescot, T.; Veber, B.; Esposito-Farese, M.; Seguin, P.; Paugam, C.; Lepape, A.; Meistelman, C.; Cousson, J.; et al. Short-course antibiotic therapy for critically ill patients treated for postoperative intra-abdominal infection: The DURAPOP randomised clinical trial. *Intensive Care Med.* **2018**, *44*, 300–310. [CrossRef] [PubMed]
17. Sartelli, M.; Chichom-Mefire, A.; Labricciosa, F.M.; Hardcastle, T.; Abu-Zidan, F.M.; Adesunkanmi, A.K.; Ansaloni, L.; Bala, M.; Balogh, Z.J.; Beltran, M.A.; et al. The management of intra-abdominal infections from a global perspective: 2017 WSES guidelines for management of intra-abdominal infections. *World J. Emerg. Surg.* **2017**, *12*, 29. [CrossRef]
18. Sartelli, M.; Catena, F.; Di Saverio, S.; Ansaloni, L.; Malangoni, M.; Moore, E.E.; Moore, F.A.; Ivatury, R.; Coimbra, R.; Leppaniemi, A.; et al. Current concept of abdominal sepsis: WSES position paper. *World J. Emerg. Surg.* **2014**, *9*, 22. [CrossRef] [PubMed]
19. Sakr, Y.; Jaschinski, U.; Wittebole, X.; Szakmany, T.; Lipman, J.; Namendys-Silva, S.A.; Martin-Loeches, I.; Leone, M.; Lupu, M.N.; Vincent, J.L.; et al. Sepsis in Intensive Care Unit Patients: Worldwide Data From the Intensive Care over Nations Audit. *Open Forum Infect. Dis.* **2018**, *5*, ofy313. [CrossRef] [PubMed]
20. Sartelli, M. A focus on intra-abdominal infections. *World J. Emerg. Surg.* **2010**, *5*, 9. [CrossRef]
21. Sartelli, M.; Weber, D.G.; Kluger, Y.; Ansaloni, L.; Coccolini, F.; Abu-Zidan, F.; Augustin, G.; Ben-Ishay, O.; Biffl, W.L.; Bouliaris, K.; et al. 2020 update of the WSES guidelines for the management of acute colonic diverticulitis in the emergency setting. *World J. Emerg. Surg.* **2020**, *15*, 32. [CrossRef]
22. Solomkin, J.S.; Mazuski, J.E.; Bradley, J.S.; Rodvold, K.A.; Goldstein, E.J.; Baron, E.J.; O'Neill, P.J.; Chow, A.W.; Dellinger, E.P.; Eachempati, S.R.; et al. Diagnosis and management of complicated intra-abdominal infection in adults and children: Guidelines by the Surgical Infection Society and the Infectious Diseases Society of America. *Clin. Infect. Dis.* **2010**, *50*, 133–164. [CrossRef] [PubMed]
23. Dindo, D.; Demartines, N.; Clavien, P.A. Classification of surgical complications: A new proposal with evaluation in a cohort of 6336 patients and results of a survey. *Ann. Surg.* **2004**, *240*, 205–213. [CrossRef] [PubMed]
24. Mangram, A.J.; Horan, T.C.; Pearson, M.L.; Silver, L.C.; Jarvis, W.R. Guideline for Prevention of Surgical Site Infection, 1999. Centers for Disease Control and Prevention (CDC) Hospital Infection Control Practices Advisory Committee. *Am. J. Infect. Control* **1999**, *27*, 97–132. [CrossRef]
25. Singer, M.; Deutschman, C.S.; Seymour, C.W.; Shankar-Hari, M.; Annane, D.; Bauer, M.; Bellomo, R.; Bernard, G.R.; Chiche, J.D.; Coopersmith, C.M.; et al. The Third International Consensus Definitions for Sepsis and Septic Shock (Sepsis-3). *JAMA* **2016**, *315*, 801–810. [CrossRef] [PubMed]
26. van den Boom, A.L.; de Wijkerslooth, E.M.L.; van Rosmalen, J.; Beverdam, F.H.; Boerma, E.G.; Boermeester, M.A.; Bosmans, J.; Burghgraef, T.A.; Consten, E.C.J.; Dawson, I.; et al. Two versus five days of antibiotics after appendectomy for complex acute appendicitis (APPIC): Study protocol for a randomized controlled trial. *Trials* **2018**, *19*, 263. [CrossRef] [PubMed]
27. van Rossem, C.C.; Schreinemacher, M.H.; van Geloven, A.A.; Bemelman, W.A. Antibiotic Duration After Laparoscopic Appendectomy for Acute Complicated Appendicitis. *JAMA Surg.* **2016**, *151*, 323–329. [CrossRef] [PubMed]
28. Sartelli, M.; Coccolini, F.; Kluger, Y.; Agastra, E.; Abu-Zidan, F.M.; Abbas, A.E.S.; Ansaloni, L.; Adesunkanmi, A.K.; Atanasov, B.; Augustin, G.; et al. WSES/GAIS/SIS-E/WSIS/AAST global clinical pathways for patients with intra-abdominal infections. *World J. Emerg Surg.* **2021**, *16*, 49. [CrossRef]
29. Duane, T.M.; Zuo, J.X.; Wolfe, L.G.; Bearman, G.; Edmond, M.B.; Lee, K.; Cooksey, L.; Stevens, M.P. Surgeons do not listen: Evaluation of compliance with antimicrobial stewardship program recommendations. *Am. Surg.* **2013**, *79*, 1269–1272. [CrossRef] [PubMed]
30. Sartelli, M.; Duane, T.M.; Catena, F.; Tessier, J.M.; Coccolini, F.; Kao, L.S.; De Simone, B.; Labricciosa, F.M.; May, A.K.; Ansaloni, L.; et al. Antimicrobial Stewardship: A Call to Action for Surgeons. *Surg Infect.* **2016**, *17*, 625–631. [CrossRef]
31. Tellado, J.M.; Sen, S.S.; Caloto, M.T.; Kumar, R.N.; Nocea, G. Consequences of inappropriate initial empiric parenteral antibiotic therapy among patients with community-acquired intra-abdominal infections in Spain. *Scand J. Infect. Dis.* **2007**, *39*, 947–955. [CrossRef]
32. Soni, N.J.; Samson, D.J.; Galaydick, J.L.; Vats, V.; Huang, E.S.; Aronson, N.; Pitrak, D.L. Procalcitonin-guided antibiotic therapy: A systematic review and meta-analysis. *J. Hosp. Med.* **2013**, *8*, 530–540. [CrossRef]
33. Harbarth, S.; Holeckova, K.; Froidevaux, C.; Pittet, D.; Ricou, B.; Grau, G.E.; Vadas, L.; Pugin, J. Diagnostic value of procalcitonin, interleukin-6, and interleukin-8 in critically ill patients admitted with suspected sepsis. *Am. J. Respir. Crit. Care Med.* **2001**, *164*, 396–402. [CrossRef] [PubMed]
34. Simon, L.; Gauvin, F.; Amre, D.K.; Saint-Louis, P.; Lacroix, J. Serum procalcitonin and C-reactive protein levels as markers of bacterial infection: A systematic review and meta-analysis. *Clin. Infect. Dis.* **2004**, *39*, 206–217. [CrossRef] [PubMed]
35. de Jong, E.; van Oers, J.A.; Beishuizen, A.; Vos, P.; Vermeijden, W.J.; Haas, L.E.; Loef, B.G.; Dormans, T.; van Melsen, G.C.; Kluiters, Y.C.; et al. Efficacy and safety of procalcitonin guidance in reducing the duration of antibiotic treatment in critically ill patients: A randomised, controlled, open-label trial. *Lancet Infect. Dis.* **2016**, *16*, 819–827. [CrossRef]
36. Spoto, S.; Valeriani, E.; Caputo, D.; Cella, E.; Fogolari, M.; Pesce, E.; Mulè, M.T.; Cartillone, M.; Costantino, S.; Dicuonzo, G.; et al. The role of procalcitonin in the diagnosis of bacterial infection after major abdominal surgery: Advantage from daily measurement. *Medicine* **2018**, *97*, e9496. [CrossRef]

37. Hochreiter, M.; Köhler, T.; Schweiger, A.M.; Keck, F.S.; Bein, B.; von Spiegel, T.; Schroeder, S. Procalcitonin to guide duration of antibiotic therapy in intensive care patients: A randomized prospective controlled trial. *Crit. Care* **2009**, *13*, R83. [CrossRef]
38. Schroeder, S.; Hochreiter, M.; Koehler, T.; Schweiger, A.M.; Bein, B.; Keck, F.S.; von Spiegel, T. Procalcitonin (PCT)-guided algorithm reduces length of antibiotic treatment in surgical intensive care patients with severe sepsis: Results of a prospective randomized study. *Langenbecks Arch. Surg.* **2009**, *394*, 221–226. [CrossRef] [PubMed]

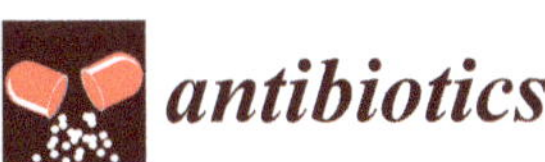

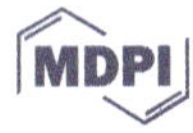

Review

Is Antibiotic Prophylaxis Necessary before Dental Implant Procedures in Patients with Orthopaedic Prostheses? A Systematic Review

Angel-Orión Salgado-Peralvo [1,2], Juan-Francisco Peña-Cardelles [2,3,4,*], Naresh Kewalramani [2,5], Alvaro Garcia-Sanchez [6], María-Victoria Mateos-Moreno [7], Eugenio Velasco-Ortega [1,2], Iván Ortiz-García [1,2], Álvaro Jiménez-Guerra [1,2], Dániel Végh [8,9], Ignacio Pedrinaci [10,11] and Loreto Monsalve-Guil [1,2]

1 Department of Stomatology, University of Seville, 41009 Seville, Spain; orionsalgado@hotmail.com (A.-O.S.-P.); evelasco@us.es (E.V.-O.); ivanortizgarcia1000@hotmail.com (I.O.-G.); alopajanosas@hotmail.com (Á.J.-G.); lomonsalve@hotmail.es (L.M.-G.)
2 Science Committee for Antibiotic Research of Spanish Society of Implants (SEI—Sociedad Española de Implantes), 28020 Madrid, Spain; k93.naresh@gmail.com
3 Department of Basic Health Sciences, Rey Juan Carlos University, 28922 Madrid, Spain
4 Fellow Oral and Maxillofacial Surgery Department and Prosthodontics Department, School of Dental Medicine, University of Connecticut Health, Farmington, CT 06030, USA
5 Department of Nursery and Stomatology, Rey Juan Carlos University, 28922 Madrid, Spain
6 Department of Oral Health and Diagnostic Sciences, School of Dental Medicine, University of Connecticut Health, Farmington, CT 06030, USA; ags.odon@gmail.com
7 Department of Clinical Specialties, Faculty of Dentistry, Complutense University of Madrid, 28040 Madrid, Spain; mateosmoreno80@hotmail.com
8 Department of Prosthodontics, Semmelweis University, 1085 Budapest, Hungary; vegh.daniel.official@gmail.com
9 Department of Dentistry and Oral Health, Division of Oral Surgery and Orthodontics, Medical University of Graz, 8010 Graz, Austria
10 Section of Graduate Periodontology, Faculty of Dentistry, Complutense University of Madrid, 28040 Madrid, Spain; ignpedri@ucm.es
11 Department of Restorative Dentistry and Biomaterials Science, Harvard School of Dental Medicine, Harvard University, Boston, MA 02115, USA
* Correspondence: juanfranciscopenacardelles@gmail.com

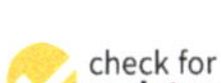

Citation: Salgado-Peralvo, A.-O.; Peña-Cardelles, J.-F.; Kewalramani, N.; Garcia-Sanchez, A.; Mateos-Moreno, M.-V.; Velasco-Ortega, E.; Ortiz-García, I.; Jiménez-Guerra, Á.; Végh, D.; Pedrinaci, I.; et al. Is Antibiotic Prophylaxis Necessary before Dental Implant Procedures in Patients with Orthopaedic Prostheses? A Systematic Review. *Antibiotics* **2022**, *11*, 93. https://doi.org/10.3390/antibiotics11010093

Academic Editor: Marc Maresca

Received: 8 December 2021
Accepted: 10 January 2022
Published: 12 January 2022

Publisher's Note: MDPI stays neutral with regard to jurisdictional claims in published maps and institutional affiliations.

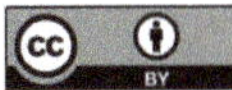

Copyright: © 2022 by the authors. Licensee MDPI, Basel, Switzerland. This article is an open access article distributed under the terms and conditions of the Creative Commons Attribution (CC BY) license (https://creativecommons.org/licenses/by/4.0/).

Abstract: As the population ages, more and more patients with orthopaedic prostheses (OPs) require dental implant treatment. Surveys of dentists and orthopaedic surgeons show that prophylactic antibiotics (PAs) are routinely prescribed with a very high frequency in patients with OPs who are about to undergo dental procedures. The present study aims to determine the need to prescribe prophylactic antibiotic therapy in patients with OPs treated with dental implants to promote their responsible use and reduce the risk of antimicrobial resistance. An electronic search of the MEDLINE database (via PubMed), Web of Science, LILACS, Google Scholar, and OpenGrey was carried out. The criteria used were those described by the PRISMA® Statement. No study investigated the need to prescribe PAs in patients with OPs, so four studies were included on the risk of infections of OPs after dental treatments with varying degrees of invasiveness. There is no evidence to suggest a relationship between dental implant surgeries and an increased risk of OP infection; therefore, PAs in these patients are not justified. However, the recommended doses of PAs in dental implant procedures in healthy patients are the same as those recommended to avoid infections of OPs.

Keywords: antibiotic prophylaxis; antibiotics; joint replacement; prosthetic joint infection; oral implantology; dental implants

1. Introduction

Today, life expectancy is higher than ever before due to the declining mortality rate of young people in developing countries [1], while "developed" countries are experiencing a large decline in mortality at older ages, with an average life expectancy of 91 years for women and 86 years for men [2]. This increases the number of people in need of orthopaedic prostheses (OPs) of any kind [3]. In 2006, around 800,000 joint replacements (hip and knee, as well as elbow, wrist, ankle, metacarpophalangeal, and interphalangeal joints) were placed in the USA [4] and it is estimated that by 2030 these numbers will increase to 4 million for hip and knee replacements alone [5]. Globally, the age group with the highest prevalence of tooth loss is 79-year-olds. Future figures may be even higher, as between 1990 and 2015, there was a 40% increase in the number of people with oral conditions such as untreated caries and/or tooth loss [6]. For these reasons, it is expected that more and more professionals will be faced with patients with OPs requiring the replacement of missing teeth with dental implants.

Infection of orthopaedic prostheses (OPIs) occurs in 0.3 to 2% of patients with OPs [7], requiring additional orthopaedic surgery, as well as the use of antibiotics for a long period [5]. Depending on the timing of their occurrence concerning orthopaedic surgery, OPIs are classified as "early", "delayed", or "late". The first two occur before three months, and between 3 and 24 months post-surgery, respectively, and are related to orthopaedic surgery. On the other hand, late OPIs often result from the late growth of bacteria accidentally inoculated during bleeding procedures or from a distant septic focus [8,9] ("hematogenous orthopaedic prosthetic infections" (HOPIs)). It is estimated that around 10% of these infections are caused by bacteria present in the oral cavity [3]. However, the frequency, duration, and intensity of bacteraemia will influence the cumulative risk [8]. In this regard, classic animal model studies have shown that high bacterial counts (>1000 colony-forming units (CFU)/mL) are required for HOPIs to occur, which is often a consequence of systemic sepsis [10,11].

Various surveys have shown that 63.4% [12] to 71.5% [13] of orthopaedic surgeons consider the prescription of prophylactic antibiotics (PAs) to be necessary indefinitely in patients with hip prostheses who are going to undergo dental treatment. A survey conducted in Canada in 2014 revealed that around 70.7% of dentists routinely prescribe Pas and 21.7% consider it essential for the rest of the patient's life [12]. Despite that, currently, antibiotic prophylaxis for patients with prosthetic joints who are undergoing dental treatment is not routinely recommended in several countries, such as Australia [14], the United Kingdom [15], Canada [16], and New Zealand [17]. Namely, a recent survey of professionals dedicated to oral implantology studied for the first time their prescription habits for PAs in patients with hip prostheses, showing that 74.3% prescribe them, as they consider these patients to be at risk [18].

Considering the current context, these data should be considered where antimicrobial resistance causes around 33,000 deaths each year in the European Union [19]. The associated healthcare costs and lost productivity are estimated to be 1.5 billion euros per year [20]. It is a naturally occurring phenomenon, and this process is being accelerated by the inappropriate and indiscriminate use of antibiotics in humans, food-producing animals, and the environment. Immediate changes in the way antibiotics are prescribed and used are urgently needed. Even if new methods are developed, resistance will continue to pose a severe threat if current prescribing patterns are not modified [21]. In this sense, a recent meta-analysis revealed that the average prescribed dose of PAs in implant surgery is approximately 5 times higher than the one recommended to healthy patients without anatomical constraints [22]. Furthermore, there is only clear scientific proof on the recommended PA dose in the clinical situation mentioned above [23] and in bone augmentation with the implant placement done in one or two phases [21], that is, 2–3 g of amoxicillin an hour before the intervention [21,23], while in allergic patients, 500 mg of azithromycin, 1 h before surgery, has recently been suggested. [24]. Regarding the remaining clinical situations, the type of antibiotic prescribed and its posology is up to the professional, who in many cases tends to over-prescribe them.

Therefore, given the data described above, it is considered necessary to carry out a literature review to determine the need for PAs in patients with OPs who are going to be treated with dental implants to promote their responsible use.

2. Materials and Methods

The criteria used are the ones described in the PRISMA® (Preferred Reporting Items for Systematic Reviews and Meta-Analyses) Declaration [25].

2.1. Focused Question

The main objective was to answer the following "PICO" (P = patient/problem/population; I = intervention; C = comparison; O = outcome) question (Table 1).

Table 1. Breakdown of the "PICO" question.

Component	Description
P (problem/population)	Patients with OPs [1] that have had a dental implant treatment
I (intervention)	PAs [2] on the day of surgery and/or extended postoperatively
C (comparison)	Not prescribing PAsPrescribing a placeboOther antibiotics or antibiotic regimensSame antibiotic with different dosage/duration
O (outcome)	Risk of infection from OPsSafety (for example, benefits for the patient, OPIs [3] prevention, resistance to antimicrobials)
PICO question	In patients with OPs who are about to undergo an implant procedure, does the prescription of PAs decrease the risk of infection of OPs versus not taking them?

[1] OPs, orthopaedic prostheses; [2] PAs, prophylactic antibiotics; [3] OPIs, orthopaedic prostheses infection.

In patients with OPs who are about to undergo an implant procedure, does the prescription of PAs decrease the risk of infection of OPs versus not taking them?

2.2. Eligibility Criteria

Before proceeding, inclusion and exclusion criteria were defined and applied to the resulting articles.

2.2.1. Inclusion Criteria

The included studies comprised (a) human studies; (b) articles published in English or Spanish (c); meta-analysis; (d) systematic reviews; (e) randomized clinical trials (RCTs); (f) clinical trials; (g) clinical studies; (h) comparative studies; (i) multicentre studies; (j) observational studies; and (k) grey literature.

2.2.2. Exclusion Criteria

The exclusion criteria determined the exclusion of the following: (a) experimental laboratory studies; (b) animal studies; (c) studies whose main topic was not the prescription of PAs before the dental procedure in patients with joint replacements; (d) duplicated articles; (e) books or chapters of books; (f) letters to the Editor; (g) commentaries; (h) literature reviews; and (i) surveys.

2.3. Information Sources and Search Strategy

A comprehensive search of the literature was conducted in the following databases: MEDLINE (via PubMed), Web of Science, Google Scholar, and LILACS. A search for unpublished studies (grey literature) was conducted on the OpenGrey database. Moreover, we examined the bibliographic references of the selected articles for publications that did not appear in the initial search and might be of interest.

The search was performed by two independent researchers (A.-O.S.-P. and J.-F.P.-C.). The search was temporarily restricted from 2 February 2011 to 2 February 2021, and was later updated on 16 February 2021.

MeSH (Medical Subject Headings) terms, keywords and other free terms were used with Boolean operators (OR, AND) to combine searches: (hip prosthesis OR hip replacement OR prosthesis joint OR joint replacement OR knee prosthesis OR knee replacement OR ankle prosthesis OR ankle replacement OR shoulder prosthesis OR shoulder replacement OR elbow prosthesis OR elbow replacement) AND (dental implant OR dental implants OR dental implantology OR oral implantology OR oral surgery OR dental OR dental treatment) AND (antibiotics OR preventive antibiotics OR antibiotic prophylaxis OR clindamycin OR amoxicillin OR erythromycin OR azithromycin OR metronidazole). The same keywords were used for all search platforms following the syntax rules for each database.

2.4. Study Records

Two researchers (A.-O.S.-P. and J.-F.P.-C.) independently compared the results to ensure completeness and removed duplicates. Then, the full title and abstracts of the remaining papers were screened individually. Finally, full-text articles included in this systematic review were selected according to the criteria described above. Disagreements over eligible studies to be included were discussed with a third reviewer (N.K.), and a consensus was reached. The reference list of the included studies was also reviewed for possible inclusion.

2.5. Risk of Bias

Data collection was conducted using a predetermined table to assess the resulting articles. Two independent reviewers (J.-F.P.-C. and A.G.-S.) evaluated the methodological quality of eligible studies following the Joanna Briggs Institute Checklist for Systematic Reviews and Research Syntheses [26], which incorporates 11 domains. The studies were classified as low-quality assessment studies (0–6) or as high-quality assessment studies (7–11).

3. Results

3.1. Study Selection

The search strategy resulted in 106 results, of which 99 remained after removing the duplicates. Then, two independent researchers (A.-O.S.-P. and J.-F.P.-C.) reviewed all the titles and abstracts and excluded 86 that were outside the scope of this review. Thus, we obtained 13 potential references. After reading the full text of those 13 papers, it was found that none answered the PICO question as they did not investigate the need to prescribe PAs in implant treatments to reduce the risk of OPIs. Six articles were included that investigated the risk of bacteraemia secondary to dental procedures with varying degrees of invasiveness, so extrapolations were made to establish clear guidelines on the need to administer PAs in implant procedures in these patients. The same situation occurred after the search in Google Scholar and the analysis of the references of the selected articles. Three articles were included in this way so that a total of four papers were analysed [5,7,27,28] (Figure 1).

3.2. Study Characteristics

Most of these studies focused on the appropriateness of the prescription of PAs in hip and/or knee prostheses [5,27] and joints in general. The main findings were described as follows.

The American Dental Association (ADA) and the American Academy of Orthopaedic Surgeons (AAOS) have collaborated on the development of Clinical Practice Guidelines (CPGs) in patients with OPs. The first collaboration was in 2013 [5], where it was determined that it was not necessary to routinely prescribe PAs for dental procedures in patients with hip or knee replacements because, although PAs have been shown to reduce bacteria associated with dental procedures, no evidence links these bacteraemias to HOPIs. Nevertheless, the authors expressed that this decision should be left to the discretion of the professional and the patient after weighing the benefits/risks. This workgroup concluded that PAs would be "rare" or "perhaps appropriate" for non-invasive treatments, meaning those that do not require gingival/mucosa manipulation/perforation, as well as for invasive treatments in healthy patients. Among severely immunocompromised patients, patients with non-controlled diabetes (with levels of glycosylated haemoglobin (HbA1c) $\geq$ 8 or blood glucose level $\geq$ 200 mg/dL) and/or patients with a history of OPI, the prescription of PAs would be considered "appropriate". Patients with severely immunosuppressed states can be classified into the following groups, according to the Center for Disease Control and Prevention (CDC) guidelines [29]: (1) patients with stage III HIV/AIDS, i.e., patients with a CD4 T-lymphocyte count < 200 or opportunistic infections; (2) patients on chemotherapy with fever (absolute neutrophil count (ANC) < 2000) (39 °C) or severe neutropenia (ANC < 500) with or without fever; (3) patients with rheumatoid arthritis (RA) on treatment with disease-modifying biologic agents, including tumour necrosis factor-alpha (TNF-α) or prednisone > 10 mg/day (4) patients who have received a solid organ transplant and are on immunosuppressants; (5) patients with hereditary immunosuppressive diseases; and (6) patients with a bone marrow transplant from the pre-transplant period until the end of immunosuppressive treatment (usually about 36 months after surgery).

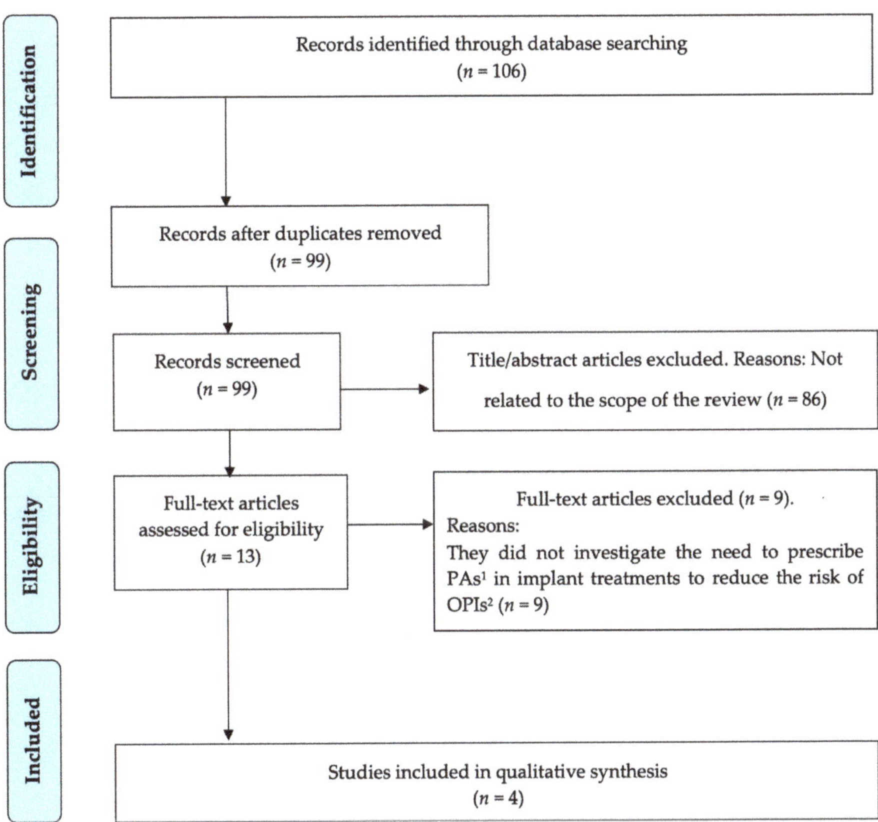

Figure 1. PRISMA® flow diagram of the search processes and results. [1] PAs, prophylactic antibiotics; [2] OPIs, orthopaedic prostheses infection.

Subsequently, the ADA [27] (2015) carried out a CPG with their workgroup following previous guidelines, not systematically recommending the PAs. Despite this, they suggest assessing the administration in diabetic or immunocompromised patients, including in the immunocompromised group those with antibiotic resistance or under treatment with systemic steroids/immunosuppressive drugs, the presence of some type of cancer, and/or with a history of chronic renal disease. The odd ratios (OR) related to the mentioned systemic alterations varied between 1.8 and 2.2 [30], although the magnitude of these values lacks clinical relevance [27]. Thus, this recommendation should be treated carefully. Also, they suggest assessing PAs on patients with a history of complications associated with joint replacement surgeries that will go through an invasive dental procedure and having an interview with the patient and a consultation with the orthopaedic surgeon. If it is favourable, the latter should recommend the adequate antibiotic prescription and, ideally, issue the pharmacological recipe.

Subsequently, the Canadian Agency for Drugs and Technologies in Health [28] (CADTH) (2016) conducted a CPG updating a previous consensus document [31] where they concluded that, although there were some cases of HOPIs after dental procedures, most of these infections were not caused by microorganisms present at the oral level and there was insufficient evidence to claim that taking PAs before a dental procedure could prevent HOPIs. Therefore, they do not recommend its prescription in patients with total joint replacements or with orthopaedic pins, plates, or screws.

In 2017, the Dutch Orthopaedic and Dental Societies [7] conducted a systematic review, concluding that there was no convincing evidence in the literature to justify PAs to avoid HOPIs. Human studies have not confirmed an increased risk of haematogenous infection in joint prostheses during the first two years after placement. Nonetheless, they did observe a higher susceptibility in those that were between two and five years old. Furthermore, the bleeding cannot be considered an isolated factor of bacteraemia, but rather that the gingival/mucosa (including chewing) manipulations cause a match between positive and negative pressures in the capillaries that could favour the diffusion of bacteria into the bloodstream [32]. Thus, positive capillary pressure could avoid the phenomenon.

3.3. Risk of Bias within Studies

Risk of bias and study quality analyses were performed independently by two review authors (J.-F.P.-C. and A.G.-S.). Using the predetermined 11 domains for the methodological quality assessment according to the JBI Prevalence Critical Appraisal Tool [26], we determined that all the papers [5,7,27,28] have a high-quality evaluation (7–11). Table 2 shows a more detailed description of the articles included.

Table 2. JBI Critical Appraisal Tool [26] for Systematic Reviews and Research Syntheses.

Questions	Rademacher et al. [7] (2017)	CADTH [28] (2016)	Sollecito et al. [27] (2013)	Watters et al. [5] (2013)
1. Is the review question clearly and explicitly stated?	+	+	+	+
2. Were the inclusion criteria appropriate for the review question?	?	+	+	+
3. Was the search strategy appropriate?	+	+	+	+
4. Were the sources and resources used to search for studies adequate?	+	+	+	+
5. Were the criteria for appraising studies appropriate?	+	+	+	+

Table 2. *Cont.*

Questions	Rademacher et al. [7] (2017)	CADTH [28] (2016)	Sollecito et al. [27] (2013)	Watters et al. [5] (2013)
6. Was critical appraisal conducted by two or more reviewers independently?	+	?	+	+
7. Were there methods to minimize errors in data extraction?	+	-	+	-
8. Were the methods used to combine studies appropriate?	?	Not applicable	+	+
9. Was the likelihood of publication bias assessed?	-	-	+	+
10. Were policy and/or practice recommendations supported by the reported data?	+	+	+	+
11. Were the specific directives for new research appropriate?	Not applicable	Not applicable	Not applicable	Not applicable

+ —Yes; - —No; ? —Unclear; ● —Not applicable.

4. Discussion

Throughout the past few years, the recommendations regarding the need to prescribe PAs in dental procedures to avoid OPIs have suffered diverse variations. In this regard, the first guidelines recommended prescribing PAs during the first two years after orthopaedic surgery [32]. Some years later, they suggested carrying it out for the rest of the individual's life [33] and, at present, some countries, such as Australia [14], the United Kingdom [15], Canada [16] and New Zealand [17], advise against its routine prescription. Undoubtedly, OPI is an important complication for the patient and with a high cost for the healthcare system, so the tendency, of oral and/or maxillofacial surgeons and orthopaedic surgeons to prescribe PAs before invasive dental procedures is understandable [8]. Despite this, their consistent use is currently not justified, as there is no evidence that bacteraemias following dental procedures are directly related to HOPIs [5,30,34]. Some authors found HOPI rates after total knee arthroplasty of 22.1%, out of which one-third occurred in immunocompromised patients, 4.2% were related to dental procedures, and 7.2% to cutaneous infections. In the remaining cases, they did not find a causal factor [35]. Thus, their incidence is very low (2.9%; 6/224) and usually related to dental abscesses [36], and often it is hard to prove the relationship between a HOPI to the carried out dental treatment. In this regard, the expected benefits do not exceed the possible adverse effects that could develop due to the consumption of antibiotics [37]. In this sense, it has been determined that the risk of suffering an OPI after a dental procedure without PAs is 0.00023 (0.00012–0.00034), while the OR associated with the PAs prescription is 0.7 [9].

Kao et al. [38] carried out a cohort study of 57,066 patients with knee or hip prostheses undergoing invasive dental treatments. They were compared to patients that had not undergone dental treatment using a ratio of 1:1, describing OPIs rates of 0.57% and 0.61%, respectively. The multivariable analysis of the COX regression did not find any relationship between the invasive dental procedures and OPIs. On the other hand, OPIs happened in 0.20% of patients of the subcohort who were prescribed with PAs and in 0.18% who were not prescribed PAs, without significant differences.

In implant surgery, there are three moments when bacteraemia can be caused: during (1) the injection of local anaesthesia, (2) the rise of mucoperiosteal flaps, and (3) the placement of the dental implant [39]. Regarding the anaesthetic technique, the infiltrative methods, which are the ones used in oral implantology, produce a significantly lower proportion of positive blood cultures than the modified and conventional intraligamentous techniques (16% vs. 50% vs. 97%, respectively)—the level of basal bacteraemia is 8% [40]. Lockhart [41] suggested that using local anaesthesia with epinephrine could decrease the transit of bacteria to the bloodstream by reducing the flow. Furthermore, the rate of secondary bacteraemia to implant surgery is very low, which was only described by Piñeiro et al. [39] The authors analysed secondary bacteraemia with the placement of implants in patients that rinsed with chlorhexidine digluconate (CLX) at 0.2% (10 mL for 1 min) (test group) before the anaesthetic injection versus a control group that did not use any type of antimicrobial. The level of bacteraemia in the control group was 2% versus 6.7% in the test group. They only observed differences between patients with positive and negative cultures concerning the intervention time (92.5 ± 24.7 min vs. 64.8 ± 20.2 min, respectively), but not so for the history of periodontal disease, the level of oral health, or the number of placed implants. These surgeries were carried out with general anaesthesia, as well as a local one, which has been related to a higher risk of bacteraemia compared to just administering local anaesthesia at 30 s (89% vs. 53%; OR = 5.04), 15 min (64% vs. 24%; OR = 5.37), and 60 min (21% vs. 4%; OR = 6.5) [42].

On the other hand, Watters et al. [5] identified bacteria associated with a higher risk of OPIs, such as *Staphylococcus* spp. (31.5%), specifically, *S. aureus* (26.0%) and *S. epidermidis* (6.5%), Gram-positives species (9.0%), and *Streptococcus* spp. (6.5%). The isolated species after secondary bacteraemia of implant placement were *Streptococcus viridans* and *Neisseria* [39], which are not directly related to OPs complications. Also, certain oral hygiene procedures carried out daily by patients have a risk of associated bacteraemia that is not inconsiderable, with higher proportions of OPI-causing bacteria than in invasive procedures related to oral implantology [5].

Noori et al. [43] (2019) established for the first time some recommendations in patients treated with foot and ankle surgeries, including total ankle arthroplasty. The bacteria implicated in post-surgery infections in hip and/or knee joint prosthesis infections are similar to those responsible for foot and ankle surgeries, so they determined that the recommendations should be the same.

If it is decided to prescribe PAs, the first-choice antibiotic would be 2 g of amoxicillin, 30–60 min before the procedure and, to those allergic to penicillin, 500 mg of azithromycin or clarithromycin [7,39]. Currently, there are only recommendations based on evidence regarding the placement of unitary implants in ordinary conditions [23] and bone regeneration with the placement of implants in one or two phases [21]. In both procedures, the recommended guideline is 2 or 3 g of amoxicillin, one hour before the intervention [21,23] and, in allergic patients, 500 mg of azithromycin one hour before surgery [24], which would be equivalent to what is recommended to prevent OPIs.

The current guidelines recommend assessing PAs in non-controlled diabetic patients, those immunocompromised, and/or in patients with a history of OPI. For a long time, it has been presumed that immunocompromised patients have a higher risk of HOPIs. Nonetheless, it has not been proved after dental procedures, since they develop comparable bacteraemia to the ones developed by healthy individuals, and with the latter, there is no evidence that there is a higher risk [7]. On the other hand, the European Association of Endodontics [44] recommends prescribing PAs in patients with OPs during the three months following orthopaedic joint surgery. Dental implants entail an elective surgery, so it does seem prudent to postpone the intervention during this time. Also, dental implant surgery is not indicated for the described systemic states until the disease has been controlled. The only scenario where the treatment could be assessed in these patients would be in those with AR being treated with biological agents modifying the disease, and despite this, different authors associated it with a higher risk of early placement failure and peri-implantitis [45,46].

The relationship between the periodontal state, or the level of hygiene, and the level of bacteraemia was not established [9,39]. Nonetheless, any implant procedure must be done in an oral cavity without any pathology. Another preventive measure is using perioperative antiseptics, such as CLX. Although ADA/AAOS was not able to conclude that rinsing with different topical antimicrobials before a dental procedure prevents HOPIs [5], further studies found that CLX rinses reduce the incidence of secondary bacteraemia in dental extractions by 12% [47–49], possibly due to a reduction of the quantity of inoculated bacteria. This is a simple preventive measure without evidence of adverse reactions. Thus, its use is recommendable despite its low efficacy [47]. Furthermore, as a chemo-preventive measure against the accumulation of biofilm, its use is recommended in the immediate post-surgery period, a time when oral hygiene procedures could experience difficulties [50].

Given that the placement of dental implants currently involves the prescription of PAs in healthy patients, future lines of research should focus on establishing the incidence of infections following implant procedures in those patients with OPs. It would also be interesting to study topical antiseptics, such as CLX, to reduce secondary bacteraemia in implant procedures.

Strengths and Limitations

This systematic review presents several strengths, such as a previous record of protocol, free search in the literature (including grey literature), the searching process of studies, data extraction, and the risk analysis bias performed in duplicate, which determined a high overall quality of the included studies.

Nonetheless, with the low number of studies available in the literature, the present systematic review has limitations, so the external validity of the results of this review should be confirmed with future studies.

5. Conclusions

No evidence suggests a relationship between dental implant surgery and a higher risk of infection of OPs. Therefore, the prescription of PAs in these patients is not justified. Nonetheless, the recommended PA dose in a dental implant procedure in healthy patients is comparable to the dose recommended to avoid infections in OPs. We should evaluate the prescription of PAs in patients with a history of infections in their OPs in second-stage implant surgeries. Furthermore, it would be wise to avoid surgeries three months after orthopaedic surgery.

Author Contributions: Conzand E.V.-O.; methodology, A.-O.S.-P. and E.V.-O.; software, A.G.-S.; validation, Á.J.-G., I.O.-G., A.G.-S. and L.M.-G.; formal analysis, M.-V.M.-M., E.V.-O., N.K. and M.-V.M.-M.; investigation, A.-O.S.-P. and J.-F.P.-C.; resources, L.M.-G. and E.V.-O.; data curation, A.-O.S.-P., J.-F.P.-C. and N.K.; writing—original draft preparation, A.-O.S.-P., J.-F.P.-C., A.G.-S., I.P. and D.V; writing—review and editing, A.-O.S.-P., E.V.-O., J.-F.P.-C., I.P. and D.V.; visualization, M.-V.M.-M., Á.J.-G. and I.O.-G.; supervision, E.V.-O.; project administration, E.V.-O. and A.G.-S. All authors have read and agreed to the published version of the manuscript.

Funding: This research received no external funding.

Institutional Review Board Statement: Not applicable.

Informed Consent Statement: Not applicable.

Data Availability Statement: Data are available in a publicly accessible repository.

Conflicts of Interest: The authors declare no conflict of interest.

References

1. Bloom, D.E. 7 Billion and Counting. *Science* **2011**, *333*, 562–569. [CrossRef] [PubMed]
2. Christensen, K.; Doblhammer, G.; Rau, R.; Vaupel, J.W. Ageing populations: The challenges ahead. *Lancet* **2009**, *374*, 1196–1208. [CrossRef]
3. Zimmerli, W.; Sendi, P. Antibiotics for Prevention of Periprosthetic Joint Infection Following Dentistry: Time to Focus on data. *Clin. Infect. Dis. Off. Publ. Infect. Dis. Soc. Am.* **2010**, *50*, 17–19. [CrossRef] [PubMed]
4. Lübbeke, A.J.; Silman, A.J.; Barea, C.; Prieto-Alhambra, D.; Carr, A.J. Mapping existing hip and knee replacement registries in Europe. *Health Policy* **2018**, *122*, 548–557. [CrossRef] [PubMed]

5. Watters, W., 3rd; Rethman, M.P.; Hanson, N.B.; Abt, E.; Anderson, P.A.; Carroll, K.C.; Futrell, H.C.; Garvin, K.; Glenn, S.O.; Hellstein, J.; et al. Prevention of Orthopaedic Implant Infection in Patients Undergoing Dental Procedures. *J. Am. Acad. Orthop. Surg.* **2013**, *21*, 180–189. [CrossRef]
6. Kassebaum, N.J.; Smith, A.G.C.; Bernabé, E.; Fleming, T.D.; Reynolds, A.E.; Vos, T.; Murray, C.J.L.; Marcenes, W.; GBD 2015 Oral Health Collaborators. Global, Regional, and National Prevalence, Incidence, and Disability-Adjusted Life Years for Oral Conditions for 195 Countries, 1990–2015: A Systematic Analysis for the Global Burden of Diseases, Injuries, and Risk Factors. *J. Dent. Res.* **2017**, *96*, 380–387. [CrossRef]
7. Rademacher, W.M.H.; Walenkamp, G.H.I.M.; Moojen, D.J.F.; Hendriks, J.G.E.; Goedendorp, T.A.; Rozema, F.R. Antibiotic prophylaxis is not indicated prior to dental procedures for prevention of periprosthetic joint infections. *Acta Orthop.* **2017**, *88*, 568–574. [CrossRef]
8. Skaar, D.D.; Park, T.; Swiontkowski, M.F.; Kuntz, K.M. Cost-effectiveness of antibiotic prophylaxis for dental patients with prosthetic joints: Comparisons of antibiotic regimens for patients with total hip arthroplasty. *J. Am. Dent. Assoc.* **2015**, *146*, 830–839. [CrossRef]
9. Moreira, A.I.; Mendes, L.; Pereira, J.A. Is there scientific evidence to support antibiotic prophylaxis in patients with periodontal disease as a means to decrease the risk of prosthetic joint infections? A systematic review. *Int. Orthop.* **2020**, *44*, 231–236. [CrossRef]
10. Zimmerli, W.; Zak, O.; Vosbeck, K. Experimental Hematogenous Infection of Subcutaneously Implanted Foreign Bodies. *Scand. J. Infect. Dis.* **1985**, *17*, 303–310. [CrossRef]
11. Blomgren, G. Hematogenous Infection of Total Joint Replacement: An Experimental Study in the Rabbit. *Acta Orthop. Scand. Suppl.* **1981**, *187*, 1–64. [CrossRef]
12. Colterjohn, T.; de Beer, J.; Petruccelli, D.; Zabtia, N.; Winemaker, M. Antibiotic Prophylaxis for Dental Procedures at Risk of Causing Bacteremia Among Post-Total Joint Arthroplasty Patients: A Survey of Canadian Orthopaedic Surgeons and Dental Surgeons. *J. Arthroplast.* **2014**, *29*, 1091–1097. [CrossRef]
13. McNally, C.M.; Visvanathan, R.; Liberali, S.; Adams, R.J. Antibiotic prophylaxis for dental treatment after prosthetic joint replacement: Exploring the orthopaedic surgeon's opinion. *Arthroplast. Today* **2016**, *2*, 123–126. [CrossRef] [PubMed]
14. Alam, M.; Bastakoti, B. Therapeutic Guidelines: Antibiotic. Version 15. *Aust. Prescr.* **2015**, *38*, 137. [CrossRef]
15. Committee, J.F. *British National Formulary 67*; BMJ Group and Pharmaceutical Press: London, UK, 2014.
16. Canadian Dental Association. New CDA position statement on dental patients with orthopedic implants. *J. Can. Dent. Assoc.* **2013**, *79*, d126.
17. New Zealand Dental Association. *Code of Practice: Antibiotic Prophylaxis for Patients with Prosthetic Joint Replacements Undergoing Dental Treatment*; New Zealand Dental Association Inc.: Auckland, New Zealand, 2018.
18. Salgado-Peralvo, A.-O.; Velasco-Ortega, E.; Peña-Cardelles, J.-F.; Kewalramani, N.; Monsalve-Guil, L.; Jiménez-Guerra, Á.; Ortiz-García, I.; Moreno-Muñoz, J.; Núñez-Márquez, E.; Cabanillas-Balsera, D. *Clinical Practice Guideline for the Prescription of Preventive Antibiotics in Oral Implantology*; Sociedad Española de Implantes: Madrid, Spain, 2021.
19. Cassini, A.; Hogberg, L.D.; Plachouras, D.; Quattrocchi, A.; Hoxha, A.; Simonsen, G.S.; Colomb-Cotinat, M.; Kretzschmar, M.E.; Devleesschauwer, B.; Cecchini, M.; et al. Attributable deaths and disability-adjusted life-years caused by infections with antibiotic-resistant bacteria in the EU and the European Economic Area in 2015: A population-level modelling analysis. *Lancet Infect. Dis.* **2019**, *19*, 56–66. [CrossRef]
20. O'Neill, J. *Tackling Drug-Resistant Infections Globally: Final Report and Recommendations. Review on Antimicrobial Resistance*; Government of the United Kingdom: London, UK, 2016.
21. Salgado-Peralvo, A.-O.; Mateos-Moreno, M.-V.; Velasco-Ortega, E.; Peña-Cardelles, J.-F.; Kewalramani, N. Preventive antibiotic therapy in bone augmentation procedures in oral implantology: A systematic review. *J. Stomatol. Oral Maxillofac. Surg.* **2021**, *22*. [CrossRef]
22. Rodríguez-Sánchez, F.; Arteagoitia, I.; Teughels, W.; Rodríguez-Andrés, C.; Quirynen, M. Antibiotic dosage prescribed in oral implant surgery: A meta-analysis of cross-sectional surveys. *PLoS ONE* **2020**, *15*, e0236981. [CrossRef]
23. Romandini, M.; De Tullio, I.; Congedi, F.; Kalemaj, Z.; D'Ambrosio, M.; Laforí, A.; Quaranta, C.; Buti, J.; Perfetti, G. Antibiotic prophylaxis at dental implant placement: Which is the best protocol? A systematic review and network meta-analysis. *J. Clin. Periodontol.* **2019**, *46*, 382–395. [CrossRef] [PubMed]
24. Salgado-Peralvo, A.-O.; Peña-Cardelles, J.-F.; Kewalramani, N.; Ortiz-García, I.; Jiménez-Guerra, Á.; Uribarri, A.; Velasco-Ortega, E.; Moreno-Muñoz, J.; Núñez-Márquez, E.; Monsalve-Guil, L. Is Penicillin Allergy a Risk Factor for Early Dental Implant Failure? A Systematic Review. *Antibiotics* **2021**, *10*, 1227. [CrossRef]
25. Moher, D.; Liberati, A.; Tetzlaff, J.; Altman, D.G.; The PRISMA Group. Preferred reporting items for systematic reviews and meta-analyses: The PRISMA Statement. *PLoS Med.* **2009**, *6*, e1000097. [CrossRef]
26. Joanna Briggs Institute. *Checklist for Systematic Reviews and Research Syntheses*; The Joanna Briggs Institute: Adelaide, Australia, 2017.
27. Sollecito, T.P.; Abt, E.; Lockhart, P.B.; Truelove, E.; Paumier, T.M.; Tracy, S.L.; Tampi, M.; Beltrán-Aguilar, E.D.; Frantsve-Hawley, J. The use of prophylactic antibiotics prior to dental procedures in patients with prosthetic joints: Evidence-based clinical practice guideline for dental practitioners—a report of the American Dental Association Council on Scientific Affairs. *J. Am. Dent. Assoc.* **2015**, *146*, 11–16.e8. [CrossRef] [PubMed]

28. Canadian Agency for Drugs and Technologies in Health. *Antibiotic Prophylaxis in Patients with Orthopedic Implants Undergoing Dental Procedures: A Review of Clinical Effectiveness, Safety, and Guidelines*; Canadian Agency for Drugs and Technologies in Health: Kanata, ON, Canda, 2016.
29. Selik, R.M.; Mokotoff, E.D.; Branson, B.; Owen, S.M.; Whitmore, S.; Hall, H.I. Control and Prevention Revised surveillance case definition for HIV infection—United States, 2014. *MMWR. Recomm. Rep.* **2014**, *63*, 1–10.
30. Berbari, E.F.; Osmon, D.R.; Carr, A.; Hanssen, A.D.; Baddour, L.M.; Greene, D.; Kupp, L.I.; Baughan, L.W.; Harmsen, W.S.; Mandrekar, J.N.; et al. Dental Procedures as Risk Factors for Prosthetic Hip or Knee Infection: A Hospital-Based Prospective Case-Control Study. *Clin. Infect. Dis. an Off. Publ. Infect. Dis. Soc. Am.* **2010**, *50*, 8–16. [CrossRef]
31. Canadian Dental Association; Canadian Orthopedic Association; Association of Medical Microbiology and Infectious Disease. *Dental Patients with Total Joint Replacement*; The Canadian Dental Association: Ottawa, ON, Canda.
32. American Dental Association; American Academy of Orthopaedic Surgeons Antibiotic prophylaxis for dental patients with total joint replacements. *J. Am. Dent. Assoc.* **2003**, *134*, 895–899. [CrossRef] [PubMed]
33. American Academy of Orthopaedic Surgeons. *Information Statement 1014: Antibiotic Prophylaxis for Bacteriemia in Patients with Joint Replacements*; American Academy of Orthopaedic Surgeons: Rosemont, IL, USA, 2009.
34. Skaar, D.D.; O'Connor, H.; Hodges, J.S.; Michalowicz, B.S. Dental procedures and subsequent prosthetic joint infections: Findings from the Medicare Current Beneficiary Survey. *J. Am. Dent. Assoc.* **2011**, *142*, 1343–1351. [CrossRef]
35. Stévignon, T.; Mouton, A.; Meyssonnier, V.; Kerroumi, Y.; Yazigi, A.; Aubert, T.; Lhotellier, L.; Le Strat, V.; Passeron, D.; Graff, W.; et al. Haematogenous prosthetic knee infections: Prospective cohort study of 58 patients. *Orthop. Traumatol. Surg. Res.* **2019**, *105*, 647–651. [CrossRef]
36. Barrere, S.; Reina, N.; Peters, O.A.; Rapp, L.; Vergnes, J.-N.; Maret, D. Dental assessment prior to orthopedic surgery: A systematic review. *Orthop. Traumatol. Surg. Res.* **2019**, *105*, 761–772. [CrossRef]
37. American Dental Association. *Management of Patients with Prosthetic Joints Undergoing Dental Procedures*; American Dental Association: Chicago, IL, USA.
38. Kao, F.-C.; Hsu, Y.-C.; Chen, W.-H.; Lin, J.-N.; Lo, Y.-Y.; Tu, Y.-K. Prosthetic Joint Infection Following Invasive Dental Procedures and Antibiotic Prophylaxis in Patients with Hip or Knee Arthroplasty. *Infect. Control. Hosp. Epidemiol.* **2017**, *38*, 154–161. [CrossRef]
39. Piñeiro, A.; Tomás, I.; Blanco, J.; Alvarez, M.; Seoane, J.; Diz, P. Bacteraemia following dental implants' placement. *Clin. Oral Implant. Res.* **2010**, *21*, 913–918. [CrossRef]
40. Roberts, G.J.; Simmons, N.B.; Longhurst, P.; Hewitt, P.B. Bacteraemia following local anaesthetic injections in children. *Br. Dent. J.* **1998**, *185*, 295–298. [CrossRef] [PubMed]
41. Lockhart, P.B. An analysis of bacteremias during dental extractions. A double-blind, placebo-controlled study of chlorhexidine. *Arch. Intern. Med.* **1996**, *156*, 513–520. [CrossRef]
42. Barbosa, M.; Carmona, I.T.; Amaral, B.; Limeres, J.; Alvarez, M.; Cerqueira, C.; Diz, P. General anesthesia increases the risk of bacteremia following dental extractions. *Oral Surg. Oral Med. Oral Pathol. Oral Radiol. Endod.* **2010**, *110*, 706–712. [CrossRef]
43. Noori, N.; Myerson, C.; Charlton, T.; Thordarson, D. Is Antibiotic Prophylaxis Necessary Before Dental Procedures in Patients Post Total Ankle Arthroplasty? *Foot Ankle Int.* **2018**, *40*, 237–241. [CrossRef] [PubMed]
44. Segura-Egea, J.J.; Gould, K.; Şen, B.H.; Jonasson, P.; Cotti, E.; Mazzoni, A.; Sunay, H.; Tjäderhane, L.; Dummer, P.M.H. European Society of Endodontology position statement: The use of antibiotics in endodontics. *Int. Endod. J.* **2018**, *51*, 20–25. [CrossRef]
45. Renvert, S.; Aghazadeh, A.; Hallström, H.; Persson, G.R. Factors related to peri-implantitis—A retrospective study. *Clin. Oral Implant. Res.* **2014**, *25*, 522–529. [CrossRef] [PubMed]
46. Nagy, R.; Szabo, K.; Szucs, A.; Ruszin, T.; Joob-Fancsaly, A. Impact of rheumatoid arthritis in oral surgery and implantology treatment based on literature. *Fogorv. Szle.* **2017**, *110*, 3–6.
47. Arteagoitia, I.; Rodriguez Andrés, C.; Ramos, E. Does chlorhexidine reduce bacteremia following tooth extraction? A systematic review and meta-analysis. *PLoS ONE* **2018**, *13*, e0195592. [CrossRef] [PubMed]
48. Canullo, L.; Laino, L.; Longo, F.; Filetici, P.; D'Onofrio, I.; Troiano, G. Does Chlorhexidine Prevent Complications in Extractive, Periodontal, and Implant Surgery? A Systematic Review and Meta-analysis with Trial Sequential Analysis. *Int. J. Oral Maxillofac. Implant.* **2020**, *35*, 1149–1158. [CrossRef]
49. Tomás, I.; Alvarez, M.; Limeres, J.; Tomás, M.; Medina, J.; Otero, J.L.; Diz, P. Effect of a Chlorhexidine Mouthwash on the Risk of Postextraction Bacteremia. *Infect. Control. Hosp. Epidemiol.* **2007**, *28*, 577–582. [CrossRef]
50. Solderer, A.; Kaufmann, M.; Hofer, D.; Wiedemeier, D.; Attin, T.; Schmidlin, P.R. Efficacy of chlorhexidine rinses after periodontal or implant surgery: A systematic review. *Clin. Oral Investig.* **2019**, *23*, 21–32. [CrossRef] [PubMed]

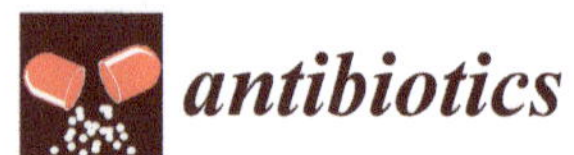

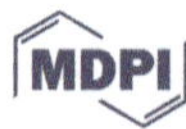

Article

Empowering Patients to Self-Manage Common Infections: Qualitative Study Informing the Development of an Evidence-Based Patient Information Leaflet

Catherine V. Hayes *, Bláthnaid Mahon, Eirwen Sides, Rosie Allison, Donna M. Lecky and Cliodna A. M. McNulty

Primary Care and Interventions Unit, Public Health England, Gloucester GL1 1DQ, UK; Blathnaid.mahon@phe.gov.uk (B.M.); Eirwen.sides@phe.gov.uk (E.S.); Rosie.allison@phe.gov.uk (R.A.); Donna.lecky@phe.gov.uk (D.M.L.); Cliodna.mcnulty@phe.gov.uk (C.A.M.M.)

* Correspondence: Catherine.hayes@phe.gov.uk

Abstract: Common self-limiting infections can be self-managed by patients, potentially reducing consultations and unnecessary antibiotic use. This qualitative study informed by the Theoretical Domains Framework (TDF) aimed to explore healthcare professionals' (HCPs) and patients' needs on provision of self-care and safety-netting advice for common infections. Twenty-seven patients and seven HCPs participated in semi-structured focus groups (FGs) and interviews. An information leaflet was iteratively developed and reviewed by participants in interviews and FGs, and an additional 5 HCPs, and 25 patients (identifying from minority ethnic groups) via online questionnaires. Qualitative data were analysed thematically, double-coded, and mapped to the TDF. Participants required information on symptom duration, safety netting, self-care, and antibiotics. Patients felt confident to self-care and were averse to consulting with HCPs unnecessarily but struggled to assess symptom severity. Patients reported seeking help for children or elderly dependents earlier. HCPs' concerns included patients' attitudes and a lack of available monitoring of advice given to patients. Participants believed community pharmacy should be the first place that patients seek advice on common infections. The patient information leaflet on common infections should be used in primary care and community pharmacy to support patients to self-manage symptoms and determine when further help is required.

Keywords: primary healthcare; general practice; community pharmacy; antibiotics; qualitative study; patient attitudes; self-care; questionnaire; behavioural science

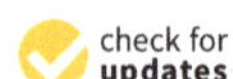

Citation: Hayes, C.V.; Mahon, B.; Sides, E.; Allison, R.; Lecky, D.M.; McNulty, C.A.M. Empowering Patients to Self-Manage Common Infections: Qualitative Study Informing the Development of an Evidence-Based Patient Information Leaflet. *Antibiotics* **2021**, *10*, 1113. https://doi.org/10.3390/antibiotics10091113

Academic Editors: Seok Hoon Jeong and Diane Ashiru-Oredope

Received: 9 August 2021
Accepted: 9 September 2021
Published: 15 September 2021

Publisher's Note: MDPI stays neutral with regard to jurisdictional claims in published maps and institutional affiliations.

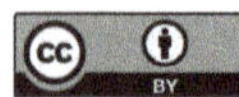

Copyright: © 2021 by the authors. Licensee MDPI, Basel, Switzerland. This article is an open access article distributed under the terms and conditions of the Creative Commons Attribution (CC BY) license (https://creativecommons.org/licenses/by/4.0/).

1. Introduction

Antimicrobial resistance (AMR) continues to be a global threat, largely driven by overuse of antibiotics [1]. Most antibiotics (70% in 2019) in England are prescribed in the community [2], with many inappropriate for self-limiting infections [3–5], and primary care continues to be a priority area for Antimicrobial Stewardship (AMS) programmes, to optimise antimicrobial use. Patient behaviour is a key target of the UK AMR national action plan (2019–2024); ambitions include preventing the need for antimicrobials and improving the publics' infection prevention behaviours [6]. The National Institute for Health and Care Excellence (NICE) and Public Health England (PHE) recommend self-care actions as first-line treatment for many common infections [7] and recommend that HCPs use patient resources to educate patients on the management of common infections [8]. Among UK primary care clinicians, 94% report using patient-facing infection-related information leaflets [9]. Interventions to facilitate shared decision-making with patients, such as leaflets, are effective at reducing antibiotic use for acute respiratory tract infections in primary care [10]. Although there are patient leaflets covering specific or childhood infections, there are no general infection self-care leaflets for use in primary care and community pharmacies to facilitate consistent advice to patients, empowering patients to manage their current and future infections.

Analysis of a large 2018/19 community cohort study in England found that most participants managed respiratory tract infection (RTI) symptoms without seeking medical attention, with only 14% leading to a GP or dental consultation and 10% antibiotic use [11]. The coronavirus disease 2019 (COVID-19) pandemic has seen an increase in GP telephone consultations, possibly resulting in more antibiotic prescriptions [12,13]. Interventions developed using behavioural science can improve antibiotic prescribing [14], and patient educational interventions developed using the TDF have high acceptability and feasibility [15,16]. A person-based approach to intervention development uses a range of qualitative research methods, evidence, and theory and puts end users at the centre of development in order to effect behaviour change [17].

This study aimed to explore patients' and HCPs' needs for providing or receiving infection self-care and safety-netting advice. Qualitative interviews and focus groups (FGs) informed by the TDF, and online questionnaires were used in this person-based approach, to inform the development of a patient and carer facing leaflet covering common infections.

2. Results

2.1. Participant Characteristics

A total of 27 patients and 7 HCPs participated in interviews and FGs and a further 5 HCPs and 25 patients (identifying from minority ethnic groups) provided feedback on a near final draft of the leaflet via questionnaires (Table 1).

Table 1. Patient and healthcare professional self-reported characteristics.

	Patients *n* = 52			Healthcare Professionals *n* = 12	
	INT and FGs (*n* = 27)	Questionnaire (*n* = 25)		INT and FGs (*n* = 7)	Questionnaire (*n* = 5)
Age			**Profession**		
16–24	1	3	Community pharmacist	3	-
25–34	3	12			
35–49	8	1	General Practitioner	2	-
50–64	8	2			
65+	7	5	Prescribing advisor	1	1
Unknown	-	2	Nurse practitioner	1	4
	Gender			**Gender**	
Female	18	13	Female	3	-
Male	9	11	Male	3	-
Unknown	-	1	Unknown	1	5
	Ethnicity				
Bangladeshi	1	5			
Black African	-	2			
Black Caribbean	1	2			
Chinese	-	5			
Indian	-	6			
Pakistani	1	2			
Sri Lankan	2	1			
White British	20	-			
White European	2	2			

INT—Interviews. FGs—Focus Groups.

2.2. Emerging Themes on Management of Common Infections

2.2.1. Patients

Patient themes regarding self-managing common infections are summarised in Table 2 (detailed in Table S1).

Table 2. Emerging themes of patients on self-management of common infections.

Theme	Sub Themes	TDF Domain(s)	Quotes	Implications for Leaflet
Preventing infections	• Healthy lifestyle • Motivations for preventing infections • Social distancing and hygiene	Knowledge; Belief about consequences; Social influences; Reinforcement	'I've suffered from urinary tract infections so drinking plenty of water is really important for me and having a lot of vegetables and fruit.' (Female, FG5) 'A lot of cleaning, a lot more cleaning. I used to clean a lot anyway but since this COVID-19, I find that it's just in my head all the time.' (Female, FG4)	• Advice on preventing infections • Focus on protecting vulnerable family members
Self-caring for infections	• Self-care actions, attitudes, and motivations • Perceived skills and confidence • Contextual barriers	Skills; Belief about consequences; Belief about capabilities; Environmental context	'Not being a child, you come across things that you've had in the past and you either using the tried and tested that you've done before . . . And if it is something that persists or goes on for longer, I go to the pharmacist.' (Male, FG4)	• Self-care advice for specific symptoms • Signpost to NHS website
Health-seeking behaviours	• Judging seriousness of symptoms • Deciding to seek help • Triaging and accessibility • Children and elderly • Community pharmacy	Memory attention and decision-making; Belief about consequences; Environmental context; Emotions	'Anything where I'm feeling this is not just an easy cold to manage. This could have quite an impact on other people, because I'm self-employed as well. So it's a really hard judgement call . . . ' (Female, FG2) 'I think after COVID I start to get a bit more anxious now thinking is it something more serious and I think if I had more of a cold now, I'd probably seek more medical attention . . . ' (Female, FG5)	• Advice on duration of symptoms and when to seek help • Serious signs of illness • Advice on use of community pharmacy
Healthcare expectations	• Experience receiving infection advice • Expectations for consultations • Beliefs about antibiotics	Reinforcement; Goals; Knowledge; Belief about consequences; Intentions	'Hopefully a way to end this illness. I don't want to come out thinking I'm none the wiser than what I was before. I'd like to know that there's an end in sight.' (Male, FG3) 'That belief that if you take antibiotics too frequently then they don't actually work as well. That's always been drummed into me, don't take antibiotics for everything.' (Female, FG3)	• Advice on when antibiotics could help an infection

TDF—Theoretical Domains Framework. FG—Focus group.

(a) Preventing and self-treating infections

Patients believed that a healthy lifestyle could prevent infections and that handwashing could stop infections from spreading. Some believed that family upbringing influenced hygiene behaviour and that if you grew up in a house 'too clean', you were more susceptible to infections. Patients interviewed at the start of the COVID-19 pandemic reported more proactive health behaviours (e.g., oral hygiene) due to a perceived lack of healthcare access and preventing COVID-19 by following social distancing and increased cleaning.

Patients reported self-care behaviours for common infections they believed their body could usually fight off, including common RTIs. Patients believed rest and hydration would help them to get better quicker. Some used over-the-counter (OTC) remedies, whilst others believed that it was important for symptoms to run their course rather than 'suppress' them with medicines and that taking any medicine too often could make them less effective. They were motivated to self-care and continued to carry out professional and social responsibilities. Behaviours were influenced by family traditions, previous successful methods, and advice from HCPs or the NHS website. Patients felt confident self-caring for familiar symptoms (e.g., cough) but less-so for perceived serious symptoms (e.g., rashes).

(b) Health-seeking behaviour

Patients reported difficulty in assessing when to consult and were guided by concerns of potentially serious or persisting symptoms. Patients' decision to consult was influenced by work, children, social pressure, and symptom tolerance. Failure to resolve symptoms through self-treatment was also a factor. Many patients expressed avoidance for seeking GP help, due to feelings of guilt about putting pressure on the NHS and their GP's time, as a habit or family culture ('we don't tend to visit the GP'), or due to inaccessibility of appointments. A minority perceived that they accessed healthcare more than necessary due to anxiety about symptoms progressing to serious illness. When booking an appointment, patients reported negative feelings about discussing symptoms with reception staff. Patients reported a lower threshold for seeking help for children or elderly family due to concerns about vulnerability, uncertainty about how the infection might progress, and an expectation that they need antibiotics due to a weaker immune system.

Many patients reported contacting community pharmacy staff for infection advice; their knowledge was trusted, and they were more accessible than GPs. Patients reported that public campaigns had increased their awareness of pharmacy services; a minority viewed pharmacies as a place to collect their medicine only. Some would not discuss certain symptoms in the pharmacy setting and were unaware of pharmacy consultation rooms, which are available in some pharmacy settings.

(c) Healthcare expectations

Expectations for the consultation included wanting to have input into decisions, a rapid solution to their symptoms, and the reassurance that their infection would resolve. Patients would also consult when they believed antibiotics were required to treat an infection, including urinary, chest, ear and skin infections, and tonsillitis. Patients were familiar with appropriate antibiotic use messages from public campaigns, but had less knowledge of antibiotic resistance; however, they believed that if they took antibiotics too much they would not work. If antibiotics were prescribed, they viewed it as important to take them as their HCP directed.

2.2.2. Healthcare Professionals

HCP themes regarding provision of advice to patients with common infections are summarised in Table 3 (detail in Table S2).

Table 3. Emerging themes of healthcare professionals on provision of advice to patients with common infections.

Theme	Sub Themes	TDF Domain(s)	Quotes	Implications for Leaflet
Roles and responsibilities	• Motivation for AMS and promoting self-care • Professional responsibilities	Belief about capabilities; Optimism; Knowledge; Skills; Social and professional role	'I'm optimistic in terms of what I can do to educate the patients, whether than then translates into a reduction in resistance is another matter. But I'm certainly confident in what I do.' (INT 4, GP, Male)	• Leaflet would support HCPs in provision of infection advice
Approaches to managing common infections	• Importance of self-care advice • Shared decision-making • Encouraging use of community pharmacy • Approaches to educating patients • Variations in practice and lack of monitoring	Belief about consequences; Belief about capabilities; Goals Social influences; Environmental context	'I personally place a huge emphasis on self-care because in this day and age of consent, shared decision-making, empowering the patient as well, culturally we've moved away from being told by healthcare professionals what to do and how to do it exactly. It is very much a collaborative process.' (FG1, pharmacist, female) '[about remote consultations] . . . can't physically assess their illnesses and [GPs] will probably prescribe more than if they were able to have that face-to-face physical assessment just to err on the side of caution unfortunately.' (FG1, pharmacist, female) 'I worked in a practice which had six partners plus extra doctors and the variation in the threshold for prescribing was enormous . . . I think if you've got that variation at a clinician level it's very difficult to expect staff to have consistent messaging.' (FG1, GP, Male)	• Self-care advice for common symptoms • Promote leaflet as a shared decision tool • Community pharmacy advice
Patient attitudes and context	• Beliefs about patient attitude/expectations • Beliefs about effect on patient behaviour • Mass media/public health campaigns • Patient contextual barriers	Belief about consequences; Belief about capabilities; Environmental context; Social influences	'It can be quite clear the patients might have a pathway in their mind about what the treatment should be like, for instance, rather than taking the information on board. I think that's probably the biggest barrier, patient expectation.' (INT 1, pharmacist, Male) 'I have prescribed paracetamol in families that I know would have struggled . . . but you have to bear in mind that if they really are struggling financially, all the self-care advice that you give is going to be difficult if they can't afford it.' (INT 2, nurse practitioner, Female)	• Information on when antibiotics are needed and consequences of using incorrectly • Align to existing campaigns and resources (Keep Antibiotics Working, TARGET antibiotics toolkit)

TDF—Theoretical Domains Framework. FG—Focus group. INT—Interview. GP—General Practitioner.

(a) Responsibilities and approaches to managing common infections

Overall, HCPs were motivated and optimistic that provision of self-care advice could help to prevent future infections and enable patients to self-care before seeking help and that these actions could reduce use of services and antibiotics. GPs discussed the benefit of shared decision-making and the importance of identifying expectations at the start of consultations and counselling against antibiotics, if not appropriate. Both GPs and pharmacists believed that community pharmacies were accessible and should be viewed as a patient's first place for advice on common infections. Pharmacists reported some hurdles to providing patients with advice, which included not being able to see the patient's record or indication and other responsibilities preventing them from having longer discussions.

GPs reported using AMS tools such as the TARGET patient leaflets [18] and reflected that they helped to reassure patients. Some used back-up prescriptions and appointments for safety-netting. A GP interviewed at the start of the COVID-19 pandemic briefly commented on the use of telephone consultations and expressed concern that this may lead to more antibiotics being prescribed. All HCPs reported that there were no systems in place to monitor advice given in community pharmacy or GP settings. For GPs, variations in antibiotic prescribing patterns at their practice were a concern and consequently their efforts to change patient's expectations could be undermined by other prescribers.

(b) Patient attitudes and context

GPs and a nurse practitioner discussed patient expectations for antibiotics as a hurdle to overcome in consultations, particularly those patients who had been prescribed them for previous infections and those consulting for children. HCPs generally believed that patients' understanding of AMR had improved somewhat in recent years due to public campaigns. In contrast, they believed that patients had less awareness of the importance of self-care but believed that campaigns and social media messaging could be effective at influencing patient behaviour.

HCPs reported difficulty in knowing whether their advice had changed patients' behaviour. There was some concern from GPs about a minority of patients who may immediately take the back-up antibiotic prescription or seek another prescriber to request antibiotics. HCPs reported barriers for patients to self-care for infections, including health inequalities and affordability of OTC medicines, literacy or language barriers, complex patients who are home bound, and those unable to take time off work.

2.3. Development of the Managing Common Infections leaflet

All participants from FGs, interviews, and questionnaires (Table 1) commented on iterations of the information leaflet.

(a) Usefulness of leaflet covering common infections

Overall, participants across the study reported that a resource was required to educate patients about managing common infections. All HCPs responding to the questionnaire reported they were likely or very likely to use the leaflet with patients; HCPs rated every section of the leaflet as very useful or useful, except for a section which included statistics on which infections were most common in the population (80%, 4/5 rated useful); this section was subsequently removed. Among the minority ethnic patients responding to the questionnaire, 88% (22/25) reported the leaflet provided all the necessary information they would need to self-manage a common infection and all agreed that the content was useful or very useful.

'Great way to get a lot of information to the patient. Will lead to less calls.'

(nurse, questionnaire)

'I think it's a very good leaflet, if the idea of this is to actually reduce the use of antibiotics when other simpler remedies could be used then I think it's a good idea.'

(Male patient, Focus Group 5)

(b) Information priorities for common infection leaflet

Priorities were similar across all participants and included information on when a GP appointment was needed, serious symptoms to look out for, average duration of illness, advice on self-care and OTC medicines for symptoms, and advice on when antibiotics are needed. Information needed to be simple with website links to further advice. Patients in FGs requested information on signs of sepsis and information to help distinguish their infection from COVID-19. Patients highlighted the need to clarify the difference between existing chronic illnesses which may present similarly to symptoms of common infection; for instance, for a urinary infection, symptoms may include passing urine more often at night. Patients also highlighted the need to include information on social distancing to protect vulnerable family members from infections.

> *'Many BAME [Black and Minority Ethnic] patients have other underlying issues, which may present the same symptoms as described in the leaflet, maybe expressing if there is some difference to the normal symptom they present?'*
>
> (patient, questionnaire)
>
> *'I think if it could be quite basic if it has links to things on the internet ... and then if you need to know more, this is where you go and look ... and that set you on the path to helping yourself by finding out other things online.'*
>
> (Female patient, Interview 1)

(c) Leaflet Design

Preferences from participants in interviews and FGs were for the leaflet to follow a logical step-by-step process for managing infections, with subtitles consisting of questions on personal actions patients could take, which could be discussed with an HCP. Suggested amendments from participants included the use of plain English, a reduction in the quantity of text, and the use of more images/icons to help understanding. Minority ethnic patients highlighted that too much text was inaccessible and intimidating, especially for patients where English was an additional language.

The final leaflet titled 'How can I manage my common infection?' (Figure 1) followed behavioural steps which helped the reader to make decisions on how to manage their own infection:

1. What are the symptoms of a common infection?
2. What if I think I have coronavirus (COVID-19)?
3. How can I treat a common infection?
4. How long could my infection last?
5. Will my infection need antibiotics to get better?
6. How can I stop my infection from spreading?
7. What symptoms of serious illness should I look out for?
8. What if I suspect signs of sepsis?

> *'[For the title] I want to say, how you can manage your common infection, question mark ... I think it will put the emphasis on empowering the person. Them at the centre of this, because that's what I think it should be about.'*
>
> (Pharmacist, focus group 1)

(d) Suggestions for implementation of leaflet

HCPs believed the leaflet would be useful as a shared decision aid to support their discussions with patients and help to educate patients in the GP and community pharmacy settings. Patients reported they would expect to receive the leaflet from a GP or pharmacist. All participants reported preferences for both printed physical and online versions of the leaflet; a GP acknowledged the latter would be useful for remote consultations. The leaflet was published as part of the TARGET antibiotics toolkit [18], including an online web version and has been translated into 26 different languages, following feedback from minority ethnic patients.

> *'Depending on where they receive the leaflet. It could be attached to their prescriptions when they collect it from the pharmacy, or handed out at the GP surgery.'*

(pharmacy staff, questionnaire)

'Unless it is translated, this would be a lot of text for an average non-English speaker. Visuals are great on this but I think there would be more required to help them better understand.'

(patient, questionnaire)

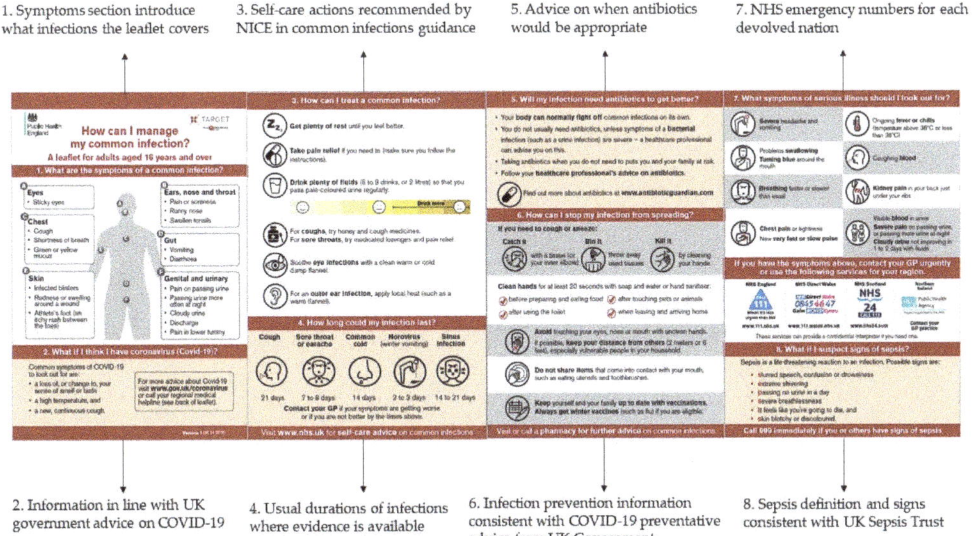

Figure 1. Labelled sections of the 'How can I manage my common infection?' leaflet. COVID-19—Coronavirus disease 2019. UK Government information on COVID-19 [19]. NICE—National Institute for Health and Care Excellence common infection guidance [8]. NHS—National Health Service. UK Sepsis Trust [20].

3. Discussion

3.1. Summary

Patients were confident about self-managing most common infections. Patients felt guilty about consulting GPs, preferring to self-care with OTC medicine, fluids, and rest unless symptoms became serious; however, they held contrasting expectations for children and elderly family members. Patients' decision to consult was based on perceived severity and concern for duration of symptoms or a belief that their symptoms were not improving through self-care; however, they struggled to judge when common infections were serious. HCPs reported patient's attitudes and expectations for antibiotics as their main hurdle to overcome in consultations where antibiotics were not necessarily needed, sometimes impacted by contradictory prescribing or advice from other prescribers. However, HCPs noted there were no systems in place to monitor patient advice, and they did not always know if their advice had influenced patients' behaviour. Both patients and HCPs valued the importance of self-care, indicated community pharmacies should be used first for advice, and recognised the need for reassurance and a focus on safety netting in consultations. Participants from the interviews, FGs, and questionnaires reported that a general infection information leaflet was useful and needed, and their priorities and feedback were used to finalise the content and design of the leaflet.

3.2. Strengths and Limitations

This study used a rigorous person-based approach [17] to develop a patient information leaflet for use in primary care and community pharmacy, underpinned by behavioural theory [21] throughout interview question development, analysis, and intervention development. Triangulation of data from patients and HCPs via multiple methods led to a large sample of participants contributing to the leaflet development, with similar themes across information and design needs.

The leaflet was designed to include general information to support HCPs' provision of advice to patients; a strength is that the leaflet may be applicable in many situations and useful when the indicated illness is not known (this is quite common in the pharmacy setting [22]). A limitation is that the leaflet cannot provide the specific advice required for some patients—for instance, those with existing conditions, where safety-netting thresholds may differ; in these contexts, the leaflet may not be suitable or HCPs may need to augment the advice provided in the leaflet.

There is potential for researcher bias in qualitative studies where preconceptions about the beliefs of participants could influence the data collection and analysis. We believe this effect was mitigated because multiple researchers collected and analysed data and met often to reflect on their role in the research and because a steering group with a range of backgrounds was involved in the design of interview schedules and interpretation of themes to inform the leaflet.

Part way through the study, interviews and FGs had to be conducted remotely and participants were encouraged to have their camera on to allow the interviewer to pick up on visual cues. The researchers consider that the input from participants and quality of data was similar with both methods.

The recruitment strategy relied on participants volunteering and may be subject to sampling biases, which could prevent transferability to other populations; however, the use of several recruitment strategies reduced this, including recruitment of minority ethnic patients. Likewise, themes may not be transferable to specific patient populations, including those with pre-existing conditions. There were a larger number of females participating in interviews/FGs than males, which is common in qualitative studies in this area [23–27] and may relate to volunteer bias; however, there was a more equal ratio in the questionnaire participants. Research studies often have low participation of minority ethnic groups [28], and where these involve designing interventions, it can reduce usability across different groups. We invited minority ethnic patients participating in another related study to complete the online questionnaire; potentially this method may have been a barrier for patients lacking access to the technology; however, we achieved views from patients identifying from a diverse range of ethnicities.

A limitation was not recruiting patients based on education/literacy level and socioeconomic status, as these aspects may affect accessibility of the leaflet. However, the leaflet was reviewed by the Plain English campaign (crystal mark 23499), and we recommend that HCPs use the leaflet in conjunction with their own advice to account for the context of patients.

3.3. Comparison with Existing Literature

In our study, patients reported being more likely to seek help for suspected infections where they expected antibiotics, one of which was UTIs, and this aligns with previous cross-sectional research where 95% of women with UTI symptoms consulted an HCP [29]. A qualitative study exploring women's process of self-care to GP consultation for UTIs described similar health-seeking behavioural influencers to our study, including perceived long duration and severity of symptoms [30]. Similarly, for RTIs, patients judged severity of symptoms on an evaluation of symptom duration, and their self-care actions were influenced by advice from their GP, pharmacy, and media [31]. In an evaluation of an AMS intervention to support community pharmacy staff advice about common infections, 20% of patients reported they did not know how long it would take them to feel better [32]. Of the literature on parents' expectations for children with common infections, a key similarity to our study was a belief of parents that consulting and being prescribed antibiotics were viewed as safer options [33,34]. Parents reported uncertainty about when to seek help for children and how to judge the seriousness of symptoms [35,36], and studies echo our implications that support is needed for patients around decision-making and self-care.

HCPs' concerns around patients' expectations for antibiotics align with previous research [37]; however, patients in our study had better knowledge of appropriate antibiotic use in comparison with the qualitative literature [23–27,38–40], which was conducted mainly before 2012. Since 2012, there has been greater emphasis on public education via national AMR campaigns, support for GPs with AMS tools [18], and incentives for Clinical Commissioning Groups around improvements in antibiotic prescribing (Quality Premiums) [41], which may have caused this attitude shift. Some patients in our study held the belief that home cleaning practices could affect immunity, which has been reported in recent public surveys [42,43]. Messages around targeted hygiene, in line with COVID-19 messaging, may help to improve these misconceptions [44]. The development of a general self-care leaflet is supported by findings of systematic reviews of shared decision-making (SDM) which have found that decision aid interventions for acute RTIs in primary care can improve patient knowledge and satisfaction and can reduce antibiotic prescribing [10,45]. HCPs concerns around the prescribing or provision of contradictory advice of other prescribers in their practice is common in the literature [16,37] and may be helped through practice-based audits and regular training. A new finding is HCPs concern around the lack of systems and processes to monitor the self-care advice given to patients, and further work may be needed to explore how this can be embedded into existing auditing.

In our study, participants views on community pharmacy concur with the literature with pharmacy staff, who view educating patients as one of their key AMS roles [22]. An evaluation of the TARGET UTI leaflet found that 25% of patients with UTI symptoms had sought help first from a pharmacist, and 65% were comfortable discussing their symptoms in private settings with a pharmacist [46]. Evaluation of a patient-facing RTI leaflet in community pharmacies led to a decrease in GP referrals for RTIs and an increase in provision of self-care advice in the intervention group [47]. This supports the use of the general infection leaflet in pharmacies, but research should explore the impact of community pharmacy staff's advice using these leaflets on patients' AMS behaviours.

3.4. Implications for Research and Practice

Patients have inherent views, expectations, and traditions around managing common infections, and HCPs should start with an honest dialogue to gauge a patient's expectations and understand their unique context. The managing common infections leaflet developed from our study can support shared decision-making and patient education in the GP and pharmacy setting, which may reduce unnecessary consultations and antibiotic use [48]. As a general information leaflet, we recommend that the patient's specific context and needs should always be considered and that appropriate tailored advice provided in addition to the leaflet as necessary. The managing common infections leaflet is freely available via the TARGET toolkit (available on the Royal College of General Practitioners (RCGP) website [18]) and will be reviewed against guidance regularly.

Patients in this study believed antibiotics were required to treat ear infections and tonsillitis, most of which are self-limiting. In a 2020 public survey of 2022 people, over two-thirds (68%) incorrectly stated that antibiotics are needed to treat most ear infections [49]. Antibiotic treatment for most ear infections opposes NICE guidelines, and it is therefore an important area for further research to understand the source of these expectations. Although we involved minority ethnic patients in the design of the leaflet, to ensure information and advice is reaching those who need it most, further work is needed with diverse minority ethnic groups and high deprivation communities to explore the accessibility and affordability of treatment for self-managed common infections and to implement and evaluate the effect of AMS educational interventions and patient-facing infection leaflets.

Implementation of patient-facing resources will become increasingly important to support carers and patients with common infections as COVID-19 social distancing measures reduce. Remote consultations are anticipated to continue [50], and future research should explore implementation of patient information leaflets in this context and evaluate their effect on antibiotic prescribing. The COVID-19 pandemic is likely to influence the themes around patient management of infections reported in our study, and further work is needed to explore the impact of the pandemic on public health-seeking behaviour and attitudes towards antibiotics and hygiene.

4. Materials and Methods

4.1. Study Design

Qualitative study using FGs, interviews, and online questionnaires with patients and HCPs to inform parallel development of a patient leaflet covering management of common infections. The qualitative schedules (Supplementary S1) for HCPs and patients included two sections: the first covered approaches to managing common infections, and the second involved reviewing and giving feedback on the leaflet under development. Questions were informed by a literature review, expert stakeholder input, and the TDF [21] in order to ensure questions covered all behavioural determinants. Iterations of the leaflet were reviewed in FGs and interviews, and participants were encouraged to think-aloud their immediate views on the information and design. Following completion of interviews and FGs, the research team decided to collect additional data from HCPs and specific patient groups via online questionnaires to finalise the leaflet. Questionnaire participants reviewed a near-final version of the leaflet towards the end of data collection. Questionnaires (Supplementary S2) were hosted on the PHE Select Survey platform and were mostly qualitative open questions, with a small number of quantitative Likert-type scale questions on usefulness and completeness of information covered in the leaflet.

The research team and study steering group (including patient and HCP representatives) were experienced in qualitative research, behavioural science, and intervention development for the primary care setting. The Consolidated Criteria for Reporting Qualitative Research (COREQ) was observed in this report (Table S3).

4.2. Intervention Development

4.2.1. Audience and Purpose of the Leaflet

The study aimed to develop a patient leaflet including general information and recommendations around common infections that could support HCPs with provision of advice to adult patients in primary care consultations and in community pharmacy settings. The leaflet was not intended to replace HCP advice, but to support it. As a general leaflet, it was not designed to account for specific patient needs, for instance, those with existing conditions who would likely need specific tailored advice from their HCP.

4.2.2. Leaflet Development

An initial leaflet draft incorporated evidence from a review of the literature on patient self-care actions for common infections, incorporating recommendations from NICE and PHE guidance and from stakeholder reviewers (different from participants in this study). The stakeholder reviewers included a range of healthcare professionals, infectious disease experts and consultants, and professionals with a background in behavioural science and knowledge and literacy. Stakeholders were identified and recruited from PHE and from a range of clinical groups and networks. Stakeholders reviewed and provided input on iterations of the leaflet throughout the study. In line with the person-based approach to intervention development [17], a log of suggested changes were kept, and leaflet drafts were revised iteratively, with support from a design team. After questionnaire feedback was incorporated, the leaflet was finally reviewed by a Plain English group to fine-tune language, and stakeholder reviewers approved final content before publication.

4.3. Setting and Participant Recruitment

Participants were recruited January–May 2020 through a range of methods. For HCPs participating in interviews and FGs, invitations were cascaded through the Gloucestershire

Clinical Commissioning Group (CCG), existing networks, mailing lists, and social media. Recruitment was purposive and aimed to recruit GPs, community pharmacists, and nurse representatives from across England. For online questionnaires, HCPs were invited to give feedback on the leaflet draft in May 2020 through the TARGET antibiotics toolkit mailing list and newsletter (sent to 750 individuals).

Patients participating in interviews and FGs were recruited through the community and known networks, including a PHE public representatives' network. Inclusion criteria for patients included being over 18 years, fluent in English, and not suffering from long term illnesses or co-morbidities, as these patients may have complex information needs that could not be captured in a general infection leaflet. Patients representing diverse minority ethnic groups, participating in another study led by members of the research team, were opportunistically invited to provide feedback on the leaflet via an online questionnaire in May 2020. Minority ethnic patients (n = 76) were recruited to this other study via purposive snowball and community sampling and were given the option to participate in an online questionnaire for the present study.

Demographic data collected from all patients included self-reported age, gender, and ethnicity. Information on socioeconomic status and health literacy and education level were not collected.

4.4. Data Collection

Initially, semi-structured interviews and FGs were conducted face-to-face in Gloucester and London; following the introduction of COVID-19 restrictions, they were undertaken remotely on Skype. Type of data collection was dependent on participant preference and availability. Participants provided written and informed consent and had the opportunity to ask questions before data collection. Discussions lasted between 45 and 80 min for the initial questions covering management of infection and between 30 and 60 min for leaflet discussion, with a break in between; FGs tended to be longer in duration than individual interviews. The leaflet was printed for face-to-face participants, and it was emailed to Skype participants, ahead of the second section of the discussion.

Data were collected by three female researchers (B.M., C.V.H., R.A.) experienced in qualitative methods and without a clinical background. Researchers made detailed field notes about participants' feedback on the leaflet. Participants were not known to researchers prior to data collection and were paid for their time according to PHE policy on public involvement in research. Data were collected until researchers agreed that data saturation had been reached [51,52], where there were no new emerging themes. Discussions were recorded, transcribed by an external agency, and checked for accuracy by researchers. Recordings or transcripts were not returned to participants. All files were handled in accordance with the Data Protection Act 2018 and General Data Protection Regulations (GDPR).

4.5. Data Analysis

Inductive thematic analysis of qualitative data followed the six stages outlined by Braun and Clarke [53]. Data were analysed in full by one researcher (C.V.H.), and 20% were double coded by a second researcher (E.S.). First, researchers became familiar with the data, and NVivo Pro-11 software was used to organise the analysis. Researchers labelled transcripts with codes, meanings, and patterns emerging from the data. Codes were subsequently arranged into themes and iteratively revised as the dataset was reviewed against the coding framework. Researchers met regularly to discuss emerging themes and insights and to discuss their own beliefs and involvement in the research process; any conflicts in coding were resolved through discussion. Following agreement of a thematic framework by the research team and steering group, the themes were mapped to the TDF for reporting, and quotes which best illustrated the meaning of the theme were identified. The quantitative Likert-type scale questionnaire data were analysed descriptively using Microsoft Excel software.

For leaflet development, two researchers collated the questionnaire findings and the field notes, emerging themes, and think-aloud feedback from the interviews and FGs. Following each data collection, key findings and suggestions were tabulated in Microsoft Excel, and discussion between the research team and steering group agreed changes or implications for the design, content, and implementation of the leaflet. This log of changes was reviewed iteratively to allow rapid changes to the leaflet ahead of subsequent interviews and FGs.

Themes from the interviews and FGs about approaches and experiences managing common infections are presented in the Results Section 3.2, while specific feedback on the leaflet (including questionnaire data) are presented in the Results Section 3.3.

5. Conclusions

A general patient information leaflet on common infections should support patients to self-manage symptoms, utilise community pharmacies for advice and empower patients to determine when GP consultation is required, especially for elderly or child dependents.

Supplementary Materials: The following are available online at https://www.mdpi.com/article/10.3390/antibiotics10091113/s1, Table S1: Patient emerging themes on self-management of common infections (additional quotes), Table S2: HCP emerging themes on provision of advice on common infections (additional quotes), Table S3: Completed COREQ checklist, Supplementary S1: Patient and HCP interview/FG schedules, Supplementary S2: HCP and minority ethnic patient questionnaires.

Author Contributions: Conceptualization, D.M.L. and C.A.M.M.; methodology, C.V.H., B.M., R.A., D.M.L. and C.A.M.M.; formal analysis, C.V.H. and E.S.; investigation, C.V.H., B.M., R.A., D.M.L. and C.A.M.M.; writing—original draft preparation, C.V.H.; writing—review and editing, C.V.H., B.M., E.S., R.A., D.M.L. and C.A.M.M.; supervision, D.M.L. and C.A.M.M.; project administration, C.V.H. and B.M. All authors have read and agreed to the published version of the manuscript.

Funding: This research received no external funding.

Institutional Review Board Statement: The study was internally reviewed by the PHE Research Ethics and Governance Group (REGG) (Reference: NR0180) and the study did not require National Research Ethics Service approval as it was classed as service evaluation.

Informed Consent Statement: Informed consent was obtained from all participants involved in the study. Written informed consent was obtained from participants for the use of anonymized quotes in reporting and publications.

Data Availability Statement: The thematic analyses generated during this study are included in full in this published article and its supplementary information files. The corresponding author can be contacted for further study materials on reasonable request.

Acknowledgments: We would like to thank the study steering group and expert advisors, including Diane Ashiru-Oredope, Tessa Lewis, Philip Howard, Carole Fry, Caroline DeBrun, Kath Hartigan, Tracey Thornley, Raj Kanth, Susan Hopkins, and Colin Brown. Thanks also to patients, healthcare professionals, expert advisors, and clinical groups who have reviewed and commented on the Managing Common Infections leaflet, including members of the Self-care Forum, Royal Pharmaceutical Society, Royal College of General Practitioners. Thank you to Julie Brooke for supporting edits to the manuscript. Thank you to Leah Jones for supporting this research, including the questionnaire with minority ethnic patients and behavioural insights into the leaflet development. Thank you to all participants for providing their time for interviews, focus groups, and questionnaires.

Conflicts of Interest: All authors have managed or provided research support for Public Health England's TARGET antibiotic toolkit.

References

1. World Health Organisation. *World Health Organisation: Antimicrobial Resistance Global Report on Surveillance*; WHO: Geneva, Switzerland, 2014. Available online: https://apps.who.int/iris/bitstream/handle/10665/112642/9789241564748_eng.pdf;jsessionid=27B57B8DEF0B3D930FA9D25FC8BD1691?sequence=1 (accessed on 15 September 2019).
2. Public Health England (PHE). *English Surveillance Programme for Antimicrobial Utilisation and Resistance (ESPAUR)*; Report 2019–2020; PHE: London, UK, 2020. Available online: https://assets.publishing.service.gov.uk/government/uploads/system/uploads/attachment_data/file/936199/ESPAUR_Report_2019-20.pdf (accessed on 20 May 2021).
3. Dolk, F.C.K.; Pouwels, K.B.; Smith, D.R.M.; Robotham, J.V.; Smieszek, T. Antibiotics in primary care in England: Which antibiotics are prescribed and for which conditions? *J. Antimicrob. Chemother.* **2018**, *73* (Suppl. 2), ii2–ii10. [CrossRef] [PubMed]
4. Pouwels, K.B.; Dolk, F.C.K.; Smith, D.R.M.; Robotham, J.V.; Smieszek, T. Actual versus 'ideal' antibiotic prescribing for common conditions in English primary care. *J. Antimicrob. Chemother.* **2018**, *73* (Suppl. 2), 19–26. [CrossRef] [PubMed]
5. Pouwels, K.B.; Dolk, F.C.K.; Smith, D.R.M.; Robotham, J.V.; Smieszek, T. Explaining variation in antibiotic prescribing between general practices in the UK. *J. Antimicrob. Chemother.* **2018**, *73* (Suppl. 2), ii27–ii35. [CrossRef] [PubMed]
6. HM Government. *UK 5-Year Action Plan for Antimicrobial Resistance 2019 to 2024*; Department of Health and Social Care: London, UK, 2019.
7. National Institute for Health Care and Excellence (NICE). *Summary of Antimicrobial Prescribing Guidance—Managing Common Infections*; NICE: London, UK, 2021; Available online: https://www.nice.org.uk/about/what-we-do/our-programmes/nice-guidance/antimicrobial-prescribing-guidelines (accessed on 20 May 2021).
8. National Institute for Health Care and Excellence (NICE). *Antimicrobial Stewardship: Changing Risk-Related Behaviours in the General Population*; NICE Guideline [NG63]; NICE: London, UK, 2017; Available online: https://www.nice.org.uk/guidance/ng63 (accessed on 20 May 2021).
9. Jones, L.F.; Verlander, N.Q.; Lecky, D.M.; Altaf, S.; Pilat, D.; McNulty, C.A.M. Self-Reported Antimicrobial Stewardship Practices in Primary Care Using the TARGET Antibiotics Self-Assessment Tool. *Antibiotics* **2020**, *9*, 253. [CrossRef]
10. Coxeter, P.; Del Mar, C.B.; McGregor, L.; Beller, E.M.; Hoffmann, T.C. Interventions to facilitate shared decision making to address antibiotic use for acute respiratory infections in primary care. *Cochrane Database Syst. Rev.* **2015**, *2015*, CD010907. [CrossRef]
11. Smith, C.M.; Shallcross, L.J.; Dutey-Magni, P.; Conolly, A.; Fuller, C.; Hill, S.; Jhass, A.; Marcheselli, F.; Michie, S.; Mindell, J.S.; et al. Incidence, healthcare-seeking behaviours, antibiotic use and natural history of common infection syndromes in England: Results from the Bug Watch community cohort study. *BMC Infect. Dis.* **2021**, *21*, 105. [CrossRef]
12. Murphy, M.; Scott, L.J.; Salisbury, C.; Turner, A.; Scott, A.; Denholm, R.; Lewis, R.; Iyer, G.; Macleod, J.; Horwood, J. Implementation of remote consulting in UK primary care following the COVID-19 pandemic: A mixed-methods longitudinal study. *Br. J. Gen. Pract.* **2021**, *71*, e166–e177. [CrossRef]
13. NHS Digital. *Appointments in General Practice. Official Statistics, Experimental Statistics*; NHS Digital: Leeds, UK, 2020. Available online: https://digital.nhs.uk/data-and-information/publications/statistical/appointments-in-general-practice (accessed on 15 July 2021).
14. McNulty, C.; Hawking, M.; Lecky, D.; Jones, L.; Owens, R.; Charlett, A.; Butler, C.; Moore, P.; Francis, N. Effects of primary care antimicrobial stewardship outreach on antibiotic use by general practice staff: Pragmatic randomized controlled trial of the TARGET antibiotics workshop. *J. Antimicrob. Chemother.* **2018**, *73*, 1423–1432. [CrossRef]
15. Jones, L.F.; Cooper, E.; Joseph, A.; Allison, R.; Gold, N.; Donald, I.; McNulty, C. Development of an information leaflet and diagnostic flow chart to improve the management of urinary tract infections in older adults: A qualitative study using the Theoretical Domains Framework. *BJGP Open* **2020**, *4*, bjgpopen20X101044. [CrossRef]
16. Lecky, D.M.; Howdle, J.; Butler, C.C.; McNulty, C.A. Optimising management of UTIs in primary care: A qualitative study of patient and GP perspectives to inform the development of an evidence-based, shared decision-making resource. *Br. J. Gen. Pract.* **2020**, *70*, e330–e338. [CrossRef]
17. Yardley, L.; Morrison, L.; Bradbury, K.; Muller, I. The Person-Based Approach to Intervention Development: Application to Digital Health-Related Behavior Change Interventions. *JMIR* **2015**, *17*, e30. [CrossRef]
18. Royal College of General Practitioners. TARGET Antibiotics Toolkit. 2021. Available online: https://www.rcgp.org.uk/clinical-and-research/resources/toolkits/amr/target-antibiotics-toolkit.aspx (accessed on 16 June 2021).
19. HM Government. Coronavirus (COVID-19). 2021. Available online: https://www.gov.uk/coronavirus (accessed on 23 July 2021).
20. UK Sepsis Trust. The UK Sepsis Trust. 2021. Available online: https://sepsistrust.org/ (accessed on 23 July 2021).
21. Atkins, L.; Francis, J.; Islam, R.; O'Connor, D.; Patey, A.; Ivers, N.; Foy, R.; Duncan, E.M.; Colquhoun, H.; Grimshaw, J.M.; et al. A guide to using the Theoretical Domains Framework of behaviour change to investigate implementation problems. *Implement. Sci.* **2017**, *12*, 77. [CrossRef]
22. Jones, L.F.; Owens, R.; Sallis, A.; Ashiru-Oredope, D.; Thornley, T.; Francis, N.A.; Butler, C.; McNulty, C.A.M. Qualitative study using interviews and focus groups to explore the current and potential for antimicrobial stewardship in community pharmacy informed by the Theoretical Domains Framework. *BMJ Open* **2018**, *8*, e025101. [CrossRef]
23. Brookes-Howell, L.; Elwyn, G.; Hood, K.; Wood, F.; Cooper, L.; Goossens, H.; Ieven, M.; Butler, C.C. 'The body gets used to them': Patients' interpretations of antibiotic resistance and the implications for containment strategies. *J. Gen. Intern. Med.* **2012**, *27*, 766–772. [CrossRef]

24. Brooks, L.; Shaw, A.; Sharp, D.; Hay, A. Towards a better understanding of patients' perspectives of antibiotic resistance and MRSA: A qualitative study. *Fam. Pract.* **2008**, *25*, 341–348. [CrossRef] [PubMed]
25. Davis, M.E.; Liu, T.L.; Taylor, Y.; Davidson, L.; Schmid, M.; Yates, T.; Scotton, J.; Spencer, M. Exploring Patient Awareness and Perceptions of the Appropriate Use of Antibiotics: A Mixed-Methods Study. *Antibiotics* **2017**, *6*, 23. [CrossRef] [PubMed]
26. Hawkings, N.J.; Butler, C.C.; Wood, F. Antibiotics in the community: A typology of user behaviours. *Patient Educ. Couns.* **2008**, *73*, 146–152. [CrossRef]
27. Hawkings, N.J.; Wood, F.; Butler, C.C. Public attitudes towards bacterial resistance: A qualitative study. *J. Antimicrob. Chemother.* **2007**, *59*, 1155–1160. [CrossRef] [PubMed]
28. George, S.; Duran, N.; Norris, K. A Systematic Review of Barriers and Facilitators to Minority Research Participation among African Americans, Latinos, Asian Americans, and Pacific Islanders. *Am. J. Public Health* **2014**, *104*, e16–e31. [CrossRef] [PubMed]
29. Butler, C.C.; Hawking, M.K.D.; Quigley, A.; McNulty, C.A.M. Incidence, severity, help seeking, and management of uncomplicated urinary tract infection: A population-based survey. *Br. J. Gen. Pract.* **2015**, *65*, e702–e707. [CrossRef]
30. Leydon, G.M.; Turner, S.; Smith, H.; Little, P. The journey from self-care to GP care: A qualitative interview study of women presenting with symptoms of urinary tract infection. *Br. J. Gen. Pract.* **2009**, *59*, e219–e225. [CrossRef]
31. McDermott, L.; Leydon, G.M.; Halls, A.; Kelly, J.; Nagle, A.; White, J.; Little, P. Qualitative interview study of antibiotics and self-management strategies for respiratory infections in primary care. *BMJ Open* **2017**, *7*, e016903.
32. Allison, R.; Chapman, S.; Howard, P.; Thornley, T.; Ashiru-Oredope, D.; Walker, S.; Jones, L.F.; McNulty, C.A.M. Feasibility of a community pharmacy antimicrobial stewardship intervention (PAMSI): An innovative approach to improve patients' understanding of their antibiotics. *JAC Antimicrob. Resist.* **2020**, *2*, dlaa089. [CrossRef]
33. Cabral, C.; Lucas, P.J.; Ingram, J.; Hay, A.D.; Horwood, J. "It's safer to … " parent consulting and clinician antibiotic prescribing decisions for children with respiratory tract infections: An analysis across four qualitative studies. *Soc. Sci. Med.* **2015**, *136–137*, 156–164. [CrossRef] [PubMed]
34. Halls, A.; Van't Hoff, C.; Little, P.; Verheij, T.; Leydon, G.M. Qualitative interview study of parents' perspectives, concerns and experiences of the management of lower respiratory tract infections in children in primary care. *BMJ Open* **2017**, *7*, e015701. [CrossRef]
35. Ingram, J.; Cabral, C.; Hay, A.D.; Lucas, P.J.; Horwood, J. Parents' information needs, self-efficacy and influences on consulting for childhood respiratory tract infections: A qualitative study. *BMC Fam. Pract.* **2013**, *14*, 106. [CrossRef]
36. Neill, S.J. Containing acute childhood illness within family life: A substantive grounded theory. *J. Child Health Care* **2010**, *14*, 327–344. [CrossRef]
37. Tonkin-Crine, S.; Yardley, L.; Coenen, S.; Fernandez-Vandellos, P.; Krawczyk, J.; Touboul, P.; Verheij, T.; Little, P. GPs' views in five European countries of interventions to promote prudent antibiotic use. *Br. J. Gen. Pract.* **2011**, *61*, e252–e261. [CrossRef] [PubMed]
38. McNulty, C.A.; Boyle, P.; Nichols, T.; Clappison, P.; Davey, P. Don't wear me out—The public's knowledge of and attitudes to antibiotic use. *J. Antimicrob. Chemother.* **2007**, *59*, 727–738. [CrossRef]
39. McNulty, C.A.M.; Collin, S.M.; Cooper, E.; Lecky, D.M.; Butler, C.C. Public understanding and use of antibiotics in England: Findings from a household survey in 2017. *BMJ Open* **2019**, *9*, e030845. [CrossRef]
40. Norris, P.; Chamberlain, K.; Dew, K.; Gabe, J.; Hodgetts, D.; Madden, H. Public Beliefs about Antibiotics, Infection and Resistance: A Qualitative Study. *Antibiotics* **2013**, *2*, 465–476. [CrossRef] [PubMed]
41. NHS England. CCG Outcomes Tools: Quality Premium. 2021. Available online: https://www.england.nhs.uk/ccg-out-tool/qual-prem/ (accessed on 16 June 2021).
42. Bloomfield, S.F.; Stanwell-Smith, R.; Crevel, R.W.R.; Pickup, J. Too clean, or not too clean: The hygiene hypothesis and home hygiene. *Clin. Exp. Allergy* **2006**, *36*, 402–425. [CrossRef]
43. Royal Society of Public Health. Too Clean or Not Too Clean? The Case for Targeted Hygiene in Home and Everyday Life. 2019. Available online: https://www.rsph.org.uk/our-work/policy/infection-control/too-clean-or-not-too-clean.html (accessed on 20 September 2019).
44. Bloomfield, S.F. The case for Targeted Hygiene. *Perspect. Public Health* **2019**, *139*, 219–221.
45. Coronado-Vázquez, V.; Canet-Fajas, C.; Delgado-Marroquín, M.T.; Magallón-Botaya, R.; Romero-Martín, M.; Gómez-Salgado, J. Interventions to facilitate shared decision-making using decision aids with patients in Primary Health Care: A systematic review. *Medicine* **2020**, *99*, e21389. [CrossRef]
46. Peiffer-Smadja, N.; Allison, R.; Jones, L.F.; Holmes, A.H.; Patel, P.; Lecky, D.L.; Ahmad, R.; McNulty, C.A.M. Preventing and Managing Urinary Tract Infections: Enhancing the Role of Community Pharmacists-A Mixed Methods Study. *Antibiotics* **2020**, *9*, 583. [CrossRef]
47. Ashiru-Oredope, D.; Doble, A.; Thornley, T.; Saei, A.; Gold, N.; Sallis, A.; McNulty, C.A.M.; Lecky, D.; Umoh, E.; Klinger, C. Improving Management of Respiratory Tract Infections in Community Pharmacies and Promoting Antimicrobial Stewardship: A Cluster Randomised Control Trial with a Self-Report Behavioural Questionnaire and Process Evaluation. *Pharmacy* **2020**, *8*, 44. [CrossRef]
48. Little, P.; Stuart, B.; Andreou, P.; McDermott, L.; Joseph, J.; Mullee, M.; Moore, M.; Broomfield, S.; Thomas, T.; Yardley, L. Primary care randomised controlled trial of a tailored interactive website for the self-management of respiratory infections (Internet Doctor). *BMJ Open* **2016**, *6*, e009769. [CrossRef]

49. McNulty, C.A.M.; Read, B.; Quigley, A.; Verlander, N.Q.; Lecky, D.M. What the public know about antibiotic use and resistance in 2020—A face-to-face questionnaire survey. *BMJ Open* **2021**. manuscript submitted.
50. Han, S.M.; Greenfield, G.; Majeed, A.; Hayhoe, B. Impact of Remote Consultations on Antibiotic Prescribing in Primary Health Care: Systematic Review. *J. Med. Internet Res.* **2020**, *22*, e23482. [CrossRef]
51. Guest, G.; Bunce, A.; Johnson, L. How Many Interviews Are Enough?:An Experiment with Data Saturation and Variability. *Field Methods* **2006**, *18*, 59–82. [CrossRef]
52. Guest, G.; Namey, E.; McKenna, K. How Many Focus Groups Are Enough? Building an Evidence Base for Nonprobability Sample Sizes. *Field Methods* **2016**, *29*, 3–22. [CrossRef]
53. Braun, V.; Clarke, V. Using thematic analysis in psychology. *Qual. Res. Psychol.* **2006**, *3*, 77–101. [CrossRef]

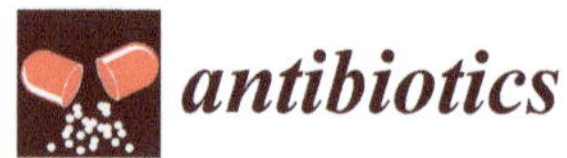

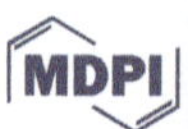

Article

Understanding Internal and External Drivers Influencing the Prescribing Behaviour of Informal Healthcare Providers with Emphasis on Antibiotics in Rural India: A Qualitative Study

Shweta Khare [1,2,*], Ashish Pathak [1,3,4,*], Cecilia Stålsby Lundborg [1], Vishal Diwan [1,5] and Salla Atkins [6,7]

1 Health Systems and Policy (HSP): Medicines, Focusing Antibiotics, Department of Global Public Health, Karolinska Institutet, Tomtebodavagen 18A, 171 77 Stockholm, Sweden; cecilia.stalsby.lundborg@ki.se (C.S.L.); vishal.diwan@icmr.gov.in (V.D.)

2 Department of Public Health and Environment, Ruxmaniben Deepchand Gardi Medical College, Ujjain 456006, Madhya Pradesh, India

3 Department of Pediatrics, Ruxmaniben Deepchand Gardi Medical College, Ujjain 456006, Madhya Pradesh, India

4 International Maternal and Child Health Unit, Department of Women and Children's Health, Uppsala University, 751 85 Uppsala, Sweden

5 Division of Environmental Monitoring and Exposure Assessment (Water and Soil), ICMR—National Institute for Research in Environmental Health, Bhopal 462030, Madhya Pradesh, India

6 Social Medicine, Infectious Diseases and Migration (SIM), Department of Global Public Health, Karolinska Institutet, Tomtebodavagen 18A, 171 77 Stockholm, Sweden; salla.atkins@tuni.fi

7 Global Health and Development, Faculty of Social Sciences, Tampere University, Arvo Ylpön Katu 34, 33520 Tampere, Finland

* Correspondence: shweta.khare@ki.se (S.K.); drashish.jpathak@gmail.com or ashish.pathak@ki.se (A.P.); Tel.: +91-98939-86241 (S.K.); +91-93022-39899 (A.P.)

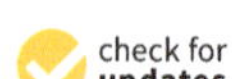

Citation: Khare, S.; Pathak, A.; Stålsby Lundborg, C.; Diwan, V.; Atkins, S. Understanding Internal and External Drivers Influencing the Prescribing Behaviour of Informal Healthcare Providers with Emphasis on Antibiotics in Rural India: A Qualitative Study. *Antibiotics* **2022**, *11*, 459. https://doi.org/10.3390/antibiotics11040459

Academic Editor: Akke Vellinga

Received: 9 February 2022
Accepted: 28 March 2022
Published: 29 March 2022

Publisher's Note: MDPI stays neutral with regard to jurisdictional claims in published maps and institutional affiliations.

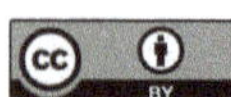

Copyright: © 2022 by the authors. Licensee MDPI, Basel, Switzerland. This article is an open access article distributed under the terms and conditions of the Creative Commons Attribution (CC BY) license (https://creativecommons.org/licenses/by/4.0/).

Abstract: Globally, Antibiotic resistance is a major public health concern, with antibiotic use contributing significantly. Targeting informal healthcare providers (IHCPs) is important to achieve universal health coverage and effective antibiotic stewardship in resource-constrained settings. We, therefore, aimed to analyse the internal and external drivers that influence IHCPs' prescribing behaviour for common illnesses in children under five, with an emphasis on antibiotic use in rural areas of India. A total of 48 IHCPs participated in focus group discussions. Thematic framework analysis with an inductive approach was used, and findings were collated in the theoretical framework based on knowledge, attitude, and practice model which depicted that the decisions made by IHCPs while prescribing antibiotics are complex and influenced by a variety of external and internal drivers. IHCPs' internal drivers included the misconception that it is impossible to treat a patient without antibiotics and that antibiotics increase the effectiveness of other drugs and cure patients faster in order to retain them. Formal healthcare providers were the IHCPs' sources of information, which influences their antibiotic prescribing. We found when it comes to seeking healthcare in rural areas, the factors that influence their choice include 'rapid cure', 'cost of treatment', 'distance' and '24 h availability', instead of qualification, which may create pressure for IHCPs to provide a quick fix. Targeted and coordinated efforts at all levels will be needed to change the antibiotic prescribing practices of IHCPs with a focus on behaviour change and to help resolve misconceptions about antibiotics.

Keywords: healthcare providers; infectious diseases; caregivers; child; prescription; antibiotics; antibiotic resistance; rural population; India

1. Introduction

Antibiotic resistance is a multi-sectoral public health risk on a global scale, posing a threat to patient safety worldwide [1]. Between 2000 and 2015, global antibiotic use increased by 65%, from 21.1 billion to 34.8 billion defined daily doses (DDDs) [2]. According to the report released by the World Health Organisation (WHO) in 2014, we are entering a 'post-antibiotic' era, in which antibiotics may no longer be effective in treating illnesses or injuries that were previously treatable [3]. Worldwide, nearly 5.4 million children under the age of five die every year, with infectious diseases accounting for approximately half of all such deaths [4]. Among the most common infections in children are acute respiratory tract infections and acute diarrhoea. Both of these are more likely to be caused by viral infections, which do not need to be treated with antibiotics [5–7]. On the other hand, antibiotics are frequently prescribed inappropriately and for illnesses that are not warranted, such as viral infections [8–10]. When antibiotic use is increased, antibiotic resistance among the bacteria that cause common infections is increased as well [11]. In many low- and middle-income countries with a high burden of infectious diseases [12] and inadequate antibiotic provision (including overuse and misuse) [13], as well as high rates of antibiotic resistance [14], the first and most severe consequences will be increased healthcare costs, which will have significant social and economic consequences [1]. Each year, an estimated 700,000 people die of diseases caused by drug-resistant pathogens, a figure that might rise to 10 million by 2050 if the current prevalence of drug resistance keeps increasing [15]. Furthermore, by 2050, the annual gross domestic product of the world is expected to decline by 3.8%. Poorer countries will be hit the hardest by the consequences of the greater prevalence of infectious diseases and the greater declines in economic growth [16].

The Indian government took action in April 2017 to combat antibiotic resistance and enacted the National Action Plan on Antimicrobial Resistance, following the approach taken by the WHO in drafting a global antimicrobial resistance action plan. The National Action Plan has numerous goals, including reducing the number of infections, strengthening surveillance, encouraging research, and improving the judicious use of antibiotics [17]. In India, antibiotics sales are regulated by the Drugs and Cosmetics Act and Rules, which provide a mandate for the identification of illegal pharmacies, unqualified doctors and regulate over-the-counter sales of antibiotics [18]. Despite the fact that these provisions exist, informal healthcare providers (IHCPs) can be found practicing in rural areas and are not forced to close down, as it is a well-known fact even to the governing authorities that they address the needs unmet by the formal healthcare system [19]. In this study, the term 'IHCP' is used for unqualified medical practitioners. IHCPs are healthcare professionals who have not acquired a formal medical degree from an institution recognised by the Medical Council of India and who are not registered with regulatory body Medical Council of India/State Medical Council(s) as healthcare practitioners [20]. Additionally, anyone qualified in another system of medicine (for example, Ayurveda, Unani, Siddha, or Homoeopathy) who practices any sort of modern system of medicine is categorised under IHCP [21]. The data from a longitudinal follow-up of caregivers' healthcare-seeking behaviour from rural areas in Ujjain, India, shows that IHCPs were first-contact providers in 73% of cases and provided 85% of the total antibiotics (mostly broad-spectrum) reported during the study [22]. In our previous study, a survey of 15,322 prescriptions given to outpatients by the IHCPs revealed that antibiotics were the most commonly prescribed drug than other medications for common illnesses in both children and adults [8].

IHCPs play important roles in rural healthcare, and their role cannot be overlooked in the effort to achieve Universal Health Coverage (UHC) and designing effective antimicrobial stewardship, especially in resource-limited settings. For them to be more efficiently involved in the provision of healthcare services, it is important to gain an understanding of their knowledge and practice—including how they interpret adequate care and rational treatment. Our aim was, therefore, to analyse the internal and external drivers that influence IHCPs prescribing behaviour for common illnesses in under-five (U-5) children, with an emphasis on antibiotic use, in rural areas of India.

2. Results

Our findings suggest that antibiotic prescribing decisions by IHCPs are complex and influenced by multiple drivers at the knowledge, attitude, and practice level. We present our themes grouped into internal and external drivers below, supported by illustrative quotes.

According to our study findings, both internal and external drivers influence IHCPs' practice, including patient behaviour and demand, availability and access to diagnostic testing, information exchange from formal healthcare providers, and referral facility and sociodemographic characteristics of the IHCPs. In order to give an illustrated overview of the internal and external factors that influence IHCPs prescription behaviours with emphasis on antibiotic prescribing, we compiled our data into a model known as knowledge, attitude, and practices (KAP), proposed by Rodrigues et al.(Figure 1) [23].

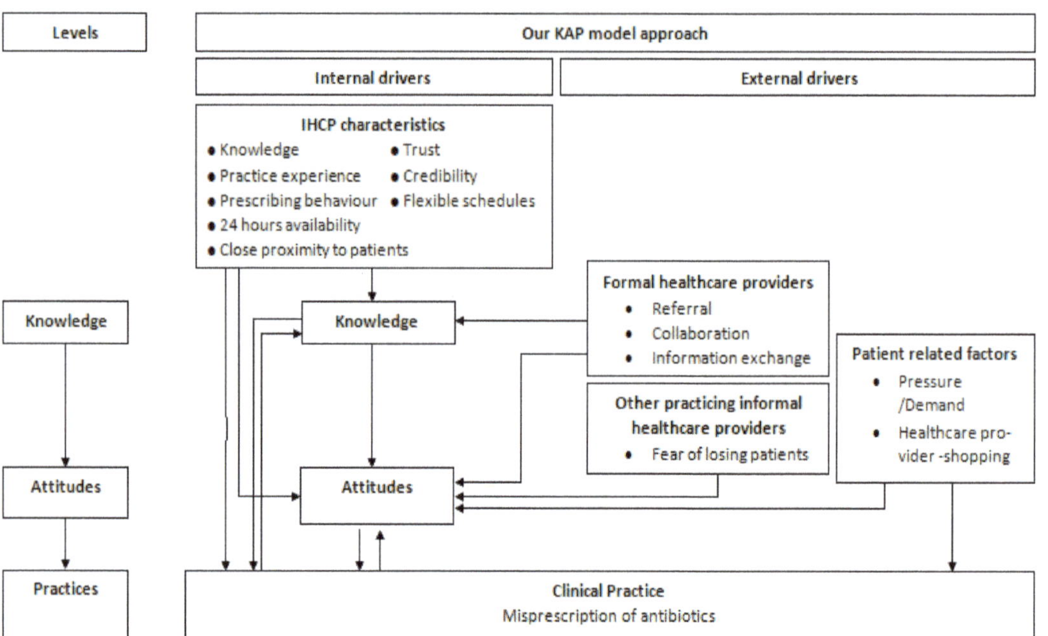

Figure 1. Overview of internal and external drivers identified, with interconnection among the drivers and impact on informal healthcare providers prescribing behaviour at all levels of the KAP model.

2.1. Internal Drivers

2.1.1. Theme 1—IHCPs' Accelerated Therapeutic Interactions with Ready Supply Antibiotics Allowed Them to Surpass Academic Credentials

IHCPs with a long history of providing care are well established and hold a decent reputation among members of their communities. There is hardly any rural community without IHCPs. They are among the vital components of the community since they tend to be less professionally distant and more social by being more interactive with the patients, always having an available source of medicine for their patients, and also adding some personal component to their approach to providing healthcare. These IHCPs and their practices are strongly supported by the villagers. Therefore, IHCPs' are the major source of healthcare and antibiotics for residents of rural areas.

> *'Like we are practicing and government try to stop us from practicing. Government officials come to the village. So villagers meet head-on with them. They will not let us stop practicing as long as the government doesn't appoint good doctors or open a government hospital in the village. Also, said that these people will work for us until and unless the government makes other arrangements'*. (Focus Group Discussion (FGD-4); Male 4)

IHCPs have been perceived as a better choice, as they were believed to accelerate therapeutic interactions. As they were primarily local to the patients, they could be more promptly available 24 h, could work a more flexible schedule, and had a readily available supply of medicines and antibiotics. Treatments were expedited as a result of these situations, so IHCPs were seen as a preferable option. Patients who arrived late at night were given antibiotics without hesitation, believing that they were a vital element of the treatment.

> *'Patient came at night and obviously, he cannot go to town at that hour so we give him primary treatment like paracetamol for fever and antibiotics for the night and tell him to go to the paediatrician in the morning'.* (FGD-3; Male 3)

Patients' paying capacity is taken into consideration by healthcare professionals working in the informal sector, which in turn affects the selection of antibiotics and their doses, resulting in a large number of inadequate doses being administered. IHCPs were supposed to provide more than just good healthcare. Low-income patients benefit from their low-cost therapy and flexible payment alternatives, which reduces their financial burden while enhancing accessibility.

> *'We write 3 days antibiotic dose properly. Actually, in rural areas, it should be at least 5–7 days dose. If we prescribe for complete 7 days, he will find it costly and so he will not take the dose'.* (FGD-2; Female 3)

Patients might easily receive credit from IHCPs for consultation fees and prescription medicines. On occasions, they would even take produce in exchange for money. People in rural areas, many of whom are employed seasonally in agriculture and farming, sometimes do not have the money to pay for healthcare. This was a distinct benefit for IHCPs, as their fees were significantly lower than those charged by traditional healthcare providers.

2.1.2. Theme 2—Beliefs Regarding Antibiotics as a Quick Fix and First Choice in 'Hit-and-Try' Prescriptions Increase Antibiotic Use

It appears that IHCPs believe antibiotics as a mandatory part of the treatment. They regarded antibiotics as vital for primary care because they believed antibiotics could heal the majority of diseases. The most common perception was that antibiotics are not for any specific disease and that it is impossible to treat a patient without antibiotics.

> *'Antibiotic is a sure-shot drug. It can cure any disease. Any kind of disease, the patient doesn't get well without antibiotics. Even if fever is there antibiotic is compulsory, for cough and a cold antibiotic is compulsory, for wounds antibiotic is compulsory, any infection of the body, immunity is enhanced by antibiotics, it is necessary for any disease'.* (FGD-4; Male 4)

Other IHCPs reiterated that antibiotics increase the effectiveness of other drugs if given along with them and enhance the immunity of the body. They also mentioned that antibiotics are already there in the human body:

> *'I mean it boosts up the body, other drugs start working in the body. They are not effective if antibiotics aren't given. If antibiotics are not included in the treatment it takes a very long time to get better and many a time there is no effect at all'.* (FGD-5; Male 4)

Another perception of some IHCPs was that more antibiotics cure faster and if any antibiotic resistance is at all present, at least one of the antibiotics in the combination or one of the antibiotics among the two or three prescribed will work:

> *'Knowledge also and they also want fast results. Like they are giving a combination of 2 antibiotics, whether it is needed or not, so accordingly he is adding and giving believing that the patient will get well fast. The patient might not get cured by giving only cefixime, so cloxacillin in combination is given or something else and he thinks that patient will get fine because cases of resistance are also coming as patients are not taking full dose'.* (FGD-4; Male 4)

One more reason for practicing more antibiotic prescribing, as mentioned by one of the IHCP, was to retain the patients. In the opinion of IHCPs, patients wanted the fastest cure possible; otherwise, they would go to other providers; hence, antibiotics were deemed absolutely necessary as part of the treatment plan:

> *'Also happens when the provider is having competition and do not want to lose his patients to another provider thinking that if the single antibiotic prescribed did not affect and the patient does not get better soon he will go to another provider and so they prescribe more than one antibiotic'.* (FGD-7; Male 1)

Antibiotics, they reasoned, were necessary for primary care since they could treat the majority of infections. The decision to use an antibiotic is not based on scientific evidence. Antibiotic selection and dose were based on IHCPs' personal experiences with the effectiveness of various antibiotics for certain illnesses. The 'hit-and-try' approach is used to choose antibiotics for a certain disease. Over time, they've come to realise which antibiotics to administer for which symptoms and diseases.

> *'Prescription of antibiotics, we do it from our experience like if the patient has a fever, in a normal way we give simple medicines many times, the fever didn't subside then second-time small antibiotic is given, Amoxicillin, MOX syrup with the fever and so we got the result. Madam, we learnt with our experience that in fever if one antibiotic is given with antipyretic then the body will get relief faster. Yes, experience teaches everything, we keep track that this was the condition, and for this condition, this medicine was better'.* (FGD-6; Male 3)

Knowledge of the cause and development of antibiotic resistance varies widely among the IHCPs. Many of the IHCPs did not know about antibiotic resistance. Some of the IHCPs identified incorrect duration and incorrect dose of the drug as causes of occurrence of antibiotic resistance.

> *'They get treatment of cough cold in the village for 2 days, but they will take treatment for only 1 day, we explain them properly, that it is very necessary to take antibiotics for 3 days and sometimes for 5 days if needed if you don't take the complete course resistance will develop and it will stop acting on you'.* (FGD-5; Male 4)

Furthermore, only a small number of IHCPs recognise that antibiotic resistance is a result of incorrect intake and that they themselves may be at fault. They justified this by stating that they do not have a thorough understanding of how and when to administer antibiotics.

> *'We are not educated in medicine; it is possible that we could be the reason for the resistance'.* (FGD-4; Male 6)

2.2. External Drivers

2.2.1. Theme 3—Mutually Beneficial Relationship between Informal and Formal Healthcare Providers Led to Available Antibiotics

The study results revealed that there was no knowledge of the different types of common acute illnesses in U-5 children among IHCPs. Their understanding of the causative organism was limited to simple inferences such as that indicated in the following statement:

> *'According to my experience, the tiny beings which we can't see from our naked eyes, they are bacteria. The ones which are tinier than bacteria, they are viruses which are dead when outside and when they reach inside the body they become alive'.* (FGD-6; Male 2)

Formal healthcare providers are the IHCPs' source of information on the treatment of illnesses which thus influence their antibiotic prescribing. IHCPs gather knowledge by working as assistants under formal healthcare providers in their clinics or pharmacies, while some have also taken one-time certificate courses organised by the government. Most of the practice of the IHCPs is based on the learning gained by studying and following the prescriptions written by formal healthcare providers or by consulting these formal healthcare providers, and in return, when needed, they refer their patients to them.

> *'I worked at the medical retail counter for 11 years so I have the knowledge of medicines and from time to time we get training from the civil hospital, welfare society, Pushpa*

Mission Hospital, etc. Apart from this whenever needed we take advice from child specialists'. (FGD-3; Male 4)

'Madam, this we have learned during 'Jan sawasthya rakshak' (Community Health Visitor) training. Also, doctors give lectures to us and tell us to come to see patients, make groups of five, and take one group every day. To study what he had diagnosed and written on a treatment pad. You have to stand there and observe'. (FGD-2; Male 1)

2.2.2. Theme 4—Patients Thought That Antibiotics Were Effective and Often Demanded Them, Leading to Prescriptions

IHCPs who participated in FGDs had varying perspectives on patients' knowledge of antibiotics; infact, it is possible that some patients have never ever heard of them; hence, there was little evidence of patients demanding antibiotics while sick. However, the majority of patients need rapid cure owing to the insecure nature of their daily wage jobs, and at a reasonable cost, which translates into a shorter course of antibiotic treatment. They relied heavily on IHCPs for healthcare and antibiotics. Additionally, several other IHCPs remarked that there are demanding patients who are difficult to convince, show dissatisfaction when they do not obtain what they desire, and frequently shift to other healthcare providers. As a result, IHCPs' decisions about whether or not to administer antibiotics are impacted. They feared that if they did not prescribe antibiotics, patients would not recover, and they would lose their patients.

'In village what happens, labour class are there, they don't have time, they come in a hurry that they have to go back for their work, for labour work, the kid should be alright instantly; if he doesn't get relief in next 2 h, they will come to me, we both are from the same village, if I am unable to give relief, they will go to him; if he is not able to provide the relief, they will go to someone else. But the kid should get relief in 1 h. Take treatment here for one day, if it gets alright, then it is ok; otherwise, we have to go to Ujjain or show to the big doctor. In such situations, we are also not able to make a decision that what type of medicine should be given'. (FGD-2; Female 5)

IHCPs noted that incredibly, some patients were able to name certain antibiotics even though they had no idea how or why they had been provided with these medications/antibiotics. This is because many patients in rural areas have been accustomed to the instant relief of symptoms with antibiotics obtained from a medical shop, without fully comprehending the hazards or uses of these medications. We also discovered that patients put pressure on their doctors to give injectables instead of oral drugs because they believe that injectables work faster.

'They purchase from medical, by directly saying give us cefixime, give us monoxil, amoxicillin. Just like zandu balm (Ayurvedic ointment for pain relief), the head is aching so give us zandu balm. They take antibiotics like that which they have learned from medical stores. If anybody goes to the store and tell them their symptoms, the medical storekeeper will make a complete dose for them and give and tell them that this is antibiotic, this is for fever, and this is for cough cold, so this is how they learn'. (FGD-4; Male 4)

3. Discussion

We identified key internal and external drivers and interconnection among drivers influencing the prescribing behaviour of IHCPs, with emphasis on antibiotic prescribing for common illnesses in U-5 children in rural areas in central India, in order to guide the implementation of a customised social marketing intervention. The study results also reflect that despite the lack of official recognition, IHCPs are part of wider rural social systems and settings, and their prescription practices are influenced by all of the different parts of this system. A KAP model was used to visualise and summarise these factors in order to better understand the complexities of prescribing behaviour of IHCPs. Such models can help to investigate and determine the healthcare providers' subjective views or the type of healthcare providers' related attitudes and knowledge [24]. While other studies have reported similar findings [24–26], our findings aligned with a recent study of antibiotic prescribing by IHCPs in rural West Bengal, India, which concluded that IHCPs must be considered as an essential part of the rural healthcare system for developing an effective antibiotic stewardship strategy and that multiple stakeholders must be targeted with a variety of regulatory, educational, and behaviour change interventions [27]. Highlighting the significance of this research even further is the fact that there is no qualitative study from this region that demonstrates the interconnection between internal and external drivers influencing the prescribing behaviour of IHCPs, especially antibiotics. Discussed below are the key findings and potential determinants for effective interventions promoting prudent antibiotic prescription in rural India and in similar contexts.

3.1. IHCPs Sociodemographic Characteristics, Awareness, Knowledge, and Misconceptions Regarding Antibiotic Use

The National Health Mission, which was implemented in 2005, envisioned the use of accredited social health activists (ASHAs) as the first point of contact for community health-related problems in order to strengthen the existing three-tier rural public health delivery system [28]. The results of our study, however, suggest that IHCPs continue to function as the initial point of contact for primary level curative healthcare and play important roles in providing healthcare and antibiotics in rural areas. Our analysis supported the findings of numerous earlier studies showing that IHCPs provide a large portion of rural populations' basic health care [29–33]. Our study results show that, among the rural population, it was not a matter of qualification of healthcare providers; when it comes to seeking healthcare, the factors which affects their selection were 'rapid cure', 'cost of treatment', 'distance', and '24 h availability', which may create pressure for IHCPs to provide a quick fix. Other comparable research also found that proximity and round-the-clock availability were the primary motivators for accessing IHCPs [33,34]. People in rural areas seek primary care that is not doctor-centric and is not given at a distant doctor's office [30].

Our study findings show that prescribing by the IHCPs was influenced by a combination of misperceptions about antibiotics as a medical requirement. This outcome is consistent with previous research indicating that IHCPs believe antibiotics are critical for patient retention and financial stability [34]. IHCPs during FGDs in our study stated that they chose antibiotic therapy based on affordability for patients and that they modify antibiotic courses based on the patient's ability to pay. Additionally, prescribe antibiotics out of fear of losing patients. Affordability, comfort, and trust [35] all also play determining roles in urban poor populations seeking care from IHCPs despite increased availability to skilled health care professionals in urban areas [36]. In order to improve the rural public healthcare system and to increase the uptake of formal healthcare providers, it is imperative that the governing bodies reform and modify the current three-tier system to better meet the demands of patients and their choices.

3.2. Influence of the Formal Healthcare Providers

Our research team also studied the prescriptions by IHCPs in the same setting in the different studies and reported that 75% of prescriptions by IHCPs contained antibiotics and were prescribed more frequently than any other medicine [8]. However, this study's findings suggest that antibiotic selection and dose patterns prescribed by the IHCPs were arbitrary, without following established treatment protocols or regulatory standards. Our study also reported that IHCPs learn from formal doctors by working at their clinics or medical shops or by following the prescriptions written by formal doctors. Therefore, IHCP practice is akin to a spillover impact from the formal system to these IHCPs, a diluted practice. Gautham et.al reported that IHCPs receive information from formal providers in return for the referral of patients to them [27]. Another study reported that the antibiotic prescribing by formal healthcare providers was 55% greater than that of IHCPs [37]; therefore, such guidance by formal providers may be a major factor in this antibiotic misprescription. In a study by our group, it was reported that IHCPs informally learn from formal providers and improve over time as they gain experience. Thus, offering educational opportunities for these IHCPs and integrating them into the official healthcare system might be some of the innovative strategies to serve the larger rural population [38].

Previous studies comparing IHCPs to formal health providers have shown that IHCPs' knowledge and methods differ, with lack of adequate training highlighted as a significant underlying issue [39]. However, other studies also reported that the quality of service provided is poor, there are knowledge gaps, and conflicting views exist on whether IHCPs should be integrated into the formal healthcare system [32,40,41]. Attracting and retaining formal providers in rural parts of low- and middle-income countries, particularly India, has proven difficult for health ministries, jeopardising rural healthcare, which forms the majority of the country's population [42]. While IHCPs fill this gap [43], the Medical Council of India still does not want IHCPs to be part of the formal healthcare system. However, the current government of India is dedicated to achieving UHC by focusing on improving the public health system and putting the needs of its citizens first. India's flagship 'skill development' programme provides short-term training or courses to improve the abilities of IHCPs [44]. The Indian government's ambitious Ayushman Bharat Scheme aims at upgrading rural sub-centres and primary health centres to health and wellness centres staffed by mid-level providers to give primary care, as one way of strengthening rural primary care [43]. However, India's huge rural population may be underserved by these figures even if they are completely operational. Therefore, in order to fully strengthen the rural public healthcare system and design effective antimicrobial stewardship, private practitioners, including IHCPs, might be included in the UHC initiative [27].

3.3. Methodological Considerations

The IHCPs were difficult to convince to participate and share details related to their practice, so the first strength of the study is that we were able to conduct these FGDs with this hard-to-reach group. Another strength of our study stems from the depth of our data. It made it possible for us to present our findings in accordance with the KAP model, where it was demonstrated that antibiotic prescribing behaviour is influenced by a plethora of internal and external drivers at all levels of the model. The FGDs provided extensive insights into IHCPs' prescribing behaviour. Though most of our respondents were male, and this represents the distribution of IHCPs in this setting, we aimed to include participants of both sexes and years of work experience. There is a possibility of information bias; respondents might be influenced to offer an answer that was either right or positive. This is a preliminary study, and our results' transferability is limited to areas with similar settings. It is vital to note that our study does not include informal pharmacists, which is critical for future studies. Further research is needed involving multiple stakeholders, such as patients and informal pharmacists, to have a deeper knowledge of individual aspects at all levels of the model. This would aid in a more thorough understanding of and response to the factors that drive antibiotic prescriptions, guiding an effective antibiotic stewardship programme.

4. Materials and Methods

4.1. Study Setting

The study was conducted in rural areas in the Ujjain District of Madhya Pradesh state, India. A vast, three-tiered rural public healthcare system exists in India, with the goal of ensuring primary care to all individuals regardless of socioeconomic status [45]. The sub-health centre (first tier) is the most remote and initial point of contact. According to population guidelines, one sub-centre is built for every 5000 people in rural areas and 3000 people in hilly/tribal/desert areas and is expected to be staffed by qualified health care professionals and auxiliary nurse midwives [46]. Primary Health Centres (second tier) serve as initial points of contact between village residents and a medical officer. According to population guidelines, one primary health centre is built for every 30,000 people in rural areas and 20,000 people in hilly/tribal/desert areas. They are to be staffed by a physician, paramedics, and other support personnel [47]. Community Health Centre (third tier) serves primarily as a referral centre for the nearby primary health centres. They are supposed to have medical experts (a surgeon, general practitioner, a gynaecologist, and a paediatrician), as well as paramedics and other support personnel, as well as 30 beds and amenities such as an operating theatre and a radiography room [48]. However, this system has not been able to provide effective care, a key reason for the failure of this healthcare system is the lack of trained physicians and nurses willing to work in rural regions, resulting in a shortage [49], as well as the absence of, appointed medical staff for a lengthy period of time [42,50]. Rural India accounts for approximately 71% of the overall population, but only 36% of all healthcare providers work in rural areas [51]. The doctor-population ratio in India is 1:1456, compared with the WHO recommendation of 1:1000, whereas the urban-to-rural doctor population ratio is wildly skewed [43,52]. IHCPs have emerged as a result of the public healthcare system's inability to deliver [45]. In 2019, 57.3% of individuals practicing allopathic medicine lack a medical degree, which, according to the WHO, is defined as IHCPs [43].

The Ujjain District is located in the Indian state of Madhya Pradesh. It has a population of 1.9 million people, with 61% residing in rural regions [53]. The district has a literacy rate of 72.3% [53] and the poverty rate of about 49%, which is higher than the national average of 21.2% [54]; the maternal mortality rate is 176 per 100,000 live births, and the infant mortality rate is 54 per 100,000 live births [55], both of which are higher than the national average. Both the public and private sectors contribute to Ujjain's healthcare system. In Ujjain, IHCPs account for 56% of all health care professionals, with the percentage being higher in rural areas [8,56].

4.2. Study Design and Participants

A qualitative approach was deemed appropriate to address our study aim. Following a literature search and gathering expert opinions, a discussion topic guide (Table S1) was developed. It was pilot tested by conducting one FGD with 8 IHCPs in March 2016 and revised accordingly. The discussion guide was first developed in English and then translated into Hindi for its use in the field. Snowball sampling was used for participants' selection [57] due to the IHCPs' reluctance to divulge their identities and details. Therefore, the first author (S.K.) contacted the eight IHCPs who had been connected with our medical college (Ruxmaniben Deepchand Gardi Medical College) with the purpose of obtaining information about treatment by attending various workshops and seminars held by the medical college, and they were willing to participate after describing the project aim. Then, the IHCPs in the first sample group were requested to help in contacting other IHCPs among their acquaintances, with the goal of obtaining a varied group of IHCPs in terms of age, gender, education, years of experience, and place of practice. This method of recruiting helped the researcher with the opportunity to communicate better with the participants who otherwise were reluctant to participate [58]. In total, 48 IHCPs took part in 7 FGDs. Age ranged from 19 to 61 years (mean $\pm$ standard deviation (SD) of 41 ($\pm$6) years); IHCPs experience ranged from 2 to 34 years (mean $\pm$ SD of 16 ($\pm$5) years) (Table 1).

4.3. Data Collection

The first author (S.K.), experienced in qualitative methods, conducted all the FGDs with the assistance of a research assistant skilled in moderating discussions, between December 2016 and February 2017. At the beginning of the FGD, IHCPs were given different case scenarios; for example, if a parent with a child U-5 years of age visits their clinic and complains about frequent watery stools since last night, how would they treat the child's illness? What treatment would they prescribe, and why would they that treatment? Then, the facilitator used a topic guide to help participants discuss their treatment experiences. The FGDs were conducted in Hindi in which the participants, as well as the data collectors, were conversant. In total, 5–8 people participated in each FGD. After the seventh FGD, we discovered that no new information had emerged, and the sampling was then closed. One

FGD was conducted with a group of female IHCPs; six were conducted with groups of male IHCPs. Audio recordings of the FGDs were performed with the participants' permission, and each discussion lasted for around 60–90 min. In addition, field notes and reflections were taken during the interviews. A light snack was provided to the attendees following the FGDs. Participants in the study were not given any additional incentives.

Table 1. Informal healthcare provider's demographic characteristics (n = 48).

Variables	Frequency, n
Age (years)	
19–28	1
29–38	7
39–48	37
49–58	2
59–68	1
Gender	
Male	43
Female	5
Education	
Secondary education (10thgrade)	14
Senior secondary education (11th–12th grade)	16
Higher education(BA/BSc/BCom) *	18
Experience as informal healthcare provider (years)	
1–10	6
11–20	36
21–30	5
31–40	1

* BA—Bachelor of Arts, BSc—Bachelor of Science, BCom—Bachelor of Commerce.

4.4. Data Analysis

Transcription was carried out in Hindi, and the content was translated into English by S.K. and research assistants. S.K. and S.A. (an experienced qualitative researcher) analysed FGD transcripts iteratively, using the thematic framework analysis with an inductive approach [59].Beginning with the first FGD, the process of analysis was initiated, allowing for the integration of results into later focus group work. To begin, transcripts were read independently multiple times and then were coded manually. Certain topics emerged from the literature research; others were identified inductively from the data through the open coding approach. This process was repeated, and finally, similar codes were grouped together and condensed into categories, then grouped into themes (Table 2). Analysis was discussed repeatedly between S.K. and S.A., and later with all co-authors until consensus was reached. Finally, findings were presented in the theoretical framework based on the KAP model [23], to depict how IHCP's practicing behaviour is influenced by processes and interactions at 3 levels: knowledge, attitude, and practice.

Table 2. Illustrative table of analysis undertaken.

Responses (Meaning Units)	Codes	Categories	Themes
"Like we are practicing and government try to stop us from practicing. Government officials come to village. So villagers meet head-on with them. They will not let us stop practicing as long as government doesn't appoint good doctors or open a government hospital in the village. Also, said that these people will work for us until and unless government makes other arrangements". (FGD 4, Male 4)	IHCPs have support from villagers which gives them the confidence to practice.	Perception of informal healthcare providers	IHCPs' accelerated therapeutic interactions with readily available antibiotics allowed them to surpass academic credentials.
"Patient came at night and obviously, he cannot go to town at that hour so we give him primary treatment like paracetamol for fever and antibiotics for the night and tell him to go to paediatrician in the morning". (FGD 3, Male 3)	IHCPs are available in the village and are available with medicines such as antibiotics, paracetamol, etc. during the wee hours.	IHCPs are approached for the treatment, as they are available for 24 h	
"They don't give us any fees; they don't give us money; they can give 200–400 rs to doctor in city but not to us that is why we do not give injections and prescribe accordingly, see I will say what is reality". (FGD 1, Male 1)	Patients ask for the treatment for which they can pay or for half of the treatment and so prescribe accordingly.	The financial condition of the caregiver affects the treatment prescribing behaviour of IHCPs	
"Antibiotic is a sure-shot drug. It can cure any disease. Any kind of disease, patient doesn't get well without antibiotic. Even if fever is there, antibiotic is compulsory, for cough and cold antibiotic is compulsory, for wounds antibiotic is compulsory, any infection of the body, immunity is enhanced by antibiotics, it is necessary for any disease". (FGD 4, Male 4)	Antibiotics boost the immune system of the body; viral will not get covered without antibiotics.	Knowledge of informal healthcare providers about antibiotic use	Beliefs regarding antibiotics as a quick fix and first choice in 'hit-and-try' prescriptions increase antibiotic use.
"I mean it boosts up the body; other drugs start working in the body. They are not effective if antibiotics aren't given. If antibiotics are not included in the treatment it takes a very long time to get better and many times there is no effect at all". (FGD 5, Male 4)	Improves the efficiency of other drugs when given along with them.	IHCPs consider antibiotics as the mandatory part of the treatment	

Table 2. *Cont.*

Responses (Meaning Units)	Codes	Categories	Themes
"Prescription of antibiotics, we do it from our experience like if patient has fever, in a normal way we give simple medicines many times, fever didn't subside then second time, small antibiotic is given, Amoxicillin, MOX syrup with the fever and so we got the result. Brother, we learnt with our experience that in fever if one antibiotic is given with antipyretic, then body will get relief faster. Yes, experience teaches everything; we keep a track that this was the condition and for this condition, this medicine was better". (FGD 6, Male 3)	Selection of antibiotics for an illness is based on 'hit-and-trial' method and learning with experience.	Antibiotics prescribing practice of IHCPs	
"I worked at medical retail counter for 11 years so I have the knowledge of medicines, and time to time, we get training from civil hospital, welfare society, Pushpa Mission Hospital, etc. Apart from this, whenever needed, we take advice from child specialists". (FGD 3, Male 4)	Gain knowledge about different treatments by assisting other formal practitioners and attending training sessions held by medical institutions.	Learning by observing and attending treatment training sessions	Mutually beneficial relationships between informal and formal healthcare providers led to available antibiotics.
"In village what happens, labour class are there, they don't have time, they come in a hurry that they have to go back for their work, for labour work, kid should be alright instantly; if he doesn't get relief in next 2 h, they will come to me, we both are from same village; if I am unable to give relief, they will go to him; if he is not able to provide relief, they will go to someone else. But kid should get relief in 1 h. Take treatment here for one day, if it gets alright then it is ok, otherwise we have to go to Ujjain or show to big doctor. In such situations, we are also not able to take decision that what type of medicine should be given". (FGD 2, Female 5)	Caregivers put pressure for quick relief.	Barriers in providing appropriate treatment	Patients thought that antibiotics were effective and often demanded them, leading to prescriptions.

5. Conclusions

We identified key drivers under the knowledge, attitude, and practice component of the model, where knowledge to practice was not always unidirectional, and the attitude of the IHCPs often affected their knowledge, as they showed interest in more training, to collect more knowledge, and improve practice. Similarly, the practice also helped to improve their knowledge, as they were untrained in medicine but with experience of working under formal healthcare providers and then with independent practice, they acquired more knowledge. By using a KAP model, we were able to discern the extent of the problem's complexity and the many implications it has for IHCPs' decisions and behaviour when it came to prescribing antibiotics. Therefore, these areas can be targeted to successfully improve IHCPs' prescribing behaviour with emphasis on antibiotics for common illnesses in U-5 children. IHCPs are a vital part of the rural healthcare system.

However, they were unable to deliver proper treatment and care due to a lack of training and knowledge. Their treatments were not always consistent with guidelines, and a number of barriers reported in the study prevented them from providing proper treatment. In addition, we found that IHCPs had a limited understanding of antibiotic resistance and the risks of irrational antibiotic use. When establishing a successful antibiotic stewardship strategy, it is critical that regulatory bodies recognise and acknowledge their role in the health system and then lawfully offer different interventions targeting the factors that affect their practices with a combination of regulatory, educational, and behaviour modification interventions. Under the Government of India's flagship 'skill development' programme, planned short-term training and courses to upgrade the skills of IHCPs can focus on improving diagnosis, enhancing IHCPs' and patients' understanding of antimicrobial resistance and rational use of antibiotics, and monitoring behavioural changes among these groups, as well as improving the referral of patients from rural areas. In addition, the services provided by IHCPs in rural areas can be supported with incentives. Finally, more study is needed to better understand the opinions and behaviour of the general public and informal pharmacists in order to develop effective intervention strategies that involve all important stakeholders.

Supplementary Materials: The following supporting information can be downloaded at: https://www.mdpi.com/article/10.3390/antibiotics11040459/s1, Table S1: Topic guide.

Author Contributions: Conceptualisation, S.K., V.D., A.P. and C.S.L.; methodology, S.K., S.A., V.D., A.P. and C.S.L.; validation, S.K.; formal analysis, S.K., S.A. and V.D.; resources, V.D. and C.S.L.; data curation, S.K.; writing—original draft preparation, S.K.; writing—review and editing, A.P., C.S.L., V.D. and S.A.; visualisation, S.K. and S.A.; supervision, S.A. and V.D.; project administration, V.D.; funding acquisition, C.S.L. All authors have read and agreed to the published version of the manuscript.

Funding: The project was funded by the Swedish Research Council (grant no 521-2012-2889 and 2017-01327).

Institutional Review Board Statement: The Institutional Ethics Committee (IEC) of RDGMC, Ujjain, approved the study (approval number DNR-311/2013).

Informed Consent Statement: The IHCPs were not obligated to participate, and they were free to quit the group at any moment without providing an explanation. Written consent was taken from participants before the discussion started, and the participants were informed about the study's aim and methodology. It was made clear that their conversation would be recorded, and the data would only be utilised for the study project.

Data Availability Statement: The data presented in this study are available on request from the authors.

Acknowledgments: We acknowledge Kailash Sharma for assistance during fieldwork, Priyank Soni for assisting during focus group discussions, and Vivek Bajpai for assistance in transcription and translation. We also thank all study participants for their participation. We also would like to thank Krushna Chandra Sahoo for his valuable comments and suggestions on the manuscript.

Conflicts of Interest: The authors declare no conflict of interest. The funders had no role in the design of the study; in the collection, analyses, or interpretation of data; in the writing of the manuscript; in the decision to publish the results.

Abbreviations

WHO	World Health Organisation
IHCPs	Informal Healthcare Providers
UHC	Universal Health Coverage
U-5	Under-Five
KAP	Knowledge, Attitude and Practices
FGD	Focus Group Discussions

References

1. World Health Organization. *Global Action Plan on Antimicrobial Resistance*; World Health Organization: Geneva, Switzerland, 2015.
2. Klein, E.Y.; Van Boeckel, T.P.; Martinez, E.M.; Pant, S.; Gandra, S.; Levin, S.A.; Goossens, H.; Laxminarayan, R. Global increase and geographic convergence in antibiotic consumption between 2000 and 2015. *Proc. Natl. Acad. Sci. USA* **2018**, *115*, E3463. [PubMed]
3. World Health Organization. Antimicrobial Resistance: Global Report on Surveillance. 2014. Available online: https://apps.who.int/iris/handle/10665/112642 (accessed on 4 December 2021).
4. Reiner, R.C., Jr.; Olsen, H.E.; Ikeda, C.T.; Echko, M.M.; Ballestreros, K.E.; Manguerra, H.; Martopullo, I.; Millear, A.; Shields, C.; Smith, A.; et al. Diseases, Injuries, and Risk Factors in Child and Adolescent Health, 1990 to 2017: Findings From the Global Burden of Diseases, Injuries, and Risk Factors 2017 Study. *JAMA Pediatr.* **2019**, *173*, e190337. [PubMed]
5. National Center for Disease Control; Directorate General of Health Services; Ministry of Health & Family Welfare, Government of India. National Treatment Guidelines for Antimicrobial Use in Infectious Diseases. 2016. Available online: http://pbhealth.gov.in/AMR_guideline7001495889.pdf (accessed on 9 February 2022).
6. Pathak, A.; Upadhayay, R.; Mathur, A.; Rathi, S.; Lundborg, C.S. Incidence, clinical profile, and risk factors for serious bacterial infections in children hospitalized with fever in Ujjain, India. *BMC Infect. Dis.* **2020**, *20*, 162. [CrossRef] [PubMed]
7. Pathak, D.; Pathak, A.; Marrone, G.; Diwan, V.; Lundborg, C.S. Adherence to treatment guidelines for acute diarrhoea in children up to 12 years in Ujjain, India–a cross-sectional prescription analysis. *BMC Infect. Dis.* **2011**, *11*, 32. [CrossRef] [PubMed]
8. Khare, S.; Purohit, M.; Sharma, M.; Tamhankar, A.J.; Lundborg, C.S.; Diwan, V.; Pathak, A. Antibiotic Prescribing by Informal Healthcare Providers for Common Illnesses: A Repeated Cross-Sectional Study in Rural India. *Antibiotics* **2019**, *8*, 139. [CrossRef] [PubMed]
9. Pathak, A.; Mahadik, K.; Dhaneria, S.P.; Sharma, A.; Eriksson, B.; Lundborg, C.S. Antibiotic prescribing in outpatients: Hospital and seasonal variations in Ujjain, India. *Scand. J. Infect. Dis.* **2011**, *43*, 479–488. [CrossRef]
10. Sharma, M.; Damlin, A.; Pathak, A.; Lundborg, C.S. Antibiotic Prescribing among Pediatric Inpatients with Potential Infections in Two Private Sector Hospitals in Central India. *PLoS ONE* **2015**, *10*, e0142317. [CrossRef] [PubMed]
11. Costelloe, C.; Metcalfe, C.; Lovering, A.; Mant, D.; Hay, A. Effect of antibiotic prescribing in primary care on antimicrobial resistance in individual patients: Systematic review and meta-analysis. *BMJ* **2010**, *340*, c2096. [CrossRef] [PubMed]
12. Vos, T.; Abajobir, A.A.; Abate, K.H.; Abbafati, C.; Abbas, K.M.; Abd-Allah, F.; Abdulkader, R.S. Global, regional, and national incidence, prevalence, and years lived with disability for 328 diseases and injuries for 195 countries, 1990–2016: A systematic analysis for the Global Burden of Disease Study 2016. *Lancet* **2017**, *390*, 1211–1259. [CrossRef]
13. Holmes, A.H.; Moore, L.S.; Sundsfjord, A.; Steinbakk, M.; Regmi, S.; Karkey, A.; Guerin, P.J.; Piddock, L.J. Understanding the mechanisms and drivers of antimicrobial resistance. *Lancet* **2016**, *387*, 176–187. [CrossRef]
14. Klein, E.Y.; Tseng, K.K.; Pant, S.; Laxminarayan, R. Tracking global trends in the effectiveness of antibiotic therapy using the Drug Resistance Index. *BMJ Glob. Health* **2019**, *4*, e001315. [CrossRef] [PubMed]
15. O'Neil, J. *Tackling Drug-Resistance Infections Globally: Final Report and Recommendations*; The Review on Antimicrobial Resistance; Wellcome Trust: London, UK, 2016. Available online: https://amr-review.org/sites/default/files/160518_Final%20paper_with%20cover.pdf (accessed on 16 March 2022).
16. The World Bank. *Drug-Resistant Infections: A Threat to Our Economic Future*; Final Report (English); The World Bank: Washington, DC, USA, 2017; Volume 2. Available online: https://documents.worldbank.org/en/publication/documents-reports/documentdetail/323311493396993758/final-report (accessed on 16 March 2022).
17. Ministry of Health & Family Welfare, Government of India. *National Action Plan on Antimicrobial Resistance (NAP-AMR) 2017–2021*; Ministry of Health & Family Welfare: New Delhi, India, 2017. Available online: https://ncdc.gov.in/WriteReadData/l892s/File645.pdf (accessed on 4 December 2021).
18. Ministry of Health & Family Welfare, Government of India. The Drugs and Cosmetics Act and Rules. 2016. Available online: https://cdsco.gov.in/opencms/export/sites/CDSCO_WEB/Pdf-documents/acts_rules/2016DrugsandCosmeticsAct1940Rules1945.pdf (accessed on 4 December 2021).
19. Chandra, S.; Bhattacharya, S. Unqualified Medical Practitioners: Their Illegal but Indispensable Role in Primary Healthcare. *Econ. Political Wkly.* **2019**, *54*, 36–44.
20. The Indian Medical Council Act. 1956. Available online: https://legislative.gov.in/sites/default/files/A1956-102_0.pdf (accessed on 30 November 2021).
21. National Medical Commission of India. *The National Medical Commission Act, 2019 NO. 30 OF 2019*; National Medical Commission of India: New Delhi, India, 2019; Available online: https://www.nmc.org.in/nmc-act/ (accessed on 30 November 2021).
22. Khare, S.; Pathak, A.; Purohit, M.R.; Sharma, M.; Marrone, G.; Tamhankar, A.J.; Lundborg, C.S.; Diwan, V. Determinants and pathways of healthcare-seeking behaviours in under-5 children for common childhood illnesses and antibiotic prescribing: A cohort study in rural India. *BMJ Open* **2021**, *11*, e052435. [CrossRef] [PubMed]
23. Rodrigues, A.T.; Roque, F.; Falcão, A.; Figueiras, A.; Herdeiro, M.T. Understanding physician antibiotic prescribing behaviour: A systematic review of qualitative studies. *Int. J. Antimicrob. Agents* **2013**, *41*, 203–212. [CrossRef]
24. Sychareun, V.; Sihavong, A.; Machowska, A.; Onthongdee, X.; Chaleunvong, K.; Keohavong, B.; Eriksen, J.; Hanson, C.; Vongsouvath, M.; Marrone, G.; et al. Knowledge, Attitudes, Perception and Reported Practices of Healthcare Providers on Antibiotic Use and Resistance in Pregnancy, Childbirth and Children under Two in Lao PDR: A Mixed Methods Study. *Antibiotics* **2021**, *10*, 1462. [CrossRef] [PubMed]

25. Liu, C.; Liu, C.; Wang, D.; Zhang, X. Intrinsic and external determinants of antibiotic prescribing: A multi-level path analysis of primary care prescriptions in Hubei, China. *Antimicrob. Resist. Infect. Control* **2019**, *8*, 132. [CrossRef] [PubMed]
26. Kotwani, A.; Wattal, C.; Katewa, S.; Joshi, P.C.; Holloway, K. Factors influencing primary care physicians to prescribe antibiotics in Delhi India. *Fam. Pract.* **2010**, *27*, 684–690. [CrossRef] [PubMed]
27. Gautham, M.; Spicer, N.; Chatterjee, S.; Goodman, C. What are the challenges for antibiotic stewardship at the community level? An analysis of the drivers of antibiotic provision by informal healthcare providers in rural India. *Soc. Sci. Med.* **2021**, *275*, 113813. [CrossRef] [PubMed]
28. May, C.; Roth, K.; Panda, P. Non-degree allopathic practitioners as first contact points for acute illness episodes: Insights from a qualitative study in rural northern India. *BMC Health Serv. Res.* **2014**, *14*, 182. [CrossRef] [PubMed]
29. Rohde, J.; Viswanathan, H. The rural private practitioner. *Health Millions* **1994**, *2*, 13–16.
30. Gautham, M.; Binnendijk, E.; Koren, R.; Dror, D.M. 'First we go to the small doctor': First contact for curative health care sought by rural communities in Andhra Pradesh & Orissa, India. *Indian J. Med. Res.* **2011**, *134*, 627–638. [PubMed]
31. George, A.; Iyer, A. Unfree markets: Socially embedded informal health providers in northern Karnataka, India. *Soc. Sci. Med.* **2013**, *96*, 297–304. [CrossRef]
32. Das, J.; Holla, A.; Das, V.; Mohanan, M.; Tabak, D.; Chan, B. In urban and rural India, a standardized patient study showed low levels of provider training and huge quality gaps. *Health Aff.* **2012**, *31*, 2774–2784. [CrossRef]
33. Anand, G.; Chhajed, D.; Shah, S.; Atkins, S.; Diwan, V. Do qualifications matter? A qualitative study of how villagers decide their health care providers in a developing economy. *PLoS ONE* **2019**, *14*, e0220316. [CrossRef]
34. Nair, M.; Tripathi, S.; Mazumdar, S.; Mahajan, R.; Harshana, A.; Pereira, A.; Jimenez, C.; Halder, D.; Burza, S. "Without antibiotics, I cannot treat": A qualitative study of antibiotic use in Paschim Bardhaman district of West Bengal, India. *PLoS ONE* **2019**, *14*, e0219002. [CrossRef]
35. Ergler, C.R.; Sakdapolrak, P.; Bohle, H.G.; Kearns, R.A. Entitlements to health care: Why is there a preference for private facilities among poorer residents of Chennai, India? *Soc. Sci. Med.* **2011**, *72*, 327–337. [CrossRef] [PubMed]
36. Priya, R.; Singh, R.; Das, S. Health Implications of Diverse Visions of Urban Spaces: Bridging the Formal-Informal Divide. *Front Public Health* **2019**, *7*, 239. [CrossRef]
37. Sulis, G.; Daniels, B.; Kwan, A.; Gandra, S.; Daftary, A.; Das, J.; Pai, M. Antibiotic overuse in the primary health care setting: A secondary data analysis of standardised patient studies from India, China and Kenya. *BMJ Glob. Health* **2020**, *5*, e003393. [CrossRef]
38. Mungai, I.G.; Baghel, S.S.; Soni, S.; Vagela, S.; Sharma, M.; Diwan, V.; Tamhankar, A.J.; Lundborg, C.S.; Pathak, A. Identifying the know-do gap in evidence-based neonatal care practices among informal health care providers—A cross-sectional study from Ujjain, India. *BMC Health Serv. Res.* **2020**, *20*, 966. [CrossRef]
39. Gautham, M.; Shyamprasad, K.M.; Singh, R.; Zachariah, A.; Singh, R.; Bloom, G. Informal rural healthcare providers in North and South India. *Health Policy Plan.* **2014**, *29*, i20–i29. [CrossRef] [PubMed]
40. Pulla, P. Are India's quacks the answer to its shortage of doctors? *BMJ* **2016**, *352*, i291. [CrossRef] [PubMed]
41. Das, J.; Chowdhury, A.; Hussam, R.; Banerjee, A.V. The impact of training informal health care providers in India: A randomized controlled trial. *Science* **2016**, *354*, aaf7384. [CrossRef]
42. De Costa, A.; Al-Muniri, A.; Diwan, V.K.; Eriksson, B. Where are healthcare providers? Exploring relationships between context and human resources for health Madhya Pradesh province, India. *Health Policy* **2009**, *93*, 41–47. [CrossRef] [PubMed]
43. Ministry of Health and Family Welfare. Press Information Bureau Government of India. FAQs on National Medical Commission (NMC) Bill; 2019. Available online: https://pib.gov.in/PressReleseDetailm.aspx?PRID=1581325 (accessed on 29 November 2021).
44. Ministry of Skill Development and Entrepreneurship. National Skill Development Mission—Pradhan Mantri Kaushal Vikas Yojana 3.0 (PMKVY) 2020–2021. Available online: https://www.msde.gov.in/en/schemes-initiatives/short-term-training/pmkvy-3.0 (accessed on 4 December 2021).
45. Chokshi, M.; Patil, B.; Khanna, R.; Neogi, S.B.; Sharma, J.; Paul, V.K.; Zodpey, S. Health systems in India. *J. Perinatol. Off. J. Calif. Perinat. Assoc.* **2016**, *36*, S9–S12. [CrossRef] [PubMed]
46. Directorate General of Health Services Ministry of Health & Family Welfare Government of India. Indian Public Health Standards (Iphs) for Sub-Centres Guidelines. March 2006. Available online: http://www.iapsmgc.org/userfiles/3IPHS_for_SUB-CENTRES.pdf (accessed on 28 November 2021).
47. Ministry of Health and Family Welfare. Primary Health Centres (PHCs). 2020. Available online: https://pib.gov.in/PressReleasePage.aspx?PRID=1656190 (accessed on 28 December 2021).
48. Directorate General of Health Services Ministry of Health & Family Welfare Government of India. Indian Public Health Standards (IPHS) Guidelines for Community Health Centres. 2012. Available online: https://nhm.gov.in/images/pdf/guidelines/iphs/iphs-revised-guidlines-2012/community-health-centres.pdf (accessed on 28 November 2021).
49. Goel, S.; Angeli, F.; Dhirar, N.; Sangwan, G.; Thakur, K.; Ruwaard, D. Factors affecting medical students' interests in working in rural areas in North India—A qualitative inquiry. *PLoS ONE* **2019**, *14*, e0210251. [CrossRef]
50. De Costa, A.; Diwan, V. 'Where is the public health sector?' Public and private sector healthcare provision in Madhya Pradesh, India. *Health Policy* **2007**, *84*, 269–276. [CrossRef] [PubMed]
51. Karan, A.; Negandhi, H.; Hussain, S.; Zapata, T.; Mairembam, D.; De Graeve, H.; Buchan, J.; Zodpey, S. Size, composition and distribution of health workforce in India: Why, and where to invest? *Hum. Resour. Health* **2021**, *19*, 39. [CrossRef]
52. Sharma, D.C. India still struggles with rural doctor shortages. *Lancet* **2015**, *386*, 2381–2382. [CrossRef]

53. Census India. Ujjain District—Census 2011. Available online: https://www.censusindia.co.in/district/ujjain-district-madhya-pradesh-435 (accessed on 1 December 2021).
54. National Bank for Agriculture and Rural Development. Potential Linked Plan. 2016–2017. 2016. Available online: https://www.nabard.org/demo/auth/writereaddata/tender/2210162338UJJAIN%20-2016-17.split-and-merged.pdf (accessed on 21 February 2022).
55. Government of India, New Delhi. Annual Health Survey Bulletin 2012–2013: Madhya Pradesh. 2013. Ministry of Home Affairs. Available online: http://www.censusindia.gov.in/vital_statistics/AHSBulletins/AHS_Factsheets_2012-13/FACTSHEET-MP.pdf (accessed on 21 February 2022).
56. UNDP. Work for Human Development. 2015. Available online: http://hdr.undp.org/sites/default/files/2015_human_development_report.pdf (accessed on 21 February 2022).
57. Naderifar, M.; Goli, H.; Ghaljaie, F. Snowball Sampling: A Purposeful Method of Sampling in Qualitative Research. *Strides Dev. Med. Educ.* **2017**, *14*, e67670. [CrossRef]
58. Polit, D.F.; Beck, C.T. *Essentials of Nursing Research: Methods, Appraisal, and Utilization*, 6th ed.; Lippincott Williams & Wilkins: Philadelphia, PA, USA, 2006.
59. Gale, N.K.; Heath, G.; Cameron, E.; Rashid, S.; Redwood, S. Using the framework method for the analysis of qualitative data in multi-disciplinary health research. *BMC Med. Res. Methodol.* **2013**, *13*, 117. [CrossRef]

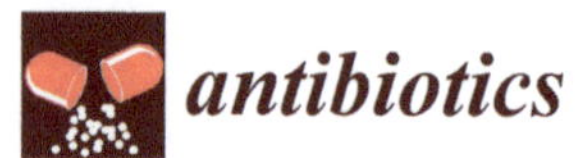

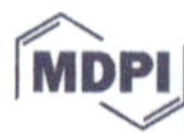

Article

Antimicrobial Prescribing in the Emergency Department; Who Is Calling the Shots?

Laura M. Hamill [1,†], Julia Bonnett [2], Megan F. Baxter [2], Melina Kreutz [2], Kerina J. Denny [3] and Gerben Keijzers [2,4,5,*]

1 Department of Emergency Medicine, Christchurch Hospital, Canterbury DHB, Christchurch 8011, New Zealand; Laura.hamill@cdhb.health.nz
2 School of Medicine, Griffith University, Gold Coast, QLD 4215, Australia; Julia.Bonnett@griffithuni.edu.au (J.B.); megan.baxter@griffithuni.edu.au (M.F.B.); melina.kreutz@griffithuni.edu.au (M.K.)
3 Department of Intensive Care, Gold Coast University Hospital, Gold Coast, QLD 4215, Australia; kerina.denny@health.qld.gov.au
4 Department of Emergency Medicine, Gold Coast University Hospital, Gold Coast, QLD 4215, Australia
5 Faculty of Health Sciences and Medicine, Bond University, Gold Coast, QLD 4215, Australia
* Correspondence: Gerben.Keijzers@health.qld.gov.au
† Previously of Department of Emergency Medicine, Gold Coast University Hospital, Gold Coast, QLD, Australia.

Abstract: Objective: Inappropriate antimicrobial prescribing in the emergency department (ED) can lead to poor outcomes. It is unknown how often the prescribing clinician is guided by others, and whether prescriber factors affect appropriateness of prescribing. This study aims to describe decision making, confidence in, and appropriateness of antimicrobial prescribing in the ED. **Methods:** Descriptive study in two Australian EDs using both questionnaire and medical record review. Participants were clinicians who prescribed antimicrobials to patients in the ED. Outcomes of interest were level of decision-making (self or directed), confidence in indication for prescribing and appropriateness (5-point Likert scale, 5 most confident). Appropriateness assessment of the prescribing event was by blinded review using the National Antibiotic Prescribing Survey appropriateness assessment tool. All analyses were descriptive. **Results:** Data on 88 prescribers were included, with 61% making prescribing decisions themselves. The 39% directed by other clinicians were primarily guided by more senior ED and surgical subspecialty clinicians. Confidence that antibiotics were indicated (Likert score: 4.20, 4.35 and 4.35) and appropriate (Likert score: 4.07, 4.23 and 4.29) was similar for juniors, mid-level and senior prescribers, respectively. Eighty-five percent of prescriptions were assessed as appropriate, with no differences in appropriateness by seniority, decision-making or confidence. **Conclusions:** Over one-third of prescribing was guided by senior ED clinicians or based on specialty advice, primarily surgical specialties. Prescriber confidence was high regardless of seniority or decision-maker. Overall appropriateness of prescribing was good, but with room for improvement. Future qualitative research may provide further insight into the intricacies of prescribing decision-making.

Keywords: antibiotics; antimicrobial stewardship; appropriateness; emergency department; prescribing

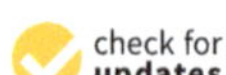

Citation: Hamill, L.M.; Bonnett, J.; Baxter, M.F.; Kreutz, M.; Denny, K.J.; Keijzers, G. Antimicrobial Prescribing in the Emergency Department; Who Is Calling the Shots? *Antibiotics* **2021**, *10*, 843. https://doi.org/10.3390/antibiotics10070843

Academic Editor: Diane Ashiru-Oredope

Received: 15 June 2021
Accepted: 8 July 2021
Published: 10 July 2021

Publisher's Note: MDPI stays neutral with regard to jurisdictional claims in published maps and institutional affiliations.

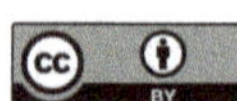

Copyright: © 2021 by the authors. Licensee MDPI, Basel, Switzerland. This article is an open access article distributed under the terms and conditions of the Creative Commons Attribution (CC BY) license (https://creativecommons.org/licenses/by/4.0/).

1. Introduction

Antimicrobial resistance (AMR) has been declared a global health crisis and if not tackled could cause up to 10 million deaths worldwide per year by 2050 [1]. While appropriate and timely antibiotic therapy saves lives [2–4] the misuse and overuse of antimicrobials accelerates the development of AMR and threatens our ability to treat infectious diseases, resulting in prolonged illness, disability, death, and increasing health care costs [5]. Overuse has harms on an individual level; from minor allergic reactions to potentially fatal infections, as well as serious medication interactions.

Errors in medication related problems are common, affecting 4–7% of medication orders [6,7]. Antimicrobial prescriptions in particular have shown greater incidence of prescription errors than other prescribing events, especially when prescribed by junior doctors. It has been estimated by the Institute of Medicine that medication errors cause 1 of 131 outpatient and 1 of 854 inpatient deaths [8]. Thus all clinicians should espouse caution and critical thinking when prescribing antimicrobials.

The Emergency Department (ED) is a uniquely challenging environment for prescribers, with high-volume care, frequent interruptions, and competing priorities. ED clinicians frequently face diagnostic uncertainty and the threat of patient deterioration whilst awaiting results of investigations [9,10]. The challenge facing ED doctors is not only one of whether to prescribe antibiotics, but also of which type, route, frequency and dose, sometimes in the absence of a clear infective source or diagnosis. Ideally, clinicians are compliant with guidelines such as the surviving sepsis campaign [11] however, most patients with infection admitted from EDs do not have sepsis, yet are frequently commenced on broad-spectrum, parenteral antibiotics [12,13].

Most patients in hospital are admitted via the ED, consequently antimicrobial prescribing in EDs impacts the patterns of antimicrobial use across the hospital [14,15]. Additionally, prescriptions started in the ED are often continued in the community setting [14], impacting outpatient antimicrobial use. However, antimicrobial stewardship initiatives rarely focus on the ED [14]. A descriptive ED-based study in 2017 showed that in 33% of all patients receiving an antimicrobial prescription, the prescription was considered inappropriate [16]. This data needs further exploration as the antimicrobial prescribing clinicians may not be the primary decision makers and may have been directed by supervising clinicians, peers or inpatient specialty teams. To get further insight in how to remediate inappropriate prescribing in ED, we need to understand who is making the prescribing decisions in ED.

This study aims to describe factors associated with overall and appropriate antibiotic prescribing in the ED, including seniority, specialty of decision-makers and level of confidence of the prescriber, in both independent and guided prescribing decisions. The overarching goal of this work will be to inform future targeted steps towards improving antimicrobial stewardship (AMS) in the ED as well as to develop novel solutions.

2. Methods

2.1. Design, Setting and Participants

This was a descriptive study using both medical record review and questionnaires. The study was conducted in two EDs within the same health service in Queensland, Australia. The first ED serves a large tertiary level 750-bed hospital, and the second ED serves a 403-bed urban district hospital. In 2019 the two sites had a combined ED attendance of around 174,000 patients (112,000 and 62,000). Both hospitals are affiliated with local university and have medical and nursing students on placement. The combined staffing of the ED included doctors with a range of experience (63 consultants, 56 registrars, 81 residents and 19 interns), as well as nurse practitioners (8). Nurse practitioners have completed additional study at Master's degree level and are senior and independent clinician with ability to prescribe antibiotics. Participants were a convenience sample of clinicians who prescribed antimicrobials to patients in the ED during data collection periods over two months in the winter of 2019. Within this health service all levels of medical practitioners can prescribe independently for all types of patients. Several guidelines, including the statewide sepsis pathway are available, which can prompt for senior medical officer input, but no formal policies or antimicrobial restrictions are enforced.

2.2. Questionnaire Design and Data Collection

The questionnaire questions were determined *a-priori* and pilot tested for face validity by three clinicians not part of the research team. After review by a qualitative research expert, questions were further refined. (Questionnaire; Appendix A).

Two research assistants collected data during six 12-h time periods (Table 1). A variety of shifts were selected including weekdays, weekends, days and nights, in order to minimize potential sample bias.

Table 1. Data Collection Periods.

Site 1	Site 2
23/08/19 20:00–08:00 (Friday–Saturday)	17/09/19 08:00–20:00 (Tuesday)
26/08/19 08:00–20:00 (Monday)	28/09/19 08:00–20:00 (Saturday)
12/09/19 08:00–20:00 (Thursday)	29/09/19 20:00–08:00 (Sunday–Monday)

All patients who presented to the ED for the six pre-determined 12-h periods were identified. The two research assistants used the integrated electronic medical record (ieMR) to manually review the medication record of every patient. If the patient had been prescribed oral or parenteral antibiotics during their ED attendance, their prescribing doctor was eligible for participation and contacted to complete the questionnaire. Prescribing events were not eligible if the prescription was for topical medication, antivirals/antifungals, or the patient did not receive the prescribed medication whilst in the ED. The medical record was reviewed to determine prescribing doctor and indication for antibiotics as well some detail on clinical variables. All eligible clinicians were invited to complete the questionnaire within the same shift (in person) or at the latest 48 h after prescribing (in person or via telephone) as to minimize recall bias. Eligible clinicians were given the explicit option to decline participation.

When a clinician did not make their own decision, this was identified as a 'guided' or 'directed' decision. This direction, guidance or advice could relate to any, some or all components (type of drug, dose, route, duration) of the prescription. We defined clinicians as *senior* (consultants and registrars), *mid-level* (senior house officers and principal house officers) and *junior* (junior house officers and interns). Some prescribing decisions were made jointly (e.g., Senior ED clinician in consultation with mid-level inpatient team). For the purposes of analysis and simplicity, the most senior person noted was considered the primary decision maker. Confidence in prescribing was measured using a 5-point Likert scale with 5 representing high confidence.

2.3. *Assessment of Appropriateness*

Antibiotic appropriateness was independently assessed by two researchers who used the National Antibiotic Prescribing Survey (NAPS) tool [16,17] (Table A1), which has been used with a high rate of inter-rater reliability and validity [17]. As no gold standard for appropriateness exists, assessments were based on interpretation of clinical record review. Prescribing which deviated from guidelines could still be classed as appropriate if clear reasons were given (such as first line medication being out of stock). The validity of this approach has been further demonstrated by the consistency of findings from nationwide hospital point-prevalence studies [18]. Each assessor allocated the antibiotic prescription as being Optimal (1), Adequate (2), Suboptimal (3), Inadequate (4), or Not Assessable (5) as per NAPS guidelines [17]. If there was no agreement, a senior researcher arbitrated the appropriateness. Ratings of 1 or 2 were given a final classification of appropriate and ratings of 3 or 4 were classified as inappropriate.

2.4. *Data Analysis*

As this is a descriptive study, no formal power calculation was performed. All data is descriptive in nature. We described the prescribers as follows; firstly, by dividing them by independent decision-makers and directed decision makers, secondly by seniority.

Ethical approval was granted by the institutional Human Research Ethics Committee (HREC/17/QGC/41). Findings are reported in accordance with the Strengthening the Reporting of Observational studies in Epidemiology (STROBE) Statement for cohort studies [19].

3. Results

The questionnaire was distributed to 128 clinicians and returned by 94 (73% response rate) of those 88 met eligibility criteria (Figure 1).

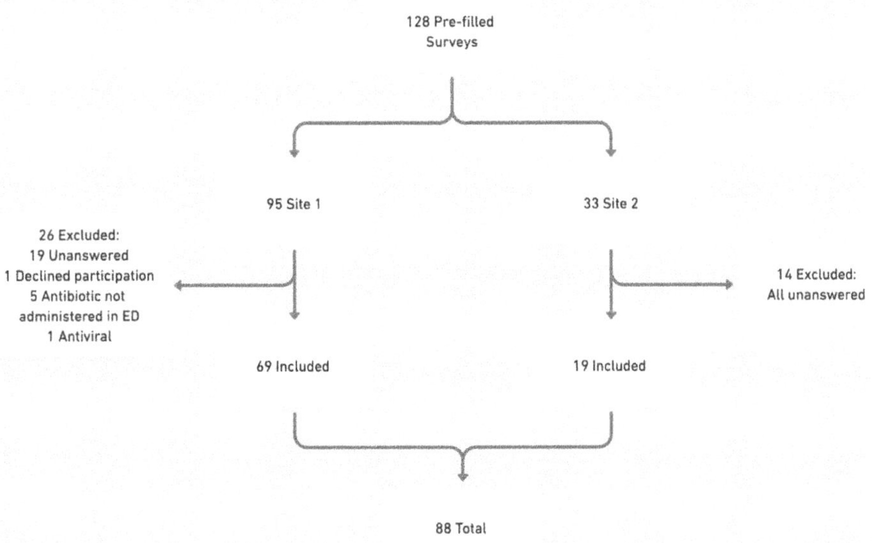

Figure 1. Flow chart of included participants.

There were few missing data (less than 3% for any variable.) Seniority of the participants are summarised in Table 2, with over three-quarters of participants classed as mid-level or senior, with the most experienced respondent practicing for 25 years. Twenty-two respondents were emergency medicine trainees. The conditions for which antibiotics were prescribed are outlined in Table A2. The three most common indications were respiratory tract infections (30%), skin and soft tissue infections (20%) and urinary tract infections (17%).

Table 2. Characteristics of Respondents.

Seniority Classification	*n* (%)	Job Role	*n* (%)	Specialty—*n* (%)
Senior	31 (35.2)	Consultant	3 (3.4)	Emergency—28 (90.3)
				Respiratory—2 (6.5)
		Registrar	28 (31.8)	Urology—1 (3.2)
Mid-level	38 (43.2)	Senior House Officer	31 (35.2)	Emergency—35 (92.1)
		Principal House Officer	7 (8.0)	Obstetrics & Gynaecology—3 (7.9)
Junior	14 (15.9)	Junior House Officer	4 (4.5)	Emergency—13 (92.9)
		Intern	10 (11.4)	Orthopaedics—1 (7.1)
Other	5 (5.7)	Nurse Practitioner	4 (4.5)	
		Unknown	1 (1.1)	

3.1. Seniority and Specialty of Prescribing Decision-Making

Almost two-thirds (61%, 54/88) of participants made the prescribing decision themselves. Of the 39% (n = 34) of clinicians who did not make their own prescribing decision, 88% (n = 30/34) reported that a senior (consultant or registrar) clinician had guided them. There were 2 interactions whereby mid-level staff advising junior or mid-level staff in their prescribing and one instance of a nurse practitioner guiding mid-level staff. No junior specialty doctor(s) advised a senior on prescribing.

In cases where the participant was not the decision maker, over half (62%) were directed by a non-ED clinician. The specialty teams involved are shown in Figure 2. Inpatient specialties were often involved when the patient had previously been under their care as an inpatient, with known microbiological sensitivities available.

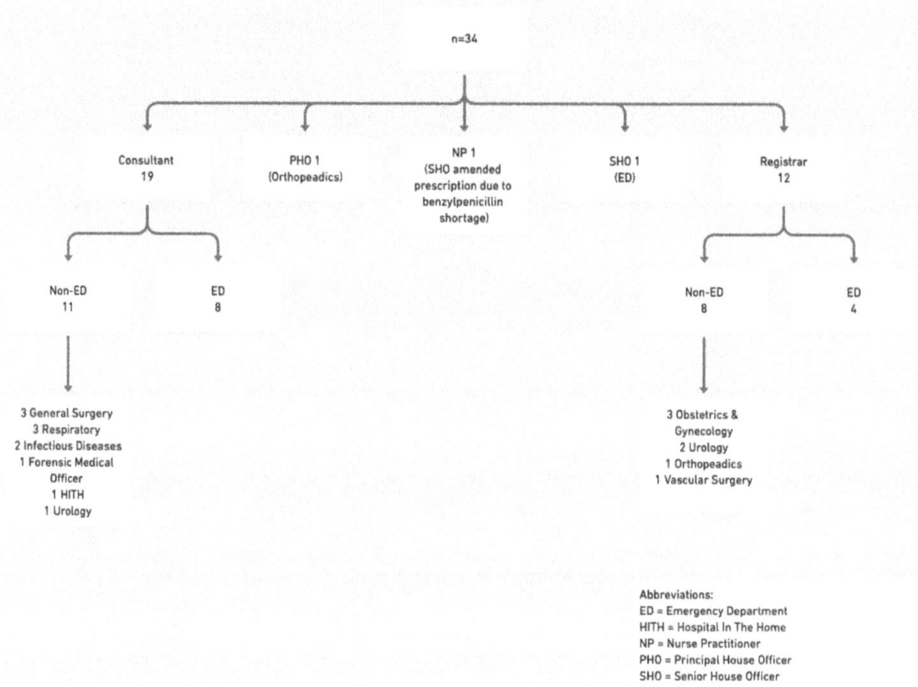

Figure 2. Antibiotic prescribing guided by other staff than prescriber (n = 34).

There were three cases where the infectious disease (ID) team was involved (3.4%). A surgical subspecialty registrar consulted ID for one patient and for the other two patients an existing ID antimicrobial plan was documented in the medical record. This plan was followed by the treating clinicians.

3.2. Resource Use

Three-quarters (74%, 40/54) of respondents who made their own decision indicated they used the national resource "Electronic Therapeutic Guidelines"™ to aid their decision making [20]. Of those who indicated they made their own decision and used eTG (35/40) 87.5% were appropriate and followed guideline recommendations. Eleven (12.5%) of respondents used other guidelines. Five (5.7%) of respondents quoted "ED experience" as the resource that they used. A quarter (23.9%) of respondents used multiple resources (n = 21) and 6.8% (n = 6) used an ED senior as a resource for direct advice.

3.3. Prescribing Confidence by Decision-Maker and Seniority

Confidence in prescribing was high across all groups. If the prescribing clinician was not the decision maker, they were less frequently 'very confident' that antibiotics were indicated or appropriate (Figure 3a,b). Confidence was similar across all groups regardless of seniority. Mean confidence on a Likert scale from 1–5 that antibiotics were indicated (4.20, 4.35 and 4.35, respectively) and appropriate (4.07, 4.23 and 4.29, respectively) was similar for juniors, mid-level and senior prescribers.

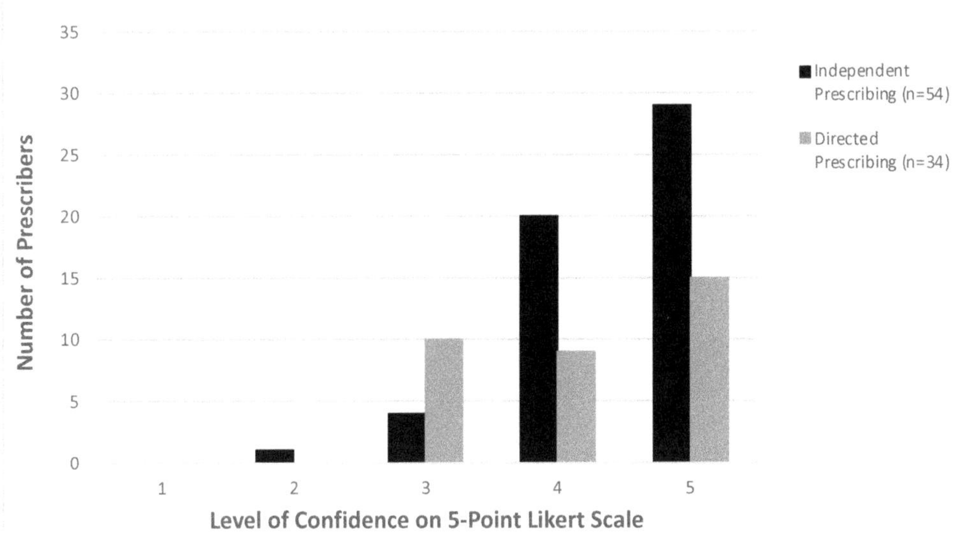

(a)

Figure 3. *Cont.*

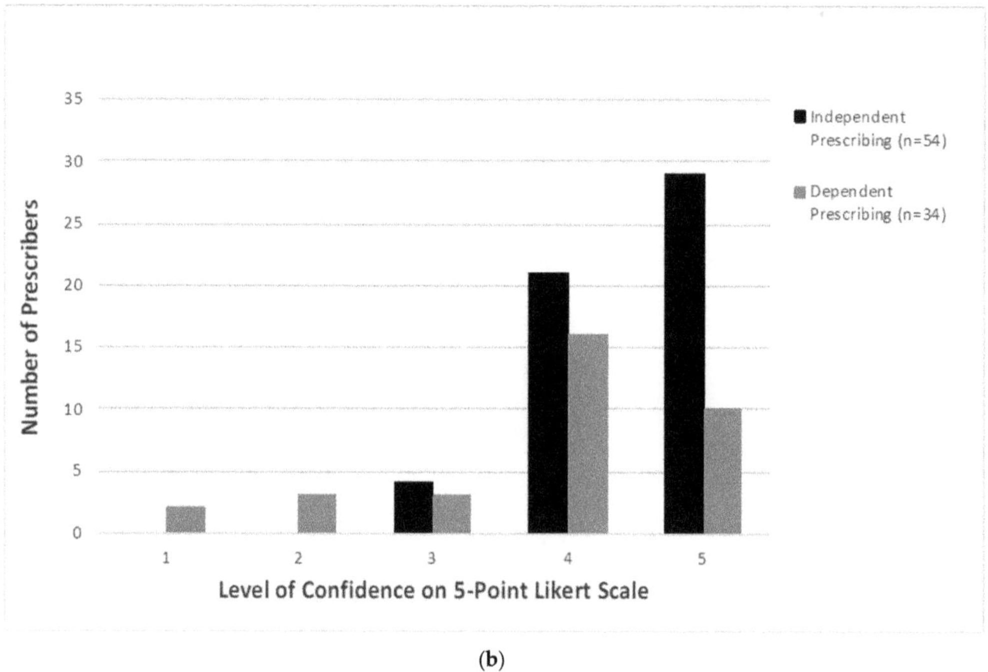

(b)

Figure 3. (**a**) Prescriber confidence if antibiotic prescription was indicated. (**b**) Prescriber confidence if antibiotic prescription was appropriate.

3.4. Appropriateness of Prescribing

Eighty-five percent (75/88) of prescribing was assessed as appropriate using the NAPS tool. Proportions of appropriate prescribing were similar, when comparing by seniority, independent vs directed prescribing or different levels of confidence (Table 3).

Table 3. Appropriateness of Prescribing.

	Seniority.	*n* (%)	Appropriate * *n* (%)
Seniority of Respondents	Senior	31 (35.2)	26 (84)
	Mid-level	38 (43.2)	33 (87)
	Junior	14 (15.9)	12 (86)
	Other	4 (4.5)	3 (75)
	Unknown	1 (1.1)	1 (100)
Seniority of decision maker	Senior	51 (60.0)	44 (86)
	Mid-level	28 (31.8)	24 (86)
	Junior	3 (3.4)	3 (100)
	Other	5 (5.7)	4 (80)
	Unknow	1 (1.1)	1 (100)

Table 3. *Cont.*

	Seniority.	*n* (%)	Appropriate * *n* (%)
Decision	Independent	54 (61.4)	47 (87)
	Directed	34 (38.6)	28 (82)
Confidence level Antibiotic Indicated—Independent	4 or 5	49 (91)	43 (88)
	1, 2 or 3	5 (9)	4 (80)
Confidence level Antibiotic Indicated—Directed	4 or 5	24 (71)	19 (79)
	1, 2 or 3	10 (29)	9 (90)
Confidence level Antibiotic Appropriate—Independent	4 or 5	50 (93)	44 (88)
	1, 2 or 3	4 (7)	3 (75)
Confidence level Antibiotic Appropriate—Directed	4 or 5	26 (76)	21 (81)
	1, 2 or 3	8 (24)	7 (88)

* Appropriateness assessed by NAPS assessment [17].

4. Discussion

This study describes the novel concept of decision-making in antibiotic prescription, in contrast with most studies which focus on the act of prescribing. We found that nearly two-thirds of clinicians who prescribe antibiotic medication decide this themselves, mostly with the support of endorsed guidelines. Over one-third of prescribing was guided or directed by senior ED clinicians or subspecialty advice. Prescriber confidence that antibiotics were indicated or appropriate was high, regardless of seniority or whether prescribing was self-directed or directed by others. Overall appropriateness of prescribing in this study was 85%, with similar proportions of appropriate prescribing when comparing seniority, decision-maker and prescriber confidence.

4.1. Seniority and Specialty of Decision-Making

Our study shows that mid-level and senior ED clinicians conduct most prescribing, with the junior cohort responsible for less than 20% of prescriptions. This is reassuring, as independent decision-making skills are still developing in this junior group. This is in contrast with a recent paper which showed that seventy percent of hospital prescribing is done by doctors in their first two years after medical school [21]. This difference may be explained by the difference in setting, where in the ED there is usually a senior clinician available for direct consultation.

Of particular interest was the decision-making process for patients who were geographically in the ED and were to be admitted under an inpatient specialty. In nearly 60%, when participants had prescribed an antibiotic and the primary decision maker was a non-ED clinician, this was directed by surgical specialties. Uncertainty about admission, institutional hierarchy, perceived urgency, and possible delays to specialty review all can influence prescribing decisions [22]. It is crucial to patient safety that there is a collaborative approach to patient care, including antimicrobial decisions, as there is an important trade-off between timely and inappropriate prescribing [21,22].

In our study, surprisingly no ED clinicians consulted with the infectious disease team. This may be due to the time constraints, but also may represent a knowledge gap on when to consult appropriately. It is possible that prescribing clinicians feel that this is core business, and they should be able to prescribe without specialist advice. The finding that 1 in 6 patients received inappropriate antibiotics suggest a more robust approach may be required. Also, after study design but before data collection, our health service ceased to have an on-call microbiology registrar, limiting consultation options.

4.2. Prescribing Details

Of note, clinicians often felt the need to further explain their decision-making process by hand-written notes on the paper questionnaire. In nine cases (10%) the clinicians stated they had deviated from guidelines due a nation-wide benzylpenicillin shortage. This demonstrates the complexities inherent in having a one-size-fits-all approach to antibiotic prescribing; nuance is required on a patient level. This is a barrier to effective guidelines, as patients will invariably have idiosyncrasies which lead to deviation. However, with developing machine learning and artificial intelligence, perhaps individualised recommendations may be the future of AMS. Decision support tools and smartphone apps have shown value in this space [23,24].

4.3. Prescribing Confidence

In our study confidence in own prescribing was high, with similar level of confidence in senior doctors and juniors, although respondents tended to be more confident in their own decisions than decision of others. Prior studies indicate that medical students and junior doctors have important shortcomings in the domain of prescribing, especially with respect to antimicrobials [25]. Despite this known weakness, there is little targeted teaching around antimicrobial choice in early clinical practice. Some junior clinicians maybe exhibiting the "unconscious incompetence" [26] of early clinical practice, which has been previously described [27,28]. However in our study appropriateness was similar for junior and senior staff.

4.4. Appropriateness

In our sample, 85% of prescriptions were deemed appropriate (NAPS 1 or 2) which compares favourably to the 67% appropriateness found in the same setting using the same methodology in 2017 [16]. This difference may be partially explained by chance (as our study was small), improved practices in our setting, or because of our design which allowed clinicians to clarify any decisions that were not strictly following guidelines. It highlights that non-compliance with guidelines cannot be entirely interpreted as inappropriate prescribing *per se*, although this finding warrants further study. Our study found similar appropriate prescribing by seniority, decision making or confidence and a larger study focusing on these factors would be required.

4.5. Limitations

This was a dual site study in a single season and findings may not be generalisable to other settings. Despite a good response rate of 73% and limited missing data, we cannot exclude selection bias. Although, we believe that as only one eligible respondent declined participation it is unlikely to have had a significant impact. Consultants only represented 3% of participants, but this is consistent with prior prescribing studies. Further, our study has limitations common to all survey-based research. Our questionnaire was purpose-made and although tested for face-validity it had limited answer options, making interpretation of more nuanced clinical situations challenging. This is highlighted by respondents using free text comments to further explain their decisions. The cross-sectional nature of this study provides a static picture of a dynamic process. This is further limited by using the terminology 'guided' or 'directed' prescribing. We acknowledge that by using this terminology certain subtleties in the decision making and prescribing etiquette cannot be commented on [29]. Furthermore, we cannot comment on what effect ED nursing or pharmacy staff may have had on prescribing habits. Response bias or recall bias may have led to erroneous or misleading answers, this was mitigated by only allowing answers up to 48 h post prescribing. Participants on night shift contributed to our non-response rates. Lastly, clinicians may be reluctant to admit that they did not use endorsed guidelines, as only two respondents stated they did not use guidelines. Given the busy nature of emergency medicine, this proportion is likely to be higher.

4.6. Recommendations

Our study has provided further insight in antimicrobial prescribing, decision-making and confidence. It provides useful information to inform future work related to individualised prescribing. Such prescribing will place the patient at the center of the decision making with a focus on areas where inappropriate prescribing is currently most common. Future qualitative research will be required to provide further insight into the intricacies of prescribing decision-making.

5. Conclusions

Nearly two-thirds of ED clinicians who prescribe antibiotic medication decide this themselves, usually supported by guidelines. In over one-third of prescribing was directed by senior ED clinicians or based on specialty advice, primarily surgical specialties. Prescriber confidence was high regardless of seniority or decision-maker. Overall appropriateness of prescribing was good with further room for improvement.

Author Contributions: K.J.D. and G.K. conceived the idea and obtained appropriate approvals, L.M.H. managed the overall study, L.M.H., J.B., M.K., M.F.B. collected and analysed data, L.M.H. drafted the first version of the manuscript. All authors have read and agreed to the published version of the manuscript.

Funding: This research received no external funding.

Institutional Review Board Statement: The study was conducted according to the guidelines of the Declaration of Helsinki, and ethical approval was granted by the institutional Human Research Ethics Committee (HREC/17/QGC/41).

Informed Consent Statement: Informed consent was obtained from all subjects involved in the study.

Data Availability Statement: The data presented in this study are available on request from the corresponding author. The data are not publicly available as this was not covered by our ethics approval.

Acknowledgments: Charlotte Steinberg and Teodora Dodic for support with survey distribution.

Conflicts of Interest: The authors declare no conflict of interest.

Appendix A. Questionnaire

Antibiotic Prescribing in ED
We are aiming to understand more about antibiotic prescribing in the ED.
There are seven (7) questions which should take <5 min to complete.
Q1. What is your role in ED?

- ○ Intern
- ○ Junior House Officer (Resident, PGY2)
- ○ Senior House Officer (Resident, PGY3 or above)
- ○ Principal House Officer (Unaccredited registrar)
- ○ ED Registrar
- ○ Consultant
- ○ Nurse practitioner
- ○ Other (please state . . . .)

In your most recent experience with antibiotic prescribing during the shift on the following date: ______________

Q2. What antibiotic was prescribed?
Antibiotic Type ____________________________
Antibiotic Dose ____________________________
Antibiotic Frequency __________________________
Q3. What condition were antibiotics prescribed for? (i.e., working diagnosis: UTI, febrile neutropenia)
____

Q4. Did you make the decision to prescribe?
○ Yes
○ No
Q5. If No, then who made the decision?
(indicate level of training and speciality)

Level of Training	Speciality
○ Intern	○ ED
○ JHO	○ General Medical
○ SHO	○ General Surgical
○ Registrar	○ ICU
○ Consultant	○ Other_____________

Q6. For your most recent experience, which of the following were used to decide on antibiotic selection? (tick all which apply)?
O Electronic Therapeutic Guidelines (eTG)
O Other guidelines (please specify ______________________)
O ED consultant recommendation (please specify if *in person* or vs *phone call*)
O Infectious disease recommendation
please specify if *registrar* or *consultant*
please specify if *in person* or *phone call*
please specify if *you* talked to ID, or *someone else*; if so, who ___________
O Microbiology recommendation
please specify if *registrar* or *consultant*
please specify if *in person* or *phone call*
please specify if *you* talked to ID, or *someone else*; if so, who ___________
O Other recommendation (please specify ________________________)
O I don't know
Q7. At time of pre-scribing, how con-fident were you on a scale of 1-5 that antibiotics were in-dicated? (please circle)
Q8. At the time of prescribing, how confident were you on a scale of 1-5 that an appropriate antibiotic was prescribed? (please circle)
Thank you for participating!

Table A1. National Antimicrobial Prescribing Survey (NAPS) tool for assessment of antibiotic appropriateness/[17].

Appropriateness			If Endorsed Guidelines Are Present	If Endorsed Guidelines Are Absent or Not Applicable
Appropriate	1	Optimal *	Antimicrobial prescription follows either the Therapeutic Guidelines ^ or endorsed local guidelines optimally, including antimicrobial choice, dosage, route and duration #, including for surgical prophylaxis	The antimicrobial prescription has been reviewed and endorsed by a clinician with expert antimicrobial prescribing knowledge $ **OR** The prescribed antimicrobial will cover the likely causative pathogen/s and there is not a narrower spectrum or more appropriate antimicrobial choice, dosage, route or duration available (including for surgical prophylaxis)
	2	Adequate	Antimicrobial prescription does not optimally follow the Therapeutic Guidelines ^ or endorsed local guidelines, including antimicrobial choice, dosage, route or duration #, however, is a reasonable alternative choice for the likely causative or cultured pathogens **OR** For surgical prophylaxis, as above and duration # is less than 24 h	Antimicrobial prescription including antimicrobial choice, dosage, route and duration # is not the most optimal, however, is a reasonable alternative choice for the likely causative or cultured pathogens

Table A1. *Cont.*

Appropriateness			If Endorsed Guidelines Are Present	If Endorsed Guidelines Are Absent or Not Applicable
Inappropriate	3	Suboptimal	Antimicrobial prescription including antimicrobial choice, dosage, route and duration # is an unreasonable choice for the likely causative pathogen/s, including: Spectrum excessively broad or an unnecessary overlap in spectrum of activity **OR** There may be a mild or non-life-threatening allergy mismatch	
	4	Inadequate	Antimicrobial prescription including antimicrobial choice, dosage, route or duration # is unlikely to treat the likely causative or cultured pathogens **OR** An antimicrobial is not indicated for the documented or presumed indication **OR** There may be a severe or possibly life-threatening allergy mismatch	
	5	Not assessable	The indication is not documented and unable to be determined from the notes **OR** The notes are not comprehensive enough to assess appropriateness **OR** The patient is too complex, due to multiple co-morbidities, allergies or microbiology results, etc.	

* Taking into account acceptable changes due to the patient's age, weight, renal function or other prescribed medications, if this information is available. ^ Antibiotic Expert Group. Therapeutic Guidelines: Antibiotic. Version 16 (2019). http://online.tg.org.au/ip/, accessed on 30 March 2021. # Duration should only be assessed if the guidelines state a recommended duration and the antimicrobial has already been dispensed for longer than this, or if there is a clear planned 'end date' documented. $ Examples including infectious disease physician, clinical microbiologist, or specialist pharmacist.

Table A2. Conditions for which antibiotic medications were prescribed.

Condition	*n*	Appropriate *n* (%)	Inappropriate *n* (%)
Aspiration pneumonitis	2	2 (2.3)	0 (0)
Bartholin's	2	0 (0)	2 (2.3)
Bronchitis	2	2 (2.3)	0 (0)
Community Acquired Pneumonia	13	12 (13.6)	1 (1.1)
C. difficile/diarrhoea	2	1 (1.1)	1 (1.1)
Cholecystitis	2	1 (1.1)	1 (1.1)
Dental abscess/infection	3	3 (3.4)	0 (0)
Diverticulitis	1	1 (1.1)	0 (0)
Dog bite prophylaxis	2	2 (2.3)	0 (0)
Ear Infection	1	1 (1.1)	0 (0)
Epididymitis	1	1 (1.1)	0 (0)
Facial bone fractures	2	0 (0)	2 (2.3)
Febrile neutropenia	1	1 (1.1)	0 (0)
Infected prosthesis	2	2 (2.3)	0 (0)
Hepatic encephalopathy	1	1 (1.1)	0 (0)
Infectious Exacerbation COPD	2	2 (2.3)	0 (0)
Mastitis	1	1 (1.1)	0 (0)
MRSA Osteomyelitis	1	1 (1.1)	0 (0)
Periorbital cellulitis	2	2 (2.3)	0 (0)
Pharyngitis	5	4 (4.5)	1 (1.1)
Pelvic Inflammatory Disease	5	5 (5.7)	0 (0)

Table A2. *Cont.*

Condition	*n*	Appropriate *n* (%)	Inappropriate *n* (%)
Post-Indwelling Catheter insertion	1	0 (0)	1 (1.1)
Post-operative infection	2	2 (2.3)	0 (0)
Pyelonephritis	3	3 (3.4)	0 (0)
Sepsis	2	2 (2.3)	0 (0)
Skin infection (cellulitis)	9	9 (10.2)	0 (0)
Sexually Transmitted Inefection	1	1 (1.1)	0 (0)
Surgical prophylaxis	1	1 (1.1)	0 (0)
Urinary tract infection (UTI)	10	10 (11.4)	0 (0)
UTI prophylaxis	1	0 (0)	1 (1.1)
Uvulitis	1	0 (0)	1 (1.1)
Wound collection	1	1 (1.1)	0 (0)
Wound prophylaxis	3	1 (1.1)	2 (2.3)
Total	88	75 (85.2)	13 (14.8)

References

1. United Nations Interagency Coordination Group on Antimicrobial Resistance (IACG). No Time to Wait: Securing the Future from Drug-Resistant Infections. Available online: https://www.who.int/antimicrobial-resistance/interagency-coordination-group/IACG_final_report_EN.pdf?ua=1 (accessed on 11 February 2021).
2. Kumar, A.; Roberts, D.; Wood, K.E.; Light, B.; Parrillo, J.E.; Sharma, S.; Suppes, R.; Feinstein, D.; Zanotti, S.; Taiberg, L.; et al. Duration of hypotension before initiation of effective antimicrobial therapy is the critical determinant of survival in human septic shock. *Crit. Care Med.* **2006**, *34*, 1589–1596. [CrossRef]
3. Kumar, A.; Ellis, P.; Arabi, Y.; Roberts, D.; Light, B.; Parrillo, J.E.; Dodek, P.; Wood, G.; Kumar, A.; Simon, D.; et al. Initiation of Inappropriate Antimicrobial Therapy Results in a Fivefold Reduction of Survival in Human Septic Shock. *Chest* **2009**, *136*, 1237–1248. [CrossRef]
4. Dellinger, R.P.; The Surviving Sepsis Campaign Guidelines Committee including The Pediatric Subgroup*; Levy, M.M.; Rhodes, A.; Annane, D.; Gerlach, H.; Opal, S.M.; Sevransky, J.E.; Sprung, C.L.; Douglas, I.; et al. Surviving Sepsis Campaign: International Guidelines for Management of Severe Sepsis and Septic Shock, 2012. *Intensiv. Care Med.* **2013**, *39*, 165–228. [CrossRef] [PubMed]
5. *Global Antimicrobial Resistance Surveillance System (GLASS) Report: Early Implementation 2016–2017*; World Health Organization: Geneva, Switzerland, 2017; p. 164. Available online: https://www.who.int/docs/default-source/searo/amr/global-antimicrobial-resistance-surveillance-system-(glass)-report-early-implementation-2016-2017.pdf?sfvrsn=ea19cc4a_2 (accessed on 11 February 2021).
6. Franklin, B.D.; O'Grady, K.; Donyai, P.; Jacklin, A.; Barber, N. The impact of a closed-loop electronic prescribing and administration system on prescribing errors, administration errors and staff time: A before-and-after study. *Qual. Saf. Heal. Care* **2007**, *16*, 279–284. [CrossRef] [PubMed]
7. Lewis, P.J.; Dornan, T.; Taylor, D.; Tully, M.P.; Wass, V.; Ashcroft, D. Prevalence, Incidence and Nature of Prescribing Errors in Hospital Inpatients. *Drug Saf.* **2009**, *32*, 379–389. [CrossRef] [PubMed]
8. Wittich, C.M.; Burkle, C.M.; Lanier, W.L. Medication Errors: An Overview for Clinicians. *Mayo Clin. Proc.* **2014**, *89*, 1116–1125. [CrossRef] [PubMed]
9. Brien, A.P.; Rawlins, M.D.; Ingram, P.R. Appropriateness and Determinants of Antibiotic Prescribing in an Australian Emergency Department. *Emerg. Med. Australas. EMA* **2015**, *27*, 83–84. [CrossRef]
10. May, L.; Gudger, G.; Armstrong, P.; Brooks, G.; Hinds, P.; Bhat, R.; Moran, G.J.; Schwartz, L.; Cosgrove, S.E.; Klein, E.Y.; et al. Multisite Exploration of Clinical Decision Making for Antibiotic Use by Emergency Medicine Providers Using Quantitative and Qualitative Methods. *Infect. Control. Hosp. Epidemiol.* **2014**, *35*, 1114–1125. [CrossRef]
11. Rhodes, A.; Evans, L.E.; Alhazzani, W.; Levy, M.M.; Antonelli, M.; Ferrer, R.; Kumar, A.; Sevransky, J.E.; Sprung, C.L.; Nunnally, M.E.; et al. Surviving Sepsis Campaign. *Crit. Care Med.* **2017**, *45*, 486–552. [CrossRef]
12. Shallcross, L.J.; Freemantle, N.; Nisar, S.; Ray, D. A cross-sectional study of blood cultures and antibiotic use in patients admitted from the Emergency Department: Missed opportunities for antimicrobial stewardship. *BMC Infect. Dis.* **2016**, *16*, 166. [CrossRef]
13. Xie, C.; Charles, P.G.; Urbancic, K. Inappropriate ceftriaxone use in the emergency department of a tertiary hospital in Melbourne, Australia. *Emerg. Med. Australas. EMA* **2013**, *25*, 94–96. [CrossRef]
14. Pulcini, C. Antimicrobial stewardship in emergency departments: A neglected topic. *Emerg. Med. J.* **2015**, *32*, 506. [CrossRef]

15. Llewelyn, M.J.; Hand, K.; Hopkins, S.; Walker, A.S. Antibiotic policies in acute English NHS trusts: Implementation of 'Start Smart–Then Focus' and relationship with Clostridium difficile infection rates. *J. Antimicrob. Chemother.* **2014**, *70*, 1230–1235. [CrossRef] [PubMed]
16. Denny, K.J.; Cotta, M.O.; Parker, S.L.; Roberts, J.A.; Lipman, J. The use and risks of antibiotics in critically ill patients. *Expert Opin. Drug Saf.* **2016**, *15*, 667–678. [CrossRef] [PubMed]
17. James, R.; Upjohn, L.; Cotta, M.; Luu, S.; Marshall, C.; Buising, K.; Thursky, K. Measuring antimicrobial prescribing quality in Australian hospitals: Development and evaluation of a national antimicrobial prescribing survey tool. *J. Antimicrob. Chemother.* **2015**, *70*, 1912–1918. [CrossRef] [PubMed]
18. Turnidge, J.D.; Thursky, K.; Chen, C.S.; McNeil, V.R.; Wilkinson, I.J. Antimicrobial use in Australian hospitals: How much and how appropriate? *Med. J. Aust.* **2016**, *205*, S16–S20. [CrossRef] [PubMed]
19. Von Elm, E.; Altman, D.G.; Egger, M.; Pocock, S.J.; Gøtzsche, P.C.; Vandenbroucke, J.P. Strobe Initiative. The Strengthening the Reporting of Observational Studies in Epidemiology (STROBE) Statement: Guidelines for reporting observational studies. *Int. J. Surg.* **2014**, *12*, 1495–1499. [CrossRef] [PubMed]
20. Therapeutic Guidelines Limited. eTG Complete. 2020. Available online: https://tgldcdp.tg.org.au/etgcomplete (accessed on 28 February 2021).
21. Alanazi, M.A.; Tully, M.P.; Lewis, P.J. Prescribing errors by junior doctors- A comparison of errors with high risk medicines and non-high risk medicines. *PLoS ONE* **2019**, *14*, e0211270. [CrossRef] [PubMed]
22. Papoutsi, C.; Mattick, K.; Pearson, M.; Brennan, N.; Briscoe, S.; Wong, G. Social and professional influences on antimicrobial prescribing for doctors-in-training: A realist review. *J. Antimicrob. Chemother.* **2017**, *72*, 2418–2430. [CrossRef] [PubMed]
23. Panesar, P.; Jones, A.; Aldous, A.; Kranzer, K.; Halpin, E.; Fifer, H.; Macrae, B.; Curtis, C.; Pollara, G. Attitudes and Behaviours to Antimicrobial Prescribing following Introduction of a Smartphone App. *PLoS ONE* **2016**, *11*, e0154202. [CrossRef] [PubMed]
24. Hamill, L.; Huynh, R.; Cross, J.; Alcorn, K.; Keijzers, G. DECIDE—Decision Support Webapp on Antimicrobial Care for Clinicians in the Emergency Department. ACEM 2019 ASM "The Changing Climate of Emergency Medicine", 36th Annual Scientific Meeting, November 2019, Hobart, Tasmania. (2019) Poster Presentations. *Emerg. Med. Australas.* **2020**, *32*, 28–72. [CrossRef]
25. Brinkman, D.J.; Tichelaar, J.; Graaf, S.; Otten, R.H.J.; Richir, M.C.; Van Agtmael, M.A. Do final-year medical students have sufficient prescribing competencies? A systematic literature review. *Br. J. Clin. Pharmacol.* **2018**, *84*, 615–635. [CrossRef] [PubMed]
26. Broadwell Martin, M. "Teaching for Learning (XVI)". (20 February 1969). Available online: https://www.businessballs.com/self-awareness/conscious-competence-learning-model///#conscious-competence-theory-origins. (accessed on 15 February 2021).
27. Lewis, P.J.; Seston, E.; Tully, M.P. Foundation year one and year two doctors' prescribing errors: A comparison of their causes. *Postgrad. Med. J.* **2018**, *94*, 634–640. [CrossRef] [PubMed]
28. Ryan, C.; Ross, S.; Davey, P.; Duncan, E.; Francis, J.J.; Fielding, S.; Johnston, M.; Ker, J.; Lee, A.J.; Macleod, M.J.; et al. Prevalence and Causes of Prescribing Errors: The PRescribing Outcomes for Trainee Doctors Engaged in Clinical Training (PROTECT) Study. *PLoS ONE* **2014**, *9*, e79802. [CrossRef] [PubMed]
29. Charani, E.; Castro-Sánchez, E.; Sevdalis, N.; Kyratsis, Y.; Drumright, L.; Shah, N.; Holmes, A. Understanding the Determinants of Antimicrobial Prescribing Within Hospitals: The Role of "Prescribing Etiquette". *Clin. Infect. Dis.* **2013**, *57*, 188–196. [CrossRef] [PubMed]

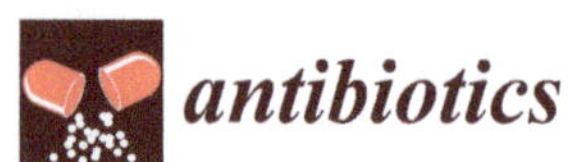

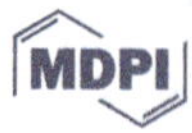

Article

Factors Affecting Antibiotic Prescription among Hospital Physicians in a Low-Antimicrobial-Resistance Country: A Qualitative Study

Ingrid Christensen [1,2,*], Jon Birger Haug [1], Dag Berild [3,4], Jørgen Vildershøj Bjørnholt [4,5], Brita Skodvin [6] and Lars-Petter Jelsness-Jørgensen [1,7]

1 Department of Infection Control, Østfold Hospital Trust, Kalnes, 1714 Graalum, Norway; jonhau@so-hf.no (J.B.H.); lars.p.jelsness-jorgensen@hiof.no (L.-P.J.-J.)
2 Faculty of Medicine, Ph.D. Program Medicine and Health Sciences, University of Oslo, 0315 Oslo, Norway
3 Department of Infectious Diseases, Oslo University Hospital, 0424 Oslo, Norway; dag.berild@medisin.uio.no
4 Faculty of Medicine, Institute of Clinical Medicine, University of Oslo, 0315 Oslo, Norway; j.v.bjornholt@medisin.uio.no
5 Department of Microbiology, Oslo University Hospital, 0424 Oslo, Norway
6 Norwegian Advisory Unit on Antibiotic Use in Hospitals, Department of Research and Development, Haukeland University Hospital, 5021 Bergen, Norway; brita.skodvin@helse-bergen.no
7 Faculty of Health and Social Studies, Østfold University College, 1671 Fredrikstad, Norway
* Correspondence: Ingrid.Christensen2@so-hf.no; Tel.: +47-9073-3113; Fax: +47-6986-4885

Abstract: Antimicrobial resistance (AMR) is a threat to hospital patients. Antimicrobial stewardship programs (ASPs) can counteract AMR. To optimize ASPs, we need to understand what affects physicians' antibiotic prescription from several contexts. In this study, we aimed to explore the factors affecting hospital physicians' antibiotic choices in a low-resistance country to identify potential targets for future ASPs. We interviewed 14 physicians involved in antibiotic prescription in a Norwegian hospital. The interviews were audiotaped, transcribed verbatim, and analyzed using thematic analysis. The main factors affecting antibiotic prescription were a high work pressure, insufficient staff resources, and uncertainties regarding clinical decisions. Treatment expectations from patients and next of kin, benevolence towards the patients, suboptimal microbiological testing, and limited time for infectious disease specialists to offer advisory services also affected the antibiotic choices. Future ASP efforts should evaluate the system organization and prioritizations to address and manage potential time-pressure issues. To limit the use of broad-spectrum antibiotics, improving microbiology testing and the routines for consultations with infectious disease specialists seems beneficial. We also identified a need among the prescribing physicians for a debate on ethical antibiotic questions.

Keywords: hospital physicians; low-resistance country; antibiotic prescription; antibiotic stewardship; antimicrobial resistance; semi-structured interviews; qualitative study

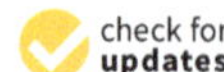

Citation: Christensen, I.; Haug, J.B.; Berild, D.; Bjørnholt, J.V.; Skodvin, B.; Jelsness-Jørgensen, L.-P. Factors Affecting Antibiotic Prescription among Hospital Physicians in a Low-Antimicrobial-Resistance Country: A Qualitative Study. *Antibiotics* **2022**, *11*, 98. https://doi.org/10.3390/antibiotics11010098

Academic Editor: Marc Maresca

Received: 19 December 2021
Accepted: 11 January 2022
Published: 13 January 2022

Publisher's Note: MDPI stays neutral with regard to jurisdictional claims in published maps and institutional affiliations.

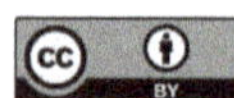

Copyright: © 2022 by the authors. Licensee MDPI, Basel, Switzerland. This article is an open access article distributed under the terms and conditions of the Creative Commons Attribution (CC BY) license (https://creativecommons.org/licenses/by/4.0/).

1. Introduction

Antibiotics are a cornerstone in the treatment of infections and critical to modern medicine [1]. However, inappropriate antibiotic use has led to increased antimicrobial resistance (AMR), threatening global health [2–4]. Antimicrobial stewardship programs (ASPs), defined as "a coherent set of actions which promote using antimicrobials responsibly" [5], are essential to combat AMR [6]. Understanding and considering the factors influencing physicians' antibiotic decisions are critical to provide tailored measures towards the stakeholders and thus the success of ASPs [7,8]. Systematic reviews on antibiotic prescribing behavior have identified some common barriers to rational prescription, including the fear of negative consequences for the patient and the belief that other professionals or other countries and health care practices, rather than themselves, are causing the problem of AMR [9–11]. ASPs are context-specific and must be adjusted to different health care environments. Exploration of key drivers from several contexts are crucial to ensure robust interventions [7,8]. Consequently, there is a need for exploratory studies across various settings [12,13].

In Norway, broad-spectrum antibiotics (BSAs) and AMR rates are lower than in most other countries. For instance, Norway has the lowest rate of methicillin-resistant staphylococcus aureus and a lower rate of other resistant bacteria, in company with Denmark and Finland, compared to southern and eastern Europe [14]. The main reasons are the historical strict national regulatory approval of new antibiotics and conservative guidelines for antibiotic use [15]. However, there has been a slight but steady increase in total and broad-spectrum antibiotic use in Norwegian hospitals, on a grander scale than the prevalence of infectious diseases suggests [16]. At the hospital where this study was conducted, BSA consumption has been relatively high compared to other Norwegian hospitals, which highlighted a need for reinforced ASPs.

The study aim of the present study was to explore factors affecting hospital physicians' antibiotic prescribing practices, in a low-resistance country, to identify potential targets for improvement of future ASPs.

2. Results

The final study population included 14 respondents: five physicians from infectious diseases; three physicians from oncology; one medical resident; and one physician from anesthesiology, gastrointestinal surgery, gastroenterology, pulmonology, and hematology. The participants' experience level and characteristics are presented in Table 1.

Table 1. Characteristics of the study participants (n = 14).

Age	**(Years)**
Median (IQR)	36.5 (14.5)
Range	29–66
Working Experience as a Physician (Years)	**(n)**
<5 years	4
5–10 years	3
10–20 years	4
>20 years	3
Gender	**(n)**
Female	9
Male	5

IQR: Interquartile range.

We identified four main themes affecting the physicians' antibiotic prescribing choices: (i) Clinical workflow pressures, (ii) Clinical uncertainty, (iii) Decision support, and (iv) Benevolence. Visualization of the themes and subthemes is shown in Figure 1. The themes, their respective subthemes, and illustrative quotes are shown in Table 2.

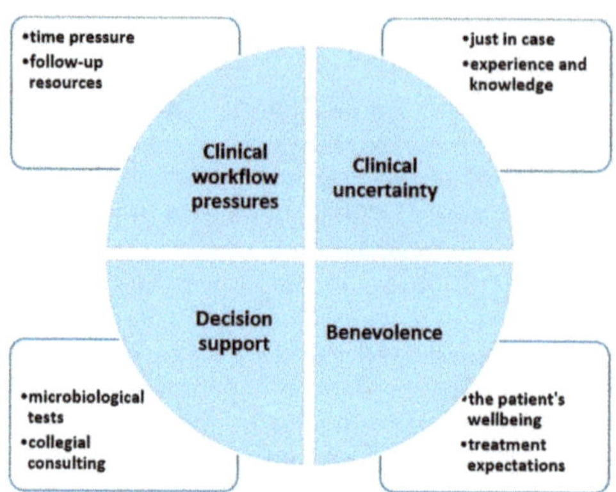

Figure 1. Visualization of the main themes (in the circle) with the consisting subthemes (squares).

Table 2. Themes, subthemes, and illustrative quotes representing the determinants of antibiotic prescription.

Theme	Subtheme	Quotes (Respondent Number, Years of Experience)
Clinical workflow pressures	Time pressure	There is too much pressure, no time to just observe the patient (. . .) so most doctors will give what they know works, which means broad-spectrum antibiotics, and the problem is that it works! (. . .) (R4, 25 years) For (patients with) chronic obstructive pulmonary disease patients and patients like that, it is difficult to know if they have an infection or not, and I feel it is more efficient just to put them on antibiotics (R14, 1 years)
	Follow-up resources	If you know the patient gets followed up, and clinical deterioration would easily get picked up, you would probably be more comfortable starting penicillin (instead of more broad-spectrum antibiotics), as opposed to a patient who gets left alone in a corridor, which is often the case (R9, 8 years) It is not the nurses' fault, but it often happens that they say no if I ask for close follow-up (of an ill patient) during night shifts. They tell me they don't have the capacity and no one to step in (R13, 4 years)
Clinical uncertainty	Just in case	9/10 doctors would, in cases of insecurity, rather ensure themselves (and give broad-spectrum antibiotics) (R9, 8 years) (Physicians continue antibiotics because) (. . .) it is the fear of doing wrong, of being appealed, both legally but also from colleagues. (R8, 23 years)
	Knowledge and experience	It is an intuition you get with clinical experience that allowed us to trust the clinical picture and withhold antibiotics (R6, 4 years) I got this idea that I wish to use narrower antibiotics, but then I don't know enough to do so (R5, 4 years)
Decision support	Microbiological tests	The most important thing is to have a resistance pattern, then I can feel safe that I use the right antibiotic (and don't need to give more broad-spectrum antibiotics) (R5, 4 years) We need to become better at sputum tests (. . .), often the patient has had a lot of productive cough and no collected sputum (. . .), which is a shame, because if you find the right microbe to target, then we will actually succeed (with narrow-spectrum antibiotics) (R11, 22 years)
	Collegial consulting	We often call up infectious medicine and ask for help (. . .) if we are in doubt. (R14, 1 years) I almost never make difficult decisions alone; I just talk to a colleague (R8, 23 years) Unfortunately, the reality is that you usually have several tasks in addition to giving consultations, and that certainly affects the quality of the advice we give (ID specialist, R4, 25 years) If you don't have time, then the advice (on antibiotics) you give may be bad and sometimes even dangerous (ID specialist, R2, 18 years)

Table 2. *Cont.*

Theme	Subtheme	Quotes (Respondent Number, Years of Experience)
Benevolence	The patient's wellbeing	If you've got an, e.g., immunosuppressed patient who is ill, then we treat with what is available in antibiotics now without worrying about the problem of resistance, sure we do (R10, 16 years) It is an analogy to peeing in one's pants; it is solving the problem now (by prescribing antibiotics), everyone know it will be uncomfortable later (...), but that is a problem for tomorrow (...) (R2, 18 years)
	Treatment expectations	In cancer and transplant patients, we often choose more broad-spectrum antibiotics, as they are immunocompromised, though you know broader spectrum means more resistance (...), and that is problematic, because patients who could have been cured from cancer could later die due the complications of the treatment (multi-resistant bacteria) (R10, 8 years) When, e.g., you are 90 years old and sick, it is probably okay to die of pneumonia. We try to tell relatives that, but they have a high level of expectations and will say, "But pneumonia is treatable", and then we start treatment anyways, and then it doesn't work, and we often try a more broad-spectrum antibiotic, and it doesn't work either, and that's a vicious circle (R4, 25 years). The family was literally praying to me, 'She must live, what can be done?' and then we continued to treat (...), but it won't be any better (R5, 5 years)

2.1. Theme (i) Clinical Workflow Pressures

The theme "Clinical workflow pressures" consists of the subthemes "time pressure" and "follow-up resources". Both subthemes represent physicians' experience of unfulfilled intentions of making thorough antibiotic decisions. The physicians constantly experienced being in a squeeze between providing optimal patient care, including making rational antibiotic decisions, and having a high workload and limited follow-up resources.

"Time pressure" reflects the pressures upon physicians' to increase patient turnover. The respondents reported experiencing a pressure mainly from nursing staff due to bed pressure. The physicians also reported putting pressure on themselves, e.g., when they observed many patients waiting in the emergency room. This strain was reported to often result in unnecessary use of broad-spectrum antibiotics to compensate for short time to observe patients and to perform adequate diagnostics:

> *"I think a lot is due to the pressure in the hospital; we hear all the time, 'Discharge, discharge, discharge' (...) We get whipped up like that, (...) and then I think the threshold (...) to give broader spectrum antibiotics is lower."* (Respondent 11, 22 years of experience).

"Follow-up resources" refers to the physicians' experience of a lack of patient follow-up resources which made them scared of patient adverse outcomes and thus led to use of more antibiotics to ensure safety. A lack of nurses (and thus capacity) was, for instance, viewed as a challenge:

> *"It is important that the patient is properly followed up; that is what's scary in an understaffed hospital full of patients: a lack of nurses. Then, it might be more rational to use broader spectrum antibiotics than in a more orderly situation (...) A typical example is that we actually shift from penicillin to cefotaxime (i.e., a more broad-spectrum antibiotic) on Fridays due to lesser capacity during weekends"* (R7, 13 years).

2.2. Theme (ii) Clinical Uncertainty

The theme "Clinical uncertainty" consisted of two subthemes: "just in case" and "knowledge and experience". Both subthemes underscored that the most important aspect for the physicians when they prescribed antibiotics was to feel certain in their decisions, both regarding a favorable outcome for their patients and to justify their decisions to their peers later.

"Just in case" reflects the finding that if the physicians were uncertain whether the clinical condition would deteriorate at home, they reported they would often continue to give antibiotics, even broad-spectrum antibiotics, to be on the safer side:

> *"We know that, theoretically, they often don't need antibiotics, but it is hard to select the patients who actually don't need antibiotics and have the courage to send them home without any (...) you are scared the patient will come back in worse shape, and you will be asked why you didn't continue antibiotics"* (R12, 10 years).

The physicians also considered their own "knowledge and experience" levels when making antibiotic decisions. The less experienced (under five years of experience) physicians more often reported that a feeling of inadequate knowledge led to less confidence to prescribe restrictively (please see Table 3 for illustrative quotes). They expressed that this lack of confidence led to an increased use of antibiotics just to be "on the safe side". In contrast, having enough experience to 'trust their gut' facilitated a more restrictive prescription:

> *"It is partly the experience level that allows you to have the guts to be restrictive"* (R7, 13 years).

2.3. Theme (iii) Decision Support

"Decision support" consists of the subthemes "microbiological tests" and "collegial consulting". These subthemes illustrated that the physicians viewed microbiological test and consultation as facilitators of rational prescription, but experienced that these facilitators were underused due to capacity constraints. Thus, they reported that underuse of available decision support negatively affected antibiotic prescription.

The physicians considered microbiological tests to aid in rational prescription as long as the sampling was correct, which was reported to not always be the case due to time pressure:

> *"Often the material is inadequate. It is an extreme pressure in the emergency ward sometimes, and you choose the easiest solution, which gives non-representative results"* (R6, 4 years).

The physicians experienced inadequate material as a lost opportunity to de-escalate to narrow-spectrum antibiotics.

"Collegial consulting" is bipartite; on one side, consultations with ID specialists were considered an important measure to facilitate more rational prescription by providing support in decision-making:

> *"What works well is to seek collegial support when you are in doubt, call an infectious disease specialist"* (R8, 23 years).

One the other side, the ID specialists highlighted that their antibiotic prescription advice was sometimes suboptimal due to limited time to engage, potentially hampering its effect on antibiotic prescription:

> *"(...) If we had time for consultation, it would be fine, but when it (the consultation phone) buzzes on top of everything else you have to do, then you don't have time (...), and the advice might be suboptimal"* (R7, 13 years).

2.4. Theme (iv) Benevolence

The theme "Benevolence" consists of the subthemes "the patient's wellbeing" and "treatment expectations". This theme addresses the physicians' benevolent efforts; they described a desire to improve their patients' health and meet the patients' or their relatives' wishes, which often would include the prescription of antibiotics. Simultaneously, they expressed a desire to limit unnecessary use of antibiotics and AMR.

"The patient's wellbeing" refers to the physicians' prioritization of the present patient's potential improvement, a possible future increase in antibiotic resistance notwithstanding, as illustrated by respondent 7:

"(...) Sometimes I think, 'Why am I doing this?' when I, e.g., give broad-spectrum antibiotics to an old patient who has dementia and has not improved on other antibiotics—it feels wrong, but at the same time, I feel I don't have a choice when I stand in front of the patient" (R7, 13 years).

The physicians expressed an unease knowing that such decisions often could result in a more inappropriate antibiotic prescription.

The "treatment expectations" subtheme represents situations when the physicians saw it as routine and expected to prescribe antibiotics, even though they often had second thoughts whether the antibiotic prescription was correct, regarding the aspect of AMR. An example some of the respondents used was oncologic or transplant patients for whom prolonged antibiotic treatment is often routine beside chemotherapeutic regimes. The physicians reported they obviously complied in offering life-extending therapy to individual patients. Nevertheless, they questioned the price to pay in terms of antibiotic resistance development:

"It is obvious that every patient, who can and wishes to get well, should receive all available treatment (...). For some patients, this would mean complicated antibiotic regimens to keep them alive during the treatment (e.g., transplant or cancer treatment). (...) This is worrisome due to the development of resistant bacteria that may kill other individuals" (R1, 12 years).

Another challenge the physicians experienced was the expectations of antibiotic treatment from the patient or the patient's family in situations when the physicians did not intend to prescribe an antibiotic:

"You often feel pressured; you know (when a relative asks), "Can you guarantee that my father doesn't have this and this condition?"—in situations like that you might push the boundaries more than you intended to" (R4, 25 years).

3. Discussion

Our main finding was the physicians report of the clinical workflow pressure to commonly facilitate excess antibiotic prescription to be on the safe side. Workflow pressure was perceived to hamper (1) correct microbiological specimens and (2) the quality of advice that the ID specialists gave, potentially facilitating unnecessary antibiotic prescriptions. We also identified a need to debate ethical dilemmas of antibiotic prescribing in specific clinical encounters, particularly with terminally ill patients.

The finding of clinical workflow pressure aligns with previous studies that have identified a high workload as a contributor to inappropriate prescriptions in hospitals [10,17,18]. In contrast, in two recent systematic reviews on determinants of physicians' antibiotic prescription decisions, time pressure was not a prominent finding [9,19]. The reason for this discrepancy may relate to the fact that the authors used frameworks for analyzing cognitive determinants of physicians' behavior. Time pressure due to high workload is mainly an external (systemic) and less of a cognitive factor and thus may not have called attention in these studies. The dominant and uniform reporting of time pressure as a barrier in our study strongly suggests that a focus on physician's behavior alone is ineffective, a notion which is in line with a recent publication by Broom et al. [20]. Based on analyses of qualitative studies over a decade, the authors argue for "no longer portraying AMR as the result of the actions of individual healthcare professionals but instead as a systemic problem (...)." Consequently, the ability of hospital administrators to analyze the work system organization and prioritizations within may be important for the success of ASPs.

Our second most prominent finding was the physicians' need for clinical certainty. This finding aligns with the findings of two systematic reviews that showed that fear of patient adverse outcomes causes' antibiotic overtreatment [9,19]. Considering the physicians' unified need to be safe, ASPs should include measures supporting prescribing physicians' sense of safety. Our study revealed several actions that could provide such support. The physicians called for improved microbiological testing, which could be achieved by reviewing sampling techniques and reinforce training [21]. Furthermore, experience and knowledge could be accelerated by systematizing consultation with ID physicians and implementing audits and feedback on antibiotic prescription, both of which are interventions that have proven effective in ASPs [13]. In particular, attention should be paid to the less experienced physicians. They expressed the highest level of insecurity in our study and potentially need more training on when and how to use expert consultations [18].

Another finding was the physicians' desire to do all they could for the present patient as a driver for an increased use of broad-spectrum antibiotics. However, the physicians sometimes had second thoughts about the benefit of their prescription (e.g., in pre-terminal patients), but they experienced that they did not have a choice when facing the patient. This sentiment echoes the 'tragedy of the commons' principle, which is known to lead to failure: If everyone thinks about themselves (misuse antibiotics now), all will suffer (increased AMR in the future) [22]. In our view, this finding highlights a need to debate when to provide and when to restrict antibiotic treatment. This topic is often too complex to be left at the discretion of the individual physician [23]. One suggestion is to develop further ethical committee services, e.g., by enabling a fast track for hospital doctors to consult with committee members. In addition, improved education on ethical topics is warranted for physicians who care for seriously ill patients, as the decision to use antibiotics is ultimately left for them [24].

In this study, we have aimed to identify factors, in a low-resistance context, that may help improve future ASPs. Factors identified in our context does not seem to diverge noteworthy from factors in other contexts [19], and thus support existing principles of ASP such as ID specialist consultation and education. However, core elements of infrastructure such as organizational structure should be reinforced [25].

Additionally, our findings of structural deficiencies may be more tangible to implement in ASPs than changes in physicians' behavior. Additionally, structure and behavior should be seen as integral to each other [20].

For more long-term gain regarding AMR ethical questions in antibiotic prescriptions should be evaluated.

The validity of our findings was strengthened as three researchers with different backgrounds (First author; IC, last author; LPJJ, and second author; JBH) read the transcripts and agreed on the themes in the analytic process [26]. To ensure adequate report of our study we used the consolidated criteria for reporting qualitative research (COREQ) (Supplementary Materials File S2).

Our study also has some limitations. First, one should always be careful to generalize the results from single center studies. Still, we believe the results from our hospital in a country with a low AMR represents a valuable supplement to similar exploratory studies from locations where AMR is far more prevalent. Several of the factors we identified may be relevant to aid in developing ASPs, particularly in settings of low antibiotic resistance rates and for high-intensity antibiotic prescribers in hospitals. Secondly, the recruitment of "frequent antibiotic prescribing physicians" resulted in a high representation of ID specialists and oncologists, indicating a potential selection bias. On the other hand, this has resulted in valuable viewpoints from two perspectives, i.e., from advice-seeking prescribers and advice-giving ID specialists. Finally, the principal investigator (IC) knew most of the respondents before the interviews, which may have affected their responses and her interpretations in the analytic process. We sought to limit such influence using reflexivity throughout the process [27].

In conclusion, future ASP efforts should evaluate the system organization and prioritizations to address and manage potential time-pressure issues. To limit the use of broad-spectrum antibiotics, improving microbiology testing and the routines for consultations with infectious disease specialists seems beneficial. We also identified a need among the prescribing physicians for a debate on ethical antibiotic questions.

4. Materials and Methods

4.1. Design and Setting

This qualitative study, using semi-structured interviews, was conducted at Østfold Hospital Trust, a 380-bed, secondary, acute care hospital with a catchment area of 320,000 inhabitants. From 2016 all Norwegian hospitals began establishing ASPs and from 2017 and at the time of the study, the study hospital had an antibiotic stewardship team consisting of an infectious disease (ID) specialist, a clinical pharmacist, and a nurse trained in infectious diseases. This team mainly conducted surveillance of antibiotic use, revised antibiotic guidelines, and conducted education promoting rational antibiotic use. The national antibiotic guidelines were made available electronically and distributed as a pocket booklet. The recommendations are based on treatment tradition and national antibiotic resistance patterns. Narrow-spectrum antibiotics are recommended in several empirical regimens, e.g., benzylpenicillin is the first choice for community-acquired pneumonia, and benzylpenicillin or ampicillin combined with gentamicin is recommended for sepsis [28].

In the study hospital, similar to most Norwegian secondary acute care hospitals, the physicians consult ID specialists by phone whenever they have complicated questions regarding infections, and antibiotic treatment.

4.2. Recruitment

To participate in the study, we sought respondents that could give rich information on the factors affecting physicians' antibiotic prescription. We purposively invited physicians that were prescribing antibiotics on a daily basis. Relevant respondents were chosen from lists over physicians in departments with high antibiotic use as documented by routine pharmacy data statistics and point-prevalence surveys of antibiotic prescriptions [29]. We made sure to include physicians representing different experience levels. A total of 17 physicians were invited by email and provided with information about the study, including the need to reserve 60–90 min of interview time. Of the 17 physicians invited to participate in the study, two did not have time to participate, and one did not respond, giving 14 potential respondents. Following the 12th interview, we identified no new themes. However, to ensure data saturation, we interviewed the two remaining physicians. The mean interview time was 52 min (range 23–74).

4.3. Interview Guide and Interviews

We developed an interview guide based on recommendations by Kallio et al. [30], and searched and used existing literature [31,32]. We designed the questions to have the respondents recall clinical situations in which they had prescribed antibiotics to obtain answers that reflected their everyday practice (Table 3). We conducted three pilot interviews with eligible candidates recruited through convenience sampling to optimize the final interview guide and technique. The data from the pilot interviews were not included in the data analysis.

The interviews were conducted in a quiet room in the study hospital from November 2018 to February 2019. The objectives of the study were presented both orally and on a written consent form. All interviews were performed by IC, a female MD and Ph.D. student trained in qualitative methods and with clinical experience in surgery and oncology. The pilot interviews were conducted together with LPJJ, a professor of health science with prior extensive experience with qualitative research, to observe and give feedback. Since interviews were performed at the same hospital as IC was employed, both interviewer and interviewees were known to each other, either in person or as colleagues. Consequently, measures were taken to minimize the risk of bias (please see data analysis).

Table 3. Summarized interview guide (full version in Supplementary Materials File S1).

1	What are your thoughts about rational antibiotic prescription?
2	What are your thoughts about antimicrobial resistance?
3	How would you describe the antibiotic prescription in this hospital, from your perspective?
4	What influences you when you prescribe antibiotics?
5	Can you please tell me about a situation where you had to decide when to start, not start, or stop antibiotics that you remember in particular?
6	Do you have any final comments on rational antibiotic prescription?

4.4. Data Analysis

The interviews were audio-recorded, transcribed verbatim, and de-identified (I.C.). In the transcripts I.C. made remarks about the physicians' body language, pauses in speech and other non-verbal communication, to provide more context to the transcripts. To minimize the risk of bias L.-P.J.-J. and J.B.H. consecutively reviewed and gave feedback on the interview transcriptions. The respondents were not automatically offered return of transcripts, unless they inquired it. One respondent did so and read and approved of the content. I.C. and L.-P.J.-J. coded the transcripts and themes derived from the data following the recommendations of Braun and Clarke [33]. NVIVO software assisted in the coding process. I.C. scanned the transcripts for illustrative quotes. Throughout this process, the possible influence of our positions and presumptions was scrutinized and documented in a project log (confer reflexivity) [27].

Supplementary Materials: The following supporting information can be downloaded at: https://www.mdpi.com/article/10.3390/antibiotics11010098/s1, File S1: Full interview guide; File S2: COREQ (COnsolidated criteria for REporting Qualitative research) Checklist.

Author Contributions: Conceptualization, I.C., J.B.H. and D.B.; Data curation, I.C. and L.-P.J.-J.; Formal analysis, I.C. and L.-P.J.-J.; Funding acquisition, J.B.H.; Methodology, I.C., J.B.H., J.V.B., B.S. and L.-P.J.-J.; Project administration, I.C. and J.B.H.; Resources, J.B.H.; Supervision, J.B.H., D.B., J.V.B. and L.-P.J.-J.; Validation, I.C., J.B.H., D.B., J.V.B., B.S. and L.-P.J.-J.; Writing—original draft, I.C.; Writing—review and editing, J.B.H., D.B., J.V.B., B.S. and L.-P.J.-J. All authors have read and agreed to the published version of the manuscript.

Funding: The study was funded by the Østfold Hospital Trust, the study hospital. Project number: AB3464.

Institutional Review Board Statement: The Regional Committees for Medical and Health Research Ethics (2018/1935 A) and the hospital data protection officer (public 18/06887) approved the study.

Informed Consent Statement: Informed consent was obtained from all subjects involved in the study.

Data Availability Statement: Extended data are available upon request to the corresponding author (I.C.).

Acknowledgments: We wish to thank all the participating physicians.

Conflicts of Interest: The authors declare no conflict of interest. The funders had no role in the design of the study; in the collection, analyses, or interpretation of data; in the writing of the manuscript, or in the decision to publish the results.

References

1. Chandler, C.I.R. Current accounts of antimicrobial resistance: Stabilisation, individualisation and antibiotics as infrastructure. *Palgrave Commun.* **2019**, *5*, 53. [CrossRef]
2. Jee, Y.; Carlson, J.; Rafai, E.; Musonda, K.; Huong, T.T.G.; Daza, P.; Sattayawuthipong, W.; Yoon, T. Antimicrobial resistance: A threat to global health. *Lancet Infect. Dis.* **2018**, *18*, 939–940. [CrossRef]
3. Podolsky, S.H. The evolving response to antibiotic resistance (1945–2018). *Palgrave Commun.* **2018**, *4*, 124. [CrossRef]
4. Antibiotic Resistance: Global Report on Surveillance. World Health Organisation. 2014. Available online: https://apps.who.int/iris/bitstream/handle/10665/112642/9789241564748_eng.pdf (accessed on 10 December 2021).

5. Dyar, O.J.; Huttner, B.; Schouten, J.; Pulcini, C. What is antimicrobial stewardship? *Clin. Microbiol. Infect.* **2017**, *23*, 793–798. [CrossRef]
6. Fridkin, S.; Baggs, J.; Fagan, R.; Magill, S.; Pollack, L.A.; Malpiedi, P.; Slayton, R.; Khader, K.; Rubin, M.A.; Jones, M.; et al. Vital signs: Improving antibiotic use among hospitalised patients. *MMWR Morb. Mortal. Wkly. Rep.* **2014**, *63*, 194–200. [PubMed]
7. Hulscher, M.; Prins, J.M. Antibiotic stewardship: Does it work in hospital practice? A review of the evidence base. *Clin. Microbiol. Infect.* **2017**, *23*, 799–805. [CrossRef]
8. Edwards, R.; Charani, E.; Sevdalis, N.; Alexandrou, B.; Sibley, E.; Mullett, D.; Loveday, H.P.; Drumright, L.N.; Holmes, A. Optimisation of infection prevention and control in acute health care by use of behaviour change: A systematic review. *Lancet Infect. Dis.* **2012**, *12*, 318–329. [CrossRef]
9. Krockow, E.; Colman, A.M.; Chattoe-Brown, E.; Jenkins, D.; Perera, N.; Mehtar, S.; Tarrant, C. Balancing the risks to individual and society: A systematic review and synthesis of qualitative research on antibiotic prescribing behaviour in hospitals. *J. Hosp. Infect.* **2019**, *101*, 428–439. [CrossRef] [PubMed]
10. Rodrigues, A.T.; Roque, F.; Falcão, A.; Figueiras, A.; Herdeiro, M.T. Understanding physician antibiotic prescribing behaviour: A systematic review of qualitative studies. *Int. J. Antimicrob. Agents* **2013**, *41*, 203–212. [CrossRef]
11. McCullough, A.; Rathbone, J.; Parekh, S.; Hoffmann, T.; Del Mar, C. Not in my backyard: A systematic review of clinicians' knowledge and beliefs about antibiotic resistance. *J. Antimicrob. Chemother.* **2015**, *70*, 2465–2473. [CrossRef]
12. Charani, E.; Edwards, R.; Sevdalis, N.; Alexandrou, B.; Sibley, E.; Mullett, D.; Franklin, B.; Holmes, A. Behaviour change strategies to influence antimicrobial prescribing in acute care: A systematic review. *Clin. Infect. Dis.* **2011**, *53*, 651–662. [CrossRef] [PubMed]
13. Davey, P.; Marwick, C.A.; Scott, C.L.; Charani, E.; McNeil, K.; Brown, E.; Gould, I.M.; Ramsay, C.R.; Michie, S. Interventions to improve antibiotic prescribing practices for hospital inpatients. *Cochrane Database Syst. Rev.* **2017**, *2*, CD003543. [CrossRef] [PubMed]
14. European Centre for Disease Prevention and Control. *Antimicrobial Resistance in the EU/EEA (EARS-Net)—Annual Epidemiological Report 2019*; ECDC: Stockholm, Sweden, 2020.
15. Hobæk, B.; Kveim Lie, A. Less Is More—Norwegian Drug Regulation, Antibiotic Policy and the Need Clause. *Milbank Q.* **2019**, *97*, 762–795. [CrossRef] [PubMed]
16. NORM/NORM-VET 2020. *Usage of Antimicrobial Agents and Occurrence of Antimicrobial Resistance in Norway*; NORM/NORM-VET: Tromsø/Oslo, The Netherlands, 2021; ISSN 1502-2307.
17. Sikkens, J.J.; Gerritse, S.L.; Peters, E.; Kramer, M.H.H.; Van Agtmael, A.M. The 'morning dip' in antimicrobial appropriateness: Circumstances determining appropriateness of antimicrobial prescribing. *J. Antimicrob. Chemother.* **2018**, *73*, 1714–1720. [CrossRef]
18. Coombes, I.; Stowasser, A.D.; Coombes, J.; Mitchell, C. Why do interns make prescribing errors? A qualitative study. *Med. J. Aust.* **2008**, *188*, 89–94. [CrossRef]
19. Warreman, E.; Lambregtsa, M.; Wouters, R.; Visser, L.; Staats, H.; van Dijk, E.; de Boer, M. Determinants of in-hospital antibiotic prescription behaviour: A systematic review and formation of a comprehensive framework. *Clin. Microbiol. Infect.* **2019**, *25*, 538–545. [CrossRef]
20. Broom, A.; Kenny, K.; Prainsack, B.; Broom, J. Antimicrobial resistance as a problem of values? Views from three continents. *Crit. Public Health* **2020**, *31*, 451–463. [CrossRef]
21. Skodvin, B.; Aase, K.; Brekken, A.L.; Charani, E.; Lindemann, P.C.; Smith, I. Addressing the key communication barriers between microbiology laboratories and clinical units: A qualitative study. *J. Antimicrob. Chemother.* **2017**, *72*, 2666–2672. [CrossRef] [PubMed]
22. Hardin, G. The tragedy of the commons. The population problem has no technical solution; it requires a fundamental extension in morality. *Science* **1968**, *162*, 1243–1248. [CrossRef]
23. Leibovici, L.; Paul, M.; Ezra, O. Ethical dilemmas in antibiotic treatment. *J. Antimicrob. Chemother.* **2012**, *67*, 12–16. [CrossRef]
24. Baker, E.F.; Geiderman, J.M.; Kraus, C.K.; Goett, R. The role of hospital ethics committees in emergency medicine practice. *J. Am. Coll. Emerg. Physicians Open* **2020**, *1*, 403–407. [CrossRef]
25. Report on the Modified Delphi Process for Common Structure and Process Indicators for Hospital Antimicrobial Stewardship Programs. Available online: https://www.cdc.gov/drugresistance/pdf/tatfar_rec1-finalreport_2015.pdf (accessed on 17 December 2021).
26. Fusch, P.; Fusch, G.E.; Ness, L.R. Denzin's Paradigm Shift: Revisiting Triangulation in Qualitative Research. *J. Soc. Chang.* **2018**, *10*, 19–32. [CrossRef]
27. Barrett, A.; Kajamaa, A.; Johnston, J. How to ... be reflexive when conducting qualitative research. *Clin. Teach.* **2020**, *17*, 9–12. [CrossRef] [PubMed]
28. The Norwegian Health Directorate. National Guidelines for Use of Antimicrobial Agents in Hospital Care. 2020. Available online: https://www.helsedirektoratet.no/retningslinjer/antibiotika-i-sykehus (accessed on 5 March 2021). (In Norwegian)
29. Point Prevalence Survey of Healthcare-Associated Infections and Antimicrobial Use in Acute Care Hospitals. *Protocol Version 5.3—Full Scale Survey*; European Centre for Disease Control and Prevention: Stockholm, Sweden, 2016; Available online: https://op.europa.eu/en/publication-detail/-/publication/39a84b73-dee0-11e6-ad7c-01aa75ed71a1 (accessed on 29 August 2019).
30. Kallio, H.; Pietilä, A.-M.; Johnson, M.; Kangasniemi, M. Systematic methodological review: Developing a framework for a qualitative semi-structured interview guide. *J. Adv. Nurs.* **2016**, *72*, 2954–2965. [CrossRef] [PubMed]

31. Skodvin, B.; Aase, K.; Charani, E.; Holmes, A.; Smith, I. An antimicrobial stewardship program initiative: A qualitative study on prescribing practices among hospital doctors. *Antimicrob. Resist. Infect. Control* **2015**, *4*, 24. [CrossRef]
32. Bate, P.; Mendel, P.; Robert, G. *Organizing for Quality: The Improvement Journey of Leading Hospitals in Europe and the United States. Nuffield Trust*; CRC Press: Boca Raton, FL, USA, 2008.
33. Braun, V.; Clarke, V. Using thematic analysis in psychology. *Qual. Res. Psychol.* **2006**, *3*, 77–101. [CrossRef]

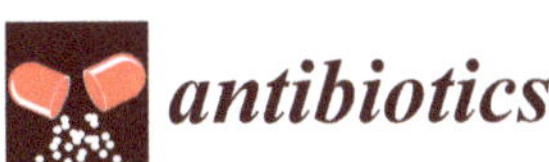 *antibiotics* MDPI

Article

Comparing Hospital and Primary Care Physicians' Attitudes and Knowledge Regarding Antibiotic Prescribing: A Survey within the Centre Region of Portugal

António Teixeira Rodrigues [1,2], João C. F. Nunes [3], Marta Estrela [1], Adolfo Figueiras [4,5,6], Fátima Roque [7,8,*] and Maria Teresa Herdeiro [1]

1 Department of Medical Sciences, iBiMED—Institute of Biomedicine, University of Aveiro, 3800 Aveiro, Portugal; at.afonso@outlook.com (A.T.R.); mestrela@ua.pt (M.E.); teresaherdeiro@ua.pt (M.T.H.)
2 Centre for Health Evaluation and Research (CEFAR), National Association of Pharmacies, 1249 Lisbon, Portugal
3 Department of Chemistry, CICECO—Aveiro Institute of Materials, University of Aveiro, 3800 Aveiro, Portugal; jcfn@ua.pt
4 Department of Preventive Medicine and Public Health, University of Santiago de Compostela, 15702 Santiago de Compostela, Spain; adolfo.figueiras@usc.es
5 Consortium for Biomedical Research in Epidemiology and Public Health (CIBER Epidemiology and Public Health—CIBERESP), 28001 Madrid, Spain
6 Health Research Institute of Santiago de Compostela (IDIS), 15706 Santiago de Compostela, Spain
7 Research Unit for Inland Development, Polytechnic of Guarda (IPG-UDI), 6300 Guarda, Portugal
8 Health Sciences Research Centre, University of Beira Interior (CICS-UBI), 6200 Covilhã, Portugal
* Correspondence: froque@ipg.pt

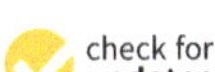

Citation: Rodrigues, A.T.; Nunes, J.C.F.; Estrela, M.; Figueiras, A.; Roque, F.; Herdeiro, M.T. Comparing Hospital and Primary Care Physicians' Attitudes and Knowledge Regarding Antibiotic Prescribing: A Survey within the Centre Region of Portugal. *Antibiotics* **2021**, *10*, 629. https://doi.org/10.3390/antibiotics10060629

Academic Editor: Seok-Hoon Jeong

Received: 13 April 2021
Accepted: 23 May 2021
Published: 25 May 2021

Publisher's Note: MDPI stays neutral with regard to jurisdictional claims in published maps and institutional affiliations.

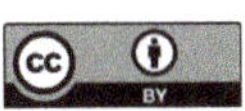

Copyright: © 2021 by the authors. Licensee MDPI, Basel, Switzerland. This article is an open access article distributed under the terms and conditions of the Creative Commons Attribution (CC BY) license (https://creativecommons.org/licenses/by/4.0/).

Abstract: Background: Antibiotic resistance is a worldwide public health problem, leading to longer hospital stays, raising medical costs and mortality levels. As physicians' attitudes are key factors to antibiotic prescribing, this study sought to explore their differences between primary care and hospital settings. Methods: A survey was conducted between September 2011 and February 2012 in the center region of Portugal in the form of a questionnaire to compare hospital (n = 154) and primary care (n = 421) physicians' attitudes and knowledge regarding antibiotic prescribing. Results: More than 70% of the attitudes were statistically different ($p < 0.05$) between hospital physicians (HPs) and primary care physicians (PCPs). When compared to PCPs, HPs showed higher agreement with antibiotic resistances being a public health problem and ascribed more importance to microbiological tests and to the influence of prescription on the development of resistances. On the other hand, PCPs tended to agree more regarding the negative impact of self-medication with antibiotics dispensed without medical prescription and the need for rapid diagnostic tests. Seven out of nine sources of knowledge's usefulness were statistically different between both settings, with HPs considering most of the knowledge sources to be more useful than PCPs. Conclusions: Besides the efforts made to improve both antibiotic prescribing and use, there are differences in the opinions between physicians working in different settings that might impact the quality of antibiotic prescribing. In the future, these differences must be considered to develop more appropriate interventions.

Keywords: hospital care; primary care; physicians; antibiotic; prescription; Portugal

1. Introduction

Antibiotic resistance is a worldwide public health problem, leading to longer hospital stays and raising medical costs and mortality levels [1–5]. Previous studies highlighted the role of the over-prescription and mis-prescription of antibiotics on the development of resistances [6–11]. Hence, promoting interventions to improve the antibiotic prescribing process is a key element to improving antibiotic use and diminishing resistances.

To improve the effectiveness of antimicrobial stewardship interventions, their design should be multifaceted, multidisciplinary and based on the characteristics of each specific setting [12–14]. However, prescribing is a complex process, usually affected by economic, demographic, clinical, cultural and social factors beyond evidence-based recommendations [6].

Attitudes are the key factors in the antibiotic prescribing process [13,15,16]. However, an in-depth understanding of how attitudes affect physicians' clinical practice in different settings is needed. To our knowledge, there are no studies assessing the differences between attitudes and knowledge of hospital physicians (HPs) and primary care physicians (PCPs). Therefore, the aim of this study was to compare both the attitudes and knowledge between PCPs and HPs with regards to antibiotic prescribing.

2. Materials and Methods

2.1. Study Design, Population and Ethics Statement

A survey was conducted in Portugal's Centre Regional Health Administration (ARS-Centro) (Population in 2011: ~1,737,059 people), from September 2011 to February 2012. Determinants of prescribing were assessed in all PCPs working in the National Health Service facilities of the ARS-Centro and hospital care physicians working in internal medicine departments within the hospitals of the ARS-Centro.

This study was approved by Portugal's Centre Regional Health Administration (Permit No. 015650/2011), by the hospital's administration and by the Portuguese Data Protection Authority (Comissão Nacional de Proteção de Dados/CNPD) (Permit No. 2886/2013). The personally addressed, reply-paid self-administered questionnaires were sent by post mail to PCPs up to four times to nonrespondents. In the case of HPs, the questionnaires were hand-delivered to the director of each hospital/medical service, who distributed them among the HPs. The answers were then collected by the administrative services of the department. The respondents did not receive any incentives. Nine hundred and fourteen questionnaires were delivered to PCPs and two hundred and twenty-seven questionnaires to HPs. All the data concerning PCPs' knowledge and attitudes has been previously published [15].

2.2. Data Collection

All physicians were asked to fill a previously validated (published elsewhere [16,17]), two-page long questionnaire, divided into 5 sections:

1. Instructions to complete the questionnaire;
2. "Antibiotics and Resistance": 17 statements regarding the knowledge and attitudes towards antibiotic prescribing, antibiotic use and antimicrobial resistance. To each of these statements, an attitude was attributed;
3. "In the treatment of respiratory infections, how would you rate the usefulness of each of these sources of knowledge?": 9 statements regarding the importance of having several sources of knowledge, which can help comprehend the sources of knowledge underlying antibiotic mis-prescription;
4. Sociodemographic and professional data (age, gender, medical specialization, workplace and workflow);
5. Open box for additional comments.

The measurement of the agreement with the questions included in Sections 2 and 3 of the questionnaire was performed through a horizontal, continuous visual analog scale, 8 cm long and unnumbered [16]. Answers were converted into a range from zero (total disagreement) to ten (total agreement). Physicians confidentiality was guaranteed.

2.3. Statistical Analysis

As the variables did not follow a normal distribution, nonparametric tests were conducted. Differences in the results between HPs and PCPs were evaluated using the Mann–Whitney U test. Differences were established as statistically significant at $p < 0.05$. The statistical analysis was performed using SPSS 25 (SPSS Inc., Armonk, NY, USA) and MS Excel (Microsoft Corporation, Redmond, WA, USA) software.

2.4. Sensitivity Analysis

In order to assess whether the differences observed were influenced by the fact that some physicians reported to work on both settings, a sensitivity analysis was conducted, in which these physicians were excluded.

3. Results

The overall response rate was 47.8%: of the PCPs; 421 answers were obtained, which corresponded to an overall response rate of 46.1%; 124 of the HPs invited accepted to participate in the study, corresponding to an overall response rate of 54.6%.

The process of distributing and collecting the questionnaires is summed up in the Figure 1 below.

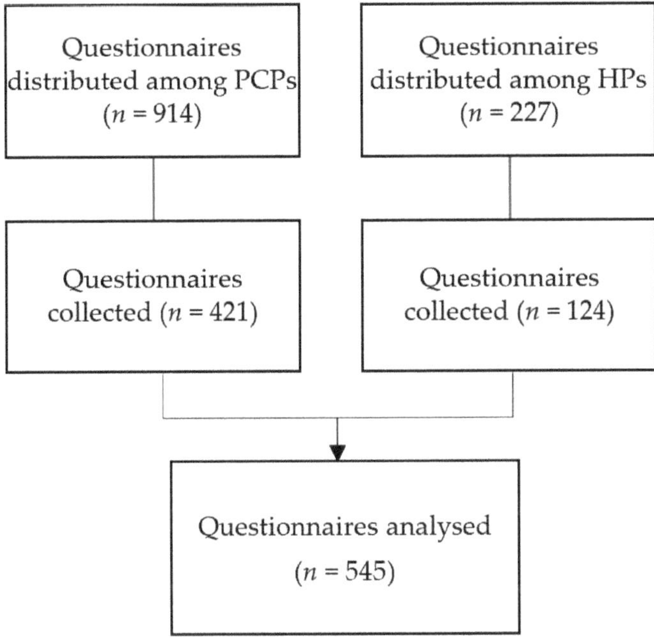

Figure 1. Questionnaire distribution and collection flowchart.

3.1. Comparison of Sociodemographic and Professional Characteristics

Table 1 presents the comparisons between the sociodemographic characteristics of PCPs and HPs.

3.2. Comparison of Knowledge and Attitudes towards Antibiotic Prescribing, Antibiotic Use and Antimicrobial Resistance

Table 2 describes and compares the results obtained for the 17 statements concerning antibiotic prescribing and resistances in both PCPs and HPs.

Statistically significant results were obtained for the attitudes such as ignorance, responsibility of others, fear, complacency and indifference statements. Regarding ignorance, hospital physicians showed a higher agreement with resistance being a public health problem (S1), the importance of microbiological tests (S2) and the influence of prescriptions on the development of resistances (S4) compared to PCPs.

Table 1. Sociodemographic and professional characteristics of both primary care and HPs.

	PCPs	HPs
Age (years)		
Median	55 (421/100%)	40 (124; 99.2%)
Gender		
Male	207/49.2%	44/35.5%
Female	214/50.8%	79/63.7%
Missing	0/0%	1/0.8%
Activity in		
Public practice	316/75.1%	99/79.8%
Public and private practice	95/22.6%	20/16.1%
Missing	10/2.4%	5/3.22%
Setting		
Primary care	309/73.4%	NA
Hospital and primary care	96/22.8%	25/20.2%
Hospital care	NA	98/79%
Missing	16/3.8%	1/0.8%
Emergency Activity		
No	133/31.6%	12/9.7%
Yes	280/66.5%	111/89.5%
Missing	8/1.9%	1/0.8%
Patients per day (25th and 75th percentile/*n*)	P25th = 20; P50th = 25; P75th = 30 *n* = 416/Missing = 5	P25th = 8; P50th = 10; P75th = 15 *n* = 124/Missing = 8
Patients in emergencies per week (25th, 50th and 75th percentile/*n*)	P25th = 15; P50th = 25; P75th = 40 *n* = 389/Missing = 32	P25th = 15; P50th = 20; P75th = 30 *n* = 124/Missing = 11
Time (min) per consultation (25th and 75th percentile/*n*)	P25th = 10; P50th = 15; P75th = 15 *n* = 385/Missing = 36	P25th = 20; P50th = 30; P75th = 30 *n* = 124/Missing = 13

About the responsibility of others, HPs appear to be less convinced that the development of new antibiotics will solve the resistance problem (S5). On the other hand, PCPs tend to agree more regarding the negative impact of self-medication with antibiotics and dispense without medical prescription (S12 and S13). Furthermore, PCPs expressed a higher agreement about the need of rapid diagnostic tests (S3).

PCPs agreed more with the prescription of antibiotics in situations of fear and uncertainty (S7 and S8), as well as about having a complacent attitude with their patients (S10).

3.3. *Comparison of the Usefulness of Different Sources of Knowledge*

Table 3 describes and compares the results regarding the usefulness of different sources of knowledge between primary care and HPs.

The differences found in the usefulness of sources of knowledge were all related to HPs considering some of the sources evaluated more helpful. Differences were found for clinical practice guidelines, documentation from the industry and from medical information officers, continuous educations, contribution of specialists, peers and the internet.

Table 2. Differences in the attitudes and knowledge regarding antibiotic prescribing between PCPs and HPs (10—completely agree; 0—completely disagree).

	PCPs Percentiles			HPs Percentiles			*p*-Value
	25th	**50th**	**75th**	**25th**	**50th**	**75th**	
S1: Antibiotic resistance is an important Public Health problem in our setting (Ignorance).	8.5	9.5	10	9.5	10	10	<0.001
S2: In a primary care context, one should wait for the microbiology results before treating an infectious disease (Ignorance).	1	3.5	5.5	1.5	5	7	0.005
S3: Rapid and effective diagnostic techniques are required for diagnosis of infectious diseases (Responsibility of others—Health-care system).	6.5	9	10	4.5	7	9	<0.001
S4: The prescription of an antibiotic to a patient does not influence the possible appearance of resistance (Ignorance).	0.5	1.5	5	0.5	0.5	1.5	<0.001
S5: I am convinced that new antibiotics will be developed to solve the problem of resistance (Responsibility of others—Research)	3.5	5.5	8	3	5	6	<0.001
S6: The use of antibiotics on animals is an important cause of the appearance of new resistance to pathogenic agents in humans (Responsibility of others)	5.5	8	9.5	5	8	9.5	0.681
S7: In case of doubt, it is preferable to use a broad-spectrum antibiotic to ensure that the patient is cured of an infection (Fear).	2.5	5.5	8	1.5	4.5	7	0.045
S8: I frequently prescribe an antibiotic in situations in which it is impossible for me to conduct a systematic follow-up of the patient (Fear).	2	4	6	0.5	2.5	5	<0.001
S9: In situations of doubt as to whether a disease might be of bacterial aetiology, it is preferable to prescribe an antibiotic (Fear).	1	3	5.5	1	4	5.5	0.183
S10: I frequently prescribe antibiotics because patients insist on it (Complacency).	0.5	0.5	1.5	0.5	0.5	1	0.011
S11: I sometimes prescribe antibiotics so that patients continue to trust me (Complacency).	0.5	0.5	1	0.5	0.5	1	0.029
S12: I sometimes prescribe antibiotics, even when I know that they are not indicated because I do not have the time to explain to the patient the reason why they are not called for (Indifference).	0.5	0.5	1	0.5	0.5	1	0.009
S13: If a patient feels that he or she needs antibiotics, he or she will manage to obtain them at the pharmacy without a prescription, even when they have not been prescribed (Responsibility of others—Other Professionals).	4.5	6.5	9	3	5.5	8.5	0.026
S14: Two of the main causes of the appearance of antibiotic resistance are patient self-medication and antibiotic misuse (Responsibility of others—Patients).	8	9.5	10	6	8.5	10	0.011
S15: Dispensing antibiotics without a prescription should be more closely controlled (Responsibility of others—Health-care system).	9.5	10	10	9.5	10	10	0.613
S16: In a primary care context, amoxicillin is useful for treating most respiratory infections (Ignorance).	5.5	8.5	9.5	5.5	8.5	9.5	0.407
S17: The phenomenon of resistance to antibiotics is mainly a problem in hospital settings (Responsibility of others—Other professionals).	1	3	6	1	3.5	7.5	0.205

Table 3. Differences in the usefulness of sources of knowledge between primary care and HPs (10—completely agree; 0—completely disagree).

	PCPs Percentiles			HPs Percentiles			p-Value
	25th	50th	75th	25th	50th	75th	
S1: Clinical practice guidelines.	7	8.5	9.5	8	9	9.5	0.003
S2: Documentation furnished by the Pharmaceutical Industry.	2.5	5	5.5	3	5	6.5	0.019
S3: Courses held by the Pharmaceutical Industry.	2.5	5	6	2.5	5	7	0.223
S4: Information furnished by Medical Information Officers.	2	3.5	5.5	2	5	6	0.024
S5: Previous clinical experience.	7.5	8.5	9.5	7.5	8.5	9.5	0.408
S6: Continuing Education Courses.	7.5	8.5	9.5	8	9	9.5	0.019
S7: Others, e.g., contribution of specialists (microbiologists, infectious disease specialists, etc.).	7	8.5	9.5	8	9	9.5	0.005
S8: Contribution of peers (of the same specialisation).	6.5	8	9	7.5	9	9.5	<0.001
S9: Data collected via the Internet.	3	5.5	7.5	5	7	8.5	<0.001

3.4. *Sensitivity Analysis*

Overall, after the sensitivity analysis, the differences between PCPs and HPs, have remained constant in almost all dimensions. However, the attitudes of fear (S7) and responsibility of others—other professionals (S13) were no longer significant. Furthermore, despite that the distribution remained the same as the one reported in Table 2, the differences between the importance attributed to Continuing Education Courses (S6) were no longer significant.

4. Discussion

This study shows that, besides an overall increasing of both apprehension and knowledge regarding health professionals and patients, there are still differences in the knowledge and attitudes that may be important to tackle in future healthcare interventions [18,19]. Furthermore, and considering that antibiotics can only be prescribed by physicians, these results provide a picture on the discrepancies between HPs and PCPs in terms of attitudes and knowledge concerning antibiotic resistances.

Regarding the attitudes underlying antibiotic prescribing, statistically significant differences were found for the responsibility of others, fear, indifference, complacency and ignorance in 12 of the 17 statements evaluated. These constitute somewhat unsettling results, as it reveals how different the attitudes concerning resistance between both settings can be.

Most HPs and PCPs agreed that antibiotic resistance is an important public health problem in their settings, reflecting the knowledge regarding antibiotic resistance is a distressing worldwide public health problem, increasing medical costs and mortality levels [3–5,20,21]. However, significant differences were found between HPs and PCPs, where the HPs showed higher agreement with the statement. This fact might be related with the challenges that HPs are facing to hamper and control the spread of resistant infections and their treatment in their setting. HPs also showed higher knowledge when considering the impact of a prescription to a patient as a factor underlying the possible appearance of resistance. Prior evidence revealed antibiotic prescriptions and use as selective pressure driving at this resistance, both on an individual [22] and community level [23].

The development of new antibiotics is also a point of discordance between PCPs and HPs: the first are more convinced that new antibiotics will be developed, and the literature shows promising lines of research [24]. However, the evidence shows the importance of conserving the molecules already available in practice, namely by using them wisely.

Significantly different answers were also obtained regarding the usefulness of the microbiology results in deciding which treatment to provide and the availability of the diagnostic techniques. The results of blood cultures help to reduce antibiotic use and narrow antibiotic therapy, thus reducing the costs [25], and there are several emerging potential technologies that can address the clinical needs [26]. Nevertheless, the differences found might be related to the availability of diagnostic techniques in time in the hospital setting, contrarywise to what is found in primary care settings, in which widespread testing is not feasible. Yet, in some specific diseases—namely, for pharyngitis—rapid antigen testing is recommended before an antibiotic prescription [27–31].

Differences were also found regarding the responsibility of patients or pharmacies, where PCPs agreed more that patients may manage to obtain antibiotics even without a prescription and/or self-medicate. This difference in physicians' perceptions might be related to the proximity between primary care and community pharmacy practices. Nevertheless, the evidence is published about the dispense without a prescription [32,33] and self-medication with antibiotics [34], which leads to antibiotic misuse and resistances.

Fear about future bacterial resistances was also an attitude where physicians showed differences. PCPs agreed more about prescribing broad-spectrum antibiotics, in the case of diagnostic uncertainty or the impossibility of following-up patients. This might be explained with the unavailability of diagnostic tools to aid physicians' diagnosis in primary care settings and is concordant with the previous research [6,35–37].

The statistically significant opinions in which physicians showed the least agreement were related to insistence from the patient, patient trust and time constraints. Again, differences were found, and PCPs seem to be more complacent with patients than the HPs. There is data indicating that both physicians consider patient satisfaction is crucial, so it is vital to manage patients' expectations [9,38], namely with emphasis on precise clarifications. As a patient's satisfaction is related to their belief of their understanding of their disease, the data shows the success of longer, patient-centered consultations with low antibiotic prescriptions [6,8,9,13,39,40]. Changing primary healthcare setting is hard, but patient empowerment and reinforcement during doctor–patient communication with a realist awareness of the patient's expectations was reveal to be essential in reducing the antibiotic prescription [41,42].

HPs tended to show higher agreement about the usefulness of the sources of knowledge. With exception to the courses promoted and organized by the pharmaceutical industry and previous clinical practices, all the other sources of knowledge evaluated were considered more useful by HPs. The reasons behind these differences are complex to understand, but the need to be continuously updated in a hospital care context might be associated with the results found. Furthermore, as the HPs tended to be younger, they might feel the need to resort to other sources of knowledge to compensate for a lower clinical practice experience when compared to PCPs, who tend to be older. Perhaps younger doctors rely more on sources of information based on scientific evidence, while older doctors rely on their clinical experience.

Considering the fact that the vast majority of antibiotics are prescribed in primary care [43], the identification of the differences in the attitudes and the underlying behaviors in antibiotic prescribing between settings allows us to tailor antibiotic stewardship interventions. As inadequate antibiotic prescriptions are an important factor for antibiotic resistances development [18,19], and high rates of inadequate antimicrobial prescribing are noted in the context of primary care [44], identifying the dimensions in which PCPs are less aware is an essential strategy toward improving these issues. Furthermore, parallel to the results in this study, in which PCPs tend to attribute more responsibility to others than HPs, and less important than the issue of antibiotic resistances, some studies have shown that PCPs do not only give less importance to the issue of antibiotic resistances but also tend to not consider themselves particularly accountable about their roles in this issue [20,21,44]. Hence, raising awareness among PCPs to tackle antimicrobial resistances should be a priority.

This study is accompanied by some limitations. Despite the statistically significant differences in attitudes, we cannot assure it triggers different antibiotic prescribing practices between settings. Considering the geographical limitations, the low response rate and specific characteristics regarding physicians' clinical practice and the Portuguese Health System, the extrapolation of the results to other countries might not be adequate, as it can compromise its external validity. Nevertheless, the internal validity has been assured, as the questionnaire has been previously validated [16,45]. The response rates obtained both with primary care and HPs are low when compared to similar studies [46–48]. However, low response rates among physicians is a recognized problem in survey research [49,50]. The fact that the questionnaires were sent by post mail to PCPs and hand-delivered to the director of each hospital/service, along with the differences in the geographical dispersion of physicians within the territory, might explain the slight discrepancy between the response rates. Still, the difference in only 8% between response rates constitutes a positive outcome in this study, as it results in a less-biased appraisal between both settings. Furthermore, at the time in which this survey was conducted, there were 4.5 physicians/1000 inhabitants, considering both the public and private sectors [51]. Considering the estimated population of the center region, we estimate that this survey is highly representative of the public sector physician population, as it included almost a third of the physicians of this region. Even though this study was conducted in 2011 to 2012, which can be considered a limitation, the data from this study remains relevant, as the attitudes are stable variables over time [20,21], and it still brings an important contribution to the knowledge on this topic.

5. Conclusions

To conclude, the results of the study revealed that there are differences in opinions between physicians working in hospital and primary care that might impact the quality of antibiotic prescribing. Therefore, interventions to improve the antibiotic prescription quality should be tailored to each setting, especially considering the more evident differences between primary care and HP attitudes (particularly, dimensions of fear, ignorance and responsibility to others) for a more effective tackling of this global concern.

Author Contributions: Conceptualization, A.F., F.R. and M.T.H.; data curation, A.T.R., F.R. and M.T.H.; formal analysis, A.T.R., J.C.F.N., M.E., A.F., F.R. and M.T.H.; funding acquisition, F.R. and M.T.H.; investigation, A.T.R., A.F., F.R. and M.T.H.; methodology, A.T.R., J.C.F.N., M.E., A.F., F.R. and M.T.H.; project administration, M.T.H.; writing—original draft, A.T.R. and writing—review and editing, J.C.F.N., M.E., A.F., F.R. and M.T.H. All authors have read and agreed to the published version of the manuscript.

Funding: This work was supported by the Foundation for Science & Technology (Fundação para a Ciência e Tecnologia—FCT), Institute of Biomedicine -iBiMED (UIDP/04501/2020) grant (UIDB/04501 /2020) and by grant PTDC/SAU-ESA/105530/2008, from the Portuguese Ministry of Science & Education, co-financed by FEDER through the COMPETE Program, and by the research project PTDC/SAU-SER/31678/2017, supported by the operational program on competitiveness and internationalization (POCI) in its FEDER/FNR component, POCI-01-0145-FEDER-031678, and by the Foundation for Science and Technology in its state budget component (OE).

Institutional Review Board Statement: The study was conducted according to the guidelines of the Declaration of Helsinki and approved by approved by Portugal's Centre Regional Health Administration (Permit No. 015650/2011), by the hospital's administration and by the Portuguese Data Protection Authority (Comissão Nacional de Proteção de Dados/CNPD) (Permit No. 2886/2013).

Informed Consent Statement: The participation of the questionnaire was a volunteer and only the participants that agree to participate fulfill the questionnaire.

Acknowledgments: We thank Tânia Magalhães Silva (iBiMED/UA) for her collaboration on the revision of the manuscript.

Conflicts of Interest: The authors declare no conflict of interest. The funders had no role in the design of the study; in the collection, analyses or interpretation of the data; in the writing of the manuscript or in the decision to publish the results.

References

1. Livermore, D. Minimising antibiotic resistance. *Lancet Infect. Dis.* **2005**, *5*, 450–459. [CrossRef]
2. Yewale, V. Antimicrobial resistance—A ticking bomb! *Indian Pediatr.* **2014**, *51*, 171–172. [CrossRef] [PubMed]
3. Kollef, M.H. Inadequate antimicrobial treatment: An Important determinant of outcome for hospitalized patients. *Clin. Infect. Dis.* **2000**, *31*, 131–138. [CrossRef]
4. Kandeel, A.; El-shoubary, W.; Hicks, L.A.; Fattah, M.A.; Dooling, K.L.; Lohiniva, A.L.; Ragab, O.; Galal, R.; Talaat, M. Patient Attitudes and Beliefs and Provider Practices Regarding Antibiotic Use for Acute Respiratory Tract Infections in Minya, Egypt. *Antibiotics* **2014**, *292*, 632–644. [CrossRef] [PubMed]
5. Kollef, M.H. The importance of appropriate initial antibiotic therapy for hospital-acquired infections. *Am. J. Med.* **2003**, *115*, 582–584. [CrossRef]
6. Ackerman, S.; Gonzales, R. The context of antibiotic overuse. *Ann. Intern. Med.* **2012**, *147*, 211–212. [CrossRef]
7. McNulty, C.A.M. European Antibiotic Awareness Day 2012: General practitioners encouraged to TARGET antibiotics through guidance, education and tools. *J. Antimicrob. Chemother.* **2012**, *67*, 2543–2546. [CrossRef]
8. Hart, A.; Pepper, G.; Gonzales, R. Balancing acts: Deciding for or against antibiotics in acute respiratory infections. *J. Fam. Pract.* **2016**, *55*, 320–325. [CrossRef]
9. Ong, S.; Nakase, J.; Moran, G.; Karras, D.; Kuehnert, M.; Talan, D. Antibiotic Use for Emergency Department Patients With Upper Respiratory Infections: Prescribing Practices, Patient Expectations, and Patient Satisfaction. *Ann. Emerg. Med.* **2007**, *50*, 213–220. [CrossRef] [PubMed]
10. Wigton, R.S.; Darr, C.A.; Corbett, K.K.; Nickol, D.R.; Gonzales, R. How do community practitioners decide whether to prescribe antibiotics for acute respiratory tract infections? *J. Gen. Intern. Med.* **2008**, *23*, 1615–1620. [CrossRef]
11. Dallas, A.; Van Driel, M.; Van De Mortel, T.; Magin, P. Antibiotic prescribing for the future: Exploring the attitudes of trainees in general practice. *Br. J. Gen. Pract.* **2014**, *64*, e561–e567. [CrossRef]
12. Roque, F.; Teixeira-Rodrigues, A.; Breitenfeld, L.; Piñeiro-Lamas, M.; Figueiras, A.; Herdeiro, M.T. Decreasing antibiotic use through a joint intervention targeting physicians and pharmacists. *Future Microbiol.* **2016**, *11*, 877–886. [CrossRef] [PubMed]
13. Lopez-Vazquez, P.; Vazquez-Lago, J.M.; Figueiras, A. Misprescription of antibiotics in primary care: A critical systematic review of its determinants. *J. Eval. Clin. Pract.* **2012**, *18*, 473–484. [CrossRef]
14. Arnold, S.; Straus, S. Interventions to improve antibiotic prescribing practices in ambulatory care. *Evid.-Based Child Health A Cochrane Rev. J.* **2006**, *1*, 623–690. [CrossRef]
15. Rodrigues, A.T.; Ferreira, M.; Piñeiro-Lamas, M.; Falcão, A.; Figueiras, A.; Herdeiro, M.T. Determinants of physician antibiotic prescribing behavior: A 3 year cohort study in Portugal. *Curr. Med. Res. Opin.* **2016**, *32*, 949–957. [CrossRef]
16. Teixeira Rodrigues, A.; Ferreira, M.; Roque, F.; Falcão, A.; Ramalheira, E.; Figueiras, A.; Herdeiro, M.T. Physicians' attitudes and knowledge concerning antibiotic prescription and resistance: Questionnaire development and reliability. *BMC Infect. Dis.* **2016**, *16*, 1–8. [CrossRef] [PubMed]
17. López-Vázquez, P.; Vázquez-Lago, J.M.; Gonzalez-Gonzalez, C.; Piñeiro-Lamas, M.; López-Durán, A.; Herdeiro, M.T.; Figueiras, A.; GREPHEPI Group. Development and validation of the knowledge and attitudes regarding antibiotics and resistance (KAAR-11) questionnaire for primary care physicians. *J. Antimicrob. Chemother.* **2016**, *71*, 2972–2979. [CrossRef]
18. Zetts, R.M.; Stoesz, A.; Garcia, A.M.; Doctor, J.N.; Gerber, J.S.; Linder, J.A.; Hyun, D.Y. Primary care physicians' attitudes and perceptions towards antibiotic resistance and outpatient antibiotic stewardship in the USA: A qualitative study. *BMJ Open* **2020**, *10*, 34983. [CrossRef]
19. Zetts, R.M.; Garcia, A.M.; Doctor, J.N.; Gerber, J.S.; Linder, J.A.; Hyun, D.Y. Primary care physicians' attitudes and perceptions towards antibiotic resistance and antibiotic stewardship: A national survey. *Open Forum Infect. Dis.* **2020**, *7*. [CrossRef] [PubMed]
20. Gonzales, R.; Bartlett, J.; Besser, R.; Cooper, R.; Hickner, J.; Hoffman, J.; Sande, M. Principles of appropriate antibiotic use for treatment of acute respiratory tract infections in adults: Background, specific aims, and methods. *Ann. Intern. Med.* **2001**, *134*, 479–486. [CrossRef]
21. Lepape, A.; Monnet, D.L. Experience of European intensive care physicians with infections due to antibiotic-resistant bacteria, 2009. *Eurosurveillance* **2009**, *14*, 9–11. [CrossRef]
22. Costelloe, C.; Metcalfe, C.; Lovering, A.; Mant, D.; Hay, A.D. Effect of antibiotic prescribing in primary care on antimicrobial resistance in individual patients: Systematic review and meta-analysis. *BMJ* **2010**, *340*, 1120. [CrossRef] [PubMed]
23. Derde, L.P.G.; Cooper, B.S.; Goossens, H.; Malhotra-Kumar, S.; Willems, R.J.L.; Gniadkowski, M.; Hryniewicz, W.; Empel, J.; Dautzenberg, M.J.D.; Annane, D.; et al. Interventions to reduce colonisation and transmission of antimicrobial-resistant bacteria in intensive care units: An interrupted time series study and cluster randomised trial. *Lancet Infect. Dis.* **2014**, *14*, 31–39. [CrossRef]
24. The Pew Charitable Trusts Tracking the Pipeline of Antibiotics in Development. Available online: https://www.pewtrusts.org/en/research-and-analysis/articles/2016/12/tracking-the-pipeline-of-antibiotics-in-development (accessed on 24 May 2021).
25. Dowell, S.F.; Marcy, S.M.; Phillips, W.R.; Gerber, M.A.; Schwartz, B. Principles of Judicious Use of Antimicrobial Agents for Pediatric Upper Respiratory tract infections. *Pediatrics* **1998**, *101*, 163–165. [CrossRef]
26. O'Brien, K.L.; Dowell, S.F.; Schwartz, B.; Marcy, S.M.; Phillips, W.R.; Gerber, M.A. Cough illness/bronchitis—Principles of judicious use of antimicrobial agents. *Pediatrics* **1998**, *101*, 178–181. [CrossRef]

27. Fraser, H.; Gallacher, D.; Achana, F.; Court, R.; Taylor-Phillips, S.; Nduka, C.; Stinton, C.; Willans, R.; Gill, P.; Mistry, H. Rapid antigen detection and molecular tests for group a streptococcal infections for acute sore throat: Systematic reviews and economic evaluation. *Health Technol. Assess.* **2020**, *24*, 1–232. [CrossRef] [PubMed]
28. Cohen, J.F.; Pauchard, J.Y.; Hjelm, N.; Cohen, R.; Chalumeau, M. Efficacy and safety of rapid tests to guide antibiotic prescriptions for sore throat. *Cochrane Database Syst. Rev.* **2020**, *2020*. [CrossRef]
29. Cohen, J.F.; Bertille, N.; Cohen, R.; Chalumeau, M. Rapid antigen detection test for group A streptococcus in children with pharyngitis. *Cochrane Database Syst. Rev.* **2016**, *2016*. [CrossRef] [PubMed]
30. Jeffrey, R. Donowitz Acute Pharyngitis—Symptoms, Diagnosis and Treatment I BMJ Best Practice. Available online: https://bestpractice.bmj.com/topics/en-gb/5 (accessed on 27 January 2020).
31. Carvalho, É.; Estrela, M.; Zapata-Cachafeiro, M.; Figueiras, A.; Roque, F.; Herdeiro, M.T. E-Health Tools to Improve Antibiotic Use and Resistances: A Systematic Review. *Antibiotics* **2020**, *9*, 505. [CrossRef]
32. Morgan, D.J.; Okeke, I.N.; Laxminarayan, R.; Perencevich, E.N.; Weisenberg, S. Non-prescription antimicrobial use worldwide: A systematic review. *Lancet Infect. Dis.* **2011**, *11*, 692–701. [CrossRef]
33. Batista, A.D.; Rodrigues, D.A.; Figueiras, A.; Zapata-Cachafeiro, M.; Roque, F.; Herdeiro, M.T. Antibiotic Dispensation without a Prescription Worldwide: A Systematic Review. *Antibiotics* **2020**, *9*, 786. [CrossRef] [PubMed]
34. Rosenstein, N.; Phillips, W.R.; Gerber, M.A.; Marcy, S.M.; Schwartz, B.; Dowell, S.F. The common cold—Principles of judicious use of antimicrobial agents. *Pediatrics* **1998**, *101*, 181–184.
35. Linder, J.A.; Schnipper, J.L.; Tsurikova, R.; Volk, L.A.; Middleton, B. Self-reported familiarity with acute respiratory infection guidelines and antibiotic prescribing in primary care. *Int. J. Qual. Health Care* **2010**, *22*, 469–475. [CrossRef] [PubMed]
36. Lee, T.H.; Wong, J.G.X.; Lye, D.C.B.; Chen, M.I.C.; Loh, V.W.K.; Leo, Y.S.; Lee, L.K.; Chow, A.L.P. Medical and psychosocial factors associated with antibiotic prescribing in primary care: Survey questionnaire and factor analysis. *Br. J. Gen. Pract.* **2017**, *67*, e168–e177. [CrossRef]
37. Allaire, A.-S.; Labrecque, M.; Giguère, A.; Gagnon, M.-P.; Grimshaw, J.; Légaré, F. Barriers and facilitators to the dissemination of DECISION+, a continuing medical education program for optimizing decisions about antibiotics for acute respiratory infections in primary care: A study protocol. *Implement. Sci.* **2011**, *6*, 3. [CrossRef]
38. Pan, D.S.T.; Huang, J.H.; Lee, M.H.M.; Yu, Y.; Chen, M.I.C.; Goh, E.H.; Jiang, L.; Chong, J.W.C.; Leo, Y.S.; Lee, T.H.; et al. Knowledge, attitudes and practices towards antibiotic use in upper respiratory tract infections among patients seeking primary health care in Singapore. *BMC Fam. Pract.* **2016**, *17*, 1–9. [CrossRef]
39. Ikai, H.; Morimoto, T.; Shimbo, T.; Imanaka, Y.; Koike, K. Impact of postgraduate education on physician practice for community-acquired pneumonia. *J. Eval. Clin. Pract.* **2012**, *18*, 389–395. [CrossRef] [PubMed]
40. Linder, J.A.; Singer, D.E. Desire for Antibiotics and Antibiotic Prescribing for Adults with Upper Respiratory Tract Infections. *J. Gen. Intern. Med.* **2003**, *18*, 795–801. [CrossRef] [PubMed]
41. Al-Homaidan, H.T.; Barrimah, I.E. Physicians' knowledge, expectations, and practice regarding antibiotic use in primary health care. *Int. J. Health Sci.* **2018**, *12*, 18–24.
42. Davey, P.; Pagliari, C.; Hayes, A. The patient's role in the spread and control of bacterial resistance to antibiotics. *Clin. Microbiol. Infect.* **2002**, *8*, 43–68. [CrossRef]
43. Llor, C.; Bjerrum, L. Antimicrobial resistance: Risk associated with antibiotic overuse and initiatives to reduce the problem. *Ther. Adv. Drug Saf.* **2014**, *5*, 229–241. [CrossRef] [PubMed]
44. Shively, N.R.; Buehrle, D.J.; Clancy, C.J.; Decker, B.K. Prevalence of Inappropriate Antibiotic Prescribing in Primary Care Clinics within a Veterans Affairs Health Care System. *Antimicrob. Agents Chemother.* **2018**, *62*. [CrossRef]
45. Terrível, J.; Terrível, J.; Teixeira Rodrigues, A.; Ferreira, M.; Ferreira, M.; Neves, C.; Neves, C.; Roque, F.; Roque, F.; Da Cruz e Silva, O.A.B.; et al. Conhecimento dos médicos relativo à prescrição de antibióticos e à resistência microbiana: Estudo piloto de comparação de questionário online vs papel. *Rev. Epidemiol. e Control. Infecção* **2014**, *3*, 93. [CrossRef]
46. Labi, A.K.; Obeng-Nkrumah, N.; Bjerrum, S.; Aryee, N.A.A.; Ofori-Adjei, Y.A.; Yawson, A.E.; Newman, M.J. Physicians' knowledge, attitudes, and perceptions concerning antibiotic resistance: A survey in a Ghanaian tertiary care hospital. *BMC Health Serv. Res.* **2018**, *18*, 126. [CrossRef] [PubMed]
47. Wester, C.W.; Durairaj, L.; Evans, A.T.; Schwartz, D.N.; Husain, S.; Martinez, E. Antibiotic resistance: A survey of physician perceptions. *Arch. Intern. Med.* **2002**, *162*, 2210–2216. [CrossRef] [PubMed]
48. Voidăzan, S.; Moldovan, G.; Voidăzan, L.; Zazgyva, A.; Moldovan, H. Knowledge, Attitudes And Practices Regarding The Use Of Antibiotics. Study on The General Population of Mureş County, Romania. *Infect. Drug Resist.* **2019**, *12*, 3385–3396. [CrossRef] [PubMed]
49. Barclay, S.; Todd, C.; Finlay, I.; Grande, G.; Wyatt, P. Not another questionnaire! Maximizing the response rate, predicting non-response and assessing non-response bias in postal questionnaire studies of GPs. *Fam. Pract.* **2002**, *19*, 105–111. [CrossRef]
50. Sibbald, B.; Addington-Hall, J.; Brenneman, D.; Freeling, P. Telephone versus postal surveys of general practitioners: Methodological considerations. *Br. J. Gen. Pract.* **1994**, *44*, 297–300.
51. PORDATA PORDATA—Médicos e Outro Pessoal de Saúde por 100 mil Habitants. Available online: https://www.pordata.pt/Portugal/Médicos+e+outro+pessoal+de+saúde+por+100+mil+habitantes-639 (accessed on 29 April 2021).

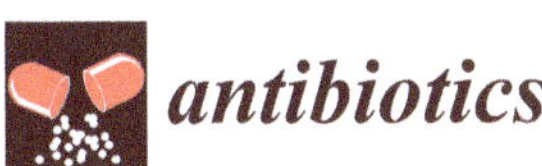 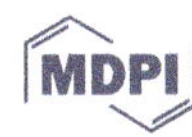

Article

Knowledge and Attitudes about Antibiotics and Antibiotic Resistance of 2404 UK Healthcare Workers

Diane Ashiru-Oredope [1,*], Ella Casale [1], Eleanor Harvey [1], Eno Umoh [1], Sagar Vasandani [1], Jacqui Reilly [2,3] and Susan Hopkins [1]

1 HCAI, Fungal, AMR, AMU & Sepsis Division, United Kingdom Health Security Agency, London SW1P 3JR, UK
2 NHS National Services Scotland, Edinburgh EH12 9EB, UK
3 Department of Nursing and Community Health, Glasgow Caledonian University, Glasgow G4 0BA, UK
* Correspondence: diane.ashiru-oredope@ukhsa.gov.uk

Abstract: Background: Using the COM-B model as a framework, an EU-wide survey aimed to ascertain multidisciplinary healthcare workers' (HCWs') knowledge, attitudes and behaviours towards antibiotics, antibiotic use and antibiotic resistance. The UK findings are presented here. Methods: A 43-item questionnaire was developed through a two-round modified Delphi consensus process. The UK target quota was 1315 respondents. Results: In total, 2404 participants responded. The highest proportion were nursing and midwifery professionals (42%), pharmacists (23%) and medical doctors (18%). HCWs correctly answered that antibiotics are not effective against viruses (97%), they have associated side effects (97%), unnecessary use makes antibiotics ineffective (97%) and healthy people can carry antibiotic-resistant bacteria (90%). However, fewer than 80% correctly answered that using antibiotics increases a patient's risk of antimicrobial resistant infection or that resistant bacteria can spread from person to person. Whilst the majority of HCWs (81%) agreed there is a connection between their antibiotic prescribing behaviour and the spread of antibiotic-resistant bacteria, only 64% felt that they have a key role in controlling antibiotic resistance. The top three barriers to providing advice or resources were lack of resources (19%), insufficient time (11%) and the patient being uninterested in the information (7%). Approximately 35% of UK respondents who were prescribers prescribed an antibiotic at least once in the previous week to responding to the survey due to a fear of patient deterioration or complications. Conclusion: These findings highlight that a multifaceted approach to tackling the barriers to prudent antibiotic use in the UK is required and provides evidence for guiding targeted policy, intervention development and future research. Education and training should focus on patient communication, information on spreading resistant bacteria and increased risk for individuals.

Keywords: anti-infective; antimicrobial; antimicrobial resistance; behaviour change; healthcare workers; antimicrobial stewardship

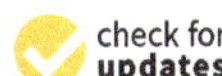

Citation: Ashiru-Oredope, D.; Casale, E.; Harvey, E.; Umoh, E.; Vasandani, S.; Reilly, J.; Hopkins, S. Knowledge and Attitudes about Antibiotics and Antibiotic Resistance of 2404 UK Healthcare Workers. *Antibiotics* **2022**, *11*, 1133. https://doi.org/10.3390/antibiotics11081133

Academic Editor: Marc Maresca

Received: 30 June 2022
Accepted: 5 August 2022
Published: 21 August 2022

Publisher's Note: MDPI stays neutral with regard to jurisdictional claims in published maps and institutional affiliations.

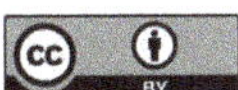

Copyright: © 2022 by the authors. Licensee MDPI, Basel, Switzerland. This article is an open access article distributed under the terms and conditions of the Creative Commons Attribution (CC BY) license (https://creativecommons.org/licenses/by/4.0/).

1. Introduction

In England, antimicrobial resistant infections increased between 2016 and 2019, peaking at an estimated 65,192 infections in 2019 [1]. Nationally and internationally, several policy papers have emphasised the need to address this globally recognised, complex threat to human health [2–5]. The UK's five-year National Action Plan (NAP) to tackle antimicrobial resistance (AMR) emphasises the importance of reducing our need for, and exposure to, antimicrobials, and optimising the use of these life-saving drugs in humans and animals. Healthcare workers' (HCWs') practices impact infections and antimicrobial use; therefore, they are vital in our efforts to tackle AMR. Moreover, HCWs play an instrumental role in implementing antimicrobial stewardship interventions, highlighting the necessity of understanding their knowledge, attitudes and behaviour towards antibiotics, antibiotic use and AMR.

To support HCWs in tackling AMR, Public Health England (PHE) published a resources toolkit aimed at healthcare workers in 2014, which outlines key actions HCWs can take to help combat AMR [6]. Studies and public health campaigns that investigate and target the general public's knowledge and understanding of antibiotics and antibiotic resistance have been conducted [7,8]. The literature reports good basic knowledge with areas for improvement, such as targeting the misunderstanding that these drugs can be used to treat viral infections [9,10]. Evidence also exists for a subset of medical prescribers and nurses. Earlier studies have reported good knowledge of antibiotics among nurse practitioners and their intention to prescribe antibiotics appropriately [11,12]. Factors impacting nurse and physician prescribing have included patient pressure, fear, complacency and time [12,13]. Although there is some evidence for medical prescribers and nurses, a gap remains in the literature regarding multidisciplinary HCWs' knowledge, attitudes and behaviours towards this topic [11–15].

The European Centre for Disease Prevention and Control (ECDC) funded the first multiprofessional study across 30 European Union (EU) and European Economic Area (EEA) countries to assess HCWs' baseline knowledge, attitudes and behaviours surrounding antibiotics in 2019. This paper presents the results for the United Kingdom and aims to:

- Assess the knowledge, attitudes and behaviour of UK HCWs (including prescribers) in regard to antibiotics and antibiotic use and resistance;
- Determine baseline data from a pre-COVID-19 pandemic landscape to allow for the future comparison of the impact of the pandemic on antimicrobial awareness and response and inform policy and interventions;
- Support the evaluation of UK communication campaigns (UK National Action Plan (NAP), Antibiotic Guardian and the Keep Antibiotics Working (KAW) campaign) and international awareness activities (World Antimicrobial Awareness Week (WAAW) and European Antibiotic Awareness Day (EAAD)) which have been targeting HCWs for over a decade.

2. Materials and Methods

This study was part of a wider 2019 ECDC-funded survey across 30 EU/EEA countries. The full methodology is described elsewhere [16,17]. Using the COM-B model of behaviour change as a framework, this study sought to understand the capabilities (C), opportunities (O) and motivations (M) which enable prudent behaviour (B) about antibiotic use amongst healthcare workers in the UK [18].

The COM-B model was selected to underpin the questionnaire and analysis because it is a comprehensive synthesis and integration of at least 19 models of behaviour change [19]. The COM-B model proposes that behaviour is an interaction involving three essential components: the 'capability' (C) to perform the behaviour and the 'opportunity' (O) and 'motivation' (M) to carry out the behaviour. Studies of the model have shown that to affect behaviour change, any introduced interventions must influence as least one of these three components, so as to reshape behaviour and minimise setbacks [18].

The final questionnaire is available in the Supplementary Materials. Perceived and actual capability were measured to assess HCWs' knowledge. Perceived capability was assessed via self-reported understanding of antibiotic use and antibiotic resistance; participants were asked 3 questions about their own understanding. Actual capability was assessed via a 7-question knowledge test, with additional questions to assess one health and hand hygiene topics. Participants were asked 3 opportunity statements to assess whether they have the opportunity to contribute to tackling AMR; these focused on access to guidelines and materials and whether they were able to provide advice to patients. Motivation statements were utilised to assess attitudes towards antibiotics and their use. Behaviour investigated included the frequency of prescribing and whether HCWs gave out resources and advice.

A Project Advisory Group (PAG) consisting of 87 nominated individuals across 51 organisations and countries within the EU and EEA was established in 2018, of these 2 were from the UK. Following a systematic review of the literature, the PAG participated in a two-round Delphi consensus process to develop the questionnaire tool. The final 43-item questionnaire was developed following a pilot of the survey across the EU/EEA, translation into 25 European languages and validation.

PAG members disseminated the validated online survey to HCWs in each of the 30 included countries. Multiple dissemination routes were used in the UK including email cascade via national AMR groups with representation from multidisciplinary professional groups asking them to cascade wider and social media, using the hashtag #ECDCAntibioticSurvey on Twitter. The information provided to survey participants is available in the Supplementary Materials. The questionnaire was live for 6 weeks, from 28 January to 4 March 2019. Participation was voluntary. Data were collected anonymously, with the option to submit contact details. Public Health England was responsible for housing all data securely and as per the General Data Protection Regulation 2016/679.

The statements used a five-point Likert score; for the purposes of this report, agreed and strongly agreed were merged in the text and reported as agreed.

The minimum survey sample size was obtained via quota sampling with the aim of generating a representative sample from different healthcare worker groups and countries and capturing different demographics, specialties, levels of experience and sectors of healthcare [16]. The sample size for the UK was calculated by determining 0.2% of practicing physicians (365/182,534), dentists (70/34,867) and pharmacists (113/56,542) and 0.1% of nursing professionals (548/548,291) available through EU/EEA healthcare personnel statistics of healthcare workers [17,20].

Data were analysed using Microsoft® Excel (2010) and STATA release 15. Descriptive statistical analysis was undertaken to analyse HCW capability, opportunity, motivation and behaviour.

The results of the UK study were shared with thirty-four attendees across the UK devolved administrations in June 2020 to inform recommendations.

Ethical statement: The data for this study were extracted from and comply with the ethical statement for the research undertaken by Ashiru-Oredope et al. [16]. Informed consent was provided prior to participation. The original study was part of an evaluation of the EU EAAD communications campaign which commenced in 2008 and included significant input in development and distribution from the PAG. The PAG officially represented all participating countries and European professional groups and organisations.

3. Results

3.1. Demographics

In the EU/EEA multicountry study, 18,365 HCWs responded to the online survey. Of these, 2404 participants were from the UK, equating to 13% of the EU/EEA total and the largest proportion among all 30 countries involved. The highest number of responses was collected from England (51%), followed by Scotland (40%), Wales (7%) and Northern Ireland (2%) (Supplementary Table S1). The highest number of participants stratified by English region were from the North West (23%), London (15%) and the South West (12%) (Supplementary Figure S1).

The UK exceeded its quota sample size by 979 responses, achieving 174% of the desired target (Supplementary Table S2). In England, Scotland and Wales, nursing professionals (nurses, nursing assistants and midwives) had the highest response rate (40%), followed by pharmacists (22%) and medical doctors (18%) (Supplementary Table S3). In Northern Ireland, pharmacists constituted the largest respondent group, followed by medical professionals and scientists. Healthcare students were not included in this sample.

Similarly to the EU/EEA survey results, most UK participants were female (77%), 21% were male and 1% preferred not to state their sex (Supplementary Table S4). UK respondents were mostly aged between 36 and 55 years (59%), 23% were under 36 years and 17% over 55 years. Respondents predominantly practised in hospitals (58%) or the community (31%).

In total, 24% of UK respondents used Facebook and 23% used Twitter for professional purposes. (Supplementary Table S5). Almost half of UK respondents (44%) did not use any social media for professional purposes.

3.2. Perceived Capability

The majority (96%) of UK respondents agreed or strongly agreed that they 'know what antibiotic resistance is' (Figure 1). Over three-quarters (78%) agreed or strongly agreed that they had sufficient knowledge on using antibiotics in their practice, and 80% agreed or strongly agreed that they know what information to provide to their patients on the prudent use of antibiotics and antibiotic resistance.

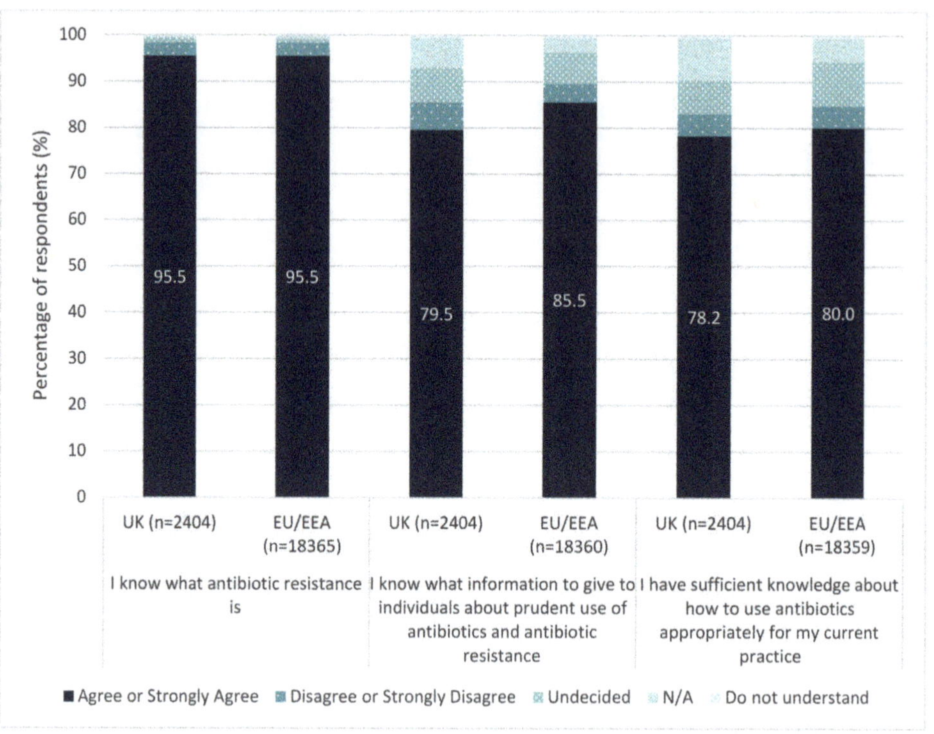

Figure 1. UK respondents' perceived capability.

3.3. Actual Capability Assessed by Seven Knowledge Test Questions

The highest proportion of correct answers in the UK were given to the true or false questions: 'Antibiotics are effective against cold and flu' (answer = false) (98% false and 2% true); 'Taking antibiotics has associated side effects or risks such as diarrhoea, colitis, allergies' (answer = true) (97% true and 3% false); and 'Unnecessary use of antibiotics make them become ineffective' (answer = true) (97% true and 3% false) (Figure 2). Over 90% of HCWs knew that healthy people can carry antibiotic-resistant bacteria.

The question that was answered incorrectly by the most respondents was 'Antibiotic resistant bacteria can spread from person to person' (answer = true) (22% of respondents incorrectly answered false), which was higher than the percentage of incorrect answers from the EU/EEA respondents (13%) for that same question. The second statement with the most incorrect answers in the UK was 'Every person treated with antibiotics is at an increased risk of antibiotic resistant infection' (answer = true) (20% incorrectly answered false); this question had a higher rate of incorrect answers from the EU/EEA respondents (25%).

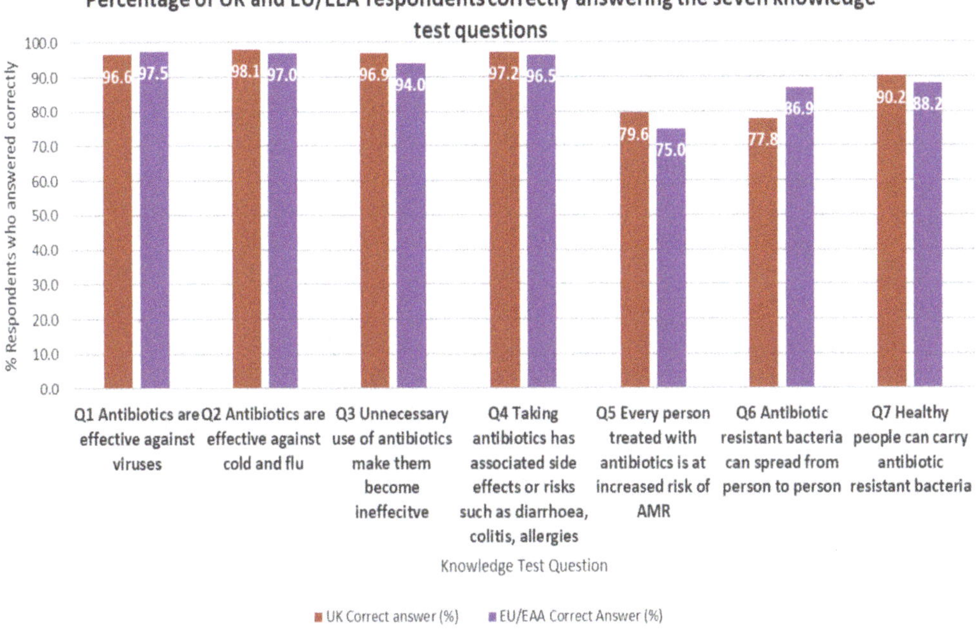

Figure 2. Percentage of UK (n = 2403) and EU/EEA respondents (n = 18,348) correctly answering the seven knowledge test questions.

In total, 59.4% of UK participants were able to answer all seven knowledge questions correctly. The EU/EEA average was 58%.

The answers to the knowledge test questions varied across professional groups. Medical doctors demonstrated the best knowledge of AMR (80% answered all questions correctly), followed by pharmacists (74%), dentists (68%) and scientists (62%) (Supplementary Figure S2). Only medical doctors had all the representatives scoring a minimum of five out of seven correct answers. Questions 5 and 6 were answered most correctly by medical doctors (86% and 96%, respectively (Supplementary Figure S3).

The percentage of respondents answering all seven questions correctly varied across the devolved administrations (54–80%). Northern Ireland had the highest proportion of respondents answering all seven questions correctly (80%, n = 41) (Supplementary Table S6). Across the EU/EEA, no country had 100% of respondents achieve 7/7 in the knowledge score.

Less than a quarter (23%) of UK participants correctly answered that the use of antibiotics to stimulate growth in farm animals is illegal in the EU (Supplementary Table S7). Almost half of respondents said they could list the WHO's five moments of hand hygiene (Supplementary Table S8).

3.4. Opportunities

Four out of five (80%) UK respondents stated having easy access to guidelines, compared to 75% of EU/EEA participants (Table 1). Only 62% of practitioners in the UK felt they have good opportunities to provide advice on prudent antibiotic use to individuals, compared to 72% of EU/EEA participants.

Table 1. Percentage of respondents who agreed or strongly agreed with the opportunity statements.

Statement	UK	EU/EEA
I have easy access to guidelines I need on managing infections (UK, n = 2291; EU/EEA, n = 14,301)	79.7%	75.1%
I have easy access to the materials I need to give advice on prudent antibiotic use and antibiotic resistance (UK, n = 2291; EU/EEA, n = 14,299)	67.5%	67.5%
I have good opportunities to provide advice on prudent antibiotic use to individuals (UK, n = 2291; EU/EEA, n = 14,296)	61.6%	72.3%

3.5. *Motivation/Attitude towards Antibiotic Resistance*

The majority (81%) of respondents who were prescribers agreed there was a connection between their prescribing and the emergence and spread of antibiotic-resistant bacteria, yet only 64% felt they have a key role in controlling antibiotic resistance (Supplementary Figure S4).

Across the devolved administrations, the percentage of survey participants agreeing with the motivation statements varied, ranging from 79% in Wales to 88% in Northern Ireland (Supplementary Figure S5).

3.6. *Behaviour (Giving out Resources or Advice) and Barriers*

In total, 59% of UK respondents had prescribed, administered or dispensed antibiotics at least once in the previous week (Supplementary Table S9), while almost 14% of the UK participants had not prescribed, administered or dispensed any antibiotics.

Of the prescribers, 21% had given out resources (e.g., leaflets or pamphlets) and 61% had given out advice on prudent antibiotic use at least once in the previous week to participating in the survey (Supplementary Figure S6).

The most common reasons respondents (n = 1671) gave for not providing resources or advice as frequently as they prescribed, administered or dispensed antibiotics were lack of resources (19%), insufficient time (11%) and the patient being uninterested in the information (7%) (Supplementary Table S10). Only 8% of HCWs stated they were able to give out advice or resources as needed.

3.7. *Awareness of National Initiatives and Campaigns, and Perceived Effectiveness*

Almost two-thirds (63%) of survey participants agreed that there has been good promotion of prudent antibiotic use and antibiotic resistance in the UK (Supplementary Figure S7). The results varied among HCWs across the devolved administrations (Supplementary Figure S8), with the most respondents agreeing from Northern Ireland (76%) and the least from Wales (54%).

Fifty-eight percent of UK respondents were aware of the National Action Plan (Figure 3). Less than half of respondents were aware of either EAAD (46% aware) or WAAW (45%), and approximately 30% felt that national campaigns had been effective. Respondents in the UK were mostly undecided (55%) on the campaign's effectiveness. Comparative data for the EU/EEA is available in Supplementary Figure S9. Focusing in on the UK constituent countries, participants from England agreed the most that national campaigns are effective (32%), whereas participants from Northern Ireland disagreed the most (24%) (Supplementary Figure S10).

Across the UK as a whole, the most commonly known resources were the National Institute for Health and Care Excellence (NICE) guidelines (49%), Treat Antibiotics Responsibly, Guidance, Education and Tools (TARGET) (31%) and Antibiotic Guardian (30%) (Figure 4). The most commonly used resources were the NICE guidelines (34%), resources other than those listed (32%) and Antibiotic Guardian (AG) (24%). Across the devolved nations results varied; however, NICE guidelines were the most commonly known and used resource across the four countries (Supplementary Figure S11).

In total, 49% percent of respondents stated they were Antibiotic Guardians; however, only 21% could recall their pledge (Supplementary Figure S12). Results varied across the four nations; England had the highest percentage of Guardians (56%) and Scotland the lowest (31%) (Supplementary Figure S12). Over three-quarters (76%) of UK HCW respondents had seen or heard the KAW advert on television (TV) or radio (Supplementary Figure S13).

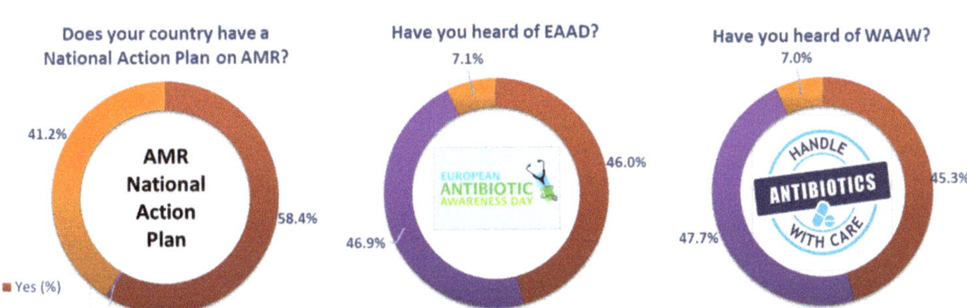

Figure 3. Awareness of campaigns in the UK; NAP (n = 2060), EAAD (n = 2070) and WAAW (n = 2054).

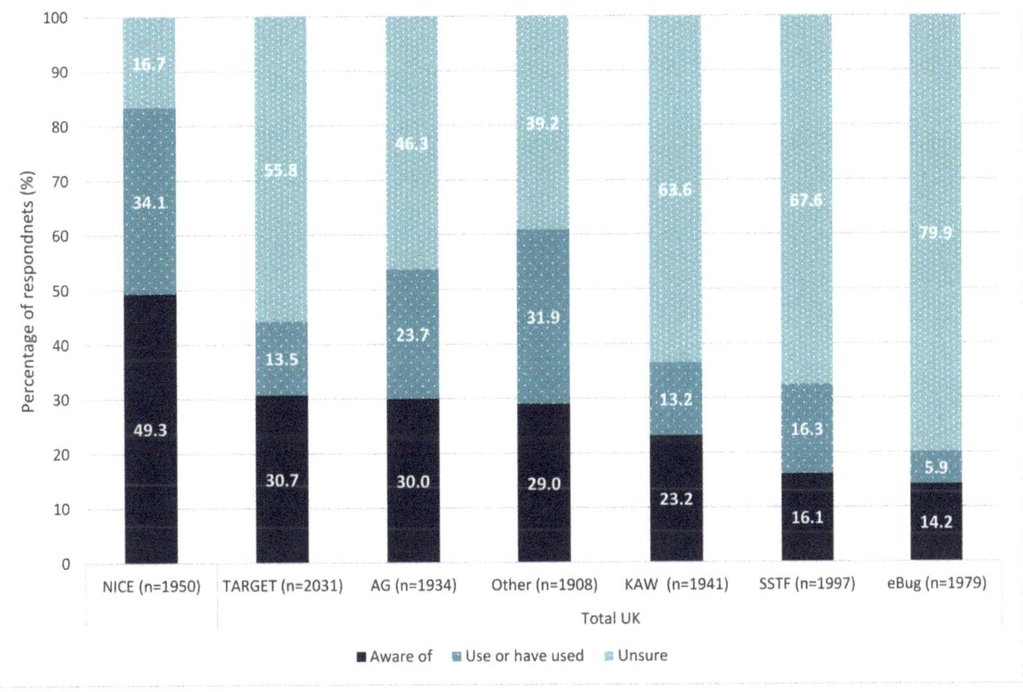

Figure 4. Awareness of campaigns, projects and platforms related to antibiotic use and AMR in the UK.

Less than a third (29%) of UK respondents stated they were prescribers of antibiotics, the majority of which were medical doctors (46%), then nurses (29%) and pharmacists (19%) (Supplementary Table S11). The majority of prescribers agreed they considered antibiotic resistance when treating a patient (92%), they have a key role to play in helping control antibiotic resistance (88%) and they are confident when making antibiotic-prescribing decisions (90%) (Table 2). Almost all prescribers were confident in the antibiotic guidelines available (96%), and they have easy access to those guidelines (94%).

Almost three-quarters (74%) of respondents agreed they feel supported not to prescribe antibiotics when they are not necessary. Over 20% of prescribers prescribed an antibiotic at least once in the past week when they would have preferred not to (Figure 5). The reasons given for this were the fear of patient deterioration or complications (34%) and uncertainty in their diagnosis (25%).

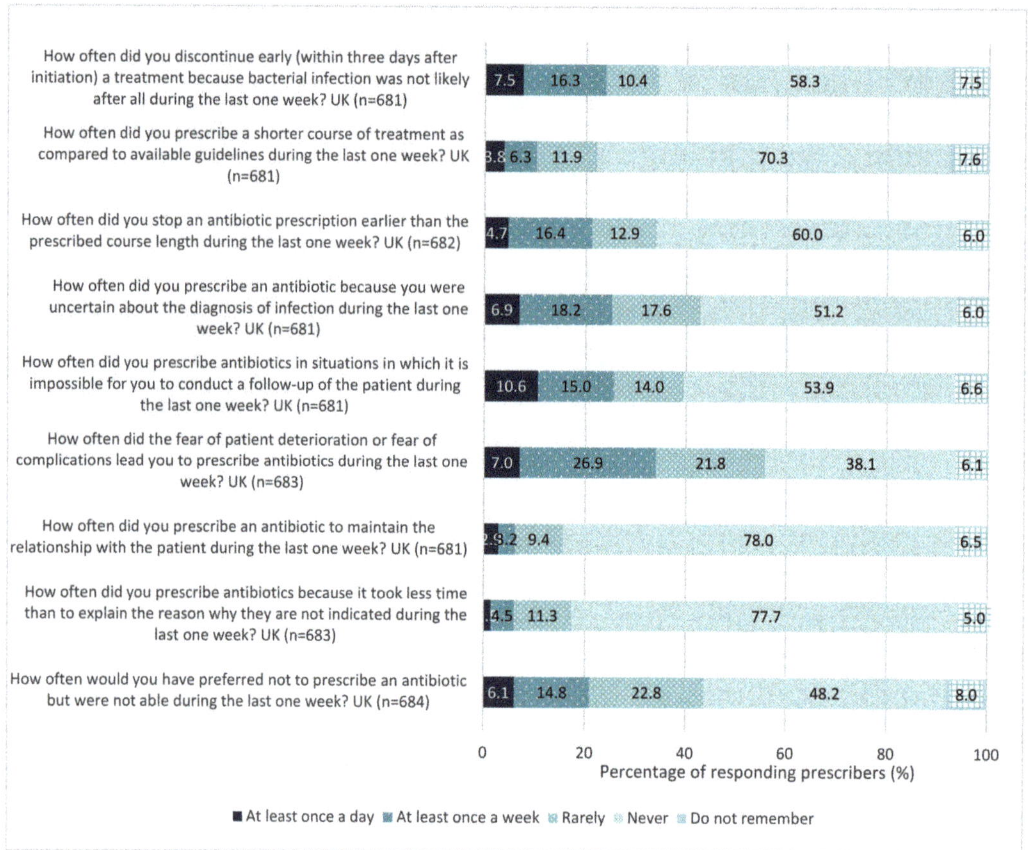

Figure 5. Reasons prescribers initiated antibiotic prescriptions when they would have preferred not to in the previous week, UK, 2019.

Table 2. Responses from UK prescribers to the motivation statements.

Motivation Statement	Agree or Strongly Agree	Disagree or Strongly Disagree	Undecided	Do Not Understand the Question
I am confident making antibiotic prescribing decisions (*n* = 682)	90.0	3.2	6.6	0.1
I have confidence in the antibiotic guidelines available to me (*n* = 681)	95.6	1.5	2.8	0.1
I have a key role in helping control antibiotic resistance (*n* = 681)	88.4	3.7	7.6	0.3
I consider antibiotic resistance when treating a patient (*n* = 681)	91.6	3.1	5.0	0.3
I have easy access to antibiotic guidelines I need to treat infections (*n* = 681)	94.0	1.9	4.0	0.1
I feel supported to not prescribe antibiotic when they are not necessary (*n* = 680)	74.3	8.4	17.1	0.3

3.8. Summary Recommendations for Action from Stakeholder Workshop

- Further analysis of the data should be undertaken to compare differences across professional groups and differences across settings.
- Sepsis messaging should be more strongly linked to antimicrobial resistance and focus on preventative measures.
- Facebook presents an opportunity to engage with UK healthcare workers. Campaigns, initiatives and interventions should be promoted on both Twitter and Facebook.
- Key organisations should be encouraged to produce a short video for WAAW outlining their AMR and AMS activities and available resources.
- All recommendations should align with the COM-B behaviour change wheel.

4. Discussion

This is the first UK-wide study assessing multidisciplinary HCWs' knowledge, attitudes and behaviour towards antibiotics, antibiotic use and resistance. As a sub-study of the multicountry EU/EEA survey, the UK results present the most comprehensive and detailed dataset for the UK so far, with responses from 2404 participants across a variety of age groups, professions and prescribing settings. All data were collected prior to the COVID-19 pandemic, providing insight into a population's baseline level prior to the widespread communication of prescribing measures that occurred throughout the pandemic. This analysis gives evidence for developing interventions targeted at HCWs, informing policy making, improving the reach and impact of public awareness campaigns and supporting HCWs with their antimicrobial stewardship.

The study exceeded its calculated quota sample by 74%, significantly increasing the generalisability and validity of the results at a country level. The UK constituted the largest proportion of respondents across the EU, equating to 13% of the total participants. However, it is worth noting that the majority of UK responses were from participants in England (50%) and Scotland (40%), limiting the direct application of these results to Northern Ireland and Wales and biasing the results to be more representative of Scotland in the context of the UK population. Volunteer bias risk is high in surveys; it is likely that those HCWs most interested in AMR completed the survey. Equally, it is possible that the wider prescribing population may not have the same level of interest and awareness of AMR. The authors also acknowledge the survey did not include the assessment of all elements of antimicrobial stewardship HCWs may utilise. Additional clinical decision and support tools, such as Electronic Health Records, and quality improvement initiatives, such as auditing, are valuable AMS strategies.

A key strength is the representation across all healthcare settings. In addition, the quota sample size was exceeded for key healthcare professional groups who prescribe, administer or dispense antibiotics such as physicians, nurses and pharmacists. [21]. In the UK, the largest groups of survey respondents were nurses and pharmacists, these two professions made up the highest percentage of the target sample size, at 175% and 462%, respectively (Supplementary Table S2). This emphasises the need to target future interventions and communications to these engaged groups and reinforces that they, along with physicians, can contribute to positive change in combating AMR. This differed to the EU/EEA in which physicians made up the greatest proportion of respondents, followed by nurses and pharmacists [16]. This is to be expected, as in mainland Europe, only medical doctors are able to prescribe.

The findings highlighted gaps in knowledge across all healthcare professional groups. Although HCWs understood the risk of side effects to the patient, fewer understood that antibiotic use increases a person's risk of AMR. Similarly, despite over 90% of HCWs understanding that healthy people can be colonised with antibiotic-resistant bacteria, one in five UK HCWs knew resistant bacteria can spread between people. It is important that prescribers understand the wider implications of AMR on patient outcomes. The positive results in the knowledge test correlate with earlier studies; in the United States,

Hamilton et al. found that 97% (n = 194) of nurse practitioners understood antibiotics can harm the patient and inappropriate use can cause resistance (97%) [11].

Overall, EU/EEA knowledge was stronger than the UK's regarding spread, but marginally weaker when it came to understanding a patient's increased risk of AMR. Future campaigns should consider including messages on the transmission of AMR, addressing the gap in knowledge identified through this study. National and local educational groups could also include these messages within their infection-related training materials.

Access to guidelines for managing infections was high in the UK (78%); however, fewer HCWs had access to the materials needed to provide advice and opportunities to provide that advice (68% and 62%, respectively). Improving opportunities to provide advice is a particular area of concern in the UK, as fewer UK respondents agreed with this statement in comparison to the EU/EEA as a whole. Increasing access to resources, as well as improving opportunities for HCWs to provide advice to patients on beneficial and judicious antibiotic use, are key to maximising HCWs' antimicrobial stewardship (AMS) capabilities. Intervention types should align with the behaviour change wheel [18] and focus on training, environmental restructuring, modelling exemplar behaviours and enablement [22] to produce durable development and improvement.

All HCWs can contribute to tackling AMR via good infection prevention and control practices; however, only 63.9% of respondents felt they had a key role in controlling AMR. As would be expected, the equivalent figure was higher in prescribers, where 88.4% felt they had a key role. Further engagement with HCWs should focus on empowering them in optimal AMS prescribing practices and reinforcing their vital role in tackling resistance. Educating HCWs on the wider context of One Health actions and impact may encourage their ensuing motivation for behaviour change, highlighting the importance prescribing behaviour can have on this global health challenge [23].

Findings from this study provide insight into the reasons why practitioners do not give AMS advice and are reinforced by the EU/EEA survey results. A lack of resources is the most frequently cited barrier (19% of respondents) to giving out advice. This can be addressed by implementing patient educational resources about antibiotics and resistance and making them easily accessible for practitioners. Resources should be accompanied by national and local campaigns to increase awareness and outline their purpose for use. These findings provide evidence of the need to further promotion and dissemination of available AMS resources such as TARGET (Treat Antibiotics Responsibly, Guidance, Education and Tools), EAAD/WAAW resources, When Should I Worry' patient brochure or 'Treating Your Infection' patient leaflet. More than half of respondents answered 'unsure' when asked if they were aware of or have used the TARGET resources; in a small evaluation of TARGET resources, participants (including HCWs) have reported these resources are useful, reinforcing the value of further dissemination [24]. A limitation of this study is that it is not known whether participants who had access to the resources were more likely to provide advice on antibiotics. It is also pertinent to understand barriers and enablers to their use. Insufficient time was cited as the second most common barrier to providing advice across both the UK and EU/EEA. This is concordant with the UK finding that only 62% of HCWs felt they had sufficient opportunity to provide advice on antibiotics (Table 1).

It is important to consider all barriers associated with prudent prescribing, taking into account the professional group, and investigate them further in order to best support HCWs to overcome these challenges. The fear of patient deterioration or complications was the foremost reason (34% of respondents), both in primary and secondary care settings, for issuing an antibiotic prescription, and uncertainty in diagnosis was the second most common reason (25%). These findings correlate with the literature; fear has been cited as a common barrier to tackling AMR amongst community healthcare providers and physicians, alongside patient pressure, time and systemic overworking [12,13,25,26].

Other factors to consider include consultation time constraints, prescriber–patient relationships and patient awareness and expectations in receiving antibiotic prescriptions.

Further qualitative research is warranted to improve our understanding of these factors and implement useful and successful interventions.

International and national campaigns provide means through which to reach more population numbers. WAAW and EAAD managed to reach nearly half of the UK respondents, with 45% stating they were aware of WAAW, and 46% were aware of EAAD. Nationally, 76% of UK HCWs had seen or heard the KAW advert on TV or radio. Conversely, in answer to a separate question, only 36% of respondents stated they were aware of or had used KAW materials.

Tackling AMR requires engagement at individual, population and government levels. The Antibiotic Guardian (AG) initiative, of which more than half of the study cohort (53.7%) are aware of or have used, includes the proactive engagement of 'pledging' [26]. The evaluation of the AG campaign demonstrated an increased commitment of healthcare workers, scientists/educators and the public in tackling AMR, increased self-reported knowledge and changed self-reported behaviour, particularly among people with prior AMR awareness [27,28]. Pledging has been identified as an effective and inexpensive driver for behaviour change relating to antibiotic use [27]. It provides individuals with concrete actions and examples of how to tackle AMR and at the same time includes them in the collective movement to drive change.

The survey identified that Facebook was the most popular social media platform used by UK HCW respondents for professional use. This communication channel presents an opportunity to disseminate information and engage with HCWs. A significant proportion (44%) of participants did not use any of the social media platforms listed. In future surveys, it would be worth expanding communication efforts beyond social media channels to engage with participants in a more inclusive manner, ultimately increasing impact.

It is important that the UK considers the findings of this study and advocates for next steps and actions to tackle the public health threat of AMR. This study provides baseline data for policy makers on AMR awareness and AMS involvement within the HCW population. It would be insightful to undertake the survey in the wake of the COVID-19 pandemic, to help assess what, if any the impact pandemic may have had (with the consistent infection prevention and control measure messages), on HCW populations and their awareness of AMR and AMS. Moreover, conducting regular surveys to evaluate ongoing initiatives would be valuable in order to measure impacts and identify areas for improvement.

The implementation of actions at both national and local levels is imperative to changing practice and behaviour. The effectiveness of interventions on improving antibiotic prescribing depends on prescribing behaviours and on perceived and actual barriers to change. Multifaceted educational interventions occurring on multiple levels will only be effective after local barriers to change are addressed [29–31]. Educational, training or communications materials for HCWs in the UK should consider the findings of this study when developing content/curriculum and embed behaviour change strategies as part of developing interventions.

5. Conclusions

These findings strengthen our understanding of UK HCWs' knowledge, attitudes and behaviours towards antibiotics and antibiotic resistance and provide an evidence base for guiding future AMS activities, interventions and research priorities. The results highlight HCWs' comprehension of AMR; however, specific knowledge gaps across professional groups should be targeted in future educational initiatives. Training materials should address the risk of AMR spread and the impact this has for individuals and the public. Resources, initiatives and future campaigns should be promoted across a variety of social media platforms to maximise engagement with UK HCWs. Further evaluation is needed to identify the most effective method for communicating with practitioners that do not use social media professionally. The findings identify potential barriers faced by HCWs. Subsequent evaluation is needed of the barriers and enablers to inform future interventions on improving awareness of and access to antibiotic resources, increasing the opportunity for HCWs to use these resources and supporting prescribers not to prescribe when they feel antibiotics are not needed. Future surveys should be undertaken to longitudinally inform and evaluate strategies in this field. Research on novel interventions should embed behaviour change strategies, aligning with the behaviour change wheel, to produce effective, long-lasting and positive behaviours relating to antibiotics and their use.

Supplementary Materials: The following supporting information can be downloaded at: https://www.mdpi.com/article/10.3390/antibiotics11081133/s1, Supplementary Material. Table S1: UK responses across the devolved administrations; Figure S1: Participation in the survey by region in England; Table S2: UK quota sample size and responses to the survey; Table S3: Percentage of UK respondents by profession; Table S4 Respondents' age, gender and professional setting; Table S5: Percentage of UK and EU/EEA respondents that use the different social media platforms; Figure S2: The percentage of respondents answering all seven knowledge test questions correctly - by profession; Figure S3a: Percentage of respondents answering question 5 correctly, by professional group; Figure S3b: Percentage of respondents answering question 6 correctly, by professional group; Table S6: Respondents answering all seven knowledge test questions correctly, by UK constituent; Table S7: Respondents answering the One Health knowledge question correctly; Table S8: Respondents answering the Hand Hygiene knowledge question correctly; Figure S4: Percentage of respondents who agree with the following motivation statements; Figure S5: Percentage of UK respondents agreeing to the motivation statements (by constituent); Table S9: The frequency of prescribing/administering/dispensing antibiotics during the last one week; Figure S6: Percentage of respondents that gave out resources or advice; Table S10: Barriers: Most common reasons why UK healthcare workers were unable to provide advice or resources to their patients in a one-week period; Figure S7: Percentage of respondents who agree with the campaign impact and effectiveness statements in the UK and EU/EEA; Figure S8: Percentage of respondents who agree with the campaign impact and effectiveness statements across the devolved administrations; Figure S9: Awareness of campaigns in a. the UK b. the EU/EEA; Figure S10: Perceived effectiveness of EAAD and WAAW in the UK; Figure S11: Awareness of campaigns, projects and platforms related to antibiotic use and AMR in the UK; Figure S12: Engagement with Antibiotic Guardian; Figure S13: Awareness of the Keep Antibiotics Working Campaign; Table S11: Professions of prescribers in the UK; Table S12: Setting of prescribers in the UK; Figure S14: Responses from UK prescribers to the motivation statements.

Author Contributions: Conceptualisation, D.A.-O. and S.H.; data curation, D.A.-O., E.U. and S.V.; formal analysis, E.C. and S.V.; funding acquisition, D.A.-O. and S.H.; methodology, D.A.-O., E.U., J.R. and S.H.; project administration, E.C., E.U. and S.V.; supervision, D.A.-O. and S.H.; writing—original draft, D.A.-O., E.C., E.U. and S.V.; writing—review and editing, D.A.-O., E.C., E.H., E.U., S.V., J.R. and S.H. All authors have read and agreed to the published version of the manuscript.

Funding: The survey was funded by the European Centre for Disease Prevention and Control (ECDC) through a specific service contract (ECD.8836) to Public Health England, London, United Kingdom. The analysis and interpretation of the findings was completed by the contractor.

Institutional Review Board Statement: The data for this study were extracted from and comply with the ethical statement for the research undertaken by Ashiru-Oredope et al. [16]. Informed consent was provided prior to participation. The original study was part of an evaluation of the EU EAAD communications campaign which commenced in 2008 and included significant input in development and distribution from the PAG. The PAG officially represented all participating countries and European professional groups and organisations.

Informed Consent Statement: Informed consent was obtained from all subjects involved in the study.

Data Availability Statement: Additional data from the study can be found via https://www.ecdc.europa.eu/en/publications-data/survey-healthcare-workers-knowledge-attitudes-and-behaviours-antibiotics (accessed on 1 April 2021).

Acknowledgments: The authors would like to thank all healthcare workers and individuals who promoted the survey locally/nationally or via social media. The authors would also like to thank the ECDC Project Advisory Group: Reinhild Strauss (Austria); Vinciane Charlier, Samuel Coenen (Belgium); Miranda Sertić, Marina Payerl-Pal (Croatia); Linos Hadjihannas, Costas A. Constantinou (Cyprus); Barbora Macková (Czech Republic); Lisa Bugge-Toft (Denmark); Pille Märtin, Mailis Hansen (Estonia); Outi Lyytikäinen, Jari Jalava (Finland); Anne Berger-Carbonne, Mélanie Colomb-Cotinat (France); Flora Kontopidou, Maria Foteinea (Greece); Martin Cormican, Audrey Lambourn (Ireland); Francesca Furiozzi, Michela Sabbatucci (Italy); Elīna Dimiņa, Kate Vulāne (Latvia); Virginija Kanapeckienė, Jolanta Kuklytė (Lithuania); Peter Zarb, Michael A. Borg (Malta); Renske Eilers (the Netherlands); Harald Pors Muniz (Norway); Waleria Hryniewicz, Beata Mazińska (Poland); Duarte Pedro De Sousa Tavares (Portugal); Livia Cioran, Alexandra Cucu (Romania); Eva Schreterova (Slovakia); Mitja Vrdelja, Maja Subelj (Slovenia); Rocío Bueno Parralo, Antonio López Navas (Spain); Agneta Andersson, Karin Carlin (Sweden); Jacqui Reilly, Diane Ashiru-Oredope (UK); Lea Pfefferle, Task Force on Antibiotics in Dentistry (Council of European Dentists); Petr Horák, Steffen Amann (European Association of Hospital Pharmacists); Andreas Trobisch, Lenneke Schrier (European Academy of Paediatrics); Tanguy Pinedo-Tora, Alyette Greiveldinger (European Dental Students' Association); Elena Carrara, Nico T. Mutters (European Committee on Infection Control); Charles Price (European Commission); Mathias Maucher (European Federation of Public Service Unions); Michele Calabrò (European Health Management Association); Pascal Garel, Laurie Andrieu (European Hospital and Healthcare Federation); Laura Alonso Irujo, María Santacreu García (European Joint Action on Antimicrobial Resistance and Healthcare-Associated Infections, EU-JAMRAI); Kitty Mohan, Sara Launio (European Junior Doctors Association); Orsolya Réka Süli (European Medical Students' Association); Ivana Silva (European Medicines Agency); Mervi Jokinen (European Midwives Association); Marta Simões, Ruben Viegas (European Pharmaceutical Students' Association); Ann Marie Borg, Sascha Marschang (European Public Health Alliance); Céline Pulcini (European Society of Clinical Microbiology and Infectious Diseases Study Group for Antimicrobial stewardship); Ber Oomen, Jeannette Verkerk (European Specialist Nurses Organisations); Ilaria Giannico, Paul Garassus (European Union of Private Hospitals); Roberto Bertollini, Melina Raso (Health First Europe); Tímea Rezi-Kató (MedTech Europe); Jan De Belie, Ilaria Passarani (Pharmaceutical Group of the European Union); Jacques de Haller, Carole Rouaud (Standing Committee of European Doctors); Jo Bosanquet, Wendy Nicholson (WHO Collaborating Centre for Nurses); Cristiana Salvi (WHO/Europe). The authors would also like to acknowledge individuals who contributed to the development of the survey tool or attended meetings of the Project Advisory Group, in particular: Jan Eyckmans, Herman Goossens, Anne Ingenbleek, Ann Vesporten (Belgium); Sven Pal, Edita Sušić (Croatia); Gideon Ertner (Denmark); Katja Sibenberg (Finland); Alise Gramatniece, Aija Vilde (Latvia); Roxana Serban (Romania); Elizabeth Beech, Leah Jones, Lyndsey Patterson, Muhammad Sartaj, Katherine Le Bosquet, Enrique Castro-Sanchez, Yvonne Dailey, Joanne Bosanquet, Penny Greenwood, Ayoub Saei (United Kingdom); Ana Maria Navarro Tamayo (European Joint Action on Antimicrobial Resistance and Healthcare-Associated Infections, EU-JAMRAI); Miriam D'Ambrosio (Standing Committee of European Doctors); Danilo Lo Fo Wong (WHO/Europe). In addition, the authors would like to pay gratitude to temporary members of the core team, especially Ola Oloyede and Aleksa Dubanowicz. The authors also thank attendees of the ECDC UK Findings Workshop that took place in June 2020: Alicia Demirjian, Anna Sallis, Aoife Hendrick, Bharat Patel, Ceri Phillips, Cliodna McNulty, Donna Lecky, Jacqui Sneddon, Jordan Charlesworth, Kiran Loi, Leah Jones, Mohamed Sadak, Natalie Gold, Nicholas Reid, Philip Howard, Sally Weston Price, Susie Singleton and Viviana Finistrella.

Conflicts of Interest: The authors declare no conflict of interest.

References

1. Public Health England. English Surveillance Programme for Antimicrobial Utilisation and Resistance (ESPAUR); 2020. Available online: https://www.gov.uk/government/publications/english-surveillance-programme-antimicrobial-utilisation-and-resistance-espaur-report (accessed on 21 June 2021).
2. Global and Public Health Group. *Tackling Antimicrobial Resistance 2019–2024*; Emergency Preparedness and Health Protection Policy Directorate, Global and Public Health Group: London, UK, 2019.
3. Global and Public Health Group. *The UK's 20-Year Vision for Antimicrobial Resistance*; Emergency Preparedness and Health Protection Policy Directorate, Global and Public Health Group: London, UK, 2019.
4. O'Neill, J. *Tackling Drug-Resistant Infections Globally: Final Rpeort and Recommendations*; Review on Antimicrobial Resistance: London, UK, 2016; Available online: https://amr-review.org/Publications.html (accessed on 21 June 2021).
5. WHO. *Global Action Plan on Antimicrobial Resistance*; WHO: Geneva, Switzerland, 2015.
6. England, P.H. World Antimicrobial Awareness Week (WAAW) & European Antibiotic Awareness Day (EAAD): Resources Toolkit for Healthcare Professionals in England in the Context of the COVID-19 Pandemic. 2020. Available online: https://www.gov.uk/government/publications/european-antibiotic-awareness-day-resources-toolkit-for-healthcare-professionals-in-england (accessed on 1 April 2021).

7. Redfern, J.; Bowater, L.; Coulthwaite, L.; Verran, J. Raising awareness of antimicrobial resistance among the general public in the UK: The role of public engagement activities. *JAC-Antimicrob. Resist.* **2020**, *2*, dlaa012. [CrossRef] [PubMed]
8. Kosiyaporn, H.; Chanvatik, S.; Issaramalai, T.; Kaewkhankhaeng, W.; Kulthanmanusorn, A.; Saengruang, N.; Witthayapipopsakul, W.; Viriyathorn, S.; Kirivan, S.; Kunpeuk, W.; et al. Surveys of knowledge and awareness of antibiotic use and antimicrobial resistance in general population: A systematic review. *PLoS ONE* **2020**, *15*, e0227973. [CrossRef] [PubMed]
9. McNulty, C.A.M.; Collin, S.M.; Cooper, E.; Lecky, D.M.; Butler, C.C. Public understanding and use of antibiotics in England: Findings from a household survey in 2017. *BMJ Open* **2019**, *9*, e030845. [CrossRef] [PubMed]
10. Mason, T.; Trochez, C.; Thomas, R.; Babar, M.; Hesso, I.; Kayyali, R. Knowledge and awareness of the general public and perception of pharmacists about antibiotic resistance. *BMC Public Health* **2018**, *18*, 711. [CrossRef] [PubMed]
11. Hamilton, R.M.; Merrill, K.C.; Luthy, K.E.; Nuttall, C. Knowledge, attitudes, and perceptions of nurse practitioners about antibiotic stewardship. *J. Am. Assoc. Nurse Pr.* **2020**, *33*, 909–915. [CrossRef] [PubMed]
12. Ness, V.; Currie, K.; Reilly, J.; McAloney-Kocaman, K.; Price, L. Factors associated with independent nurse prescribers' antibiotic prescribing practice: A mixed-methods study using the Reasoned Action Approach. *J. Hosp. Infect.* **2021**, *113*, 22–29. [CrossRef] [PubMed]
13. Teixeira Rodrigues, A.; Roque, F.; Falcão, A.; Figueiras, A.; Herdeiro, M.T. Understanding physician antibiotic prescribing behaviour: A systematic review of qualitative studies. *Int. J. Antimicrob. Agents* **2013**, *41*, 203–212. [CrossRef] [PubMed]
14. Ness, V.; Price, L.; Currie, K.; Reilly, J. Influences on independent nurse prescribers' antimicrobial prescribing behaviour: A systematic review. *J. Clin. Nurs.* **2016**, *25*, 1206–1217. [CrossRef] [PubMed]
15. Nuttall, D. Nurse prescribing in primary care: A metasynthesis of the literature. *Prim. Health Care Res. Amp. Dev.* **2018**, *19*, 7–22. [CrossRef] [PubMed]
16. Ashiru-Oredope, D.; Hopkins, S.; Vasandani, S.; Umoh, E.; Oloyede, O.; Nilsson, A.; Kinsman, J.; Elsert, L.; Monnet, D.L. Healthcare workers' knowledge, attitudes and behaviours with respect to antibiotics, antibiotic use and antibiotic resistance across 30 EU/EEA countries in 2019. *Eurosurveillance* **2021**, *26*, 1900633. [CrossRef] [PubMed]
17. European Centre for Disease Prevention and Control & Public Health England. *Survey of Healthcare Workers' Knowledge, Attitudes and Behaviours on Antibiotics, Antibiotic Use and Antibiotic Resistance in the EU/EEA*; European Centre for Disease Prevention and Control: Stockholm, Sweden, 2019.
18. Michie, S.; Van Stralen, M.M.; West, R. The behaviour change wheel: A new method for characterising and designing behaviour change interventions. *Implement. Sci.* **2011**, *6*, 42. [CrossRef] [PubMed]
19. Cane, J.; O'Connor, D.; Michie, S. Validation of the theoretical domains framework for use in behaviour change and implementation research. *Implement. Sci.* **2012**, *7*, 37. [CrossRef] [PubMed]
20. Eurostat. Healthcare Personnel Statistics. Available online: https://ec.europa.eu/eurostat/statisticsexplained/index.php/Healthcare_personnel_statistics_-_physicians#Healthcare_personnel (accessed on 2 August 2021).
21. United Kingdom Health Security Agency. *English Surveillance Programme for Antimicrobial Utilisation and Resistance (ESPAUR) Report 2020 to 2021*; United Kingdom Health Security Agency: London, UK, 2021.
22. Public Health England. Achieving Behaviour Change: A Guide for National Government. Available online: https://www.gov.uk/government/publications/behaviour-change-guide-for-local-government-and-partners (accessed on 27 July 2021).
23. McEwen, S.A.; Collignon, P.J. Antimicrobial Resistance: A One Health Perspective. *Microbiol. Spectr.* **2018**. [CrossRef] [PubMed]
24. Jones, L.F.; Hawking, M.K.D.; Owens, R.; Lecky, D.; Francis, N.A.; Butler, C.; Gal, M.; McNulty, C.A.M. An evaluation of the TARGET (Treat Antibiotics Responsibly; Guidance, Education, Tools) Antibiotics Toolkit to improve antimicrobial stewardship in primary care-is it fit for purpose? *Fam. Pr.* **2018**, *35*, 461–467. [CrossRef] [PubMed]
25. Ellen, M.E.; Shach, R.; Perlman, S. Exploring community healthcare providers' perceptions on antimicrobial resistance. *J. Glob. Antimicrob. Resist.* **2019**, *18*, 215–222. [CrossRef] [PubMed]
26. Kesten, J.M.; Bhattacharya, A.; Ashiru-Oredope, D.; Gobin, M.; Audrey, S. The Antibiotic Guardian campaign: A qualitative evaluation of an online pledge-based system focused on making better use of antibiotics. *BMC Public Health* **2017**, *18*, 5. [CrossRef] [PubMed]
27. Chaintarli, K.; Ingle, S.M.; Bhattacharya, A.; Ashiru-Oredope, D.; Oliver, I.; Gobin, M. Impact of a United Kingdom-wide campaign to tackle antimicrobial resistance on self-reported knowledge and behaviour change. *BMC Public Health* **2016**, *16*, 393. [CrossRef] [PubMed]
28. Public Health England. Antibiotic Guardian. Available online: https://antibioticguardian.com/ (accessed on 27 July 2021).
29. Charani, E.; Edwards, R.; Sevdalis, N.; Alexandrou, B.; Sibley, E.; Mullett, D.; Franklin, B.D.; Holmes, A. Behavior change strategies to influence antimicrobial prescribing in acute care: A systematic review. *Clin. Infect. Dis.* **2011**, *53*, 651–662. [CrossRef] [PubMed]
30. Arnold, S.R.; Straus, S.E. Interventions to improve antibiotic prescribing practices in ambulatory care. *Cochrane Database Syst. Rev.* **2005**, *2005*, Cd003539. [CrossRef] [PubMed]
31. Public Health England. Behaviour Change and Antibiotic Prescribing in Healthcare Settings: Literature Review and Behavioural Analysis. 2015. Available online: https://www.gov.uk/government/publications/antibiotic-prescribing-and-behaviour-change-in-healthcare-settings (accessed on 1 April 2021).

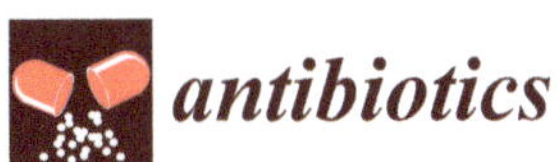

Article

Parental Knowledge, Attitude, and Practices on Antibiotic Use for Childhood Upper Respiratory Tract Infections during COVID-19 Pandemic in Greece

Maria-Eirini Oikonomou †, Despoina Gkentzi *,†, Ageliki Karatza, Sotirios Fouzas, Aggeliki Vervenioti and Gabriel Dimitriou

Department of Paediatrics, Medical School, University of Patras, Rion 26504, Greece; mareiroik@yahoo.gr (M.-E.O.); akaratza@hotmail.com (A.K.); sfouzas@upatras.gr (S.F.); aggelikivervenioti@gmail.com (A.V.); gdim@upatras.gr (G.D.)

* Correspondence: gkentzid@upatras.gr or gkentzid@gmail.com

† These authors contributed equally to this work.

Abstract: This cross-sectional study aims to assess parents' knowledge, attitude, and practices on antibiotic use for children with URTIs symptoms in Greece in the era of the COVID-19 pandemic. We distributed a questionnaire to a random sample of parents who visited primary health care centers in Patras, Greece. Out of 412 participants, 86% believed that most infections with common cold or flu symptoms were caused by viruses, although 26.9% believed that antibiotics may prevent complications. Earache was the most common symptom for which antibiotics were needed. Most of them (69%) declare being considerably anxious about their children's health during the COVID-19 pandemic. The majority (85%) knew that COVID-19 was of viral origin, yet half of them declared uncertain whether antibiotics were needed. All demographic characteristics, except for gender, were found to have a significant effect on parents' knowledge, attitude, and practices on antibiotic use for URTIs and COVID-19. Factor analysis revealed six groups of parents with common characteristics associated with misuse of antibiotics. Our findings highlight the need to decrease misconceptions regarding antibiotic use by providing relevant education for parents targeting particular characteristics, especially during the COVID-19 pandemic. Continuous education of healthcare providers in the field is also of paramount importance.

Keywords: upper respiratory tract infections; antibiotics; antimicrobial resistance; parental knowledge; attitudes; practices; child; Greece; COVID-19

Citation: Oikonomou, M.-E.; Gkentzi, D.; Karatza, A.; Fouzas, S.; Vervenioti, A.; Dimitriou, G. Parental Knowledge, Attitude, and Practices on Antibiotic Use for Childhood Upper Respiratory Tract Infections during COVID-19 Pandemic in Greece. *Antibiotics* **2021**, *10*, 802. https://doi.org/10.3390/antibiotics10070802

Academic Editor: Albert Figueras

Received: 4 June 2021
Accepted: 29 June 2021
Published: 1 July 2021

Publisher's Note: MDPI stays neutral with regard to jurisdictional claims in published maps and institutional affiliations.

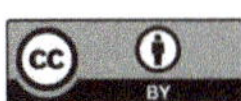

Copyright: © 2021 by the authors. Licensee MDPI, Basel, Switzerland. This article is an open access article distributed under the terms and conditions of the Creative Commons Attribution (CC BY) license (https://creativecommons.org/licenses/by/4.0/).

1. Introduction

Upper respiratory tract infections (URTIs) in children account for more than 10% of the total outpatient and emergency department visits and are considered the main cause of children's absenteeism from school as well as parents' from the workplace [1,2]. The discovery of antibiotics is a very important achievement of the 20th century, and their proper and judicious use reduces mortality and morbidity [3]. However, antibiotics are often used inappropriately, especially for the treatment of URTIs in children, even though there is sufficient evidence to support the viral origin of these conditions and the fact that this practice does not change the duration and severity of symptoms [4,5]. Many issues have been raised because of overuse or misuse of antibiotics, such as the high cost of health services, rise of side effects such as diarrhea, and increased antibacterial resistance [6–8]. There is a strong association between antibiotic overuse and the development of resistance, and countries with high rates of antibiotic consumption have reported a high incidence of resistant pathogens [9,10]. As a result, over the past decade, the World Health Organization (WHO) recognized the emergence of antibiotic resistance as one of the 10 top global public health threats facing humanity [11]. Based on numerous reports, factors leading to antimicrobial overuse in children are complex, involving easy access to antibiotics for self-medication [12], overprescribing by physicians due to diagnostic uncertainty [13], or parents' wish, which is mainly driven by lack of knowledge and misperceptions [14–17]. A recent review demonstrated that one-third of the population of low and middle-income countries have significant knowledge gaps in the field [18]. The quality of communication between parents and pediatricians plays an important role in the decision of prescribing [19]. Associations between demographic characteristics and parental knowledge, attitude, and practices towards antibiotic use in URTIs have also been described [13,20–24].

Coronavirus infectious disease 2019 (COVID-19), declared as a pandemic on the 11th of March of 2020, may cause URTI symptoms and, in the majority of children, warrants only symptomatic treatment [25–27]. No studies on parents' knowledge, attitude, and practices on antibiotic use have been thus far conducted during the pandemic. Despite numerous national educational activities in Greece on judicious antibiotic use, antibiotic consumption in the community has been found to be the highest amongst 31 European countries [28–30]. A nationwide study conducted in 2010 demonstrated that Greek parents understand the benign course of URTIs, rarely give antibiotics without medical advice, and contribute less than expected to antibiotic misuse [31]. The present study aims to explore parental knowledge, attitude, and practices (KAP) regarding antibiotic use for URTIs and COVID-19 infection in Greece, during the COVID-19 pandemic, with the view of designing educational strategies focusing on those parents who are prone to antibiotic misuse.

2. Results

2.1. Parents' Demographic Characteristics

Out of the 499 questionnaires distributed, 412 were returned (response rate 82.5%). Table 1 shows the demographics of our studied population. Of note, the majority of our study participants were women (77.2%), aged between 31–50 years old (88.1%), of Greek nationality (85.7%), and with good self-perceived access to the health care system (65.8%).

Table 1. Demographic characteristics of the study participants.

Demographic Characteristics	Total Frequency (n = 412)	Percent (%)
Gender		
Female	318	77.2
Male	91	22.1
N/A *	3	0.7
Parental age (years)		
18–30	26	6.3
31–50	363	88.1
51–60	20	4.9
N/A	3	0.7
Ethnicity		
Greek	353	85.7
Non—Greek	59	14.3
Education		
Primary school	6	1.5
Secondary school	20	4.9
High school	76	18.4
College	42	10.2
University	170	41.3
Postgraduate-doctoral degree	59	14.3
N/A	39	9.5
Occupation		
Unemployed	87	21.1
Student	2	0.5
Part-time	34	8.3
Full-time	287	69.7
Retired	2	0.5

Table 1. *Cont.*

Demographic Characteristics	Total Frequency (*n* = 412)	Percent (%)
Medical Insurance		
Public	358	86.9
Private	13	3.2
Both	19	4.6
None	22	5.3
Family income		
Low	75	18.2
Middle	311	76.9
High	20	4.9
Age of child		
0–5 years	121	29.4
6–11 years	166	40.3
12–16 years	122	29.6
N/A	3	0.7
Single-parent family		
Yes	36	8.7
No	376	91.3
Chronic disease in child		
Yes	19	4.6
No	393	95.3
Access to the healthcare system		
Low	40	9.7
Moderate	101	24.5
Good	271	65.8
Pediatrician		
Public	259	62.9
Private	153	37.1

* N/A: not answered.

2.2. Parental Knowledge on Antibiotic Use in Children with URTIs

The vast majority of parents (81.6%) knew that infections with signs of cold or flu symptoms were caused by viruses. Most of them acknowledged that antibiotics were not necessary, and (69%) answered that symptomatic treatment was only needed for viral infections. Of note, 48.5% of parents thought that antibiotics were needed for bacterial infections while 50.7% for viral ones. Earache was the most common symptom for which parents thought that antibiotics were needed (25.2%), followed by a runny nose (9.5%). More than half of the parents (52.2%) declared that antibiotics were always needed for their child's tonsillitis and 47.1% for otitis. The majority of parents (73.6%) identified successfully antibiotics between other drugs. Half of them did not believe that antibiotic use may protect them from complications of the common cold or the flu. Most of the parents (80.8%) knew that imprudent use of antibiotics reduces their efficacy and may cause antibiotic resistance, and two-thirds of them were familiar with the fact that antibiotics may have some side effects. Most parents (73.3%) declared to be adequately informed about judicious use of antibiotics, and 91.7% of them declared that an educational program about the proper use of antibiotics would be useful.

2.3. Parental Attitude and Practices towards Antibiotic Use in Children with URTIs

Nearly half of the parents (48.8%) declared that they did not know whether their child needed an antibiotic before visiting the pediatrician. Most of the responders (69.4%) would not feel more satisfied if their pediatrician were to prescribe antibiotics for their child's cold symptoms. Moreover, 93% of the participants always comply with their pediatrician's recommendations. When asked if they would visit another pediatrician for a second opinion in case their own would not prescribe antibiotics, 82% disagreed. In addition, the majority (86.6%) would not change pediatrician because they would not prescribe antibiotics as frequently as they desired. Most of them never used leftover antibiotics, while 13.6% sometimes did. A total of 84% of the participants never insisted that their pediatrician prescribe antibiotics, and most of them (90.3%) answered that their pediatrician did not prescribe antibiotics because they insisted, while 7.8% declared that this happens frequently. A total of 85% did not purchase antibiotics for their child's cold or flu symptoms over the counter, while 15% of them adopted this practice sometimes, often, or always. Moreover, 61.4% of the parents answered that their pediatrician never recommended antibiotics over the phone, while 32.5% answered that this had happened sometimes. If their child was unwell, parents always (50.5%) or most of the time (27.6%) consulted their pediatrician, followed by previous experience where they referred to sometimes (27.9%) or often (19.7%). Moreover, 23.1% sometimes asked their relatives, while 14.6% sought advice from the internet.

2.4. *Parental Knowledge Attitude, and Practices towards Antibiotic Use in Children with COVID-19 Infection*

Most parents (85%) declared that COVID-19 infection was of viral origin, and 72.3% answered that it may cause flu and cold symptoms in children. Most parents (68.4%) declared being anxious for their child's health during the COVID-19 pandemic. Approximately half of the parents (49.8%) declared unaware whether antibiotics were needed for COVID-19, and 47.8% did not know whether their child would be sick for a longer time if they would not receive antibiotics for COVID-19. Half of the parents (51.5%) declared more satisfied if their pediatrician would not recommend antibiotics for their child's cold or flu symptoms. The vast majority of parents (93.2%) answered that their pediatrician did not recommend antibiotics over the phone for their child's cold or flu symptoms during the pandemic.

2.5. *Effect of Demographic Characteristics and Knowledge, Practice, and Attitude on Antibiotic Use*

The correlations between sociodemographic characteristics and KAP on antibiotic use during the COVID-19 pandemic are shown in Table 2. Of note, KAP on antibiotic use during COVID-19 was not associated with parental age and gender, chronic disease in the child, and number of children in the family. Various other associations have been demonstrated between KAP and other sociodemographics. The relevant correlations between KAP and URTIs in general (not only for COVID-19) are available as Supplemental Tables S1 and S2.

Table 3 shows the results of factor analysis. We found six groups of parents who misused antibiotics, which in total accounts for 76.6% of the variation of the answers given on KAP in our study (meaning that 76.6% of our study participants belong to at least one of these groups).

Table 2. Association of demographic characteristics with knowledge/attitude/practice statements on COVID-19.

Statement/Question	Correct	Incorrect	*p*-Value (Chi-Square Test)							
			Nationality	Education	Occupation	Insurance	Income	Age of Child	Single Parent	Access on Health System
COVID-19 is caused by a virus.	85%	14.3%	0.000 I **: Other	0.000 I: primary school	0.020 I: retired	0.000 I: None	0.005 I: low	NS *	NS	0.021 I: low
COVID-19 in children causes cold or flu symptoms.	72.3%	26.5%	0.010 I: Other	0.000 I: High school	0.000 I: unemployed	0.006 I: None	0.000 I: low	0,005 I:6–11 years	0.009 I: Yes	NS
Antibiotics are always needed for my child's COVID-19.	31.6%	67.3%	0.006 I: Other	0.027 I: primary school	0.000 I: student	0.007 I: None	0.000 I: low	0.006 I:12–16 years	NS	NS
My child will be sick for a longer time if it doesn't get treated with antibiotics for its cold or flu symptoms.	36.9%	62.1%	0.013 I: Other	0.000 I: primary school	0.013 I: retired	0.007 I: None	0.002 I: low	NS	NS	
I am more satisfied if my pediatrician assures me that my child doesn't need antibiotics for its cold or flu symptoms.	13.8%	85.7%	NS	NS	NS	NS	0.038 I: low	NS	NS	0.000 I: low
How often did your pediatrician recommend antibiotics for your child's cold or flu symptoms by phone during COVID-19 pandemic?	93.2%	6.3%	0.000 I: Other	0.008 I: Primary school	NS	0.001 I: None	NS	NS	0.001 I: Yes	0.019 I: low

* NS: not statistically significant. ** For statistically significant associations for each statement, the subgroup of parents who answered incorrectly (I) in a higher percentage are noticed in parentheses.

Table 3. Factor analysis of parental characteristics associated with antibiotic misuse *.

Group 1 (Eigenvalue 3.6/24% of variation)	
Knowledge of no use for viral infections	−0.656
Education	−0.642
Income	−0.507
Feeling of adequate information	0.491
Second opinion	0.488
Group 2 (eigenvalue 1.52/10.2% of variation)	
Father	0.577
Second opinion	0.431
Knows if child needs antibiotics	0.430
Education	0.365
Income	0.347
Group 3 (eigenvalue 1.31/8.8% of variation)	
Father	0.623
Knows when child needs antibiotics	−0.571
Education	0.344
Second opinion	0.370
Feeling of adequate information	0.303
Group 4 (eigenvalue 1.26/8.4% of variation)	
Knowledge of no use for viral infections	0.500
Feeling of adequate information	0.419
Age	0.403
Income	−0.360
Group 5 (eigenvalue 1.1/7.3% of variation)	
Age	0.617
Knows when the child needs antibiotics	−0.396
Group 6 (eigenvalue 1.05/7% of variation)	
Knowledge of no use for viral infections	0.415
Second opinion	−0.415
Knows when the child needs antibiotics	0.400
Age	0.317

* Exploratory dichotomous factor analysis (promax oblique rotation and least-squares extraction method) of parental characteristics associated with antibiotic misuse. Only parameters with a factor loading >0.300 are shown.

3. Discussion

This is the first study on knowledge, attitude, and practices from parents in Greece regarding antibiotic use in young children with URTIs in the era of the COVID-19 pandemic. The response rate was 82.4%, which is rather satisfactory, especially taking into account the COVID-19 strict restrictions during visits in primary health care.

According to the results of this study, parents have a satisfactory level of knowledge on antibiotic use for URTIs, however some incorrect perceptions have been revealed. The majority of parents (81.6%) correctly answered that most URTIs are viral in origin, in contrast to parents from a similar study from Northern Ethiopia who scored lower percentages of correct answers (31.4%) [15]. In the latter study, 30% of the responders believed incorrectly that antibiotics were needed for viral infections, and 20.6% declared to be uncertain. Of note, this percentage is even smaller than other studies in China and Pakistan (79% and 83%, respectively) [32,33]. Almost 70% of parents were aware that common cold and flu need only supportive care, although 26.9% falsely believed that antibiotic use may protect from complications while 26.9% declared uncertain, which are similar percentages to those previously reported [32–39]. A total of 15.6% answered that their children's disease will get complicated in the case of not using antibiotics in contrast to similar surveys in China [32], Cyprus [14], and the Republic of Macedonia [18], in which the percentages were higher, 50%, 48%, and 44%, respectively. In our study, most responders were familiar with antibiotics and able to distinguish them among other drugs similar to Palestinian parents [38]. In particular, 61% were worried about antibiotics' side effects, and the majority knew that imprudent use drives antimicrobial resistance, as previously depicted in similar studies worldwide [8,14,16,23].

The results of this study regarding parents' attitudes and practices towards antibiotic use for children's URTIs are of great interest. Parents do not seek antibiotics as 83% of them do not insist on this practice, and 69% are not more satisfied if this happens. Less than 10% believed that their pediatrician prescribes antibiotics due to their insistence, which is less than Palestinian parents (28%) but more than the percentage of parents from Cyprus [8,14]. Of note, only 8% of Australian parents asked their pediatrician for antibiotics (8%), whereas 82% of Chinese parents mentioned that they would not get displeased if their pediatrician rejected their demand for antibiotics [22,32]. In general, parents expect physical examination and adequate consultation for the nature of the disease and the need for antibiotics [37–40]. These findings emphasize the vital role of communication between parents and pediatricians.

The findings of the survey also demonstrate that Greek parents do not treat their children without medical advice. Only 12.6% of the participants reported that they have sometimes purchased antibiotics without medical prescription by the drug store. This finding is lower than in other countries such as Peru (23.5%) and Lebanon (22.5%) [34–38]. Of note, 16.3% have sometimes used leftover antibiotics in contrast with Saudi Arabia and the Republic of Macedonia, where higher percentages were recorded, 66%, 60.8%, respectively [16,18]. Moreover, it appears that Greek parents trust their pediatricians as the vast majority would neither visit another pediatrician for a second opinion (81.3%) if their pediatrician would not prescribe antibiotics for their child's cold or flu, nor change their pediatrician in case they did not prescribe antibiotics as often as they believed that they should (86.4%). In addition, 93% always comply with their pediatrician recommendations in regards to their child's cold or flu symptoms. These findings are similar to a similar study in Palestine but differ from a study in Jordan where 39.3% of the parents answered that they would indeed change pediatrician if they prescribed antibiotics less frequently than they desired [23,39]. The pediatrician remains the main source of information for the ill child, followed by previous experience, pharmacist, relatives, and the internet. Finally, more than one-third of the parents obtained antibiotics for their child following a telephone consultation, and the same percentages have been reported in Jordan and Cyprus [14,23].

It is of interest to note that we did not find many differences in comparison with a similar survey conducted in our country a decade ago [31]. Earache was the most common symptom for which parents anticipated receiving antibiotics. Whereas in both studies, most parents declared to be aware of antimicrobial resistance due to antibiotic misuse (88% in the previous and 81% in our study), a similar percentage of parents (24.7% in the previous and 24% in our study) would administer antibiotics in case their child got flu or cold symptoms in order to recover sooner. Moreover, similar percentages of parents (42% in the previous and 38% in the current study) got a medical recommendation for antibiotics over the phone. As a result, the development and implementation of parental education measures to improve antibiotic use are crucial and still warranted at a national level.

This is the first study on parental knowledge, attitude, and practices towards antibiotic use on COVID- 19 infection in children in our country. The majority of parents (68.4%) declared to be extremely anxious as far as their children's health is concerned due to the pandemic. Most parents knew that COVID-19 causes flu or cold symptoms and is of viral origin. However, half of them declared to be uncertain as to whether antibiotics were needed for its treatment, and a third of them were not aware if their child's illness would last for longer if no antibiotics are used. These results were predictable as COVID-19 was a new infection, and parents were not adequately informed, especially in the beginning of the pandemic. Therefore, pediatricians should invest more time in order to inform parents about COVID-19. As far as over the telephone diagnosis and recommendation of antibiotics are concerned, the vast majority of parents (93%) replied that this never happened during the pandemic, whereas 63% replied that this was never practiced by their pediatrician before. Parents expect physical examination and recommendation of the appropriate treatment. Given the circumstances during the pandemic, this might not always be feasible. Healthcare providers should therefore have a low threshold of antibiotic prescribing and continue to adhere to the antimicrobial stewardship principles during the pandemic to combat further development of resistant pathogens.

Factor analysis revealed six groups of parents with common characteristics that were associated with antibiotic misuse. Group 1 that accounts for 24% of the variation includes parents that do not have an adequate background on judicious antibiotic use. Even worryingly, group 2 (10.2% of the variation) includes parents that are confident in antibiotic use yet misuse them. For these two groups, more time needs to be invested by prescribers in educating parents in the field. On the other hand, groups 3, 4, 5, and 6 (31.5% of the variation) are parents that do not use antibiotics prudently but do listen to their pediatricians. The latter highlights the need for interventions on antibiotic prescribers, including continuing education. Educational activities for prescribers should start early on in their career, as research thus far has highlighted gaps in medical training in the field [41,42]. Novel and effective training methods on all aspects of antimicrobial stewardship and antimicrobial resistance should be incorporated in the Medical Curricula worldwide. In addition to education, better prescribing requires expert personnel, practice guideline drafting, and implementation aids, as well as setting clear goals and quantitative targets for quality in prescribing [43]. All the above have been used with apparent success in some Northern European countries and should guide relevant interventions in Greece [43].

It is of interest to highlight that our study population included a small percentage of parents with low cultural and economic levels. In particular, more than half of our study participants were urban with a university education. As the problem of antimicrobial misuse is a social issue, it demands a relevant approach from that perspective [44]. Hence, a good level of knowledge on antibiotics use could be partially related to the high socioeconomic status of our participants. The involvement of social scientists in the field is crucial to address the multiple dimensions of the problem, such as socio-cultural, economic, and political. In addition to the above, given the dynamic and constantly changing nature of human behavior, social media could also play an important role in public health interventions to combat antimicrobial resistance, and their role is yet to be further established [44,45].

We acknowledge that our study as a pragmatic one has strengths and limitations. One of its strengths is that data were collected through self-administered questionnaires. This methodology was preferred more than face-to-face or telephone interviews in order to avoid the chance of the interviewer influencing the parent's response as well as the likelihood that interviewers respond in accordance with what is believed to be the expected answer. With regards to study limitations, firstly, the distribution of the questionnaires took place in the summer months of 2020 (during precautionary measures to prevent the spread of COVID-19) with a low number of primary care visits. Secondly, it was difficult for parents with low socioeconomic status or belonging to special population groups (e.g., Roma) to take part in the study because they might have been incapable of reading or understanding the questionnaire. Moreover, the study enrolled parents who only sought care at health care centers, which limits the generalizability of the results. Finally, data were collected from a large city in Greece and thus mainly represent the urban but not necessarily the rural population of the area.

4. Materials and Methods

We performed a cross-sectional study including parents of children aged 0–16 years and attending the primary pediatric healthcare services in the city of Patras during a period of 4 months (May–August 2020). Patras is the third-largest city in Greece after Athens and Thessaloniki. All parents/guardians of children attending the primary care clinics were informed in detail with a written information sheet about the study aims, as well as data confidentiality. Parents who agreed to take part in the study were asked to complete an anonymous self-administered questionnaire regarding their KAP on the use of antibiotics for childhood URTIs and COVID-19. The questionnaire was written in Greek and consisted of 2 parts. Part A included 13 questions on demographics (age, gender, nationality, level of education, occupation, health insurance status, single-family status, child's chronic disease, access to the healthcare system). Part B included 23 questions on the parent's knowledge, attitudes, and practices on antibiotic use for URTIs and COVID-19. Answers were given on a 5-point Likert scale ("strongly agree", "agree", "uncertain", "disagree", "strongly disagree", or "never", "sometimes", "often", "most of the time", "always"). Statistics were performed using the SPSS v.21 software (IBM Corp, Armonk, NY, USA). The level of significance was set to 0.05 for all analyses. Descriptive statistics were used to summarize data on demographic characteristics, knowledge, attitude, and practices towards antibiotic use. Chi-square test was used to test for significant association between demographic characteristics and parents' knowledge, attitude, and practices. Unsure responses were scored as incorrect. Factor analysis was used in order to identify groups of parents with common characteristics that were at high risk of inappropriate antibiotic use.

5. Conclusions

This study is an important step towards a better understanding of the knowledge, attitude, and practices regarding antibiotic use in URTIs in children during the COVID-19 pandemic. It revealed that there was a diversity of parental awareness about antibiotics and antimicrobial resistance on the basis of social-demographic factors. Of note, the pandemic does not seem to have influenced parental views on antibiotic use for their offspring. Educational campaigns targeting high risk groups to decrease misconceptions about antibiotic use and to increase awareness regarding the risks of inappropriate use are warranted. Targeted education on the particularities of COVID-19 is also vital for parents. In addition, continuous training of pediatricians about effective communication with parents and prudent prescribing of antibiotics is essential. Ideally, this study should be conducted with a large country-representative sample and during the consequent phases of the pandemic in order to assess for possible changes. It would also be useful to assess attitudes pre and post-training, specifically designed for that purpose, for both parents and pediatricians. Furthermore, studies assessing country-specific determinants of antibiotic misuse, such as country wealth and health care system particularities, would also be useful for the implementation of multilevel interventional programs aimed at limiting the spread of antibiotic resistance. Despite multiple efforts to achieve that in Greece during the last decades, there is still room for further development. Public health interventions at a national level should be constant and sustainable following the successful examples of other European countries. Finally, antimicrobial stewardship activities and interventions should not be neglected during the COVID-19 pandemic.

Supplementary Materials: The following are available online at https://www.mdpi.com/article/10.3390/antibiotics10070802/s1, Table S1: Association of demographic characteristics with knowledge statements about URTIs, Table S2: Association of demographic characteristics with attitude/practice statements about URTIs.

Author Contributions: Conceptualization, D.G., G.D.; methodology, D.G., G.D.; software D.G., M.-E.O. and G.D.; validation, D.G. and G.D.; formal analysis, S.F. and M.-E.O.; investigation, M.-E.O. and A.V.; resources, M.-E.O. and A.V.; data curation, M.-E.O., A.K., and A.V.; writing—original draft preparation, M.-E.O. and D.G.; writing—review and editing, M.-E.O., D.G., A.K., A.V., S.F.,

G.D.; visualization, D.G.; supervision, D.G., G.D.; project administration, M.-E.O. and A.V.; funding acquisition N/A. All authors have read and agreed to the published version of the manuscript.

Funding: This research received no external funding.

Institutional Review Board Statement: The study was conducted according to the guidelines of the Declaration of Helsinki and approved by the Institutional Review Board of Research and Ethics Committee of Patras Medical School (decision number 5919/25.05.2020).

Informed Consent Statement: Informed consent was obtained from all parents involved in the study.

Data Availability Statement: The data presented in this study are available on request from the corresponding author.

Conflicts of Interest: The authors declare no conflict of interest.

References

1. West, J.V. Acute upper airway infections: Childhood respiratory infections. *Br. Med. Bull.* **2002**, *61*, 215–230. [CrossRef]
2. Linder, J.A. Improving care for acute respiratory infections: Better systems, not better microbiology. *Clin. Infect. Dis.* **2007**, *45*, 1189–1191. [CrossRef] [PubMed]
3. Mazinska, B.; Struzycka, I.; Hryniewicz, W. Surveys of public knowledge and attitudes with regard to antibiotics in Poland: Did the European Antibiotic Awareness Day campaigns change attitudes? *PLoS ONE* **2017**, *12*, e0172146. [CrossRef]
4. Earnshaw, S.; Monnet, D.L.; Duncan, B.; O'Toole, J.; Ekdahl, K.; Goossens, H. European antibiotic awareness day technical advisory committee; European antibiotic awareness day collaborative group. European antibiotic awareness day, 2008-the first Europe-wide public information campaign on prudent antibiotic use: Methods and survey of activities in participating countries. *Eurosurveillance* **2009**, *14*, 19280.
5. Harnden, A.; Perera, R.; Brueggemann, A.B.; Mayon-White, R.; Crook, D.W.; Thomson, A.; Mant, D. Respiratory infections for which general practitioners consider prescribing an antibiotic: A prospective study. *Arch. Dis. Child.* **2007**, *92*, 594–597. [CrossRef]
6. Vandepitte, W.; Ponthong, R.; Srisarang, S. Treatment outcomes of the uncomplicated upper respiratory tract infection and acute diarrhea in preschool children comparing those with and without antibiotic prescription. *J. Med. Assoc. Thail.* **2015**, *98*, 974–984.
7. Finkelstein, J.A.; Dutta-Linn, M.; Meyer, R.; Goldman, R. Childhood infections, antibiotics, and resistance: What are parents saying now? *Clin. Pediatr.* **2014**, *53*, 145–150. [CrossRef] [PubMed]
8. Zyoud, S.H.; Abu Taha, A.; Araj, K.F.; Abahri, I.A.; Sawalha, A.F.; Sweileh, W.M.; Al-Jabi, S.W. Parental knowledge, attitudes and practices regarding antibiotic use for acute upper respiratory tract infections in children: A cross-sectional study in Palestine. *BMC Pediatr.* **2015**, *15*, 176. [CrossRef]
9. Costelloe, C.; Metcalfe, C.; Lovering, A.; Mant, D.; Hay, A.D. Effect of antibiotic prescribing in primary care on antimicrobial resistance in individual patients: Systematic review and meta-analysis. *BMJ* **2010**, *340*, c2096. [CrossRef]
10. Yagupsky, P. Selection of antibiotic-resistant pathogens in the community. *Pediatr. Infect. Dis. J.* **2006**, *25*, 974–976. [CrossRef]
11. WHO Report on Antimicrobial Resistance. Available online: https://www.who.int/news-room/fact-sheets/detail/antimicrobial-resistance (accessed on 12 March 2021).
12. Grigoryan, L.; Haaijer-Ruskamp, F.M.; Burgerhof, J.G.M.; Mechtler, R.; Deschepper, R.; Tambic-Andrasevic, A.; Andrajati, R.; Monnet, D.L.; Cunney, R.; Di Matteo, A.; et al. Self-medication with antimicrobial drugs in Europe. *Emerg. Infect. Dis.* **2006**, *12*, 452–459. [CrossRef]
13. Horwood, J.; Cabral, C.; Hay, A.D.; Ingram, J. Primary care clinician antibiotic prescribing decisions in consultations for children with RTIs: A qualitative interview study. *Br. J. Gen. Pract.* **2016**, *66*, e207–e213. [CrossRef] [PubMed]
14. Rousounidis, A.; Papaevangelou, V.; Hadjipanayis, A.; Panagakou, S.; Theodoridou, M.; Syrogiannopoulos, G.; Hadjichristodoulou, C. Descriptive study on parents' knowledge, attitudes and practices on antibiotic use and misuse in children with upper respiratory tract infections in Cyprus. *Int. J. Environ. Res. Public Health* **2011**, *8*, 3246–3262. [CrossRef]
15. Zeru, T.; Berihu, H.; Buruh, G.; Gebrehiwot, H.; Zeru, M. Parental knowledge and practice on antibiotic use for upper respiratory tract infections in children, in Aksum town health institutions, Northern Ethiopia: A cross-sectional study. *Pan Afr. Med. J.* **2020**, *35*, 142. [CrossRef]
16. Al-Ayed, M. Parents' Knowledge, Attitudes and Practices on Antibiotic Use by Children. *Saudi J. Med. Med Sci.* **2019**, *7*, 93–99. [CrossRef]
17. Paredes, J.L.; Navarro, R.; Riveros, M.; Picon, V.; Conde, F.; Suito-Ferrand, M.; Ochoa, T.J. Parental Antibiotic Use in Urban and Peri-Urban Health Care Centers in Lima: A Cross-Sectional Study of Knowledge, Attitudes, and Practices. *Clin. Med. Insights Pediatr.* **2019**, *13*. [CrossRef] [PubMed]
18. Alili-Idrizi, E.; Dauti, M.; Malaj, L. Validation of the parental knowledge and attitude towards antibiotic usage and resistance among children in Tetovo, he Republic of Macedonia. *Pharm. Pract.* **2014**, *12*, 467. [CrossRef]
19. Mangione-Smith, R.; Zhou, C.; Robinson, J.D.; Taylor, J.A.; Elliott, M.N.; Heritage, J. Communication practices and antibiotic use for acute respiratory tract infections in children. *Ann. Fam. Med.* **2015**, *13*, 221–227. [CrossRef]

20. Gualano, M.R.; Gili, R.; Scaioli, G.; Bert, F.; Siliquini, R. General population's knowledge and attitudes about antibiotics: A systematic review and meta-analysis. *Pharmacoepidemiol. Drug Saf.* **2015**, *24*, 2–10. [CrossRef]
21. Siddiqui, S.; Cheema, M.S.; Ayub, R.; Shah, N.; Hamza, A.; Hussain, S.; Khan, M.H.; Raza, S.M. Knowledge, attitudes and practices of parents regarding antibiotic use in children. *J. Ayub Med. Coll. Abbottabad* **2014**, *26*, 170. [PubMed]
22. Biezen, R.; Grando, D.; Mazza, D. Dissonant views-GPs' and parents' perspectives on antibiotic prescribing for young children with respiratory tract infections. *BMC Fam. Pract.* **2019**, *20*, 46. [CrossRef]
23. Hammour, K.A.; Jalil, M.A.; Hammour, W.A. An exploration of parents' knowledge, attitudes and practices towards the use of antibiotics in childhood upper respiratory tract infections in a tertiary Jordanian Hospital. *Saudi Pharm. J. SPJ Off. Publ. Saudi Pharm. Soc.* **2018**, *26*, 780–785. [CrossRef] [PubMed]
24. Cantarero-Arévalo, L.; Hallas, M.P.; Kaae, S. Parental knowledge of antibiotic use in children with respiratory infections: A systematic review. *Int. J. Pharm. Pract.* **2017**, *25*, 31–49. [CrossRef]
25. Up to Date. Coronavirus Disease 2019 (COVID-19). Clinical Manifestations and Diagnosis in Children. Available online: https://www.uptodate.com/contents/coronavirus-disease-2019-covid-19-clinical-manifestations-and-diagnosis-inchildren?topicRef=126981&source=related_link (accessed on 7 January 2021).
26. WHO. Director General's Opening Remarks at the Media Briefing on Covid-19. Available online: https://www.who.int/director-general/speeches/detail/who-director-general-s-opening-remarks-at-the-media-briefing-on-covid-19---11-march-2020 (accessed on 7 January 2021).
27. Up to Date. Coronavirus Disease 2019 (COVID-19). Management in Children. Available online: https://www.uptodate.com/contents/coronavirus-disease-2019-covid-19-management-in-children?topicRef=127488&source=see_link (accessed on 7 January 2021).
28. National Institution of Public Health. Judicious Use of Antibiotics. Available online: https://eody.gov.gr/tag/antiviotika (accessed on 13 March 2021).
29. European Centre for Disease Prevention and Control. European Antibiotic Awareness Day. Available online: https://www.ecdc.europa.eu/en/news-events/european-antibiotic-awareness-day-eaad-2020 (accessed on 10 March 2021).
30. European Centre For Disease Prevention and Control. Rates by Country. Available online: https://www.ecdc.europa.eu/en/antimicrobial-consumption/database/rates-country (accessed on 12 March 2021).
31. Panagakou, S.G.; Spyridis, N.; Papaevangelou, V.; Theodoridou, K.M.; Goutziana, G.P.; Theodoridou, M.N.; Hadjichristodoulou, C.S. Antibiotic use for upper respiratory tract infections in children: A cross-sectional survey of knowledge, attitudes, and practices (KAP) of parents in Greece. *BMC Pediatr.* **2011**, *11*, 60. [CrossRef] [PubMed]
32. Yu, M.; Zhao, G.; Stålsby Lundborg, C.; Zhu, Y.; Zhao, Q.; Xu, B. Knowledge, attitudes, and practices of parents in rural China on the use of antibiotics in children: A cross-sectional study. *BMC Infect. Dis.* **2014**, *14*, 112. [CrossRef]
33. Atif, M.; Sadeeqa, S.; Afzal, H.; Latif, S. Knowledge, attitude and practices regarding antibiotic use among parents for their children. *IJPSR* **2018**, *9*, 2140–2148.
34. Lucas, P.; Cabral, C.; Hay, A.; Horwood, J. A systematic review of parent and clinician views and perceptions that influence prescribing decisions in relation to acute childhood infections in primary care. *Scand. J. Prim. Health Care* **2015**, *33*, 11–20. [CrossRef]
35. Mustafa, M.; Wood, F.; Butler, C.C.; Elwyn, G. Managing expectations of antibiotics for upper respiratory tract infections: A qualitative study. *Ann. Fam. Med.* **2014**, *12*, 29–36. [CrossRef] [PubMed]
36. Fletcher-Lartey, S.; Yee, M.; Gaarslev, C.; Khan, R. Why do general practitioners prescribe antibiotics for upper respiratory tract infections to meet patient expectations: A mixed methods study. *BMJ Open* **2016**, *6*, e012244. [CrossRef]
37. McKay, R.; Mah, A.; Law, M.; McGrail, K.; Patrick, D. Systematic review of factors associated with antibiotic prescribing for respiratory tract infections. *Antimicrob. Agents Chemother.* **2016**, *60*, 4106–4118. [CrossRef]
38. Mallah, N.; Badro, D.A.; Figueiras, A.; Takkouche, B. Association of knowledge and beliefs with the misuse of antibiotics in parents: A study in Beirut (Lebanon). *PLoS ONE* **2020**, *15*, e0232464. [CrossRef]
39. Parimi, N.; Pinto Pereira, L.M.; Prabhakar, P. Caregivers' practices, knowledge and beliefs of antibiotics in pediatric upper respiratory tract infections in Trinidad and Tobago: A cross-sectional study. *BMC Fam. Pract.* **2004**, *5*, 28. [CrossRef]
40. Di Gennaro, F.; Marotta, C.; Amicone, M.; Bavaro, D.F.; Bernaudo, F.; Frisicale, E.M.; Kurotschka, P.K.; Mazzari, A.; Veronese, N.; Murri, R.; et al. Italian young doctors' knowledge, attitudes and practices on antibiotic use and resistance: A national cross-sectional survey. *J. Glob. Antimicrob. Resist.* **2020**, *23*, 167–173. [CrossRef] [PubMed]
41. Efthymiou, P.; Gkentzi, D.; Dimitriou, G. Knowledge, Attitudes and Perceptions of Medical Students on Antimicrobial Stewardship. *Antibiotics* **2020**, *9*, 821. [CrossRef] [PubMed]
42. Kern, W.V. Organization of antibiotic stewardship in Europe: The way to go. *Wien. Med. Wochenschr.* **2021**, *171* (Suppl. 1), 4–8. [CrossRef]
43. Lu, J.; Sheldenkar, A.; Lwin, M.O. A decade of antimicrobial resistance research in social science fields: A scientometric review. *Antimicrob. Resist. Infect. Control* **2020**, *9*, 178. [CrossRef]
44. Acharya, K.P.; Subedi, D. Use of Social Media as a Tool to Reduce Antibiotic Usage: A Neglected Approach to Combat Antimicrobial Resistance in Low and Middle Income Countries. *Front. Public Health* **2020**, *8*, 558576. [CrossRef] [PubMed]
45. Davis, M.; Whittaker, A.; Lindgren, M.; Djerf-Pierre, M.; Manderson, L.; Flowers, P. Understanding media publics and the antimicrobial resistance crisis. *Glob. Public Health* **2018**, *13*, 1158–1168. [CrossRef] [PubMed]

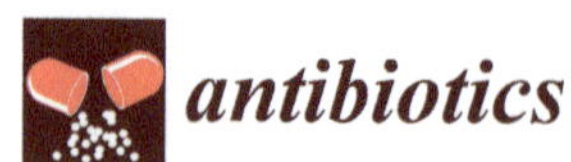

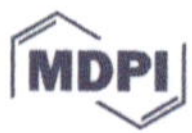

Article

Factors Associated with Antimicrobial Stewardship Practices on California Dairies: One Year Post Senate Bill 27

Essam M. Abdelfattah [1,2,3], Pius S. Ekong [1], Emmanuel Okello [1,3], Deniece R. Williams [1], Betsy M. Karle [4], Terry W. Lehenbauer [1,3] and Sharif S. Aly [1,3,*]

1 Veterinary Medicine Teaching and Research Center, School of Veterinary Medicine, University of California, Davis, Tulare, CA 93274, USA; eabdelfattah@ucdavis.edu (E.M.A.); pekong@ucdavis.edu (P.S.E.); eokello@ucdavis.edu (E.O.); dvmwilliams@ucdavis.edu (D.R.W.); tlehenbauer@ucdavis.edu (T.W.L.)
2 Department of Animal Hygiene and Veterinary Management, Faculty of Veterinary Medicine, Benha University, Moshtohor 13736, Egypt
3 Department of Population Health and Reproduction, School of Veterinary Medicine, University of California, Davis, CA 95616, USA
4 Cooperative Extension, Division of Agriculture and Natural Resources, University of California, Orland, CA 95963, USA; bmkarle@ucanr.edu
* Correspondence: saly@ucdavis.edu

Abstract: Background: The current study is aimed at identifying the factors associated with antimicrobial drug (AMD) use and stewardship practices on conventional California (CA) dairies a year after CA Senate Bill 27. Methods: Responses from 113 out of 1282 dairies mailed a questionnaire in 2019 were analyzed to estimate the associations between management practices and six outcomes including producer familiarity with medically important antimicrobial drugs (MIADs), restricted use of MIADs previously available over the counter (OTC), use of alternatives to AMD, changes in on-farm management practices, changes in AMD costs, and animal health status in dairies. Results: Producers who reported having a veterinarian–client–patient relationship (VCPR) and tracking AMD withdrawal intervals had greater odds of being familiar with the MIADs. Producers who began or increased the use of preventive alternatives to AMD in 2019 had higher odds (OR = 3.23, $p = 0.04$) of decreased use of MIADs previously available OTC compared to those who did not. Changes in management practices to prevent disease outbreak and the use of diagnostics to guide treatment were associated with producer-reported improved animal health. In addition, our study identified record keeping (associated with familiarity with MIADs), use of alternatives to AMD (associated with management changes to prevent diseases and decreased AMD costs), and use of diagnostics in treatment decisions (associated with reported better animal health) as factors associated with AMD stewardship. Conclusions: Our survey findings can be incorporated in outreach education materials to promote antimicrobial stewardship practices in dairies.

Keywords: antimicrobial drug use; antimicrobial stewardship; dairy cattle; knowledge; logistic regression models; machine learning; survey

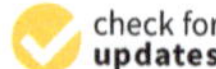

Citation: Abdelfattah, E.M.; Ekong, P.S.; Okello, E.; Williams, D.R.; Karle, B.M.; Lehenbauer, T.W.; Aly, S.S. Factors Associated with Antimicrobial Stewardship Practices on California Dairies: One Year Post Senate Bill 27. *Antibiotics* **2022**, *11*, 165. https://doi.org/10.3390/antibiotics11020165

Academic Editor: Marc Maresca

Received: 16 December 2021
Accepted: 25 January 2022
Published: 27 January 2022

Publisher's Note: MDPI stays neutral with regard to jurisdictional claims in published maps and institutional affiliations.

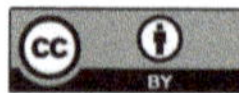

Copyright: © 2022 by the authors. Licensee MDPI, Basel, Switzerland. This article is an open access article distributed under the terms and conditions of the Creative Commons Attribution (CC BY) license (https://creativecommons.org/licenses/by/4.0/).

1. Introduction

Antimicrobial drugs (AMD) are important compounds used in humans and livestock for the prevention, control, and treatment of bacterial infections. Medically important antimicrobial drugs (MIADs) are AMD considered as essential or otherwise important for therapeutic purposes in humans. In the United States, MIADs are AMDs that are important for treating human disease and includes all critically important, highly important, and important drugs according to the Federal Food and Drug Administration's Guidance for Industry #152 [1]. According to the U.S. Food and Drug Administration [1], for the 2019 calendar year, the cattle industry was involved with 41% of the total sales and distribution of MIADs approved for use in food-producing animals. Likewise, the FDA estimated for the 2019 sales and distribution data that 81% of cephalosporins, 65% of sulfas, 45% of aminoglycosides, and 42% of tetracyclines were associated with cattle. However, AMD use comes with the risk of antimicrobial resistance (AMR) in humans and livestock [2–5].

In January 2017, the FDA fully implemented the Veterinary Feed Directive (VFD) final rule requiring approval and oversight by a licensed veterinarian for MIADs administered for therapeutic purposes via animal feed to food-producing animals and eliminated non-therapeutic uses for both growth promotion and feed efficiency [6]. The FDA also concurrently applied the same requirement for MIADs administered in drinking water for food-producing animals. Beyond these national regulations, in January 2018, California (CA) implemented Senate Bill 27 (SB 27; codified as the Food and Agricultural Code, FAC 14400-14408, here onwards referred to as SB 27), becoming the first state to require a veterinary prescription, under a valid veterinarian–client–patient relationship (VCPR), for all other dosage forms (e.g., injectables and boluses) of MIADs used for livestock [7]. The SB 27 removed all MIADs from over the counter (OTC) sales for livestock. In addition, SB 27 mandated the development of antimicrobial stewardship (AMS) guidelines and resources that support the collection of information on livestock management practices, the monitoring of AMD sales, and AMD use to provide relevant information to producers and other stakeholders. Similar legislation was passed in other states to increase AMS through the judicious use of AMD, such as Maryland SB 471 [8] and Oregon SB 920 [9]. The implementation of effective AMS practices is critical to reducing the threat AMR poses to animal and public health [10]. Similarly, worldwide AMD use in food-producing animals is increasingly being regulated with the goal of adopting AMS practices. Such regulations have included the ban on the preventive use of AMD in the feed of food-producing animals in the European Union [11], benchmarking AMD use between farms in the Netherlands [12], documenting AMD use on individual farms through electronic connection with billing in Denmark [13] and setting up national targets for a reduction of AMD use in Belgium [14].

Ekong et al. [15] conducted a survey immediately after the implementation of SB 27 to identify the factors associated with the adoption of AMS practices in CA conventional dairies. Amongst the survey findings were that dairy producers who reported keeping written or computerized animal health protocols, keeping a drug inventory log, being aware that the use of MIADs required a prescription, involving a veterinarian in the AMD treatment duration and determination, and using on-farm diagnostics to guide AMD therapy were associated with good AMS practices. Our hypothesis was that factors that were associated with AMS immediately after the implementation of SB 27 were still important a year later. Our objective was to identify the factors associated with AMS practices in adult cows in conventional dairies one year post implementation of SB 27 in CA and to compare them to those identified immediately after SB 27.

2. Results

2.1. Descriptive Statistics

A total of 131 (10.2%) out of 1282 CA licensed grade A conventional and organic dairies responded to our survey. For the current study, AMS was investigated using responses from only conventional dairies, specifically a total of 113 survey responses. Herd demographics of the dairies included in the survey analyses are summarized in Supplementary Materials Table S1. The majority of dairies were from Northern San Joaquin Valley (NSJV; 46.9%) and Greater Southern California (GSCA; 46.0%) compared to Northern California (NCA; 7.1%). The distribution of breeds in respondent dairies was primarily Holstein (56.3%), mixed herds of Holstein and Jersey breeds (35.7%), crossbreed (5.4%), and Jersey (2.4%).

2.2. Logistic Regression Models

For each of the six logistic regression models, the NCA and NSJV regions were combined due to limited sample size and collectively compared to the GSCA region. With a few exceptions, region, herd size, and breed were not significantly associated with the model outcomes.

2.2.1. Predictors Concerning Familiarity of Dairies with the FDA "MIADs" Term

Among the dairies that completed the survey, a total of 73 respondents (65.8%) reported familiarity with FDA's term 'MIADs', while 38 respondents (34.2%) were not familiar with this term. Table 1 summarizes the final logistic regression model for the association between the survey factors and familiarity with MIADs. Dairy producers who reported tracking both milk and meat withdrawal intervals, amongst other information such as date, dose, or route of AMD treatment, had greater odds (OR = 10.6, $p < 0.01$) of being familiar with MIADs compared to those who did not track either. Among the dairies in our study, 94 dairies (84%) selected milk and/or meat withdrawal intervals as information they tracked during AMD treatment and 18 dairies (16.1%) reported tracking either date, dose, or route of AMD treatment. Responses to the related question of "Do you keep track of AMD withdrawal intervals for treated cows?" confirmed a similarly high response rate with 99% of respondents reporting that they keep track of AMD withdrawal intervals, with more than half (58%) using computer software while the remaining (41%) use either paper records, white/chalk board, memory, or markings on animals. In addition, dairy producers who reported having a VCPR had greater odds (OR = 15.3, $p = 0.03$) of being familiar with MIADs than those who reported they did not have a VCPR.

Table 1. Estimated coefficients and odds ratios from a multilevel mixed-effects logistic regression model for the association between survey factors and familiarity with the U.S. Food and Drug Administration's term "medically important antimicrobial drugs".

Variables	Coefficient	SE	Odds Ratio	95% CI		*p*-Value [2]
				Lower	Upper	
Region [1]						
GSCA	Referent					
NCA + NSJV	−0.49	0.51	0.61	0.22	1.63	0.32
Herd size, milking cows						
<1304	Referent					
≥1304	−1.10	0.63	0.33	0.09	1.17	0.09
Breed						
Holstein	Referent					
Jersey	−0.82	1.41	0.44	0.02	7.01	0.56
Crossbreed	1.75	1.25	5.74	0.49	66.25	0.16
Mix/Other	−0.37	0.59	0.69	0.21	2.22	0.54
Which AMD treatment information do you track or record?						
No milk or meat withdrawal interval	Referent					
Included milk and meat withdrawal interval	2.36	0.69	10.57	2.73	40.94	<0.01
Included milk or meat withdrawal interval	−0.34	0.99	0.71	0.10	5.01	0.74
Do you have a veterinarian–client–patient relationship (VCPR)?						
No	Referent					
Yes	2.73	1.24	15.29	1.34	173.53	0.03

[1] Northern California (NCA), Northern San Joaquin Valley (NSJV), and Greater Southern California (GSCA).
[2] Factors are statistically significant at $p \leq 0.05$.

2.2.2. Predictors Concerning the Use of MIADs That Were Restricted from OTC Sales Beginning in January 2018

In our survey, 81 of the 113 respondent dairies reported use of OTC MIADs before 2018. However, of the 81 respondents, only 78 dairies responded to a survey question regarding the changes (decreased, no change, or increased) they made for use of OTC MIADs after SB 27 became effective. Of those 78 dairies, 37 (47.4%) reported decreased use of MIADs federally labeled for OTC sale, while 41 dairies (52.6%) reported increased or no change of this category of MIADs. The final model for the associations between the survey factors and the change in use of MIADs that were previously available OTC is summarized in Table S2. Large dairies (≥1304 cows) had six-times greater odds for the decreased use of OTC MIADs compared to small dairies (<1304 cows; $p < 0.01$). In addition, our model showed that producers who began using or increased the use of preventive alternatives to AMD in their dairies in 2019 had higher odds (OR = 3.2, $p = 0.04$) of a decreased use of MIADs that were previously available OTC compared to those who did not. For producers who reported the use of preventive alternatives to AMD in our study, 58.3% reported the use of vaccines, herbal remedies (36.1%), vitamins (66.7%), and/or minerals (38.9%).

An analysis of the survey responses from producers who began or increased their use of preventive alternatives to AMD in 2019 showed that a higher percentage of such producers made changes in management to prevent disease outbreaks or spread compared to those who neither began nor increased their use of such alternatives (44.8% ± 9.4 vs. 23.8% ± 4. 8; $p = 0.03$). Furthermore, a higher percentage of such producers vaccinated their animals against coliform mastitis compared to those who neither began nor increased their use of AMD alternatives (92.6% ± 5.13 vs. 74.3% ± 5.11; $p = 0.04$).

2.2.3. Predictors Concerning the Use of Preventive Alternatives to AMD on Dairy Farms

Among the dairies who completed the survey, a total of 30 respondents (26.8%) reported an increased use of preventive alternatives to AMD in their dairies during 2019. Table 2 summarizes the final model for the survey factors associated with the use or increased use of preventive alternatives to AMD.

Table 2. Estimated coefficients and odds ratios from a multilevel mixed-effects logistic regression model for the association between survey factors and use or increased use of preventive alternatives to AMD.

Variables	Coefficient	SE	Odds Ratio	95% CI		p-Value [2]
				Lower	Upper	
Region [1]						
GSCA	Referent					
NCA + NSJV	−0.79	0.64	0.45	0.13	1.61	0.22
Herd size						
<1304	Referent					
≥1304	−0.75	0.77	0.47	0.10	2.13	0.32
Breed [3]						
Holstein	Referent					
Others (Jersey, crossbreed, and mix)	0.68	0.68	1.97	0.51	7.61	0.32
Participate in any dairy quality assurance programs?						
No	Referent					
Yes	1.26	0.65	3.55	0.98	12.80	0.05
Changes made by farm regarding MIADs previously available OTC since 2018						
Increased/no changes	Referent					
Decreased	1.79	0.74	5.99	1.38	25.84	0.01

[1] Northern California (NCA), Northern San Joaquin Valley (NSJV), and Greater Southern California (GSCA). [2] Factors are statistically significant at $p \leq 0.05$. [3] Breed was categorized into two levels, namely Holstein and others (Jersey, crossbreed, and mixed herds), due to small sample size.

Our model showed that producers who received training or participated in any dairy quality assurance programs during 2019 had greater odds (OR = 3.6, $p = 0.05$) of using or increasing the use of AMD preventive alternatives compared to those who did not participate in such programs. In addition, our survey revealed that conventional dairies that reported a decreased use of MIADs previously available OTC had higher odds (OR = 6.0, $p = 0.01$) of usage or an increase in the use of AMD preventive alternatives compared to dairies that reported increased or no change in the use of MIADs previously available OTC.

2.2.4. Predictors Concerning Changes in Management Practices to Prevent Spread or Outbreaks of Disease on Dairies

Among the dairies who completed the survey, a total of 32 respondents (29.4% ± 4.4) reported they had made changes in management to prevent disease outbreaks or spread in their dairies, while 77 respondents (70.6% ± 4.4) reported they had made no changes in management. In our study, 22% of respondents reported a change in management in the form of vaccination programs to prevent disease, 4.6% reported a change in management in the form of improved biosecurity (e.g., restricted traffic on operation, better isolation of sick animals, or designated separate equipment for feed and manure handling), 1.8% reported a change in management in the form of prepurchase testing of animals before being added to the herd, and 0.9% reported a change in management in the form of quarantining of purchased/returning animals from offsite locations.

Table S3 summarizes the final model for the survey factors associated with changes in management to prevent outbreaks. Our model showed that producers who included veterinarians in the revision of animal health protocols for cows had greater odds (OR = 13.5, $p = 0.01$) of reporting changes in management practices in their dairies compared to those who did not include veterinarians in protocol reviews. In addition, producers who reported better animal health on their farms during 2019 had greater odds (OR = 4.7, $p < 0.01$) of having made management changes to prevent disease spread or outbreaks compared to those who reported no changes to their animal health. Finally, producers who reported the use or increased use of alternatives to AMD in their dairies, such as vitamins, minerals, and vaccines, to reduce the use of MIADs were at greater odds (OR = 2.7, $p = 0.04$) of having made management changes to prevent disease spread or outbreaks compared to those who did not use any alternatives to AMD.

2.2.5. Predictors Concerning Change in a Dairy's AMD Costs

Changes in a dairy's drug costs were dichotomized as "decreased AMD costs" vs. "increased/no change" in AMD costs. Among the dairies who completed the survey, a total of 29 respondents (26.6% ± 4.3) reported decreased farm AMD costs since January 2018, while 80 respondents (73.4% ± 4.3) reported increased or no change in farm AMD costs. Table S4 summarizes the final model for the survey factors associated with decreased farm AMD costs.

Our model showed that producers who reported the use or increased use of AMD preventive alternatives reported decreased AMD costs in their dairies compared to those who did not use AMD preventive alternatives (OR = 7.89; $p \leq 0.01$). In addition, our study showed that producers who indicated better animal health in their farms also reported decreased AMD costs in their dairies compared to those who reported no change or worse animal health (OR = 5.48; $p \leq 0.01$).

2.2.6. Predictors Concerning Change in Reported Farm Animal Health

The response to a survey question regarding the farm animal health status as an outcome was dichotomized as "better animal health" vs. "worse/no change". Among the dairies who completed the survey, a total of 47 respondents (44.3% ± 4.9) reported better animal health since January 2018, while 59 respondents (55.7% ± 4.9) reported worse or no change on the farm's animal health. Table 3 summarizes the final model for the survey factors associated with better animal health in the dairy farms.

Our results showed that producers who included the veterinarian in the decision as to which AMD were used to treat sick cows had lower odds of reporting better animal health in their dairies compared to those who did not include the veterinarian in their treatment decision (OR = 0.31; $p = 0.01$).

Table 3. Estimated coefficients and odds ratios from a multilevel mixed-effects logistic regression model for the association between antimicrobial drugs (AMD) survey factors and better farm animal health.

Variables	Coefficient	SE	Odds Ratio	95% CI		p-Value [2]
				Lower	Upper	
Region [1]						
GSCA	Referent					
NCA + NSJV	−0.30	0.51	0.76	0.28	2.10	0.59
Herd size						
<1304	Referent					
≥1304	−0.33	0.53	0.72	0.25	2.10	0.54
Breed [3]						
Holstein	Referent					
Other (Jersey, crossbreed, and mix)	−0.02	0.55	0.97	0.32	2.90	0.96
Who decides AMD to treat sick cows?						
Dairy personnel only	Referent					
Veterinarian involved	−1.20	0.51	0.31	0.12	0.84	0.02
Have you used on-farm diagnostic techniques to guide AMD treatment?						
No	Referent					
Yes	1.51	0.52	4.53	1.61	12.71	<0.05
Have you made changes in management to prevent disease outbreak/spread?						
No	Referent					
Yes	1.10	0.52	2.91	1.10	8.10	0.04
Farm's AMD costs						
Increased/no change	Referent					
Decreased	1.30	0.54	3.68	1.30	10.78	0.01

[1] Northern California (NCA), Northern San Joaquin Valley (NSJV), and Greater Southern California (GSCA). [2] Factors are statistically significant at $p \leq 0.05$. [3] Breed was categorized into two levels, namely Holstein and others (Jersey, crossbreed, and mixed herds), due to small sample size.

Producers who indicated using on-farm diagnostic techniques to guide AMD treatment decisions had greater odds of reporting better animal health on their dairies compared to those who did not use diagnostic techniques (OR = 4.53; $p < 0.01$).

In addition, the current model indicated that producers who reported management changes in their dairies to prevent disease spread or outbreaks had greater odds (OR = 2.91, $p < 0.01$) of having better animal health in their farms during 2019 compared to those who reported no changes in management practices. Similarly, producers who reported decreased AMD costs in their dairies had greater odds (OR = 3.68, $p = 0.01$) of having better animal health in their farms during 2019 compared to those reported increased/no change in their AMD costs.

2.2.7. Predicting Factors Associated with Dairy Producers' Perceptions Regarding the Importance of AMS Practices on Dairies Using Machine Learning Classification Models

The distribution of CA dairy producers (n = 113) with respect to five statements on the importance of AMS practices is presented in Figure 1. Based on the number of the AMS practices that the dairy producers scored as very important, we found that 41.3%, 37.6%, 19.3%, 0.9%, and 0.9% of producers were given a score of 5, 4, 3, 2, and 1, respectively. By classifying producers as having "good to excellent = score of 4 and 5" AMS knowledge or as having "limited-moderate = score of 3 or less" AMS knowledge, we found that 78.9% (86/109) of producers had "good to excellent" knowledge, while 21.1% (23/109) of producers were classified as having "limited-moderate" knowledge based on their responses.

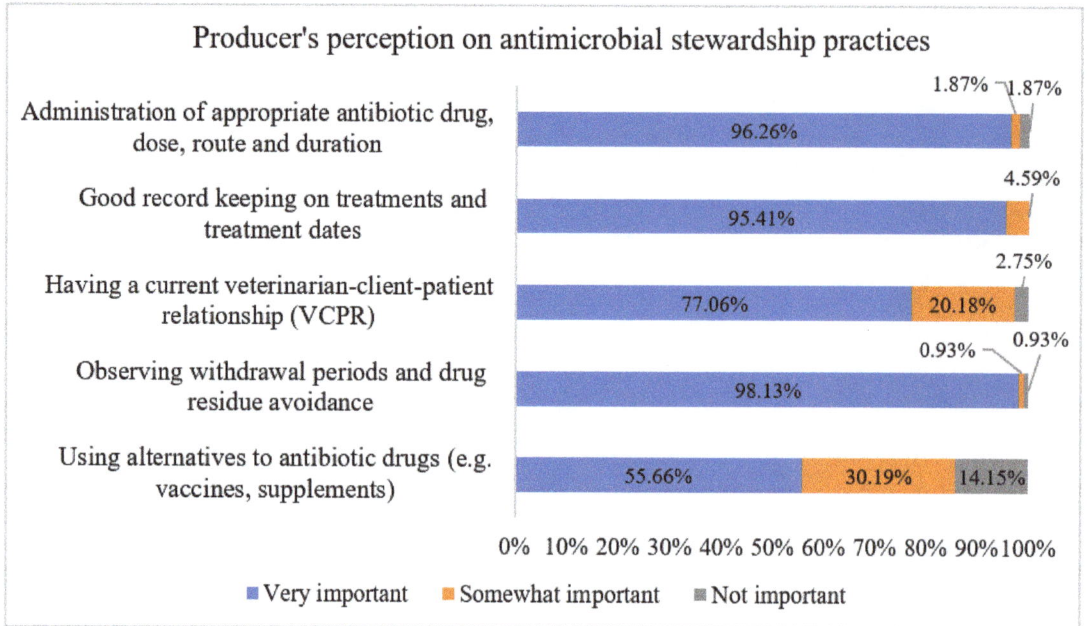

Figure 1. Distribution of responses from Californian conventional dairy producers to five statements on importance of antimicrobial stewardship practices. Bars represent proportion of responses by level of importance. The plot summarizes survey responses from 113 conventional dairy respondents.

A descriptive analyses of responses based on their knowledge of AMS practices (Table S5) showed that a greater percentage of respondents classified as having good to excellent AMS knowledge kept drug inventory logs compared with respondents classified as having limited–moderate knowledge (81.4% ± 5.9 vs. 18.6% ± 5.9; $p < 0.01$). Similarly, results showed that a greater percentage of respondents classified as having good to excellent AMS practices knowledge were familiar with FDA's term "MIADs" compared with respondents classified as having limited–moderate knowledge (90.1% ± 3.5 vs. 9.85% ± 3.5; $p < 0.01$).

Table S6 summarizes the performance of three different classification algorithms. The three models had similar specificity; however, the highest sensitivity was achieved by the gradient boosting (GB) model. The three classification models identified herd size and familiarity with MIADs as the top two important predicting variables for classifying dairy producers' AMS knowledge. The decision tree (DT) model showed that a higher percentage of dairy producers who were familiar with the FDA term MIAD were classified as producers with "good-excellent" AMS knowledge compared to producers with "limited-moderate" AMS knowledge. In addition, the DT model further classified dairies of a herd size >1737 milking cows/herd as dairies with "good-excellent "AMS practices compared with dairies of a herd size ≤1737 cows/herd.

Despite the moderate sensitivity (46.5%), random forest had the greatest precision (88.9%) compared to the remaining ML models. In general, the best classification performance as measured using the AUC was obtained using the GB model (AUC = 96). The top ten GB-identified predicting variables included herd size, familiarity with the FDA term "MIADs", annual RHA for milk production, location of herd in CA, veterinarian input on parenteral AMD purchases, willingness to treat animals with AMD alternatives, use of on-farm diagnostic techniques to guide AMD treatment decisions, producer agreement with the statement that antibiotics use in livestock may cause problems in humans, and the basis for the mastitis treatment decision (abnormal milk, California Mastitis Test, microbiologic culture of milk samples, drug sensitivity testing or treatment while culture results are pending) and producer agreement that current antibiotic use in livestock will make it harder to treat future infections (Supplementary Materials Figure S1).

3. Discussion

The response rate obtained in this survey was relatively low; however, our response rate is consistent with other mailed surveys conducted in CA [16,17] and with other surveys of both Canadian [18] and UK dairies [19]. Furthermore, response rates stratified by region in our survey were like the regional distribution of herds as reported in a California Department of Food and Agriculture report [20]. The current survey respondents reported a greater proportion of mixed-breed herds compared to a previous survey, indicating either a different population of respondents or a shift in the state dairy herd breed make-up [21]. Earlier surveys also reported higher estimates for the Holstein herd composition (65% in Aly et al. [22]; 77% in Love et al. [16]; and 66% in Ekong et al. [23]) compared to our survey. Such variability may be due to inherent differences in producers responding to such a wide range of surveys (beef quality assurance, bovine respiratory disease, and antimicrobial stewardship), which could be influenced by their interests.

3.1. Predictors Concerning Familiarity of Dairies with the FDA "MIADs" Term

Our results showed that dairy producers who reported tracking both milk and meat withdrawal intervals during AMD treatment or those who reported having a VCPR were more familiar with the FDA's term "MIADs" than those who did not report. These findings agree with findings from the survey conducted the year SB 27 was implemented [15]. However, our survey showed that 34.2% of the dairy respondents were not familiar with or not sure how the FDA's term "MIADs" related to their dairies. Similarly, a survey that was conducted to identify the common perceptions of Tennessee cattle producers regarding the VFD [24] found that 13% and 25% of dairy producers were not familiar at all or were slightly familiar with VFD, respectively. Hence, more educational outreach is needed to increase producers' knowledge and familiarity with the judicious use of MIADs in maintaining the health of cattle and reducing the pressure for AMR. The veterinarians can play an important role in communicating and educating farmers on concepts of AMR and the judicious use of AMD at the farm level. The survey conducted in the UK [19] found that the dairy farmers who had greater awareness of AMR were those that had more visits from and contact with their vets.

The majority of respondents (94.6%) in our survey confirmed they had a VCPR, while the remaining respondents (5.4%) indicated they did not; however, the latter also indicated that a veterinarian was involved in AMD treatment decisions, which may refer to the need for outreach on what establishes a valid VCPR. Veterinarians can play a major role in educating dairy producers to ensure that they have knowledge of AMR threat and AMS. Alternatively, producers may gain knowledge of MIADs independent of their herd veterinarian due to their own education and inquisition. Nevertheless, under the recently adopted VFD final rule and SB 27 regulations, veterinarians are expected to work alongside livestock producers as well as feed manufacturers and distributors to assume a greater role and increased responsibility for the use of MIADs. The VFD final rule specifies that the veterinarian must work with their client and assume responsibility for making clinical judgments about animal health; must have sufficient knowledge of the animals by virtue of examinations and/or visits to the farm where the animals are located; and must provide for any necessary follow-up evaluation or care, which are necessary components of a VCPR [6].

3.2. Predictors Concerning the Use of MIADs That Were Restricted from OTC Sales Beginning in January 2018

On January 2018, SB 27 moved all MIADs that were federally labeled for OTC sale, such as penicillin, oxytetracycline, and tylosin, to prescription status in CA. Our model showed that herd size and the use of preventive AMD alternatives were important predictors for dairy producers reporting a decreased use of OTC AMD in their dairies. The reported decrease in the use of OTC MIADs by large dairies compared to smaller dairies could be attributed to the differences in management practices, presence of computerized health protocols, and familiarity with MIADs or the use of preventive alternatives to MIADs. Our machine learning models also showed that the majority (84%) of the large dairy producers were classified as producers with "good to excellent" AMS knowledge compared with producers of small dairies. Similarly, the survey by Ekong et al. [15] found that large dairies producers were more familiar with MIADs, reported a greater use of alternatives to AMD, and reported better animal health compared to small dairy producers after implementation of SB 27.

The use of preventive alternatives to AMD may have filled the gap in the decreased use of OTC MIADs; however, it is not known whether the increased use of alternatives preceded or followed the decrease in the use of AMD previously available OTC. Similarly, Ekong et al. [15] found that producers of large dairies and producers who began using AMD alternatives had higher odds for reporting a decreased use of MIADs that were previously available OTC compared to producers of small dairies or producers who did not use alternatives to AMD.

In addition, most producers (53%) who reported a decreased use of OTC MIADs also reported that they strongly agreed that current AMD use practices in animal agriculture will make it harder to treat future livestock infections compared to producers who did not report a decreased use of AMD. Such findings indicate that producers who believe that current AMD use practices will make it harder to treat future livestock infections may have also employed good management strategies that include disease prevention and outbreak investigations, and the use of preventive alternatives, which may result in decreased AMD use on dairy farms. A study that surveyed the New York State dairy veterinarians' perceptions of AMD use [25] reported that veterinarians in their study believed that AMD use could be reduced through improved herd management strategies. However, the veterinarians also stated that the biggest barrier to implementing these changes were financial. Gerber et al. [26] found that dairy producers who implemented preventive management changes for udder and uterine health significantly reduced the use of systemic AMD for both udder and uterine health while maintaining animal health compared to producers that did not implement improvements in herd health management.

3.3. *Predictors Concerning the Use of Preventive Alternatives to AMD on Dairy Farms*

Our results showed that dairy producers who reported a decreased use of OTC AMD and reported participation in dairy quality assurance programs were more likely to report the use or increased use of preventive alternatives to AMD in their dairies. Dairy quality assurance programs are voluntary programs that promote quality animal care practices, food safety and quality assurance, as well as enhanced consumer confidence in dairy products (CDRF, 2011). These programs, including CDQAP (California Dairy Quality Assurance Program), the National Dairy FARM (Farmers Assuring Responsible Management) program, cooperative extension outreach education, creamery-led programs, and on-farm training, provide training and standards for quality animal care to promote best management practices for AMS and public health. Most of these programs have specific modules about AMS which provide ongoing education for the dairy community on the judicious and responsible use of MIADs, including avoidance of drug residues in milk and meat.

Similar results were obtained by Ekong et al. [15] who found that producers who reported a decreased use of OTC MIADs had 5.2-times greater odds of having initiated the use or increased use of alternatives to AMD in their dairies compared to producers who made no change or increased use of OTC MIADs. Antimicrobial drug preventive alternatives may have replaced MIADs that were previously available OTC, as evident by the reported decrease in the use of AMD for therapeutic purposes by producers who used or increased the use of alternatives. Alternatively, producers could have increased their use of AMD alternatives due to other reasons including changes in costs of MIADs that may have favored a shift in use of such alternatives. Therefore, further research is needed to verify our findings and determine the success of such preventive measures as alternatives to AMD.

3.4. Predictors Concerning Changes in Management Practices to Prevent the Spread or Outbreak of Disease in Dairies

Our results showed that dairy producers who reported the inclusion of veterinarians in the revision of health protocols were more likely to report changes in management practices. Herd veterinarians are professionals with experience in animal health and direct knowledge of their herds, and hence are capable of identifying the successful interventions to control and prevent diseases. The survey conducted in New York exploring dairy farmers' attitudes [27] indicated that dairy farmers are more receptive to the opinions of fellow farmers and veterinarians regarding AMD use compared to scientists/researchers and government regulators. A valid VCPR between the dairy producer and herd veterinarian can improve the health and welfare of animals by identifying shared concerns and adopting action plans [28]. For example, Jansen et al. [29] found that the communication between farmers and veterinarians helped in the adoption of practices that reduced mastitis.

Our survey findings also showed that changes in management practices were associated with better animal health. Implementing a disease prevention plan that includes good hygiene, isolation of sick or new animals, and a regular vaccination program are associated with improved animal health and productivity [30]. Good management practices help in reducing disease incidence through inhibiting the proliferation of, exposure, or susceptibility to pathogens [31]. Good management practices for biosecurity focus on efforts to prevent the entry of diseases onto the farm (external biosecurity) as well as to prevent disease transmission within the farm (biocontainment) [32,33]. Ohlson et al. [34] found an association between the lower prevalence of BRD infections with better biosecurity at the herd level. There is strong evidence that high standards of both biocontainment and external biosecurity may lead to improved animal health and, in turn, to a reduction of AMD use [30,35].

Producers who reported making changes in management to prevent disease outbreaks or spread in their dairies also reported an increased usage of alternative preventive measures to reduce the use of AMD. Preventive alternatives may work by improving animal health and hence reducing the need for AMD. However, more research is needed to identify alternatives with the same effectiveness and safety for dairy cattle in comparison to AMD [36].

3.5. Predictors Concerning Change in Dairy's AMD Costs

Producers reported that better animal health and use or increased use of AMD alternatives were important predictors of decreased AMD costs in their dairies. Increased use of preventive alternatives to AMD in livestock production has been associated with improved animal health and reduction in both AMD use and AMR [31,37]. The use of vaccines and other preventive measures can help minimize the need for AMD by preventing and controlling infectious diseases in animal populations [31]. Several studies have demonstrated that the use of various bacterial as well as viral vaccines in animals can result in a significant reduction in AMD consumption [31,38,39]. Furthermore, improved animal health may be associated with decreased AMD use and consequently reduced AMD cost. Maximizing the management practices that promote animal health and reduce the incidence of diseases may decrease the use of MIADs in dairy cattle, which is an important factor in reducing the pressure for AMR [40]. In agreement with our results, Ekong et al. [15] found that the reported use or increased use of AMD preventive alternatives was a predictor for a reported decrease in farm AMD cost, their study also reported that inclusion of veterinarian in decision to use AMD, decreasing use of MIADs previously available OTC, participation in dairy quality assurance programs were positively associated with reporting decreased farm AMD cost.

3.6. Predictors Concerning Farm's Animal Health Compared to 2018

Our findings showed that the use of on-farm diagnostic techniques reduced AMD cost and adopting changes in management to prevent disease outbreak/spread were positively associated with better animal health. In agreement with the findings reported by Ekong et al. [15], our survey producers who reported decreased AMD costs on their dairies had greater odds (OR = 4.57, p = 0.01) of having better animal health in their farms during 2019 compared to those who reported increased/no change in their AMD costs. Both surveys also identified the use of on-farm diagnostic techniques to guide AMD treatment and improved management practices to prevent both disease outbreak and spread as predictors of producers who reported better animal health. The use of diagnostic techniques such as laboratory culture, auscultation, and lung ultrasound to guide treatment decisions for cows is an important practice to facilitate the judicious use of AMD [41,42]. The availability of affordable diagnostic tools that can detect animals at early stages of disease is important to prevent the high financial costs derived from lost productivity and the treatment of diseased animals [43]. Testing animals for disease can boost herd health and cut costs associated with AMD treatment [44]. A UK survey of dairy herds reported that both farmers and veterinarians recognized there was substantial room for improvement of current diagnostic tools for the detection of mastitis and metabolic disease in dairy cows, particularly with regard to early disease detection [44].

3.7. Comparing Survey Findings Immediately Post SP 27 (2018) and One Year Later (2019)

A detailed comparison of the associations explored over the two AMS surveys conducted in CA post SB 27 shows specific shared predictors with similar magnitudes of associations (Figure S2). Predictors common between the current survey (2019) and a year prior (2018) include the reported decreased use of AMD, increased use of AMD alternatives, having a VCPR, tracking AMD treatment information, on-farm record keeping, the use of on-farm diagnostic techniques to guide AMD treatment, participation in dairy quality assurance programs, the inclusion of veterinarians in decisions for the selection of AMD to treat sick cows, and implementation of management practices to prevent disease introduction and spread. In agreement with the current survey (2019), surveys conducted on Illinois dairies [45] and Ohio dairies [46] identified appropriate antimicrobial treatment selection; the use of health protocols; on-farm record keeping; and the application of herd-specific veterinary written protocols, education, and training of farm personnel on diagnostic criteria for the initiation of AMD treatments as important areas for the improvement of AMS in dairies.

3.8. Factors Associated with Dairy Producers' Perceptions Regarding the Importance of AMS Practices on Dairies

Our main goal for machine learning (ML) classification models was to identify factors that can assign dairy producers with good–excellent AMS knowledge. Machine learning models have been used in human medicine to predict AMS intervention in hospitals [47]; however, their use lacks prediction of AMS in veterinary medicine. Using such tools can be helpful for the prediction of AMS interventions in the dairy industry. Machine learning models can be developed to predict which dairies require a stewardship intervention. However, further work is required to develop models with adequate discriminatory power to be applicable to the real-world dairy industry. Our ML models classified producers of large dairies (>1737 milking cows/herd) as producers with "good-excellent" AMS knowledge compared with producers of small dairies ($\leq$1737 cows/herd). A recent Australian study [48] surveyed livestock veterinary practices and identified a lack of access to education, training, and AMS resources as key barriers to the implementation of AMS practices in veterinary practices. Jones et al. [49] suggested that the scientific advice to convey to dairy farmers to achieve responsible AMD use would include advice on best farm practice to minimize the risk of disease and data on cost savings that might be obtained from reduced AMD. In agreement with Ekong et al. [15], our classification ML models also showed that the knowledge of dairy producers about AMS and the adoption of AMS programs may be improved using continuing education and outreach specifically to producers of small and medium-sized dairies. Our results identified that herd size, familiarity with MIADs, RHA, the location of the dairy in CA, tracking AMD treatment, having a written computerized protocol, the somatic cell count, vaccination of animals against mastitis, keeping a drug inventory log, and awareness that MIADs require prescription were the common predictors for classifying dairy producer knowledge regarding AMS practices.

The majority of conventional dairy producers in our study (>95%) indicated that the administration of the appropriate AMD dose, the route, good record keeping on AMD treatment, and observing AMD withdrawal periods are very important AMS practices. This agrees with a previous study that has suggested that improvement in dairy farmers' AMD use practices can be achieved by using written treatment protocols [50] and the appropriate use of AMD through antimicrobial testing to guide the AMD treatment [51]. Therefore, more extension and outreach efforts should focus on those components to improve antimicrobial stewardship in California dairies.

3.9. Study Limitations

The response rate of the current survey was relatively low; however, it is similar to other surveys conducted in California. Furthermore, it is possible that only the producers most interested in AMS responded to this survey, therefore our survey could be subject to different selection bias. As with any survey, our findings are limited by the responses obtained through a questionnaire mailed to CA conventional dairy producers, which may be subject to information bias. However, we piloted the questionnaire using in-person interviews with extension and outreach specialists and veterinarians in CA [21] and used both multiple-point scales and ordinal Likert scales. The actual AMD usage or treatment practices and the health status of the cows on respondent dairies were not measured and hence findings based on related questions should be interpreted with caution. Finally, AMS practices cannot be characterized by the current survey's responses alone. Therefore, further studies are needed to directly measure the associations between AMD use and AMS practices based on management protocols and an evaluation of both health and production records.

4. Materials and Methods

A survey instrument was developed to collect information on AMD use in adult cows in CA dairies during 2019, one year post full implementation of SB 27. The survey was mailed to 1282 grade A dairies in CA during the period from May to December 2019. A list of all licensed grade A dairies in California in 2017 was obtained from the California Department of Food and Agriculture and served as a sampling frame for our survey. The survey development, descriptive statistics, and cluster analyses of the 2019 survey are described in detail in Abdelfattah et al. [21]. Briefly, the survey questionnaire consisted of 44 questions partitioned into three main sections. The first section included variables about herd demographics including the respondent's role, the county where the dairy was located, the herd's breed(s), number of milking cows, annual rolling herd average (RHA) milk production, and previous month's average bulk tank somatic cell count. The second section included questions about dairy cow health management and AMD use including protocols for dry-off, vaccination, disease prevention and diagnosis, sources of information on AMD, who makes decisions on the AMD purchased and used, whether producers had written or computerized animal health protocols, use of a drug inventory, and the presence of a VCPR in dairies. The third section inquired about the dairy practices including enrollment in the animal welfare audit and/or dairy quality assurance programs, producer's familiarity with MIADs and changes made since 2018 with regard to MIADs previously available OTC, AMD costs, the use of AMD alternatives, disease prevention, and the herd's health status. An optional comments section was included in the survey to allow respondents to provide feedback about their concern regarding AMD use and AMR in dairies. Multiple-point scales and ordinal Likert scales were used to capture the participant responses to the survey questions.

4.1. Statistical Analyses

4.1.1. Descriptive Statistics

For the 113 conventional survey responses, proportions and their standard errors were computed for categorical and ordinal variables, while means and standard errors were computed for continuous variables. Data on the location of dairies in CA were categorized into three regions, namely Northern California (NCA), Northern San Joaquin Valley (NSJV), and Greater Southern California (GSCA), based on the distinct differences among the three regions in dairy infrastructure and management practices [16]. For the purposes of model building, milking herd size was categorized as ≤1304 or >1304 milking cows based on the CA mean herd size while RHA was categorized as <10,880 kg/cow or >10,880 based on the CA mean herd milk production [20].

4.1.2. Logistic Regression Models

Six survey questions related to AMD use and AMR in CA dairies were selected and analyzed as outcome (dependent) variables. These outcome questions included:

(1) Familiarity of dairy producers with the FDA's MIADs term. The familiarity of dairy producers with MIADs was identified if the survey respondent recognized the FDA classification of MIADs as important, highly important, or critically important drugs, and/or that MIADs are available for livestock only via prescription or veterinary feed directive pursuant to VCPR with a licensed veterinarian. Familiarity with MIADs was dichotomized into 2 levels: "familiar" and "not familiar."

(2) Changes made since January 2018 regarding the use of injectable, bolus, and/or intramammary dosage forms of OTC MIADs. This outcome was classified as "decreased OTC MIADs use" or "increased or no change in the use of OTC MIADs".

(3) Initiation or increased use of alternatives to AMD since January 2018. This third outcome was dichotomized as "yes" (use AMD alternatives) or "no" (do not use AMD alternatives).

(4) Changes in management practices to prevent disease outbreak or spread since January 2018. This fourth outcome was dichotomized as "yes" (made changes in management practices in the form of improvement in vaccination programs, quarantined purchased and returned animals from offsite locations, improvements of farm biosecurity measures, or testing of pre-purchased animals for infectious diseases before joining the herd) and "no" (no changes in management practices).

(5) Description of the farm's AMD costs since January 2018. This fifth outcome modeled the changes in the farm AMD drug costs in 2019 and was dichotomized as "decreased AMD cost" or "increased/no change AMD cost".

(6) Description of the farm's animal health conditions since January 2018. This sixth outcome modeled the changes in farm animal health and was dichotomized as "better animal health" or "worse/no change in animal health".

Logistic regression models were specified for each outcome. Univariate models were used to assess the association between the survey variables described in Abdelfattah et al. [21] and each of the six outcomes of interest. Predictors associated with an outcome of interest at $p \leq 0.20$ were considered for further modeling. A manual forward model building approach was used while assessing confounding by the breed, herd size, RHA, and region using the method of change in estimates [52]. Previously excluded variables were offered into the model again and retained at $p \leq 0.05$. All biologically meaningful interaction terms were explored using significance testing. Collinearity of all the potential explanatory variables was checked using the spearman rank correlation statistic. The diagnostics were performed, and plots of residuals were examined, confirming the goodness of fit of each model. Final model selection and fit were assessed using the Akaike Information Criterion (AIC). The coefficients, odds ratios (OR), and their associated 95% confidence intervals were estimated in the final logistic model for factors statistically significant ($p \leq 0.05$) with the outcome. All statistical analyses were performed using Stata 15 (Stata Corp, College Station, TX, USA).

4.1.3. Machine Learning Classification Models

Machine learning algorithms were used to predict dairy producers who considered AMS practices as important to preserve the efficacy of AMD and reduce AMR in dairy farms. In this study, three widely used machine learning algorithms were evaluated, including decision tree (DT), random forest (RF), and gradient boosting (GB) algorithms. The responses of 113 conventional dairy producers to survey questions about AMS practices were used as a target for the three predictive models. The question requested respondents to classify the following five AMS practices as very important, somewhat important, or not important: (1) administration of appropriate AMD dose, route, and duration; (2) good record keeping on treatment and treatment dates; (3) having a current VCPR; (4) observing withdrawal periods and drug residue avoidance; and (5) using alternatives to AMD such as vaccines and supplements. The respondents were given a score of one to five based on the number of the AMS practices that they scored as very important. For example, if one respondent indicated that all five previously mentioned AMS practices are very important, they would be given a score of 5 and so on. A score of 5 was ranked "excellent", 4 as "good", 3 as "moderate", and 2 or 1 as "limited" knowledge of AMS practices. Then, dairy respondents were reclassified as having "good to excellent" AMS knowledge based on a score of ≥4 or as having "limited-moderate" knowledge based on a score of ≤3. Having "good to excellent" vs. "limited-moderate" AMS knowledge was the outcome of the three predictive models (target variable). Each model was offered a set of 27 survey factors (predictor variables) that contributed to most of the variability in the survey responses, as identified using multiple factor analysis, as reported by Abdelfattah et al. [21]. The predictor variables included herd demographics (herd size, location, annual rolling herd average milk production, and somatic cell count); good general practices (feed newborn calves colostrum from fresh cows, have a separate calving pen, and vaccinate against different diseases); AMD usage information (sources of information about AMD, inclusion of veterinarian in the decision to purchase and treat cows with AMD, tracking of AMD withdrawal periods, and having a written/computerized health protocol); mastitis management practices (basis for treatment of mastitis with AMD, AMD treatment choice, and class of AMD used to treat mastitis); metritis management practices (basis for treatment of metritis and AMD treatment choice); treatment choice for pneumonia in adult cows (oral or injectable AMD); familiarity of producers with the FDA's term "MIADs" and that MIADs require prescription; and the level of agreement (strongly agreed/agreed, neutral, or strongly disagree/disagree) of dairy producers on the following statements: current antibiotic use practices in animal agriculture will make it harder to treat future livestock infections, antibiotic use in livestock does not cause problems in humans, antibiotic use in livestock leads to bacterial infections in people that are more difficult to treat, any use of antibiotics may result in infections that are more difficult to treat in the future, and willingness to treat animals with alternatives to antibiotics if they were equally effective and comparable in price. The original dataset was partitioned into training and testing data sets using a random split ratio of 70: 30 (training: test). Each model was trained with the training dataset and evaluated by assessing their predictive performance on the testing dataset using Salford Predictive Modeler 8.0 software (https://www.minitab.com/en-us/products/spm/ accessed on 15 July 2021). For the DT algorithm, we used a 10-fold cross-validation method for testing, Gini as the optimization method, and the minimum cost tree as the choice for the best tree [53]. The RF method is based on multiple decision trees: it builds several individual classification trees using a random subsample of the data and then selects the most popular class [54]. For the RF model, we used the out-of-bag testing method with 500 classification trees. Meanwhile, for the GB model, we used a 10-fold cross-validation method, a tree size of 500, balanced sample weights, and the best model chosen by cross-entropy [54]. Evaluation of model performance was based on accuracy, sensitivity, specificity, F1 score, and the Area Under Curve (AUC) estimated from receiver operator characteristic (ROC) curve analyses [55]. The probability threshold at which a classification was made was initially set at a standard 0.5. Then, the obtained results were explored, and the optimal predictive threshold was determined to select the highest specificity [56].

5. Conclusions

The majority of survey producers agreed that the administration of the appropriate AMD dose, the route, keeping good records on AMD treatment, and observing AMD withdrawal periods are very important AMS practices. Our results showed that better cow health was positively associated with management changes to prevent disease spread and the use of on-farm diagnostic techniques to guide AMD treatment decisions. In addition, the use or increased use of preventive alternatives to AMD was positively associated with the decreased use of OTC AMD and decreased farm AMD cost. Our findings identified that factors that were associated with antimicrobial stewardship practices in conventional CA dairies immediately after implementation of SB 27 are still important one year later. These factors included a valid veterinarian–client–patient relationship, a reduction in the use of MIADs that were previously available OTC before implementation of SB 27, a decreased farm AMD cost, and the use or increased use of AMD alternatives. In addition, herd size, familiarity with MIADs, location of the dairy in CA, tracking AMD treatment, having a written computerized protocol, keeping drug inventory logs, and awareness that MIADs require prescription were the common predictors between the survey of 2018 and 2019 that identified dairy producers with "good to excellent" antimicrobial stewardship knowledge using machine learning. The findings of our survey should be interpreted with caution due to biases related to surveys.

Findings from this survey may benefit extension outreach efforts by offering education and training on identified areas associated with improved antimicrobial stewardship practices in CA dairies. Future research is needed to study the association between the implementation of antimicrobial stewardship practices and the reduction in the prevalence of AMR in food-producing animals. In addition, further research is needed to identify the barriers that prevent the implementation of the identified components of antimicrobial stewardship practices in CA dairies.

Supplementary Materials: The following supporting information can be downloaded at: https://www.mdpi.com/article/10.3390/antibiotics11020165/s1. Table S1: Summary of herd characteristics from 113 responses received from conventional dairies to a mailed questionnaire on antimicrobial drug (AMD) use in adult cows in California during 2019; Table S2: Estimated coefficients and odds ratios from a multilevel mixed-effects logistic regression model for the association between survey factors and decreased use of antimicrobial drugs (AMD) that were previously available over the counter; Table S3: Estimated coefficients and odds ratios from a multilevel mixed-effects logistic regression model for the association between survey factors and having farm-made changes in management to prevent spread of disease; Table S4: Estimated coefficients and odds ratios from a multilevel mixed-effects logistic regression model for the association between survey factors and decreased AMD cost compared to 2018; Table S5: Summary of descriptive analysis of dairy producers' respondents classified as having "limited-moderate knowledge" or "good-excellent knowledge" in antimicrobial stewardship practices based on responses obtained from 113 conventional California dairies; Table S6: Performance metrics of three classification models used to study the association between good–excellent antimicrobial stewardship practices and survey responses in 113 conventional California dairies during 2019; Figure S1: Predictive variables importance plot showing the ranking of variables' relative importance for predicting dairies with good to excellent antimicrobial stewardship practices based on survey responses from 113 conventional California dairies during 2019. "MIADs" are medically important antimicrobial drugs. "AMD" is antimicrobial drug; and Figure S2: Web diagram showing the magnitude and direction of the associations between six antimicrobial stewardship outcomes and predictors from logistic regression models based on surveys of conventional California dairies during 2018 (black arrows) and 2019 (red arrows). Associations with both black and red arrows identify common associations between surveys.

Author Contributions: Conceptualization, E.M.A., E.O., D.R.W., B.M.K., T.W.L. and S.S.A.; methodology, E.M.A., P.S.E. and S.S.A.; software, E.M.A., P.S.E. and S.S.A.; validation, E.M.A., D.R.W., B.M.K., T.W.L. and S.S.A.; formal analysis, E.M.A. and S.S.A.; investigation, E.M.A. and S.S.A.; resources, E.M.A. and S.S.A.; data curation, E.M.A. and S.S.A.; writing—original draft preparation, E.M.A. and S.S.A.; writing—review and editing, E.M.A., E.O., D.R.W., B.M.K., T.W.L. and S.S.A.; visualization, E.M.A., P.S.E. and S.S.A.; supervision, S.S.A., E.O. and T.W.L.; project administration, S.S.A., E.O. and T.W.L.; funding acquisition, S.S.A., E.O., B.M.K. and T.W.L. All authors have read and agreed to the published version of the manuscript.

Funding: This research study was funded by the California Department of Food and Agriculture, the University of California Davis's School of Veterinary Medicine, and the Office of Research's Principal Investigator Bridge Program. The funders had no role in the study design, data collection and analysis, decision to publish, or preparation of the manuscript.

Institutional Review Board Statement: The study was reviewed by the University of California, Davis Institutional Review Board, and was granted exemption approval as our research did not involve human subjects (IRB number: 1537295-1; approval date: 9 January 2020).

Informed Consent Statement: Not applicable.

Data Availability Statement: This study was sponsored by the California Department of Food and Agriculture, and is subject to California Food and Agriculture Code (FAC) Sections 14400 to 14408. FAC Section 14407 requires that the data collected be kept confidential to prevent individual identification of a farm or business; as such, raw data from this study are not able to be shared.

Acknowledgments: The authors are grateful for survey producers, herd managers, and veterinarians.

Conflicts of Interest: The funders had no role in the design of the study; in the collection, analyses, or interpretation of data; in the writing of the manuscript, or in the decision to publish the results.

References

1. FDA (Food and Drug Administration), Center for Veterinary Medicine. Summary Report on Antimicrobials Sold or Distributed for Use in Food-Producing Animals. Food and Drug Administration; Center for Veterinary Medicine Website. 2019. Available online: https://www.fda.gov/media/144427/download (accessed on 7 July 2021).
2. McManus, M.C. Mechanisms of bacterial resistance to antimicrobial agents. *Am. J. Health-Syst. Pharm.* **1997**, *54*, 1420–1433. [CrossRef] [PubMed]
3. Cuny, C.; Wieler, L.H.; Witte, W. Livestock-associated MRSA. The impact on humans. *Antibiotics* **2015**, *4*, 521–543. [CrossRef] [PubMed]
4. CDC (U.S. Centers for Disease Control and Prevention). Biggest Threats and Data: 2019 AR Threats Report; Centers for Disease Control and Prevention Website. Available online: https://www.cdc.gov/drugresistance/biggest-threats.html (accessed on 28 April 2020).
5. WHO (World Health Organization). Global Action Plan on Antimicrobial Resistance. 2015. Available online: http://www.who.int/antimicrobial-resistance/publications/global-action-plan/en/ (accessed on 9 July 2020).
6. FDA (Food and Drug Administration). Fact Sheet: Veterinary Feed Directive Final Rule and Next Steps. 2017. Available online: https://www.fda.gov/animal-veterinary/development-approval-process/fact-sheet-veterinary-feed-directive-final-rule-and-next-steps (accessed on 12 July 2021).
7. FAC (Food and Agricultural Code); Sacramento, C.A. Livestock: Use of Antimicrobial Drugs [14400–14408]. 2015. Available online: https://leginfo.legislature.ca.gov/faces/codes_displaySection.xhtml?sectionNum=14401.&lawCode=FAC (accessed on 9 July 2021).
8. Hogan, L.J., Jr. Senate Bill 471. Agriculture–Use of Antimicrobial Drugs—Limitations and Reporting Requirements. Chapter 679. 2019. Available online: https://legiscan.com/MD/text/SB471/2019 (accessed on 10 December 2020).
9. Anderson, M.; Buckley, G.; Hayward, S. Oregon Senate Bill 920. 78th Oregon Legislative Assembly—2015 Regular Session. 2015. Available online: https://olis.oregonlegislature.gov/liz/2015R1/Downloads/MeasureDocument/SB920 (accessed on 26 January 2022).

10. Tang, K.L.; Caffrey, N.P.; Nóbrega, D.B.; Cork, S.C.; Ronksley, P.E.; Barkema, H.W.; Polachek, A.J.; Ganshorn, H.; Sharma, N.; Kellner, J.D.; et al. Restricting the use of antibiotics in food-producing animals and its associations with antibiotic resistance in food-producing animals and human beings: A systematic review and meta-analysis. *Lancet Planet. Health* **2017**, *1*, e316–e327. [CrossRef]
11. EC (European Commission). New EU Rules on Veterinary Medicinal Products and Medicated Feed; European Commission Website. 2019. Available online: https://ec.europa.eu/food/sites/food/files/animals/docs/ah_vet-med_feed_factsheet-2018_en.pdf (accessed on 9 July 2021).
12. Speksnijder, D.C.; Mevius, D.J.; Bruschke, C.J.M.; Wagenaar, J.A. Reduction of veterinary antimicrobial use in The Netherlands. The Dutch success models. *Zoonoses Public Health* **2015**, *62* (Suppl. 1), 79–87. [CrossRef] [PubMed]
13. Jensen, V.F.; de Knegt, L.V.; Andersen, V.D.; Wingstrand, A. Temporal relationship between decrease in antimicrobial prescription for Danish pigs and the "Yellow Card" legal intervention directed at reduction of antimicrobial use. *Prev. Vet. Med.* **2014**, *117*, 554–564. [CrossRef] [PubMed]
14. More, S.J. European perspectives on efforts to reduce antimicrobial usage in food animal production. *Ir. Vet. J.* **2020**, *73*, 2. [CrossRef]
15. Ekong, P.S.; Abdelfattah, E.M.; Okello, E.; Williams, D.R.; Lehenbauer, T.W.; Karle, B.M.; Rowe, J.D.; Aly, S.S. 2018 Survey of factors associated with antimicrobial drug use and stewardship practices in adult cows on conventional California dairies: Immediate post-Senate Bill 27 impact. *PeerJ* **2021**, *9*, e11596. [CrossRef]
16. Love, W.J.; Lehenbauer, T.W.; Karle, B.M.; Hulbert, L.E.; Anderson, R.J.; Van Eenennaam, A.L.; Farver, T.B.; Aly, S.S. Survey of management practices related to bovine respiratory disease in preweaned calves on California dairies. *J. Dairy Sci.* **2016**, *99*, 1483–1494. [CrossRef]
17. Martins, J.P.N.; Karle, B.M.; Heguy, J.M. Needs assessment for cooperative extension dairy programs in California. *J. Dairy Sci.* **2019**, *102*, 7597–7607. [CrossRef]
18. Denis-Robichaud, J.; Cerri, R.L.A.; Jones-Bitton, A.; LeBlanc, S.J. Study of reproduction management on Canadian dairy farms. *J. Dairy Sci.* **2016**, *99*, 9339–9351. [CrossRef]
19. Higham, L.E.; Deakin, A.; Tivey, E.; Porteus, V.; Ridgway, S.; Rayner, A.C. A survey of dairy cow farmers in the United Kingdom: Knowledge, attitudes and practices surrounding antimicrobial use and resistance. *Vet. Rec.* **2018**, *183*, 746. [CrossRef] [PubMed]
20. CDFA (California Department of Food and Agriculture); Sacramento, C.A. California Agricultural Statistics Review 2017–2018. 2018. Available online: https://www.nass.usda.gov/Statistics_by_State/California/Publications/Annual_Statistical_Reviews/2019/2018cas-all.pdf (accessed on 12 July 2021).
21. Abdelfattah, E.M.; Ekong, P.S.; Okello, E.; Williams, D.; Karle, B.; Rowe, J.; Marshall, E.; Lehenbauer, T.W.; Aly, S. 2019 Survey of Antimicrobial Drug Use and Stewardship Practices in Adult Cows on California Dairies: Post Senate Bill 27. *Microorganisms* **2021**, *9*, 1507. [CrossRef] [PubMed]
22. Aly, S.S.; Rossow, H.A.; Acetoze, G.; Lehenbauer, T.W.; Payne, M.; Meyer, D.; Maas, J.; Hoar, B. Survey of Beef Quality Assurance on California dairies. *J. Dairy Sci.* **2014**, *97*, 1348–1357. [CrossRef] [PubMed]
23. Ekong, P.S.; Abdelfattah, E.M.; Okello, E.; Williams, D.R.; Lehenbauer, T.W.; Karle, B.M.; Rowe, J.D.; Marshall, E.S.; Aly, S.S. 2018 Survey of antimicrobial drug use and stewardship practices in adult cows on California dairies: Post-Senate Bill 27. *PeerJ* **2021**, *9*, e11515. [CrossRef]
24. Ekakoro, J.E.; Caldwell, M.; Strand, E.B.; Okafor, C.C. Perceptions of Tennessee cattle producers regarding the Veterinary Feed Directive. *PLoS ONE* **2019**, *14*, 1–19. [CrossRef]
25. Padda, H.; Wemette, M.; Safi, A.G.; Beauvais, W.; Shapiro, M.A.; Moroni, P.; Ivanek, R. New York State dairy veterinarians' perceptions of antibiotic use and resistance: A qualitative interview study. *Prev. Vet. Med.* **2021**, *194*, 105428. [CrossRef] [PubMed]
26. Gerber, M.; Dürr, S.; Bodmer, M. Reducing Antimicrobial Use by Implementing Evidence-Based, Management-Related Prevention Strategies in Dairy Cows in Switzerland. *Front. Vet. Sci.* **2021**, *7*, 611682. [CrossRef]
27. Vasquez, A.K.; Foditsch, C.; Dulièpre, S.-A.C.; Siler, J.D.; Just, D.R.; Warnick, L.D.; Nydam, D.V.; Sok, J. Understanding the effect of producers' attitudes, perceived norms, and perceived behavioral control on intentions to use antimicrobials prudently on New York dairy farms. *PLoS ONE* **2019**, *14*, e0222442. [CrossRef]
28. Sumner, C.L.; von Keyserlingk, M.A.G.; Weary, D.M. Perspectives of farmers and veterinarians concerning dairy cattle welfare. *Anim. Front.* **2018**, *8*, 8–13. [CrossRef]
29. Jansen, J.; Renes, R.J.; Lam, T.J.G.M. Evaluation of two communication strategies to improve udder health management. *J. Dairy Sci.* **2010**, *93*, 604–612. [CrossRef]
30. Laanen, M.; Persoons, D.; Ribbens, S.; de Jong, E.; Callens, B.; Strubbe, M.; Maes, D.; Dewulf, J. Relationship between biosecurity and production/antimicrobial treatment characteristics in pig herds. *Vet. J.* **2013**, *198*, 508–512. [CrossRef] [PubMed]
31. Buchy, P.; Ascioglu, S.; Buisson, Y.; Datta, S.; Nissen, M.; Tambyah, P.A.; Vong, S. Impact of vaccines on antimicrobial resistance. *Int. J. Infect. Dis.* **2020**, *90*, 188–196. [CrossRef] [PubMed]
32. Moore, D.; Adaska, J.; Higginbotham, G.; Castillo, A.; Collar, C.; Sischo, W. Testing new dairy cattle for disease can boost herd health, cut costs. *Calif. Agric.* **2009**, *63*, 29–34. [CrossRef]
33. Buhman, M.; Dewel, G.; Griffen, D. Biosecurity Basics for Cattle Operations and Good Management Practices (GMP) for Controlling Infectious Diseases. Nebraska Cooperative Extension G00–1411-A. 2000. Available online: http://extensionpublications.unl.edu/assets/pdf/g1411.pdf (accessed on 5 July 2021).

34. Ohlson, A.; Emanuelson, U.; Tråvén, M.; Alenius, S. The relationship between antibody status to bovine corona virus and bovine respiratory syncytial virus and disease incidence, reproduction, and herd characteristics in dairy herds. *Acta Vet. Scand.* **2010**, *52*, 1–7. [CrossRef]
35. Ribbens, S.; Dewulfa, J.; Koenenb, F.; Mintiensc, K.; De Sadeleera, L.; de Kruifa, A.; Maes, D. A survey on biosecurity and management practices in Belgian pig herds. *Prev. Vet. Med.* **2008**, *83*, 228–241. [CrossRef] [PubMed]
36. Kurt, T.; Wong, N.; Fowler, H.; Gay, C.; Lillehoj, H.; Plummer, P.; Scott, H.M.; Hoelzer, K. Strategic Priorities for Research on Antibiotic Alternatives in Animal Agriculture—Results from an Expert Workshop. *Front. Vet. Sci.* **2019**, *6*, 1–6. [CrossRef] [PubMed]
37. Hoelzer, K.; Bielke, L.; Blake, D.P.; Cox, E.; Cutting, S.M.; Devriendt, B.; Erlacher-Vindel, E.; Goossens, E.; Karaca, K.; Lemiere, S.; et al. Vaccines as alternatives to antibiotics for food producing animals-part 2: New approaches and potential solutions. *Vet. Res.* **2018**, *49*, 141. [CrossRef]
38. Buckley, B.S.; Henschke, N.; Bergman, H.; Skidmore, B.; Klemm, E.J.; Villanueva, G. Impact of vaccination on antibiotic usage: A systematic review and meta-analysis. *Clin. Microbiol. Infect.* **2019**, *25*, 1213–1225. [CrossRef]
39. Murphy, D.; Ricci, A.; Auce, Z.; Beechinor, J.G.; Bergendahl, H.; Breathnach, R.; Bureš, J.; Da Silva, D.; Pedro, J.; Hederová, J. EMA and EFSA Joint Scientific Opinion on measures to reduce the need to use antimicrobial agents in animal husbandry in the European Union, and the resulting impacts on food safety (RONAFA). *EFSA J.* **2017**, *15*, 4666.
40. Lam, T.J.G.M.; Jansen, J.; Wessels, R.J. The RESET Mindset Model applied on decreasing antibiotic usage in dairy cattle in the Netherlands. *Ir. Vet. J.* **2017**, *70*, 1–9. [CrossRef]
41. Ollivett, T.L. Thoracic ultrasound to monitor lung health and assist decision making in preweaned dairy calves. *AABP Proc.* **2018**, *51*, 185–187.
42. Lago, A.; Godden, S.M.; Bey, R.; Ruegg, P.L.; Leslie, K. The selective treatment of clinical mastitis based on on-farm culture results: I. Effects on antibiotic use, milk withholding time, and short-term clinical and bacteriological outcomes. *J. Dairy Sci.* **2011**, *94*, 4441–4456. [CrossRef] [PubMed]
43. Macrae, A.; Esslemont, R. The prevalence and cost of important endemic diseases and fertility in dairy herds in the UK. In *Bovine Medicine*, 3rd ed.; Crockfort, P.D., Ed.; John Wiley & Sons Ltd.: Hoboken, NJ, USA, 2015.
44. Donadeu, F.X.; Howes, N.L.; Esteves, C.L.; Howes, M.P.; Byrne, T.J.; Macrae, A.I. Farmer and Veterinary Practices and Opinions Related to the Diagnosis of Mastitis and Metabolic Disease in UK Dairy Cows. *Front. Vet. Sci.* **2020**, *7*, 127. [CrossRef]
45. Ramirez, C.R.; Dumas, S.E.; Schlist, K.L.; French, D.D.; Bichi, E.; Rivero, B.R.C.; Aldridge, B.M.; Lowe, J.F. Evidence in support of veterinary involvement in antimicrobial stewardship training programs in the dairy industry: A preliminary study. *Bov. Pract.* **2017**, *51*, 200–204.
46. Habing, G.; Djordjevic, C.; Schuenemann, G.M.; Lakritz, J. Understanding antimicrobial stewardship: Disease severity treatment thresholds and antimicrobial alternatives among organic and conventional calf producers. *Prev. Vet. Med.* **2016**, *130*, 77–85. [CrossRef]
47. Bystritsky, R.; Beltran, A.; Young, A.; Wong, A.; Hu, X.; Doernberg, S. Machine learning for the prediction of antimicrobial stewardship intervention in hospitalized patients receiving broad-spectrum agents. *Infect. Control. Hosp. Epidemiol.* **2020**, *41*, 1022–1027. [CrossRef] [PubMed]
48. Hardefeldt, L.Y.; Gilkerson, J.R.; Billman-Jacobe, H.; Stevenson, M.A.; Thursky, K.; Bailey, K.E.; Browning, G.F. Barriers to and enablers of implementing antimicrobial stewardship programs in veterinary practices. *J. Vet. Intern. Med.* **2018**, *32*, 1092–1099. [CrossRef]
49. Jones, P.J.; Marierb, E.A.; Trantera, R.B.; Wub, G.; Watsonb, E.; Tealeb, C.J. Factors affecting dairy farmers' attitudes towards antimicrobial medicine usage in cattle in England and Wales. *Prev. Vet. Med.* **2015**, *121*, 30–40. [CrossRef]
50. Friedman, D.B.; Kanwat, C.P.; Headrick, M.L.; Patterson, N.J.; Neely, J.C.; Smith, L.U. Importance of Prudent Antibiotic Use on Dairy Farms in South Carolina: A Pilot Project on Farmers' Knowledge, Attitudes and Practices. *Zoonoses Public Health* **2007**, *54*, 366–375. [CrossRef]
51. USDA. *Health and Management Practices on U.S. Dairy Operations; USDA–APHIS–VS–CEAH–NAHMS*; National Animal Health Monitoring System: Fort Collins, CO, USA, 2014. Available online: https://www.aphis.usda.gov/aphis/ourfocus/animalhealth/monitoring-and-surveillance/nahms/NAHMS_Dairy_Studies (accessed on 30 October 2020).
52. Aly, S.S.; Anderson, R.J.; Adaska, J.M.; Jiang, J.; Gardner, I.A. Association between Mycobacterium avium subspecies paratuberculosis infection and milk production in two California dairies. *J. Dairy Sci.* **2010**, *93*, 1030–1040. [CrossRef]
53. Slob, N.; Catal, C.; Kassahun, A. Application of machine learning to improve dairy farm management: A systematic literature review. *Prev. Vet. Med.* **2021**, *187*, 105237. [CrossRef] [PubMed]
54. Breiman, L. Random Forests. *Mach. Learn.* **2001**, *45*, 5–32. [CrossRef]
55. Hyde, R.M.; Down, P.M.; Bradley, A.J.; Breen, J.E.; Hudson, C.; Leach, K.A.; Green, M.J. Automated prediction of mastitis infection patterns in dairy herds using machine learning. *Sci. Rep.* **2020**, *10*, 4289. [CrossRef] [PubMed]
56. Kuhn, M. Building Predictive Models in R Using the caret Package. *J. Stat. Softw.* **2008**, *28*, 1–26. [CrossRef]

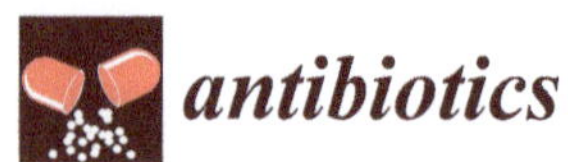

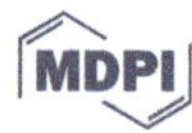

Review

Scoping Review of National Antimicrobial Stewardship Activities in Eight African Countries and Adaptable Recommendations

Nduta Kamere [1], Sandra Tafadzwa Garwe [1], Oluwatosin Olugbenga Akinwotu [1], Chloe Tuck [1], Eva M. Krockow [2], Sara Yadav [1], Agbaje Ganiyu Olawale [1], Ayobami Hassan Diyaolu [1], Derick Munkombwe [1,3], Eric Muringu [1,4], Eva Prosper Muro [1,5], Felix Kaminyoghe [1,6], Hameedat Taiye Ayotunde [1], Love Omoniyei [1], Mashood Oluku Lawal [1,7], Shuwary Hughric Adekule Barlatt [1,8], Tumaini J. Makole [1], Winnie Nambatya [1,9], Yvonne Esseku [1,10], Victoria Rutter [1] and Diane Ashiru-Oredope [1,*]

1 Commonwealth Partnerships Programme on Antimicrobial Stewardship, Commonwealth Pharmacists Association, London E1W 1AW, UK
2 Department of Neuroscience, Psychology and Behaviour, University of Leicester, Leicester LE1 7RH, UK
3 Pharmacy Department, University of Zambia, Lusaka P.O. Box 50110, Zambia
4 Projects Department, Pharmaceutical Society of Kenya, Nairobi P.O. Box 44290-00100, Kenya
5 Department of Pharmacology, Kilimanjaro Christian Medical University, Kilimanjaro P.O. Box 2240, Tanzania
6 Pharmaceutical Society of Malawi, Lilongwe P.O. Box 2240, Malawi
7 Pharmaceutical Society of Nigeria, Lagos P.O. Box 531, Nigeria
8 Drug Information Services & Quality Assurance Unit, Directorate of Pharmaceutical Services, Freetown P.O. Box 232, Sierra Leone
9 Pharmacy Department, College of Health Sciences, Makerere University, Kampala P.O. Box 7062, Uganda
10 Ghana College of Pharmacists, Accra P.O. Box CT 10740, Ghana
* Correspondence: diane.ashiru-oredope@commonwealthpharmacy.org

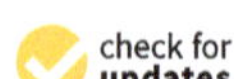

Citation: Kamere, N.; Garwe, S.T.; Akinwotu, O.O.; Tuck, C.; Krockow, E.M.; Yadav, S.; Olawale, A.G.; Diyaolu, A.H.; Munkombwe, D.; Muringu, E.; et al. Scoping Review of National Antimicrobial Stewardship Activities in Eight African Countries and Adaptable Recommendations. *Antibiotics* **2022**, *11*, 1149. https://doi.org/10.3390/antibiotics11091149

Academic Editor: Gabriella Orlando

Received: 14 July 2022
Accepted: 17 August 2022
Published: 25 August 2022

Publisher's Note: MDPI stays neutral with regard to jurisdictional claims in published maps and institutional affiliations.

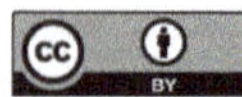

Copyright: © 2022 by the authors. Licensee MDPI, Basel, Switzerland. This article is an open access article distributed under the terms and conditions of the Creative Commons Attribution (CC BY) license (https://creativecommons.org/licenses/by/4.0/).

Abstract: Antimicrobial resistance (AMR) is a global health problem threatening safe, effective healthcare delivery in all countries and settings. The ability of microorganisms to become resistant to the effects of antimicrobials is an inevitable evolutionary process. The misuse and overuse of antimicrobial agents have increased the importance of a global focus on antimicrobial stewardship (AMS). This review provides insight into the current AMS landscape and identifies contemporary actors and initiatives related to AMS projects in eight African countries (Ghana, Kenya, Malawi, Nigeria, Sierra Leone, Tanzania, Uganda, and Zambia), which form a network of countries participating in the Commonwealth Partnerships for Antimicrobial Stewardship (CwPAMS) programme. We focus on common themes across the eight countries, including the current status of AMR, infection prevention and control, AMR implementation strategies, AMS, antimicrobial surveillance, antimicrobial use, antimicrobial consumption surveillance, a one health approach, digital health, pre-service and in-service AMR and AMS training, access to and supply of medicines, and the impact of COVID-19. Recommendations suitable for adaptation are presented, including the development of a national AMS strategy and incorporation of AMS in pharmacists' and other healthcare professionals' curricula for pre-service and in-service training.

Keywords: antibiotic resistance; CwPAMS; national action plans; pharmacy; One Health

1. Background

Antimicrobial resistance (AMR) is a worldwide public health threat of global dimensions. The 2016 Review on AMR commissioned by the UK Government estimated that, by 2050, antimicrobial-resistant infections could be responsible for 10 million deaths globally each year. This is more than cancer, road traffic accidents, diabetes, and diarrhoeal diseases, with developing countries and large emerging nations bearing the brunt of this problem [1]. The impact of this will be felt in all healthcare provisions, with routine surgeries and minor infections becoming life-threatening once again. In 2019, it was estimated that the highest rates of AMR burden were in sub-Saharan Africa, among all regions [2]. However, in sub-Saharan Africa, inadequate surveillance and regulation make it challenging to define the accurate status of AMR and to implement effective and sustainable programmes to address it [3].

According to country-specific situational analyses, joint external evaluation reports, and other studies from hospital to the national level, worsening AMR trends have been identified in many low- and middle-income countries (LMICs) within the African continent. Coupled with the burden of infectious diseases, such as tuberculosis (TB), respiratory infections, and diarrhoeal diseases, emerging resistance to treatments for these diseases has a potentially devastating impact on healthcare in these countries [4,5]. AMR has been exacerbated in these contexts by the irrational use of medicines and national guidelines have identified the need to address inadequate AMR surveillance and enable legislation to monitor the rise in AMR [6,7].

This paper presents findings from a rapid scoping review to assess national antimicrobial stewardship (AMS) activities (including those following a One Health approach) in eight African countries (Ghana, Kenya, Malawi, Nigeria, Sierra Leone, Tanzania, Uganda and Zambia) that were carried out as part of the Commonwealth Partnerships for Antimicrobial Stewardship (CwPAMS) programme [8]. CwPAMS provided the useful setting for the review of existing AMS activities because the programme had established an infrastructure that enabled the easy identification of relevant national stakeholders to be included in the scoping process. Given the CwPAMS partnerships' efforts in running AMS interventions in LMICs, the project further provided the ideal context for assessing existing AMS and infection prevention and control (IPC) structures (including the One Health approach), as well as national policies and guidelines in place.

This review addresses three main research questions in relation to the eight African CwPAMS countries:

1. What is the current status of AMR?
2. What programmes of AMS and IPC are currently in place for human and animal health?
3. What national policies and guidelines exist to support these programmes?

By addressing these questions, the review aims to critically review and compare existing AMS approaches in sub-Saharan Africa and outline gaps or areas for improvement. We conclude by proposing a number of actionable recommendations to support ongoing efforts to tackle AMR in LMICs of the African continent and beyond.

2. Methods

The CwPAMS scoping, Figure 1, involved a literature search using topics and keywords (detailed further in Box S1) relating to AMS conducted on the Medline database from 2015 to 2021 for each CwPAMS country. References to relevant articles were reviewed to identify any additional literature. This timeframe was chosen to ensure the timeliness and current relevance of the research. A total of 2197 articles were identified and screened for relevance against the scoping review objectives. A total of 267 articles were selected and reviewed in full. Citation and references were found in selected articles. An additional search using keywords was conducted for One Health literature for each country, resulting in 204 articles being identified and screened for relevance. Overall, 66 articles were included in the review [9–74]. With English being an official language in all eight African countries included in this review, only publications in English were screened.

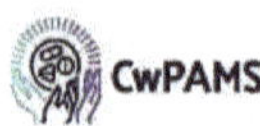

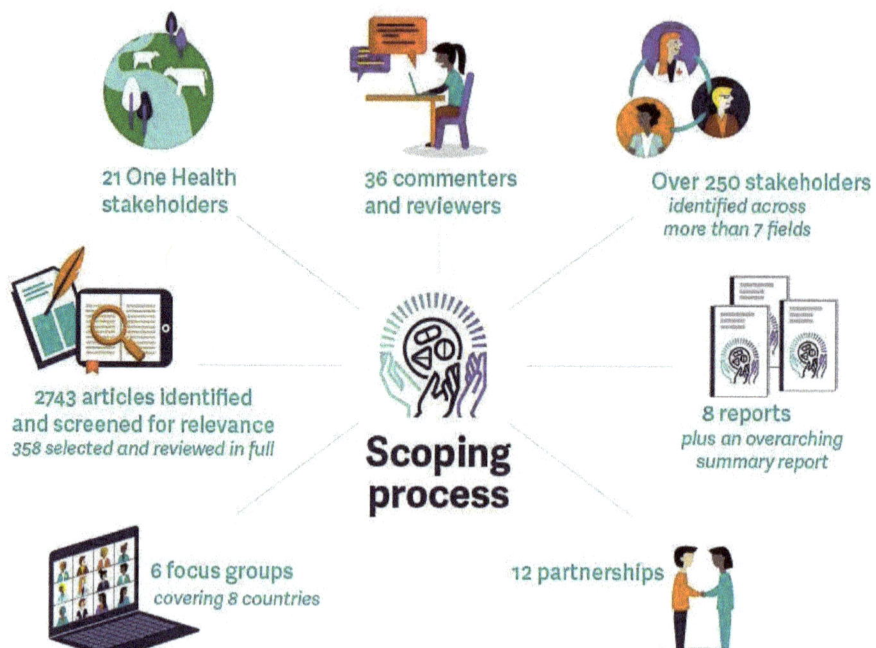

Figure 1. Summary of CwPAMS scoping process.

Additionally, purposive searches of key organisational websites, such as respective government websites and World Health Organization, were conducted for reports and policy documents. This was supported by local expert correspondence to identify additional relevant literature from stakeholders and acting bodies in each country. This identified 342 relevant articles for the scoping review.

The study findings informed the discussion guide for a series of focus group discussions with participants and stakeholders in each country.

Between April and May 2021, workshops, key stakeholders and personal interviews, (Table S1), were conducted with a total of 55 experts with representation from National AMR Committees, Antimicrobial Stewardship, Ministries of Health, One Health, Animal and Environmental Health, Infection Prevention and Control, Medicine, Nursing and Pharmacy.

3. Findings

3.1. *The Current Status of Antimicrobial Resistance*

All the eight assessed countries previously participated in the WHO Joint External Evaluations (JEE), which informed the development of national action plans (NAPs) to implement international health regulations (IHR). A summary of recommended priority actions for AMR, which are currently under implementation, is explained further in the Box S2 [9–13].

Several studies in these countries have shown resistance to the most commonly used antimicrobials, such as penicillin, tetracyclines, ciprofloxacin, and cotrimoxazole [14]. Resistance to frequently used antimicrobials has been identified in multiple common microbial organisms, including *Staphylococcus aureus* and other Staphylococci (including Methicillin-resistant *Streptococcus pneumoniae, Salmonella typhi, Shigella* spp., *Escherichia coli*, and *Vibrio Cholerae* [6,7,15]. In addition, several studies suggest various drivers of AMR, mostly due to gaps in health systems' capacity, supply, and regulation of antimicrobials across multiple sectors. These are detailed further in the Box S3 [7,15].

3.2. *Antimicrobial Use, Monitoring, and Stewardship*

Evidence suggests inappropriate use of antimicrobials in hospitals, community settings, and veterinary treatment [10–13,16–18]. As a result, AMR prevention interventions have targeted healthcare facilities, communities, and the animal industry. There are variations in the status of AMS programme implementation in the eight countries and, despite recent strides, many face challenges, including leadership commitment to AMS, clinical pharmacy expertise, reporting, education, and accountability. Only one of the countries, Kenya, had specific national AMS guidelines for healthcare settings.

Country-specific studies at the hospital level further reported suboptimal compliance with treatment guidelines in healthcare-associated infections (HCAIs); lack of clarity in documentation in AMS; prolonged surgical antibiotic prophylaxis; extensive misuse of antibiotics (particularly in treating uncomplicated infections) and a lack of awareness among health workers.

3.3. *Infection Prevention and Control (IPC)*

IPC is a central precondition for reducing the need for antimicrobials. Our scoping search evidenced the existence of national IPC plans, policies, and documents to support IPC and water sanitation and hygiene (WASH) in healthcare facilities across the eight countries. However, IPC appears to be a neglected area at the healthcare facility level, and it is evident that there is a need for strengthening activities to address this.

There are little data on the incidence of (HCAIs), although it is a widely recognised priority issue to address. The actual burden of HCAIs in many LMICs is unknown due to microbiological data scarcity, inaccurate patient records, lack of electronic medical records, and inadequate surveillance systems to track HCAIs. However, studies indicate urinary tract infections (UTIs), surgical site infections (SSI), and healthcare-associated pneumonia (HAP) as common HCAIs in the eight African countries included in this review [19].

Effective IPC practices require training and monitoring of the health workforce. Barriers to IPC include a lack of adherence to training guidelines. Several studies were conducted on IPC knowledge, awareness, and practice by healthcare workers in the eight countries of interest. Results of the studies showed poor hygiene compliance due to inadequate training, poor infrastructure, and lack of personal protective equipment (PPE) in hospitals [20–23].

3.4. *Use of WHO Tools and Participation in Assessments*

Several WHO guidance and policy documents are available to inform national policy and decision-makers by providing data and guidelines on the burden of AMR, IPC and WASH, among other critical areas.

A range of WHO tools and guidelines used by the eight countries are summarised in Table 1.

Table 1. Summary of range of WHO tools used by the focus countries.

	Enrolment to GLASS-AMR	WHO Joint External Evaluation (JEE)	WHO Methodology for PPS	National Action Plans	WHO WASH FIT	WHO Global Plan on AMR	Global TrACSS
Ghana	x	x		x		x	x
Kenya	x	x	x	x	x	x	x
Malawi	x	x	x	x	x	x	
Nigeria	x	x		x	x		x
Sierra Leone		x		x		x	x
Tanzania	x	x		x		x	x
Uganda	x	x	x	x	x	x	
Zambia	x	x		x	x		x

These tools serve different purposes in providing guidance for the participating countries. Global antimicrobial resistance and use surveillance system (GLASS)-AMR provides a standardized approach to the collection, analysis, and sharing of AMR data by countries and seeks to support capacity development and monitor the status of existing or newly developed national AMR surveillance systems. The joint external evaluation (JEE) is a voluntary, collaborative, multisectoral process to comprehensively assess a country's capacity to prevent, detect, and rapidly respond to public health risks in the framework of the international health regulations (IHR). The WHO point prevalence survey (PPS) methodology collects basic information from medical records and associated patient documentation on all hospitalized patients, which is of relevance for the treatment and the management of infectious diseases regardless of whether these patients are on antibiotic treatment at the time of data collection.

The national action plan (NAP) is a government document and is aligned with government policies, laws, regulations, and structures as necessary or relevant to AMR. Water and sanitation for health facility improvement tool (WASH FIT) is a risk-based approach for improving and sustaining water, sanitation and hygiene, and healthcare waste management infrastructure and services in healthcare facilities in LMICs. The global action plan (GAP) provides a framework for developing national action plans, including key actions that the various actors should take within 5–10 years to combat AMR. The tripartite AMR country self-assessment survey (TrACSS) is an annual evaluation jointly administered by the Food and Agriculture Organization (FAO), World Organisation for Animal Health (OIE), and WHO to monitor a country's progress in the implementation of NAPs.

3.5. *National AMR Strategies and Their Status of Implementation*

National AMR action plans or strategies were available in all eight countries and included some or all of the necessary elements for effective AMS. These plans and strategies are led by an AMR coordinating committee (AMRCC) or a platform of multi-sector stakeholders who coordinate implementation activities. They represent a promising advancement in the form of increased policy awareness and commitment to tackle AMR. However, national AMR strategies varied in their degrees of implementation. Significant barriers remained, including gaps in operationalizing One Health interventions and a lack of monitoring processes for implementation. Additionally, input from in-country consultants indicated a lack of financial resources to effectively measure and establish the impact of AMR, e.g., through measuring cost-efficiency, quality-adjusted life years (QALYs), disability-adjusted life years (DALYs), mortality rates, costs associated with infectious disease, bed space, drugs, and treatment.

3.6. Notable Themes in National Action Plans

All eight countries adopted a multi-stakeholder approach to developing NAPs based on the country-specific Global Antibiotic Resistance Partnership (GARP) situation analysis recommendations. The stakeholders included WHO, FAO, Fleming Fund and respective government line ministries. Out of the eight assessed countries, the Malawi NAP was not readily available to stakeholders but was under review to improve implementation strategies.

Across all countries, representatives from different pharmaceutical bodies and pharmacists were involved in the drafting of the NAP. One of the NAP principles in all eight countries was using a One Health approach. There was a common understanding that AMR requires collective actions from all One Health components, including human and animal production, crop agriculture, and environmental activities.

Most of the countries' NAPs contain clear implementation plans with monitoring and evaluation (M&E) indicators. However, there was limited documented evidence on the status of implementation of the NAPs. Fleming Fund country grant activities were implemented to support NAP development, along with an M&E plan to track progress in its implementation.

3.7. Surveillance of Antimicrobial Use (Including Point Prevalence Survey)

Most of the data that support treatment guidelines come from studies and surveillance systems from high-income countries (HICs). However, even in HICs, gaps still exist in the surveillance of bacterial pathogens that cause animal and human infections [24]. In addition, reports have shown that LMICs' capacity for AMR laboratory testing is centralized, with minimal capacity at district level.

Several country-specific examples [24–28] are outlined in the Box S4.

3.8. Guidelines on Antimicrobial Use

The national clinical guidelines across all eight countries inform the prescription and dispensing of antimicrobials. However, Kenya was the only country out of the eight with dedicated national AMS guidelines for healthcare settings. In contrast, the rest of the countries have several updated guidelines, such as Standard Treatment Guidelines and Essential Medicines Lists, where AMS principles have been integrated. All countries have a broad legal framework for medicines control, including antimicrobials. However, there is currently limited literature on the implementation status of these guidelines.

3.9. Behavioural Barriers to AMS

Although policies on tackling AMR are available, they are often not implemented in practice due to resource limitations [29]. In addition, AMS activities are affected by the behaviour of health workers, individuals, and service providers. It was noted that structural barriers may result in additional behavioural barriers. Box 1 highlights behavioural barriers (including structural barriers) to tackling AMR in the eight countries [29–33]:

3.10. Initiatives to Improve AMS

Focus group discussions highlighted the urgent need for progress with regard to AMS interventions. In addition to behavioural barriers to implementation, a lack of financial resources and competing national priorities often result in AMS work being side-lined.

Examples of current initiatives to improve AMS in the eight countries include:

- The African Institute for Development Policy (AFIDEP) developed awareness materials, such as comic strips and fact and information sheets, in the local Chichewa language in Malawi [34].
- The Drivers of Resistance in Uganda and Malawi (DRUM) consortium is a multi-stakeholder project working in Malawi and Uganda, researching AMR in humans, animals, and the environment [35].
- Nigeria utilises social media to promote AMS awareness and has an AMR Awareness Facebook page, where information is shared to support the implementation of the

Global Action Plan on Antimicrobial Resistance and minimise the impact of AMR on human health, animal health, and the environment [36].

- A project was conducted to increase the awareness of AMR from February 2nd to May 13th, 2019, in Nigeria. The project used community outreach and social media to raise awareness about AMR and address issues, such as misconceptions and knowledge gaps. The student-led project had over 200,000 likes on Facebook, demonstrating how social media can be a powerful tool to reach the masses [37].
- In collaboration with relevant ministries, departments, and agencies in the animal and human health sectors, Nigeria's Centre for Disease Control participates in World Antimicrobial Awareness Week activities every year. In 2020, under the theme 'Antimicrobials: Handle with care', several activities were conducted. These included a webinar regarding operationalising One Health interventions on AMS, engagement with livestock farmers, and training with Fleming Fund Fellows on AMR and antimicrobial use (AMU) surveillance [38].
- ReAct Africa assists countries, such as Zambia and Ghana, by bringing together experts and key stakeholders to form technical working groups on AMR. They ensure a multi-sectoral, holistic approach to AMR, targeting the general public, as well as the health, veterinarian, agricultural, and environmental sectors. Their role is to also increase collaboration with other relevant networks and organisations [39].
- In Kenya, both public and private hospitals, such as the Kenyatta National Hospital, Aga Khan University Hospital, and The Nairobi Hospital, have developed and implemented AMS programmes. They have observed significant adherence to AMU guidelines in surgical prophylaxis, restricted carbapenem, and other reserve antibiotic use, resulting in a decline in multi-drug resistant infections and candidemia. Other hospitals are in the process of establishing AMS teams with mentorship from hospitals that have implemented AMS programmes. Insights from the focus group discussions showed initiatives and unpublished documentation on AMS in the country. There is ongoing work with the United States Agency for International Development - Medicines, Technologies, and Pharmaceutical Services (MTaPS) Program (USAID-MTaPS), Fleming Fund, ReAct, CDC, WHO, FAO, and OIE.
- In 2017, Mbeya Zonal Referral Hospital (MZRH) and the University of South Carolina (UofSC) agreed on a collaborative project to strengthen antimicrobial prescribing in the southern highlands of Tanzania and train a new generation of clinicians in responsible AMU and adherence to national guidelines [40].

3.11. *Guidelines on Infection Prevention and Control*

Multiple partners, such as US CDC implementing partners, USAID-MTaPS, WHO, and ReAct, have been supporting countries to improve IPC. At the national level, in Kenya, they have provided technical assistance to the National Infection Prevention and Control Advisory Committee and the MoH Patient and Health Worker Safety Division to review the existing policies for health care workers. The National IPC Advisory and Coordination Committee supports and improves adherence to hand hygiene and waste management practices.

Several documents have been developed and implemented across all eight countries to facilitate IPC procedures and policies at the national and hospital level. They include but are not limited to: IPC plan; Infection Control and Waste Management plan; Standard Treatment guidelines; National Communication Strategy for IPC; National IPC Guidelines & Pocket Guides; Quality Improvement—IPC Orientation Guide for Participants; National IPC Standards; National Health Care Waste Management Policy Guidelines; HCWM Standards and Procedures; HCWM Monitoring Plan; National Catalogue for National HCWM Equipment and Facility Options; Essential Medicine List.

Box 1. Behavioural barriers (including structural barriers) to tackling AMR [29–33].

- Unrestricted access to antimicrobial medicines without prescription due to limited enforcement of legisla-tion;
- Individuals use antimicrobials to try to prevent infection, rather than using for treatment;
- Unaffordability of antimicrobials results in purchasing less than prescribed and patients tend not to finish their prescribed courses;
- Self-medication is common with medicines from market vendors, pharmacies, and drugs shared between friends and family;
- There is a lack of medical supplies, and long distances to health facilities;
- Poor attitudes of medical professionals towards patients;
- The misuse of antibiotics in hospitals, while not well documented, is evident, and there are no national guidelines for the use of antibiotics in intensive care unit (ICUs);
- Guidelines are not adhered to and hardly used, which may be due to a lack of faith in the advice;
- Up-to-date information on AMR is limited and not circulated or collated to be available from one source, so it does not influence clinical practice. This has led to the prescription of antibiotics being a matter of trial and error;
- Financial incentives exist through privately selling antibiotics in hospitals;
- Polypharmacy, including antimicrobials, and the use of fixed-dose combinations;
- Poor enforcement of laws and regulations on the handling of medicines. In addition, many drug shops and private clinics do not conform to the required standards and remain operational in many districts;
- Lack of diagnostic tests in medical decision-making, increasing or decreasing the probability of infection in a patient based on the result;
- Poor education on IPC and AMR;
- Characteristics of the facility and the healthcare worker, such as the healthcare worker's knowledge and the availability of supplies, suggest that improvements will require a broader focus on behavioural change. Findings also emphasise the need to create hospital leadership buy-in in order to overcome challenges in effective AMS programme implementation, in the response to AMR.

3.12. One Health Initiative in Relation to Antimicrobial Stewardship

3.12.1. One Health Approach

Currently, in Ghana, Kenya, Nigeria, Tanzania, and Zambia, One Health collaboration is established within multi-sectoral working groups that operate using clear terms of reference and defined activities and follow arrangements pertaining to reporting and accountability [41]. By contrast, in Sierra Leone, One Health initiatives are established but did not have clear terms of reference and defined activities.

In Uganda, national strategic plans were reviewed by key stakeholders in the relevant ministries (Ministries of Health, Agriculture and Environment) to include the AMS/AMR agenda as part of their deliverables for further implementation. These efforts are expected to promote AMS activities at sub-national, district, and individual farmer levels. In Malawi, only a concept note exists on the One Health approach to date.

The FAO, WHO, and OIE have played a strong role in promoting intersectoral co-ordination and collaboration at the country level, particularly in Ghana, Sierra Leone, and Tanzania through One Health intersectoral groups and committees [42]. The Fleming Fund also signed an MoU with relevant ministries, departments, and agencies (MDAs) to implement a One Health approach to respond to public health threats through health promotion, early detection, timely response, and post-outbreak management [43].

3.12.2. Raising Awareness of AMR in The Animal Health Sector

The FAO's awareness-raising activities have targeted a range of stakeholders from food producers and medicine sellers to veterinarians and para-veterinarians in some of the countries included in the review [42]. However, despite the evidence of nationwide, government-supported AMR awareness campaigns in some countries [41], there is a need for more awareness targeting the animal, food, and environmental health sectors in all eight countries.

3.12.3. Antimicrobial Use and Stewardship in Farms

Antibiotics are used in the animal health sector for the treatment and prevention of infections, among other purposes. In addition, they are used in sub-therapeutic doses in livestock feeds to enhance growth and improve feed efficiency in intensive livestock farming [44]. The situation on AMU/AMS [17,41,42,45–54] across the agricultural sector in the eight countries are depicted in Table S2.

3.12.4. Veterinarians and AMS

In Ghana, there are agencies responsible for monitoring the use of antibiotics and surveillance of resistance in animals. Ad hoc AMR training courses are available for veterinary-related professionals in Ghana, Nigeria, and Sierra Leone [41]. In addition, plans to strengthen the capacity gaps in veterinary services are currently being developed in Sierra Leone [41].

Continued professional training on AMR/AMU exists for veterinary-related professionals in Tanzania and Zambia [41]. In Sierra Leone, the monitoring of veterinary services performance is carried out regularly, e.g., through Performance of Veterinary Services (PVS) Evaluation follow-up missions [41]. No regular training is provided to farmers in Nigeria because it is challenging to engage with them easily. In Malawi, the development of AMS guidelines in the animal sector is still underway.

3.12.5. Antimicrobial Surveillance in Animal and Environmental Sectors

In Kenya, all laboratories performing antimicrobial sensitivity testing are integrated into the AMR surveillance system [41]. Some AMR data are collected locally and fed into the national surveillance system for AMR in livestock and aquaculture.

In the other countries, there are national surveillance systems for AMR in the animal, food, and environmental health sectors. The surveillance plans for AMR in animal health sectors have been approved in Kenya, while the surveillance plans for AMC/AMU in animal health and environmental health sectors are under review in Malawi and Ghana. However, in some countries, the animal health and food safety sectors are not integrated into the national AMR laboratory network. As a result, the antimicrobial sensitivity testing conducted in those labs is not included in the national AMR surveillance system [41]. In Ghana and Tanzania, there are IPC programmes in the animal and plant health services, while in the other countries, there is no evidence of national IPC guidelines covering the animal, food, environment, and agriculture sectors [41].

3.13. Stakeholder and AMR Coordinating Committee (AMRCC) Engagement

The eight assessed countries have well established AMRCC committees to facilitate AMR-NAP implementation, with the names of these differing across countries. For example, in Kenya, it is referred to as the 'National Antimicrobial Stewardship Interagency Committee' while in Sierra Leone, it is the 'National Multi-Sectoral Coordinating Group'. The AMRCC oversees and provides overall coordination of the AMR National Action Plan (AMR-NAP) implementation. The activities of the AMRCC are supported by national technical working groups in the implementation of each of the strategic objectives. These technical working groups are composed of technical experts from key stakeholders, representing animal health, food and animal production, human health, the environment, public, private institutions, and civil society.

Currently, the AMRCC in all eight countries has been conducting:

- Assessment of various curricula to determine the extent of inclusion of AMR content;
- Situation analysis of sanitary and phytosanitary measures, IPC, and biosecurity;
- Periodic studies on the efficacy of antimicrobials.

3.14. Digital Health

The penetration of mobile phones and other digital technologies has provided an opportunity for digital health initiatives. There has been an increased use of digital health, mirroring global trends fuelled by the COVID-19 pandemic. Additionally, our review demonstrated increased development and implementation of mobile health applications.

Countries, such as Ghana, Kenya, Malawi, and Zambia, have adopted national e-Health strategies whilst Nigeria, Sierra Leone, Tanzania, and Uganda are yet to do so [55].

District Health Information Software-2 (DHIS-2), a digital interface designed initially for collecting and using district health information, has been implemented in seven countries. Sierra Leone has not yet implemented the use of DHIS-2 [56].

3.14.1. Advances in the Use of E-Prescribing

Medical apps for healthcare professions have been developed to support adverse event monitoring, prescribing, and quality assurance. These applications are used for various purposes, including point-of-care reference tools, physician consultation, monitoring adherence to therapy, inter-professional interaction, etc.

As part of the CwPAMS programme, the Commonwealth Pharmacists Association (CPA) developed an antimicrobial-prescribing app, to support antimicrobial-prescribing and AMS activities conducted by health partnerships through the programme in Ghana, Tanzania, Uganda, and Zambia by providing guidance, resources, and training documents. The use of apps to aid AMS and inform practice has been well implemented in hospitals [57]. In addition, the UK-led telemedicine initiatives, such as Virtual Doctors have also supported healthcare workers in rural areas in Zambia [58]. However, several barriers to using digital health existed in LMICs, including unavailability of digital tools and connectivity issues [59].

Electronic health services, such as prescribing, are becoming increasingly popular in LMICs. Some examples include the MyDawa app in Kenya [60]; the Surveillance Programme of In-patients and Epidemiology (SPINE) and the MicroGuide app [61,62], implemented in Malawi; and the electronic health records system, 'Stre@mline' in Uganda [63].

3.14.2. Use of Medicines Supply Apps or Software

Mobile applications have eased service provision to local hospitals, enabling more efficient and effective distribution of essential medical supplies. However, in some cases, there was no evidence to support whether hospitals had widely implemented the apps [64]. Additional studies on clinical usability and the workflow fit of digital health systems are needed to ensure efficient system implementation. However, this requires support from critical stakeholders, including the government, international donors, and regional health informatics organisations [64].

A study on improving access to antimicrobial prescribing guidelines in four African countries noted initial barriers to uptake that were addressed using a behaviour change approach [59].

3.15. *Coverage of AMR and AMS in Pharmacy Training*

There is a critical shortage of pharmacy personnel, especially in government health centres in all assessed countries. This shortage leads to unqualified personnel managing medicines and supply chains and dispensing medicines to patients, impacting patient care and medicine availability. Countries, such as Kenya, Malawi, Nigeria, Tanzania and Zambia, train pharmacy assistants and technicians for 2–3 years, while pharmacists undergo higher education by completing a 5–6 year Bachelor or Doctor of Pharmacy, respectively. Both the pharmacy technician and pharmacist qualifications require a pre-registration placement [65]. Most of the eight countries have some form of continuing professional development (CPD), designed to update pharmacists' knowledge and enable them to keep abreast of advancements in pharmaceutical development and modern trends in pharmacy [66]. The uptake of CPD is currently low in countries where it is not mandated, requiring personal motivation to engage [67,68]. The number and role of pharmacists in the eight countries are detailed further in the Table S3.

3.16. Access to Antimicrobials, Supply of Medicines

The CwPAMS programme running from 2018 to 2021 highlighted that, in some cases, medicine supply issues led to challenges in achieving AMS. Many African countries are regularly impacted by shortages, substandard/falsified medicines, and supply issues due to COVID-19 and heavy import dependency, especially in the pharmaceutical sector [1,69–72].

The medicine supply chains of the eight countries in focus have commonalities and variables between them, relating to factors, such as procurement agency type and authority in place. All eight countries procure, source funding from, and distribute essential medicines from a combination of government (Ministries of Health), non-government/not-for-profit organisations, and private sectors. The systems in place are categorised as tier systems, single agency, or devolved.

3.17. Access to Medicines via Community Pharmacy

Several studies [17,59] have documented the over-the-counter supply of antibiotics in community pharmacies and enable patient self-medication and misuse of antibiotics. The additional drivers of misuse [73,74] in community pharmacies are highlighted in Box 2

Box 2. Key drivers of antimicrobial misuse in community pharmacies [73,74].

Further findings that highlight the key drivers of antimicrobial misuse in community pharmacies include;

- Poor and inefficient public health systems;
- Lack of policies nor strict enforcement;
- Dispensing of antimicrobials in partial doses;
- Sub-optimal AMR knowledge and attitudes among pharmacy personnel;
- Lack of antimicrobial sensitivity knowledge in patients and clients.

3.18. Impact of COVID-19

Understandably, COVID-19 has radically shifted the focus of public health agendas. It is, therefore, important to consider how COVID-19 might be impacting the emergence and spread of drug-resistant pathogens through the overuse of medication for the treatment of COVID-19 and secondary infections. COVID-19 has affected the assessed countries' strides in tackling AMR. The eight countries included in this review operate with several COVID-19 guidelines, and IPC measures are included in these as an integral part of the clinical management of patients. The guidelines highlight the need to ensure standard precautions in all areas of healthcare facilities, including hand hygiene and the use of PPE to avoid direct contact with patients. None of the guidelines mention AMR.

COVID-19 also diverted personnel and resources away from priority diseases, such as HIV/AIDS, TB, malaria, and routine healthcare services, such as antenatal care and vaccination programmes. The full impact of this is yet to be realized.

4. Conclusions

This scoping review provides a current overview and assessment of national AMS activities, including IPC programmes and One Health approaches, by eight countries in sub-Saharan Africa: Ghana, Kenya, Malawi, Nigeria, Sierra Leone, Tanzania, Uganda, and Zambia. Notably, all countries have existing NAPs that were developed with the inclusion of pharmacists and reflect the prominence of AMR on the political agenda. Our review further highlighted a significant number of IPC and WASH activities in the eight countries and a notable increase in digital health approaches. However, we also identified a number of shortcomings in national AMS activities, including a lack of documented evidence on AMR and AMU surveillance, AMS activities, and evaluation of NAP implementation. Additionally, there is a need to match increased political motivation to tackle AMR with sufficient investment in technical workforce capacity and expertise in spite of competing healthcare agendas (e.g., around the management of COVID-19). Below, we suggest adaptable recommendations to improve existing AMS practices and increase the sustainability of interventions in the eight countries that were part of this study and beyond.

5. Recommendations

The following recommendations for promoting AMS activities are based on the scoping review and focus group discussions with local and national stakeholders in the eight focus countries. They should be adapted to ensure relevance for context and take into account available resources, barriers, and facilitators.

- Develop national AMS plans or guideline documents to facilitate the implementation of national action plans on AMR.
- Increase the number of AMS programmes in healthcare facilities through national roll-outs of successful pilot programmes.
- Incorporate AMS in the curricula for pre-service and in-service training of pharmacists and other healthcare professionals in the national health budget to increase human resources for the in-country implementation of national AMR programmes.
- Identify National Action Plan indicators that need to be improved or upgraded.
- Increase capacity and recognition of technical working groups on AMS.
- Provide technical support to increase the workforce and streamline processes to improve monitoring and evaluation (M&E) for NAPs (Most countries did not have enough literature on the status of AMS implementation).
- Update hospital/healthcare clinical guidelines to include AMS principles and integration of the Access, Watch and Reserve (AWaRe) classification of antibiotics. These customisable guidelines can also be incorporated into existing digital and e-health applications, such as DHIS-2 to optimise prescriptions. The shift towards digitisation can potentially improve antimicrobial prescribing through easy access to information and records.
- Improvement and enforcement of regulations regarding sales of prescription-only antibiotics (There were notable gaps in the policies that govern the sale of antibiotics, especially in community pharmacies. It is important to harness advances in digital technology where possible).
- Streamlining and strengthening national medicine supply chain systems to ensure the consistent availability of quality-assured antimicrobials.
- Encouraging more policies and government regulatory frameworks on the distribution and manufacturing of quality-assured health products at the national level.
- Incorporate bottleneck analysis of national supply chains to identify root causes and human behaviour influencing them.
- The establishment of AMS programmes that incorporate medical supply chain management to facilitate rational antimicrobial selection, procurement, use, monitoring, storage, distribution, and supply.
- The improvement of national quality control and assurance systems of pharmaceuticals to reduce the prevalence of substandard and falsified antimicrobials within the country's distribution systems and channels.
- The provision of incentives to support AMS programmes and further inclusion/collaboration into/with IPC, WASH, TB and other health programmes in all healthcare facilities.
- The prioritisation of institutionalising and subsequent decentralisation of One Health activities to the sub-national level for implementation, fostering operation, and capacity building.
- Expanding national AMU and AMR surveillance programmes and AMR/AMS awareness campaigns targeted at the stakeholders and MDAs in the animal, food processing, agriculture, and environmental health sectors to enhance coverage.
- The involvement of pharmacists and pharmacy associations further in the implementation of national AMS activities.

- At every opportunity, strengthen and foster partnerships and opportunities that ensure the inclusion of all relevant stakeholders/actors (nationally and internationally) in the implementation of AMS activities.
- The encouragement of more AMR and/or One Health-driven research collaborations between government and non-government stakeholders, with the aim of enhancing the implementation of NAPs.
- Conduct a comprehensive ethnographic study on the use and misuse of antimicrobial drugs in human and animal health, agriculture, and the environment to adequately inform antimicrobial stewardship initiatives.
- Use of digital health tools to support AMS. In Kenya, Sierra Leone, Zambia, and Malawi, it was noted that there is a need for easy access to prescribing information through an app.

Supplementary Materials: The following are available online at https://www.mdpi.com/article/10.3390/antibiotics11091149/s1, Box S1: Keywords/Search Terms Box S2: Recommended priority actions for AMR, Box S3: AMR drivers, Box S4: Country-specific examples of AMU, Table S1: Workshops, Key Stakeholders, and Personal Interview Schedule, Table S2: The situation on AMU/AMS in the eight countries for agriculture and animal health, Table S3: The number and role of pharmacists in the eight countries.

Author Contributions: Conceptualization, D.A.-O.; Methodology, D.A.-O., C.T., N.K., S.T.G., O.O.A.; Data curation, N.K., S.T.G., O.O.A., C.T., A.G.O., A.H.D., H.T.A., L.O., T.J.M.; Writing—Original draft preparation, N.K., S.T.G., O.O.A., C.T., A.G.O., A.H.D., H.T.A., L.O., T.J.M., S.Y.; Writing—Review and editing, N.K., S.T.G., O.O.A., C.T., A.G.O., A.H.D., E.M.K., H.T.A., L.O., T.J.M., S.Y., D.M., E.M., E.P.M., F.K., M.O.L., S.H.A.B., W.N., Y.E.; Project administration, S.Y.; Funding acquisition, D.A.-O., V.R. All authors have read and agreed to the published version of the manuscript.

Funding: This project and partnership was part of the Commonwealth Partnerships for Antimicrobial Stewardship (CwPAMS) managed by the Tropical Health and Education Trust (THET) and Commonwealth Pharmacists Association (CPA). CwPAMS is a global health partnership programme funded by the Department of Health and Social Care (DHSC) using UK aid funding, managed by the Fleming Fund. The Fleming Fund is a GBP 265 million UK aid investment to tackle AMR by supporting low- and middle-income countries to generate, use, and share data on AMR and is managed by the UK Department of Health and Social Care. The views expressed in this publication are those of the author(s) and not necessarily those of the Department of Health and Social Care, the UK National Health Service, the Tropical Health and Education Trust, or The Commonwealth Pharmacists Association.

Institutional Review Board Statement: Not applicable.

Acknowledgments: The authors acknowledge the Commonwealth Partnerships for Antimicrobial Stewardship (CwPAMS) Commonwealth Pharmacists Association Team not on authorship: Fran Garraghan, Sarah Cavanagh, Wei Ping Khor, Nikki D'Arcy, Tola Ogunnigbo, Pauline Roberts, Ifunanya Ikhile, Beth Ward, Emma Foreman, Manjula Halai, Jolaade Taiwo, Vanessa Carter, Tatiana Hardy and the Tropical Health and Education Trust (THET) Team: Will Townsend; Richard Skone-James; Beatrice Waddingham; Jessica Fraser. Focus group discussion attendees and reviewers from Ghana, Kenya, Malawi, Nigeria, Sierra Leone, Tanzania, Uganda and Zambia.

Conflicts of Interest: The authors declare no conflict of interest. The funders had no role in the design of the study; in the collection, analyses, or interpretation of data; in the writing of the manuscript; or in the decision to publish the results. Participants in the focus group discussions came from a diverse background and recommendations were created by consensus. They, therefore, may not represent the individual views of all those who participated.

References

1. Elton, L.; Thomason, M.J.; Tembo, J.; Velavan, T.P.; Pallerla, S.R.; Arruda, L.B.; Vairo, F.; Montaldo, C.; Ntoumi, F.; Hamid, M.M.A.; et al. Antimicrobial resistance preparedness in sub-Saharan African countries. *Antimicrob. Resist. Infect. Control* **2020**, *9*, 145. [CrossRef] [PubMed]
2. Murray, C.J.; Ikuta, K.S.; Sharara, F.; Swetschinski, L.; Aguilar, G.R.; Gray, A.; Han, C.; Bisignano, C.; Rao, P.; Wool, E.; et al. Global burden of bacterial antimicrobial resistance in 2019: A systematic analysis. *Lancet* **2022**, *399*, 629–655. [CrossRef]
3. The Review on Antimicrobial Resistance Review. 2016. Available online: https://amr-review.org/ (accessed on 15 June 2022).
4. Commonwealth Pharmacists Association. Commonwealth Partnership for Antimicrobial Stewardship (CwPAMS) Toolkit. 2020. Available online: https://commonwealthpharmacy.org/cwpams-toolkit/ (accessed on 15 June 2022).
5. Masich, A.M.; Vega, A.D.; Callahan, P.; Herbert, A.; Fwoloshi, S.; Zulu, P.M.; Chanda, D.; Chola, U.; Mulenga, L.; Hachaambwa, L.; et al. Antimicrobial usage at a large teaching hospital in Lusaka, Zambia. *PLoS ONE* **2020**, *15*, e0228555. [CrossRef] [PubMed]
6. National Action Plan on Prevention and Containment of Antimicrobial Resistance, 2017–2022. WHO Regional Office for Africa. Available online: https://www.afro.who.int/publications/national-action-plan-prevention-and-containment-antimicrobial-resistance-2017-2022 (accessed on 23 June 2021).
7. *Infection and Prevention Control & WASH Guidelines for Malawi*; Ministry of Health Malawi: Lilongwe, Malawi, 2020.
8. Commonwealth Pharmacists Association. Commonwealth Partnership for Antimicrobial Stewardship (CwPAMS). Available online: https://commonwealthpharmacy.org/cwpams/ (accessed on 28 March 2022).
9. World Health Organization. *Joint External Evaluation of IHR Core Capacities of the Republic of Uganda: Mission Report: 26–30 June 2017*; World Health Organization: Geneva, Switzerland, 2017; License: CC BY-NC-SA 3.0 IGO; Available online: https://apps.who.int/iris/handle/10665/259164 (accessed on 15 June 2022).
10. World Health Organization. *Joint External Evaluation of IHR Core Capacities of the Republic of Uganda: Executive Summary, 26–30 June 2017*; World Health Organization: Geneva, Switzerland, 2017; License: CC BY-NC-SA 3.0 IGO; Available online: https://apps.who.int/iris/handle/10665/258730 (accessed on 15 June 2022).
11. World Health Organization. *Joint External Evaluation of IHR Core Capacities of the Republic of Zambia: Mission Report, 7–11 August 2017*; World Health Organization: Geneva, Switzerland, 2017; License: CC BY-NC-SA 3.0 IGO; Available online: https://apps.who.int/iris/handle/10665/259675 (accessed on 15 June 2022).
12. Khuluza, F.; Haefele-Abah, C. The availability, prices and affordability of essential medicines in Malawi: A cross-sectional study. *PLoS ONE* **2019**, *14*, e0212125. [CrossRef]
13. World Health Organization. *Joint External Evaluation of IHR Core Capacities of the Republic of Malawi: Mission Report: 11–15 February 2019*; World Health Organization: Geneva, Switzerland, 2019; License: CC BY-NC-SA 3.0 IGO; Available online: https://apps.who.int/iris/handle/10665/325321 (accessed on 15 June 2022).
14. Antimicrobial Use and Resistance in Nigeria: Situation Analysis and Recommendations. 2017. Available online: https://www.proceedings.panafrican-med-journal.com/conferences/2018/8/2/abstract/ (accessed on 15 June 2022).
15. World Health Organization. *Joint External Evaluation of IHR Core Capacities of the United Republic of Tanza-nia-Zanzibar: Mission Report, 22–28 April 2017*; World Health Organization: Geneva, Switzerland, 2017; License: CC BY-NC-SA 3.0 IGO; Available online: https://apps.who.int/iris/handle/10665/258696 (accessed on 15 June 2022).
16. *Water, Sanitation and Hygiene in Health Care Facilities: Practical Steps to Achieve Universal Access*; World Health Organization: Geneva, Switzerland, 2019; Licence: CC BY-NC-SA 3.0 IGO; Available online: http://apps.who.int/iris (accessed on 15 June 2022).
17. Lyus, R.; Pollock, A.; Ocan, M.; Brhlikova, P. Registration of antimicrobials, Kenya, Uganda and United Republic of Tanzania, 2018. *Bull. World Health Organ.* **2020**, *98*, 530–538. [CrossRef] [PubMed]
18. Gates Foundation Project. Alliance for the Prudent Use of Antibiotics. Antibiotic Resistance Situation Analysis and Needs Assessment (ARSANA) in Uganda and Zambia. 2022. Available online: https://apua.org/gates-foundation-project (accessed on 15 June 2022).
19. WHO Guidelines on Hand Hygiene in Health Care: First Global Patient Safety Challenge Clean Care Is Safer Care. Geneva: World Health Organization. The Burden of Health Care-Associated Infection. 2019. Available online: https://www.ncbi.nlm.nih.gov/books/NBK144030/ (accessed on 15 June 2022).
20. Bedoya, G.; Dolinger, A.; Rogo, K.; Mwaura, N.; Wafula, F.; Coarasa, J.; Goicoechea, A.; Das, J. Observations of infection prevention and control practices in primary health care, Kenya. *Bull. World Health Organ.* **2017**, *95*, 503–516. [CrossRef]
21. Ashinyo, M.E.; Dubik, S.D.; Duti, V.; Amegah, K.E.; Ashinyo, A.; Asare, B.A.; Ackon, A.A.; Akoriyea, S.K.; Kuma-Aboagye, P. Infection prevention and control compliance among exposed healthcare workers in COVID-19 treatment centers in Ghana: A descriptive cross-sectional study. *PLoS ONE* **2021**, *16*, e0248282. [CrossRef]
22. *Global Antimicrobial Resistance Surveillance System (GLASS) Report: Early Implementation 2016–2017*; World Health Organization: Geneva, Switzerland, 2017. Licence: CC BY-NC-SA 3.0 IGO. Available online: http://apps.who.int/iris. (accessed on 15 June 2022).
23. Horumpende, P.G.; Sonda, T.B.; Van Zwetselaar, M.; Antony, M.L.; Tenu, F.F.; Mwanziva, C.E.; Shao, E.R.; Mshana, S.E.; Mmbaga, B.T.; Chilongola, J. Prescription and non-prescription antibiotic dispensing practices in part I and part II pharmacies in Moshi Municipality, Kilimanjaro Region in Tanzania: A simulated clients approach. *PLoS ONE* **2018**, *13*, e0207465. [CrossRef]
24. *Global Antimicrobial Resistance Surveillance System (GLASS) Report: Early Implementation*; World Health Organization: Geneva, Switzerland, 2020; Licence: CC BY-NC-SA 3.0 IGO; Available online: http://apps.who.int/iris (accessed on 15 June 2022).

25. *Global Antimicrobial Resistance Surveillance System (GLASS) Report: Early Implementation 2017–2018*; World Health Organization: Geneva, Switzerland, 2018; Licence: CC BY-NC-SA 3.0 IGO; Available online: http://apps.who.int/iris (accessed on 15 June 2022).
26. World Health Organization. *WHO Report on Surveillance of Antibiotic Consumption: 2016–2018 Early Implementation*; World Health Organization: Geneva, Switzerland, 2018; License: CC BY-NC-SA 3.0 IGO; Available online: https://apps.who.int/iris/handle/10665/277359 (accessed on 15 June 2022).
27. UNAS; CDDEP; GARP-Uganda; Mpairwe, Y.; Wamala, S. Antibiotic Resistance in Uganda: Situation Analysis and Recommendations (pp. 107). Kampala, Uganda: Uganda National Academy of Sciences; Center for Disease Dynamics, Economics & Policy. 2015. Available online: https://www.cddep.org/wp-content/uploads/2017/06/uganda_antibiotic_resistance_situation_reportgarp_uganda_0-1.pdf (accessed on 15 June 2022).
28. Seale, A.C.; Hutchison, C.; Fernandes, S.; Stoesser, N.; Kelly, H.; Lowe, B.; Turner, P.; Hanson, K.; Chandler, C.I.; Goodman, C.; et al. Supporting surveillance capacity for antimicrobial resistance: Laboratory capacity strengthening for drug resistant infections in low and middle income countries. *Wellcome Open Res.* **2017**, *2*, 91. [CrossRef]
29. African Journal of Clinical and Experimental Microbiology. (n.d.). Antimicrobial Stewardship Implementation in Nigerian Hospitals: Gaps and Challenges. Available online: https://www.ajol.info/index.php/ajcem/article/view/203077 (accessed on 15 June 2022).
30. Mehtar, S.; Wanyoro, A.; Ogunsola, F.; Ameh, E.A.; Nthumba, P.; Kilpatrick, C.; Revathi, G.; Antoniadou, A.; Giamarelou, H.; Apisarnthanarak, A.; et al. Implementation of surgical site infection surveillance in low- and middle-income countries: A position statement for the International Society for Infectious Diseases. *Int. J. Infect. Dis.* **2020**, *100*, 123–131. [CrossRef]
31. Sambakusi, C.S. Knowledge, attitudes and practices related to self-medication with antimicrobials in Lilongwe, Malawi. *Malawi Med. J.* **2019**, *31*, 225–232. [CrossRef] [PubMed]
32. Antimicrobial Resistance—AMR Awareness. Facebook. Available online: https://www.facebook.com/amr.nigeria/. (accessed on 15 June 2022).
33. Adebisi, Y. Lesson learned from student-led one hundred days awareness on antimicrobial resistance in Nigeria. *Int. J. Infect. Dis.* **2020**, *101*, 66. [CrossRef]
34. Raising Public Awareness on Antibiotic Resistance in Malawi: Antibiotic Awareness Week 2019. African Institute for Development Policy—AFIDEP. Available online: https://www.afidep.org/raising-public-awareness-on-antibiotic-resistance-in-malawi-antibiotic-awareness-week-2019/ (accessed on 28 March 2022).
35. Drivers of Resistance in Uganda and Malawi. African Institute for Development Policy—AFIDEP. Available online: https://www.afidep.org/publication/info-sheet-drivers-of-resistance-in-uganda-and-malawi/ (accessed on 28 March 2022).
36. Nigeria Centre for Disease Control. AMR Situation Analysis. Available online: https://ncdc.gov.ng/diseases/guidelines (accessed on 15 June 2022).
37. ReAct Africa—A global network. ReAct. Available online: https://www.reactgroup.org/about-us/a-global-network/react-africa/ (accessed on 15 June 2022).
38. Hall, J.W.; Bouchard, J.; Bookstaver, P.B.; Haldeman, M.S.; Kishimbo, P.; Mbwanji, G.; Mwakyula, I.; Mwasomola, D.; Seddon, M.; Shaffer, M.; et al. The Mbeya Antimicrobial Stewardship Team: Implementing Antimicrobial Stewardship at a Zonal-Level Hospital in Southern Tanzania. *Pharmacy* **2020**, *8*, 107. [CrossRef] [PubMed]
39. Global Database for the Tripartite Antimicrobial Resistance (AMR) Country Self-Assessment Survey (TrACSS). Available online: http://amrcountryprogress.org/ (accessed on 8 June 2021).
40. FAO. Evaluation of FAO's Role and Work on Antimicrobial Resistance (AMR).Thematic Evaluation Series, 03/2021. Rome . 2021. Available online: http://www.fao.org/documents/card/en/c/cb3680en/ (accessed on 15 June 2022).
41. Sierra Leone. Fleming Fund. Available online: https://www.flemingfund.org/countries/sierra-leone/ (accessed on 15 June 2022).
42. Ghana National Action Plan on Antimicrobial Resistance 2017–2021.pdf. Available online: https://www.who.int/publications/m/item/ghana-national-action-plan-for-antimicrobial-use-and-resistance (accessed on 15 June 2022).
43. Andoh, L.A.; Dalsgaard, A.; Obiri-Danso, K.; Newman, M.J.; Barco, L.; Olsen, J.E. Prevalence and antimicrobial resistance of *Salmonella* serovars isolated from poultry in Ghana. *Epidemiol. Infect.* **2016**, *144*, 3288–3299. [CrossRef] [PubMed]
44. Donkor, E.S.; Newman, M.J.; Yeboah-Manu, D. Epidemiological aspects of non-human antibiotic usage and resistance: Implications for the control of antibiotic resistance in Ghana. *Trop. Med. Int. Health* **2012**, *17*, 462–468. [CrossRef]
45. Lakoh, S.; Adekanmbi, O.; Jiba, D.F.; Deen, G.F.; Gashau, W.; Sevalie, S.; Klein, E.Y. Antibiotic use among hospitalized adult patients in a setting with limited laboratory infrastructure in Freetown Sierra Leone, 2017–2018. *Int. J. Infect. Dis.* **2019**, *90*, 71–76. [CrossRef]
46. Global Antibiotic Resistance Partnership—Tanzania Working Group. Situation Analysis and Recommendations: Anti-biotic Use and Resistance in Tanzania. Washington, DC and New Delhi: Center for Disease Dynamics, Economics & Policy. 2015. Available online: https://cddep.org/wp-content/uploads/2017/06/garp-tz_situation_analysis-1.pdf (accessed on 15 June 2022).
47. Pharmacy Assistant Training Program—VillageReach. Available online: https://www.villagereach.org/impact/pharmacy-assistant-training-program/ (accessed on 15 June 2022).
48. Alhaji, N.B.; Isola, T.O. Antimicrobial usage by pastoralists in food animals in North-central Nigeria: The associated socio-cultural drivers for antimicrobials misuse and public health implications. *One Health* **2018**, *6*, 41–47. [CrossRef]

49. Adesokan, H.K.; Akanbi, I.O.; Akanbi, I.M.; Obaweda, R.A. Pattern of antimicrobial usage in livestock animals in south-western Nigeria: The need for alternative plans. *Onderstepoort J. Veter- Res.* **2015**, *82*, 6. [CrossRef]
50. Sierra Leone. Terms of Reference for Request for Proposals. Available online: https://1doxu11lv4am2alxz12f0p5j-wpengine.netdna-ssl.com/wp-content/uploads/7135a0cec08f827c92300d81b0c2e002.pdf (accessed on 15 June 2022).
51. Kimera, Z.I.; Mshana, S.E.; Rweyemamu, M.M.; Mboera, L.E.G.; Matee, M.I.N. Antimicrobial use and resistance in food-producing animals and the environment: An African perspective. *Antimicrob. Resist. Infect. Control* **2020**, *9*, 37. [CrossRef]
52. Multi-sectoral National Action Plan on Antimicrobial Resistance 2017–2027. Government of the Republic of Zambia. Available online: https://www.who.int/publications/m/item/zambia-multi-sectoral-national-action-plan-on-antimicrobial-resistance (accessed on 15 June 2022).
53. NAFDAC—National Agency for Food & Drug Administration & Control. Available online: https://www.nafdac.gov.ng/ (accessed on 15 June 2022).
54. Dacombe, R.; Bates, I.; Gopul, B.; Owusu-Ofori, A. Overview of the Antimicrobial Resistance Surveillance Systems for Ghana, Ma-lawi, Nepal and Nigeria. Available online: https://www.flemingfund.org/wp-content/uploads/b1ef6816d1e94134427b27f4c118ebae.pdf (accessed on 15 June 2022).
55. Sub-Saharan Africa, The Mobile Economy. Available online: https://www.gsma.com/mobileeconomy/sub-saharan-africa/ (accessed on 28 March 2022).
56. District Health Information System 2 (DHIS2). Open Health News. Available online: https://www.openhealthnews.com/resources/district-health-information-system-2-dhis2 (accessed on 15 June 2022).
57. Olaoye, O.; Tuck, C.; Khor, W.P.; McMenamin, R.; Hudson, L.; Northall, M.; Panford-Quainoo, E.; Asima, D.M.; Ashiru-Oredope, D. Improving Access to Antimicrobial Prescribing Guidelines in 4 African Countries: Development and Pilot Implementation of an App and Cross-Sectional Assessment of Attitudes and Behaviour Survey of Healthcare Workers and Patients. *Antibiotics* **2020**, *9*, 555. [CrossRef]
58. Technology & Medicine. Telemedicine Charity. The Virtual Doctors. Available online: https://www.virtualdoctors.org/ (accessed on 15 June 2022).
59. Omotosho, A.; Emuoyibofarhe, J.; Ayegba, P.; Meinel, C. E-Prescription in Nigeria: A Survey. *J. Glob. Pharma Technol.* **2018**, *10*, 58–64. Available online: https://www.researchgate.net/publication/330825533_E-Prescription_in_Nigeria_A_Survey (accessed on 15 June 2022).
60. MyDawa Brand the First ever Retail License for an e-Retailing Pharmacy in Kenya. CIO East Africa. Available online: https://www.cio.co.ke/mydawa-brand-the-first-ever-retail-license-for-an-e-retailing-pharmacy-in-kenya/ (accessed on 15 June 2022).
61. SanJoaquin, M.A.; Allain, T.J.; Molyneux, M.E.; Benjamin, L.; Everett, D.B.; Gadabu, O.; Rothe, C.; Nguipdop, P.; Chilombe, M.; Kazembe, L.; et al. Surveillance Programme of IN-patients and Epidemiology (SPINE): Implementation of an Electronic Data Collection Tool within a Large Hospital in Malawi. *PLoS Med.* **2013**, *10*, e1001400. [CrossRef] [PubMed]
62. Antimicrobial Stewardship Improved by MicroGuide No 1 Medical Guidance. Available online: http://www.test.microguide.eu/ (accessed on 15 June 2022).
63. Liang, L.; Wiens, M.O.; Lubega, P.; Spillman, I.; Mugisha, S. A Locally Developed Electronic Health Platform in Uganda: Development and Implementation of Stre@mline. *JMIR Form. Res.* **2018**, *2*, e20. [CrossRef] [PubMed]
64. Kariuki, J.; Njeru, M.K.; Wamae, W.; Mackintosh, M. Local Supply Chains for Medicines and Medical Supplies in Kenya: Under-standing the Challenges. Africa Portal. African Centre for Technology Studies (ACTS). 2015. Available online: https://www.africaportal.org/publications/local-supply-chains-for-medicines-and-medical-supplies-in-kenya-understanding-the-challenges/ (accessed on 15 June 2022).
65. Kalungia, A.C.; Muungo, L.T.; Marshall, S.; Apampa, B.; May, C.; Munkombwe, D. Training of pharmacists in Zambia: Developments, curriculum structure and future perspectives. *Pharm. Educ.* **2019**, *19*, 69–78. Available online: https://pharmacyeducation.fip.org/pharmacyeducation/article/view/638 (accessed on 15 June 2022).
66. Librarian, I. Assessment of the Pharmaceutical Human Resources in Tanzania and the Strategic Framework. Available online: https://www.hrhresourcecenter.org/node/3269.html (accessed on 15 June 2022).
67. Partnership between Korle-Bu Teaching Hospital and North Middlesex University Hospital NHS Trust. Fleming Fund. Available online: https://www.flemingfund.org/publications/about-the-partnership-between-korle-bu-teaching-hospital-and-north-middlesex-university-hospital-nhs-trust/ (accessed on 15 June 2022).
68. Blogs—The Medicines, Technologies, and Pharmaceutical Services (MTaPs) Program. Available online: https://www.mtapsprogram.org/news-type/blogs/ (accessed on 15 June 2022).
69. Banga, K.; Keane, J.; Mendez-Parra, M.; Pettinotti, L.; Sommer, L. Africa Trade and COVID-19. Available online: https://cdn.odi.org/media/documents/Africa_trade_and_Covid19_the_supply_chain_dimension.pdf (accessed on 15 June 2022).
70. Manji, I.; Manyara, S.M.; Jakait, B.; Ogallo, W.; Hagedorn, I.C.; Lukas, S.; Kosgei, E.J.; Pastakia, S.D. The Revolving Fund Pharmacy Model: Backing up the Ministry of Health supply chain in western Kenya. *Int. J. Pharm. Pract.* **2016**, *24*, 358–366. [CrossRef]
71. Shaban, H.; Maurer, C.; Willborn, R.J. Impact of Drug Shortages on Patient Safety and Pharmacy Operation Costs. *Fed. Pract.* **2018**, *35*, 24–31.
72. Shafiq, N.; Pandey, A.K.; Malhotra, S.; Holmes, A.; Mendelson, M.; Malpani, R.; Balasegaram, M.; Charani, E. Shortage of essential antimicrobials: A major challenge to global health security. *BMJ Glob. Health* **2021**, *6*, e006961. [CrossRef]

73. Awosan, K.J.; Ibitoye, P.K.; Abubakar, A.K. Knowledge, risk perception and practices related to antibiotic resistance among patent medicine vendors in Sokoto metropolis, Nigeria. *Niger. J. Clin. Pract.* **2018**, *21*, 1476–1483.
74. Bonniface, M.; Nambatya, W.; Rajab, K. An Evaluation of Antibiotic Prescribing Practices in a Rural Refugee Settlement District in Uganda. *Antibiotics* **2021**, *10*, 172. [CrossRef]

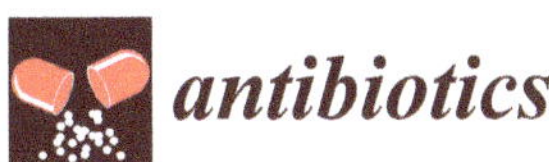

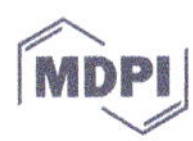

Article

Exploring the Antimicrobial Stewardship Educational Needs of Healthcare Students and the Potential of an Antimicrobial Prescribing App as an Educational Tool in Selected African Countries

Omotola Ogunnigbo [1], Maxencia Nabiryo [1], Moses Atteh [2], Eric Muringu [3], Olatunde James Olaitan [4], Victoria Rutter [1] and Diane Ashiru-Oredope [1,*]

1 Commonwealth Pharmacists Association, London E1W 1AW, UK; omotola.ogunnigbo@commonwealthpharmacy.org (O.O.); maxencia.nabiryo@commonwealthpharmacy.org (M.N.); victoria.rutter@commonwealthpharmacy.org (V.R.)
2 Grand Erie District School Board, Brantford, ON N3T 5V3, Canada; moses.atteh@granderie.ca
3 Pharmaceutical Society of Kenya, Hurlingham, Jabavu Lane, Nairobi P.O. Box 44290-00100, Kenya; emuringu158@gmail.com
4 Department of Pharmaceutical and Medicinal Chemistry, Faculty of Pharmacy, Olabisi Onabanjo University, Ago Iwoye P.O. Box 2002, Nigeria; olatunde.olaitan@oouagoiwoye.edu.ng
* Correspondence: diane.ashiru-oredope@commonwealthpharmacy.org

check for updates

Citation: Ogunnigbo, O.; Nabiryo, M.; Atteh, M.; Muringu, E.; Olaitan, O.J.; Rutter, V.; Ashiru-Oredope, D. Exploring the Antimicrobial Stewardship Educational Needs of Healthcare Students and the Potential of an Antimicrobial Prescribing App as an Educational Tool in Selected African Countries. *Antibiotics* **2022**, *11*, 691. https://doi.org/10.3390/antibiotics11050691

Academic Editor: Seok Hoon Jeong

Received: 7 April 2022
Accepted: 12 May 2022
Published: 19 May 2022

Publisher's Note: MDPI stays neutral with regard to jurisdictional claims in published maps and institutional affiliations.

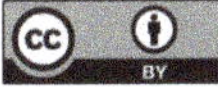

Copyright: © 2022 by the authors. Licensee MDPI, Basel, Switzerland. This article is an open access article distributed under the terms and conditions of the Creative Commons Attribution (CC BY) license (https://creativecommons.org/licenses/by/4.0/).

Abstract: Antimicrobial resistance (AMR) is a global health threat and one of the top 10 global public health threats facing humanity. AMR contributes to 700,000 deaths annually and more deaths, as many as 10 million are projected to happen by 2050. Antimicrobial stewardship (AMS) activities have been important in combating the ripple effects of AMR and several concerted efforts have been taken to address the issues of antimicrobial resistance. The Commonwealth Pharmacists Association through the Commonwealth Partnerships for Antimicrobial Stewardship (CwPAMS) programme has been enhancing the capacity of health institutions in Low-Middle-Income Countries (LMIC) to combat AMR. Through such efforts, an antimicrobial prescribing app (CwPAMS app) was launched and delivered to support antimicrobial prescribing and improve AMS practice in four African countries; Ghana, Uganda, Zambia, and Tanzania. The app provides easy access to infection management resources to improve appropriate use of antimicrobials in line with national and international guidelines. This study aimed to identify and explore the potential for the usability of the CwPAMS app among healthcare students across selected African countries that are part of the Commonwealth. The study equally evaluated the healthcare students' understanding and attitudes towards antimicrobial resistance and stewardship. Despite 70% of the respondents indicating that they had been taught about prudent use of antibiotics, diagnosis of infections and their management using antibiotics in their universities, notable knowledge gaps were discovered: 52.2% of the respondents had no prior information on the term AMS, 50.6% of them reported a lack of resources for accessing up-to-date information on drugs, for instance only 36% had had an opportunity to access an app as a learning resource even when 70% of the respondents thought that a mobile app would support in increasing their knowledge. Those challenges reveal an opportunity for the CwPAMS App as a potential option to address AMR and AMS gaps among healthcare students.

Keywords: antimicrobial resistance; CwPAMS; prescribing app; antimicrobial surveillance; antibiotics; antimicrobials; antimicrobial stewardship

1. Introduction

Resistance to antimicrobials threatens the effective prevention and treatment of an ever-increasing range of infections [1]. Antimicrobial resistance is a current global health and development threat and the World Health Organization declared it as one of the top 10 global public health threats facing humanity [1]. The overarching issue is that antimicrobial resistance threatens the very core of modern medicine and the sustainability of an effective global public health response [2]. Each year, 700,000 people lose their lives to AMR, and more deaths.As many as 10 million deaths are projected to happen by 2050 with a 3.8 percent reduction in the annual gross domestic product (GDP) if action is not taken [3]. AMR significantly affects the economy through prolonging illness, thus causing longer hospital stays and the need for more expensive medicines, which pose financial challenges for the national health systems and the affected individuals [1,4].

Whilst resistance to existing antibiotics is increasing, the development of new antibiotics is low. In 2019, the WHO identified only six antibiotics of the 32 antibiotics that were in clinical development that address the WHO list of priority pathogens [1]. Misuse and overuse of antimicrobials are the main drivers in the development of drug-resistant pathogens [1]. Existing literature commonly highlights that health care providers especially those in LMIC have inadequate knowledge on use of antimicrobials and antimicrobial resistance [5,6]. As a result, the challenge of inappropriate prescription of antimicrobials continues to prevail, thus worsening antimicrobial resistance [5–7].

Antimicrobial stewardship alongside infection prevention and control have been the mainstay in tackling the challenge of AMR. As a global response, antimicrobial stewardship, which is the systematic, coordinated effort that promotes the appropriate use of antimicrobials was launched through several collaborations and concerted efforts of governments and healthcare bodies and organisations [8,9]. It is important that prescribers ensure "the right antibiotic, at the right dose at the right time" [10] Antimicrobial stewardship programmes should take into consideration monitoring and evaluation of antimicrobial prescribing, regular feedback to prescribers, education and training for health and social care staff, and integrating audits into existing quality improvement programmes [11].

The UK aid Fleming Fund funded a new programme in 2018, the Commonwealth Partnerships for Antimicrobial Stewardship programme (CwPAMS), managed by the Commonwealth Pharmacists Association (CPA) and Tropical Health and Education Trust (THET) and supports improvement of antimicrobial prescribing, surveillance and stewardship [12]. As part of the CwPAMS antimicrobial stewardship interventions, an Antimicrobial Prescribing app (CwPAMS app) was launched in 2019 and delivered to improve antimicrobial prescribing practice in four African countries; Ghana, Uganda, Zambia, and Tanzania [13]. The app provides easy access to infection management resources and improves the appropriate use of antimicrobials according to national and international guidelines.

Following the launch of the CwPAMS app in the four African countries, there were 530 downloads of the app and 2795 guides opened within 12 months. Ghana received more downloads (50.3 percent) than Uganda (31 percent), Tanzania (13 percent), Zambia (1.9 percent), and others (3.8 percent) [13]. Relatedly, Olaoye et al. [13] reported that the CwPAMS app improved the health care providers' awareness on AMS and prescribing practices. Further, the health care providers found the CwPAMS app easily accessible as its usability is not internet dependent [13]. To respond to one of the recommendations of this study, which was further dissemination of the CwPAMS app; identifying and addressing the educational needs of health care students (future healthcare professionals) was considered paramount to effecting long term and sustainable changes in antimicrobial stewardship. By taking stewardship activities to the grassroots, i.e., healthcare students, they can be better informed on antimicrobial prescribing and more empowered healthcare providers as professionals. The importance of smartphones in healthcare training and education cannot be underestimated. Smartphones are described as a resource called "Learn Anywhere" [14].

In this context, this study aimed to understand the potential use of the CwPAMS app to guide antimicrobial prescribing, and specifically to serve as an educational tool for healthcare students in Commonwealth countries within the African continent. The study was also planned to evaluate knowledge and attitudes of healthcare students towards antimicrobial resistance and stewardship activities.

2. Materials and Methods

2.1. Survey Development

A survey- based approach was adopted, using a 59-item questionnaire (Supplementary Materials) developed from two existing validated surveys in the literature; European survey of healthcare workers' knowledge, attitudes and behaviours with respect to antibiotics, antibiotic use and antibiotic resistance [15] and healthcare students' survey assessing the knowledge, attitudes and behaviors of human and animal health students towards antibiotic use and resistance [16]. The survey was hosted on Survey Monkey, a web-based survey platform. A pilot survey was initially conducted in Nigeria and Uganda with seventeen [17] health care students. The survey was updated based on feedback and disseminated to healthcare students across ten African countries. Time taken to fill the survey and other suggestions for improvement were noted during the pilot. Pilot data was excluded from the final analysis. All questions were presented to respondents in English language. The questions were a mixture of Likert-scale, True or False, and choice format. The questionnaire included study information about respondents, inclusion of antimicrobial stewardship as part of their learning, existence of educational content focusing on AMR and stewardship, and explored perspectives to understand the potential benefits of a mobile application that guides antimicrobial prescribing. It also focused on information about individuals who had participated in a prudent antibiotic use campaign in the past three years. The survey was reviewed and refined by discussing with the CwPAMS project team and CPA's global AMR lead.

2.2. Target Respondents and Data Collection Procedure

The target population were undergraduate health care students from universities in Africa. Promotion was primarily to eight countries that are part of the original and extension phase of CwPAMS programme—Ghana, Kenya, Malawi, Nigeria, Uganda, Tanzania, Zambia. Healthcare students from diverse academic backgrounds were eligible to participate in this survey. Participation was voluntary, with the survey being open for responses over a 6-week period (12 April until 20 May 2021).

The survey was promoted through the support of CwPAMS representatives to health students in the selected African countries. The survey was also promoted through social media platforms amongst students and university leads.

2.3. Data Analysis

Descriptive statistics on the frequency distributions and percentages were used to analyse the responses and IBM SPSS Statistics 25 and Microsoft Excel 2016 were used to analyse the data.

2.4. Ethics

Formal ethics approval was not required because this study was classified as a service evaluation of CPA's activities. Informed consent was obtained from all the respondents to participate in the study (100%). No personal and identifiable data was collected and respondents were assured that the information provided would be kept confidential. Participation in this study was optional, and they had the option to withdraw their consent if they no longer agreed to any aspect. The data were held securely and in-line with the General Data Protection Regulation 2016/679.

3. Results

3.1. Demographics of Respondents and Countries Involved

The study included responses from 483 health care students from 44 universities across 10 Commonwealth countries; Nigeria (313), Kenya (111), Uganda (34), Tanzania (16), Zambia (2), Malawi (2), India (1), Democratic Republic of Congo, Rwanda (1 student each). The respondents were studying a range of health related courses 250 pharmacy, 84 pharmacology, 66 medicine, 42 pharmacy technicians, 31 biomedical sciences, 5 nursing, 1 dentistry,

1 veterinary medicine and 3 others, which are part of the aforementioned courses). Most of the respondents had at least 4 years and above for their chosen undergraduate degree (90.2). The majority of respondents were already in their penultimate and final year of undergraduate degree; third year (23.6%) and fourth year of education (31.1%) (Table 1).

Table 1. Demographics of respondents and countries involved (across 10 Commonwealth countries).

	Variables	Frequency	Percentage (%)
The undergraduate degree being studied	Pharmacy	250	51.8
	Pharmacology	84	17.4
	Medicine	66	13.7
	Pharmacy Technician	42	8.7
	Health sciences (biomedical sciences)	31	6.4
	Nursing	5	1
	Others (Veterinary Medicine, Dentistry, Clinical Pharmacology & Therapeutics, Clinical Medicine)	5	1
	Total	**483**	**100.0**
Years of the undergraduate degree for the chosen career	3 years	47	9.7
	4 years	158	32.7
	5 years	213	44.1
	6 years	6	1.2
	>6 years	59	12.2
	Total	**483**	**100.0**
Country	Nigeria	313	10.1
	Kenya	111	20.1
	Uganda	34	23.6
	Tanzania	16	31.1
	Ghana, Rwanda, Congo, Malawi, Zambia and Others	9	11.2
	Total	**483**	**100.0**

3.2. *Knowledge of Antimicrobials, Antimicrobial Use and Stewardship*

3.2.1. Teachings on Antibiotic Treatment and Usage

Most of the respondents reported that they received lectures about antibiotics during their undergraduate degree programme. More than two thirds of the respondents had teaching on prudent antibiotic use (70.4%), diagnosis of infections (74.3%), and antibiotic treatment (77.2%). Few were not taught about the prudent use of antibiotics (18.4%), diagnosis of infections (14.3%) and treatment with antibiotics (14.3%). Small percentages were not sure if they had been taught about the prudent use of antibiotics (11.2%), diagnosis of infections (11.4%) and treatment with antibiotics (8.5%) (Supplementary Material Table S1).

3.2.2. Examination Questions on Antibiotic Use

Most of the respondents reported having had exam questions on antibiotics. More than half of them had exam questions on: prudent antibiotics (60.2%); diagnosis of infections (66.0%) and antibiotic treatment (70.0%). Only a few had no exam questions on prudent use of antibiotics (25.9%), diagnosis of infections (21.5%) and antibiotic treatment (18.8%). A small percentage was not sure if they had exam questions on prudent use of antibiotics (13.9%), diagnosis of infections (12.4%) and antibiotic treatment (11.2%) (Supplementary Material Table S2).

3.2.3. Students' Participation in Public Health Campaigns on Prudent Antibiotic Use

Many of the respondents (69.6%) reported that they had not been involved in a campaign linked to prudent antibiotic use in the previous three years, 18% stated they had participated in campaigns and 12.4% could not remember whether they had participated or not. Of the 87 respondents that participated in a prudent antibiotic use campaign, 39.1% provided education on antimicrobial resistance, 20.7% reported they shared their knowledge about antimicrobial resistance on social media, others participated in Antimicrobial Resistance Seminar (10.3%), engaged in rallies and campaigns (9.2%), joined debates and conferences (4.6%), and (4.6%) helped to raise community awareness in a rally (Table 2).

Table 2. Students' participation in public health campaigns on prudent antibiotic use.

	Variables	Frequency	Percentage (%)
Participation in a campaign on the prudent use of antibiotics over the last three years	Yes	87	18.0
	No	336	69.6
	Cannot remember	60	12.4
Means of participation	Through rallies and campaigns	8	9.2
	Surveys on AMR and Surveys on AMR and data collection (4.5%)	4	4.5
	Social media awareness on antimicrobial resistance	18	20.7
	SARS committee member MKU chapter	2	2.3
	Outreach program to secondary schools in Ilala Tanzania	2	2.3
	In debate and conferences	4	4.6
	I wrote a poem on antimicrobial resistance for the world health students' alliance.	2	2.3
	Educating people about antimicrobial resistance	34	39.1
	Community awareness rally	4	4.6
	Attended an AMR seminar	9	10.3
	Total	**87**	**100.0**

3.2.4. Teaching Methods for Prudent Antibiotic Use

The most common method used for teaching the majority of the respondents on prudent antibiotic use was lecturing to more than 15 people (61.7%). Another teaching/learning technique frequently used was active learning tasks such as reading articles, group work, preparing an oral presentation (53.4%), e-learning (52.8%), discussion of clinical cases and vignettes (40.0%), peer or near-peer teachings such as classes led by other students or recently qualified doctors (39.3%), and digital resources such as apps (36.0%). On the other hand, unpopular learning methods included small group teachings with less than 15 people and clinical microbiology placement as reported by almost half of the respondents (Table 3).

3.2.5. Reference Sources for Information on Antimicrobials

Almost half of the students stated they did not know of any source of information on antimicrobials (47.0%) Those who had an antimicrobial reference source represented 40.8%, and 12.2% could not decide whether they knew or not. There were mixed responses on the reference sources that respondents were using with the highest proportion (13.5%) stating antimicrobial textbooks, followed by 8.9% who stated internet research and 7.2% who stated Emdex. Less than 5% referred to other sources including the BNF and the World Health Organization handbook on antimicrobial stewardship. Almost half (48.9%) did not specify the reference sources they currently use (Supplementary Material Table S3).

Table 3. Teaching methods used to teach students about prudent use of antibiotics/antibiotic treatment.

Statements	Yes	No	Unsure
Lectures (with >15 people)	295 (61.1%)	95 (19.7%)	93 (19.3%)
Small group teaching (with <15 people)	96 (19.9%)	217 (44.9%)	170 (35.2%)
Discussions of clinical cases and vignettes	193 (40.0%)	143 (29.6%)	147 (30.4%)
Active learning assignments (e.g., article reading, group work, preparing an oral presentation)	258 (53.4%)	109 (22.6%)	116 (24.0%)
E-learning	255 (52.8%)	115 (23.8%)	113 (23.4%)
Role play or communication skills sessions dealing with patients demanding antibiotic training	147 (30.4%)	183 (37.9%)	153 (31.7%)
Infectious diseases clinical placement (i.e., clinical rotation or training in infectious diseases, involving patients)	131 (27.1%)	185 (38.3%)	131 (27.1%)
Microbiology clinical placement	117 (24.2%)	216 (44.7%)	150 (31.1%)
Peer or near peer-teaching (i.e., teaching led by other students or recently qualified doctors)	190 (39.3%)	159 (32.9%)	134 (27.7%)
Use of digital resources such as apps	174 (36.0%)	169 (35.0%)	140 (29.0%)

An online learning platform was the most popular reference source of information used by the students. Half of the students mainly used online libraries for their medical reference (48.0%), 35% used textbooks, 8% used the BNF and 9% used other sources.

3.2.6. Antimicrobial Stewardship Awareness amongst Students

Slightly more than half (52.2%) of participants reported that they had no prior knowledge of the term antimicrobial stewardship (AMS); 42% stated they had heard of AMS and 5.8% were unsure.

3.2.7. Barriers to Up-to-Date Information about Drugs amongst Students

About half of the respondents indicated that one of the challenges in obtaining up-to-date information on drugs was lack of resources (50.6%). Other factors highlighted included internet access (29.8%), power outages (17.9%), reliable sources (0.7%) and laxity (0.2%). Only 0.9% had no challenges in obtaining current information (Supplementary Material Table S4).

3.2.8. Social Media Channels Used Mostly amongst Students

When asked "What social media channel do you think students relate with the most?"; the most common channels selected by the respondents were Twitter (33.5%), Instagram (23.6%), Facebook (17.2%) and WhatsApp (16.8%). Others included YouTube (0.4%), Zoom (0.2%), the Internet (0.2%) and Google (0.2%) (n = 483). There was no response from 6.8% of the respondents (Supplementary Material Table S5).

3.3. *Students' Perspectives on Antimicrobial Resistance and Stewardship*

3.3.1. Students' Perspectives on Antibiotics Use

The majority (73.5%) of respondents believed that: unnecessary use of antibiotics makes them ineffective, that taking antibiotics is associated with side effects or risks, such as diarrhoea, colitis and allergies (66.7%), that healthy people can carry antibiotic-resistant bacteria (55.3%), and that any person treated with antibiotics is at increased risk of antibiotic-resistant infection (49.9%) (Table 4). About half of the respondents reported that antibiotics are not effective against viruses (53.6%), cold, and flu (42.4%). Approximately a quarter of the respondents (23.6%) could correctly answer that the use of antibiotics for growth promotion in farm animals is not legal in the EU.

Table 4. Students' responses to statements on antibiotics.

Statement (Correct Answers—False (F); True (T))	True	False	Unsure	Do Not Know
Antibiotics are effective against viruses (F)	118 (24.4%)	259 (53.6%)	81 (16.8%)	25 (5.2%)
Antibiotics are effective against cold and flu (F)	176 (36.4%)	205 (42.4%)	72 (14.9%)	30 (6.2%)
Unnecessary use of antibiotics makes them become ineffective (T)	355 (73.5%)	43 (8.9%)	56 (11.6%)	29 (6.0%)
Taking antibiotics have associated side effects or risks such as diarrhea, colitis, allergies (T)	322 (66.7%)	39 (8.1%)	90 (18.6%)	32 (6.6%)
Every person treated with antibiotics is at an increased risk of antibiotic-resistant infection (T)	241 (49.9%)	111 (23.0%)	91 (18.8%)	40 (8.3%)
Bacteria that are resistant to antibiotics spread easily from person to person (T)	224 (46.4%)	95 (19.7%)	118 (24.4%)	46 (9.5%)
Healthy people can carry antibiotic resistant bacteria (T)	267 (55.3%)	68 (14.1%)	101 (20.9)	47 (9.7%)
The use of antibiotics to stimulate growth in farm animals is legal in the EU (F)	114 (23.6%)	69 (14.3%)	216 (44.7%)	84 (17.4%)

More than three quarters of the students (82%) agreed or strongly agreed that prescribing, dispensing or administering inappropriate or unnecessary antibiotics was professionally unethical. A similar proportion of students strongly agreed or agreed that antibiotic resistance is both a national problem (73%) and one that would be a problem for their future individual practice (71%) (Table 5).

Table 5. Level of agreement or disagreement with antibiotic prescribing patterns.

Statements	Strongly agree	Agree	Neutral	Strongly Disagree	Disagree	No Response
Most coughs, colds and sore throats get better on their own without the need for antibiotics	162 (33.5%)	156 (32.3%)	85 (17.6%)	13 (2.7%)	23 (4.8%)	44 (9.1%)
Prescribing, dispensing, or administering inappropriate or unnecessary antibiotics is professionally unethical	315 (65.2%)	81 (16.8%)	26 (5.4%)	7 (1.4%)	7 (1.4%)	47 (9.7%)
There are enough antibiotics under development worldwide to keep up with the problem of resistance	99 (20.5%)	103 (21.3%)	116 (24.0%)	49 (10.1%)	67 (13.9%)	49 (10.1%)
Antibiotic resistance is a national problem	228 (47.2)	128 (26.5%)	60 (12.4%)	9 (1.9%)	9 (1.9%)	49 (10.1%)
I think the antibiotic resistance will be a problem for my future individual practice	240 (49.7%)	100 (20.7%)	63 (13.0%)	9 (1.9%)	19 (3.9%)	52 (10.8%)

3.3.2. Students' Perspectives on Indiscriminate Antimicrobial Use in Respondents' Countries

The majority of the respondents (74.9%) thought that the rate of the indiscriminate use of antimicrobials in their countries was alarming; 13% chose maybe, 6% respectively disagreed or were unsure.

3.3.3. Students' Perspectives on Education about Antimicrobial Resistance and Antimicrobial Stewardship

There were mixed responses to the statements measuring students' perspectives on antimicrobial resistance and stewardship as shown in Table 6. More than a quarter (40.6%) of the respondents indicated that antimicrobial resistance (AMR) is a recurrent theme in their teaching and 40.8% reported that there is not enough educational content about AMR/AMS at their institution. More than half of the students thought that more AMR and stewardship learning content should be offered (56.1%) and 55.9% stated that an application that provides essential information about antimicrobials would be helpful for their learning. More than half also highlighted that increasing national campaigns on the prudent use of antimicrobials would help disseminate information about antimicrobial resistance and 54.7% agreed that social media would help increase awareness of antimicrobial stewardship. Those who would likely engage with an educational tool such as a phone app to learn more about antimicrobials accounted for 50.1%. Slightly more than half (52.1%) believed a medical information app offline and on the go will help them make more informed decisions about antibiotics. However, 52.2% of respondents believed antimicrobial resistance is not really as it seems, with new antibiotics being developed by scientists every year.

Table 6. Students' perspectives on antimicrobial resistance and stewardship.

Variables	Strongly Agree	Agree	Neutral	Strongly Disagree	Disagree	No Response
Antimicrobial resistance (AMR) is a recurring theme in my learning	71 (14.7%)	126 (26.1)	97 (20.1)	94 (19.5)	50 (10.4)	45 (9.3%)
There is enough educational content around AMR/AMS in my institution	24 (5.0%)	84 (17.4%)	129 (26.7%)	61 (12.6%)	136 (28.2%)	49 (10.1%)
I think more learning content about AMR and stewardship opportunities should be made available	172 35.6%)	99 (20.5%)	43 (8.9%)	108 (22.4%)	18 (3.7%)	43 (8.9%)
An App that provides important information about antimicrobials will be useful for my personal learning	172 (35.6%)	98 (20.3%)	45 (9.3%)	106 (21.9%)	20 (4.1%)	42 (8.7%)
Reinforcement of national campaigns around prudent antimicrobial use will help spread information about antibiotic resistance	155 (32.1%)	110 (22.8%)	47 (9.7%)	106 (21.9%)	17 (3.5%)	48 (9.9)
Social media handles among student health professionals will help to raise more awareness of antimicrobial stewardship.	138 (28.6%)	126 (26.1%)	53 (11.0%)	91 (18.8%)	25 (5.2%)	50 (10.4%)
Antimicrobial resistance is not really as it seems because new antibiotics are developed yearly by scientists	26 (5.4)	47 (9.7%)	99 (20.5%)	125 (25.9%)	127 (26.3%)	59 (12.2%)
I am likely to engage with an educational tool such as an App on my phone to learn about antimicrobials	117 (24.2%)	125 (25.9%)	71 (14.7%)	90 (18.6%)	23 (4.8%)	57 (11.8%)
Having an offline and on-the-go medical information app will help me make more informed choices about antibiotics	147 (30.4%)	105 (21.7%)	55 (11.4%)	102 (21.1%)	20 (4.1%)	54 (11.2%)

3.4. Factors Contributing to AMR

There was a mixed response on the highest implicating factor in antimicrobial resistance. Approximately one-third of respondents reported that the factor contributing most to AMR was not completing the full course of antibiotics (36.6%) or an inappropriate prescription of antibiotics (34.8%). Other respondents thought the highest implicating factor was poor management of antibiotic residues (9.3%), lack of infection control (5.6%), and poor hygiene (4.8%) (Supplementary Material Table S6).

3.5. Responsibility for Antimicrobial Stewardship

Most respondents stated that health professionals (61.8%) have the greatest responsibility for antimicrobial stewardship, followed by the Ministry of Health (26.5%), medical institutions (9.7%), all individuals (1.1%), the community (0.2%), and patients themselves (0.4%) (Supplementary Material Table S7).

3.6. Topics Students Would like more Information about and Educational Tools Students Would Use if Available

There was a mixed response on the topics healthcare students would like to receive more information about (Figure 1). The medical conditions for which antibiotics are used ranks as the primary topic students want to know more about (37.5%). Others include resistance to antibiotics (31.8%), methods of antibiotic use (14.9%), hygiene and infection control measures (14.4%), and 0.2% each for a systematic review of antibiotics and a complete library of diseases. Of all respondents, less than 1% (0.9%) stated that they would like more information on all the topic options provided.

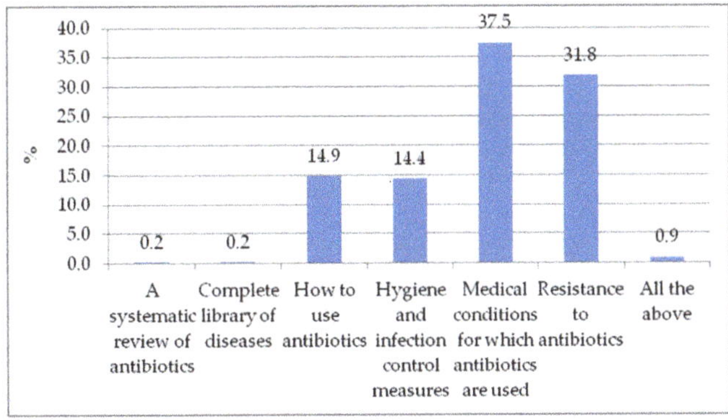

Figure 1. The topics on which to receive more information about.

The majority of the respondents would like to use an antimicrobial app as an educational tool that is part of their regular learning, if available (68.7%). Printed guidelines on antibiotics would be an alternative for 19.1% of them, and antimicrobial journals were of interest to 11.7%. A combination of antimicrobial app and journals was found appealing by 0.2%, as shown in Figure 2.

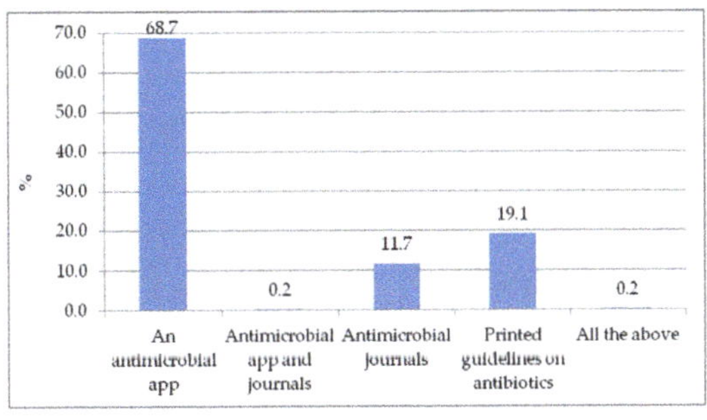

Figure 2. Educational tools that will be part of my regular learning, if available.

4. Discussion

This is the first service assessment to consider the possibility of rolling out the CwPAMS Antimicrobial prescribing app to undergraduate students as an educational and learning tool. The study also aimed to assess the knowledge and perspectives of health care students towards AMR and stewardship.

4.1. Knowledge and Students' Perceptions on Antimicrobial Stewardship

The study demonstrated that education on antimicrobials is highly considered in universities; more than 70% of the study respondents agreed that they had been taught about prudent use of antibiotics, diagnosis of infections and their management using antibiotics (Supplementary Material Table S1). This is important as, previously highlighted in a knowledge, attitude and practice study conducted among medical students in Colombia, university training improved knowledge of students on antimicrobials and their use [17]. In that study and a similar one conducted in China it was revealed that the knowledge level on antimicrobials increased as students progressed to higher academic years of study within their respective programmes [16–18].

Various educational strategies were used to educate students on prudent use of antimicrobials with the most common being lectures of at least 15 people (61.1%), oral presentation (53.4%) and e-learning (52.8%) (Table 3). These methods are not unique to the current study participants; the literature shows they have been used elsewhere, for example, in European settings, with lectures also being the most commonly used strategy [19,20].

While close to 70% of the respondents thought that a mobile application app would be essential in increasing their knowledge on the prudent use of antimicrobials, at the time the study was conducted, less than half (36.0%) of the participants previously had an opportunity to use digital resources such as apps for learning (Figure 2). As access to smart phones increases, several studies recommend the usage of mobile applications for medical education, as they have been shown to facilitate quick and timely access to information, flexible learning and peer interactions, thus improving efficiency and patient care [21–24]. Despite the advantages that come with using apps in patient care, some studies have noted that these can be sources of disruptions while providing patient care, as clinicians' attention may be drawn to notifications from other personal mobile apps [22]. Furthermore, usage of phone could also be perceived negatively by patients as demonstrated in previous studies [13,25].

Earlier research findings have shown that usage of mobile applications in medical education can be facilitated by affordable cost and the ability to use the phone in an offline mode, thus not requiring internet connectivity and also reducing interference from other mobile apps [21,22]. Those facilitators were considered when developing the CwPAMS app as it is freely accessible without cost and, once downloaded, there is no need for internet connectivity to use it [13].

Despite this study reflecting a high consideration of prudent use of antimicrobials as part of the education system, the study also revealed notable gaps in the knowledge and access to information on antimicrobial usage. For instance, more than half of the participants had no prior knowledge on the term antimicrobial stewardship (AMS) and reported a lack of resources for obtaining up to date information on drugs (Supplementary Material Table S4). This is similar to a research finding among physicians in Nigerian Hospitals [26]. Relatedly, almost 70% of the study participants reported not participating in a campaign that included prudent antibiotic use in the previous three years (Table 2) and close to 50% of them did not know any source of information about antimicrobials. These findings indicate that besides the formal educational curriculum, there are opportunities for engaging and empowering students in Africa in antimicrobial stewardship. This is also evident in the study participants' perspectives, where more than half of the students noted their need for more AMR and stewardship content, and suggested that increasing national campaigns on the prudent use of antimicrobials would help disseminate information about antimicrobial resistance. Previous studies also recommend the usage of various educational strategies to improve access to information on antimicrobial resistance and stewardship among students [27–29]. In that regard, interventions such as the CwPAMS app, which has been proven to provide easy access to infection management resources and to improve the appropriate use of antimicrobials according to national and international guidelines, can be an important tool in empowering students in Africa [13]. This study revealed that if an intervention like a prescribing app is availed, more than half of the students could potentially use it to as an educational tool (Figure 2).

Additionally, 54.7% of the study participants thought that social media could help as part of improving their knowledge on antimicrobial resistance and stewardship. Here, the most preferred social media channels were Twitter, Instagram, Facebook and WhatsApp. With about 47% of the global population having access to the internet via mobile phones, the usage of social media has increased and this should be taken as an opportunity to increase awareness about disease prevention, and rational use of antibiotics and antibiotic resistance among the population and health workers [3,30,31]. An earlier research study about usage of social media in LMICs demonstrated that social media can be used as a platform to promote various educational interventions such as videos, games, and images [3]. As such, social media can be leveraged for promoting the usage of interventions such as the CwPAMS app that has proven to be an essential tool for enhancing antimicrobial stewardship in Africa.

With most of the study respondents (61.8%) indicating that health professionals have the greatest responsibility for antimicrobial stewardship (Supplementary Material Table S6), it suggests that as health care students, they are aware that students have an important role to play. Thus, if empowered and given the opportunity, they can contribute to the reduction in the burden of AMR, as recommended in another study that increasing the knowledge of healthcare students, especially pharmacists who will have frequent interactions with antimicrobial users in the future, is key [32]. Students who participated in this study felt the need for more knowledge in some of the following areas: medical conditions for which antibiotics are used, resistance to antibiotics, methods of antibiotic use, hygiene, and infection control measures (Figure 1). The CwPAMS app can be an appropriate intervention for those needs as it hosts national and international guidelines with instructions on antimicrobial usage and infection prevention and control [13].

4.2. Strengths and Limitations

Although the survey includes responses from several respondents in Low-Middle-Income-Countries (LMIC) within the Commonwealth, the number of respondents for some countries was low, and only selected African countries participated in the survey. In addition, the number of medical students who responded to the survey was disproportionately lower than that of students from the pharmacy profession; however some of our findings such as knowledge of AMS amongst health students is similar to a study conducted amongst physicians in Nigeria, which reported that although physicians are familiar with AMR they have limited knowledge of AMS [26]. The results do not provide in-depth details of the issues within each country or across educational institutions, hence we cannot determine the local learning needs across regions. Further evaluation, perhaps using follow-up surveys, would be required to explore this. Nevertheless, the survey provides useful data on healthcare students' knowledge and perspectives towards AMR and provides insights into the potential use of mobile applications such as the CwPAMS app for educating health students.

5. Conclusions

While progress has been made through collaborative programs to optimize the appropriate use of antimicrobials, more concerted effort is required to understand the needs of healthcare students and channel educational resources to improve their knowledge and involvement in antimicrobial stewardship. The study findings highlight that university education provides an avenue for health care students to learn about prudent antimicrobial usage. However, the study also revealed several opportunities for strengthening the knowledge and engagement of students in antimicrobial stewardship. The demonstration of poor knowledge of the term antimicrobial stewardship and limited access to related information shows that there could be value in the use of mobile applications such as CwPAMS app as an educational tool for AMR and AMS amongst healthcare students in LMICs. The strength of successful usage of the CwPAMS app lies in the fact that it can be used in an offline mode and is freely accessible. It is important that global health organisations such as the Commonwealth Pharmacists Association (CPA), leading on AMS interventions, consider expanding their support beyond qualified healthcare professionals to include the education and training of health care students; working in collaboration with international health student bodies such as the International Pharmaceutical Students' Federation and International Federation of Medical Students' Associations. This approach can potentially establish embedding use of evidence based guidelines in preparation for their professional careers.

Supplementary Materials: The following supporting information can be downloaded at: https://www.mdpi.com/article/10.3390/antibiotics11050691/s1, Table S1: Teaching about antibiotic treatment and prudent antibiotic use during my studies; Table S2: My examinations included questions on antibiotic treatment or prudent use of antibiotics; Table S3: Reference sources being used; Table S4: Challenges encountered in obtaining current information about drugs; Table S5: Social media channels students relate with the most; Table S6: The highest implicating factor in AMR; Table S7: Who has the highest responsibility for antimicrobial stewardship?.

Author Contributions: Conceptualization, O.O. and D.A.-O.; Data curation, O.O., E.M. and O.J.O.; Formal analysis, M.A.; Funding acquisition, V.R. and D.A.-O.; Methodology, O.O., E.M., O.J.O. and D.A.-O.; Project administration, O.O.; Supervision, D.A.-O.; Validation, D.A.-O.; Writing—original draft, O.O., M.N., D.A.-O. and M.A.; Writing—review & editing, O.O., M.N., E.M., O.J.O., V.R. and D.A.-O. All authors have read and agreed to the published version of the manuscript.

Funding: This project and partnership was part of the Commonwealth Partnerships for Antimicrobial Stewardship (CwPAMS) managed by the Tropical Health and Education Trust (THET) and Commonwealth Pharmacists Association (CPA). CwPAMS is a global health partnership programme funded by the Fleming Fund using UK aid funding. The Fleming Fund is a UK aid programme supporting up to 25 countries across Sub-Saharan Africa and Asia to tackle antimicrobial resistance. The Fund is managed by the UK Department of Health and Social Care and invests in strengthening surveillance systems through a portfolio of country and regional grants, global projects and fellowship schemes. The views expressed in this publication are those of the authors and not necessarily those of the UK Department of Health and Social Care, the NHS, the represented NHS Trusts, CPA or THET.

Institutional Review Board Statement: Formal ethics approval was not required because this is a service needs assessment and evaluation. Informed consent was obtained from all the respondents to participate in the study (100%). Respondents were assured that the information provided would be kept confidential and that they would not be harmed in any way by the study and could not be associated with it. They were also informed that all information provided belonged to the CwPAMS. Participation in this study was optional, and they had the option to withdraw their consent if they no longer agree to any question. The data were held securely and in-line with the General Data Protection Regulation 2016/679.

Informed Consent Statement: Informed consent was obtained from all participants involved in the study.

Data Availability Statement: Data is contained within the article or Supplementary Material.

Acknowledgments: The authors are grateful to respondents in the different Commonwealth countries and especially the CPA members and in-country consultants in these countries that actively promoted the survey.

Conflicts of Interest: The authors declare no conflict of interest. The funders had no role in the design of the study; in the collection, analyses, or interpretation of data; in the writing of the manuscript, or in the decision to publish the results.

References

1. World Health Organization. Antimicrobial Resistance: Key Facts. 2020. Available online: https://www.who.int/news-room/fact-sheets/detail/antimicrobial-resistance (accessed on 21 June 2021).
2. World Health Organization. Global Action Plan on Antimicrobial Resistance. 2016. Available online: https://www.who.int/publications/i/item/9789241509763 (accessed on 8 March 2022).
3. Acharya, K.P.; Subedi, D. Use of Social Media as a Tool to Reduce Antibiotic Usage: A Neglected Approach to Combat Antimicrobial Resistance in Low and Middle Income Countries. *Front. Public Health* **2020**, *8*, 558576. [CrossRef] [PubMed]
4. ReAct. Antibiotic Resistance Is Costly, Both for the Individual and for Society. 2022. Available online: https://www.reactgroup.org/toolbox/understand/why-should-i-care/economic-losses/ (accessed on 8 March 2022).
5. Kagoya, E.K.; Royen, K.V.; Waako, P.; Royen, P.V.; Iramiot, J.S.; Obakiro, S.B.; Kostyanev, T.; Anthierens, S. Experiences and views of healthcare professionals on the prescription of antibiotics in Eastern Uganda: A qualitative study. *J. Glob. Antimicrob. Resist.* **2021**, *25*, 66–71. [CrossRef] [PubMed]
6. Thakolkaran, N.; Shetty, A.V.; D'Souza, N.D.R.; Shetty, A.K. Antibiotic prescribing knowledge, attitudes, and practice among physicians in teaching hospitals in South India. *J. Fam. Med. Prim. Care* **2017**, *6*, 526–532.
7. Mittal, A.K.; Bhardwaj, R.; Mishra, P.; Rajput, S.K. Antimicrobials Misuse/Overuse: Adverse Effect, Mechanism, Challenges and Strategies to Combat Resistance. *Open Biotechnol. J.* **2020**, *14*, 107–112. [CrossRef]
8. MacDougall, C.; Polk, R.E. Antimicrobial stewardship programs in health care systems. *Clin. Microbiol. Rev.* **2005**, *18*, 638–656. [CrossRef] [PubMed]
9. Liaskou, M.; Duggan, C.; Joynes, R.; Rosado, H. Pharmacy's role in antimicrobial resistance and stewardship. *Clin. Pharm.* **2018**, *10*. [CrossRef]
10. Dryden, M.; Johnson, A.P.; Ashiru-Oredope, D.; Sharland, M. Using antibiotics responsibly: Right drug, right time, right dose, right duration, J Antimicrob. *Chemotherapy* **2018**, *66*, 2441–2443. [CrossRef]
11. National Institute for Health and Care Excellence. Antimicrobial Stewardship: Systems and Processes for Effective Antimicrobial Medicine Use. 2015. Available online: https://www.nice.org.uk/guidance/NG15 (accessed on 23 June 2021).
12. Commonwealth Pharmacists Association. Commonwealth Partnerships for Antimicrobial Stewardship. 2022. Available online: https://commonwealthpharmacy.org/cwpams/ (accessed on 16 June 2021).
13. Olaoye, O.; Tuck, C.; Khor, W.P.; McMenamin, R.; Hudson, L.; Northall, M.; Panford-Quainoo, E.; Asima, D.M.; Ashiru-Oredope, D. Improving Access to Antimicrobial Prescribing Guidelines in 4 African Countries: Development and Pilot Implementation of an App and Cross-Sectional Assessment of Attitudes and Behaviour Survey of Healthcare Workers and Patients. *Antibiotics* **2020**, *9*, 555. [CrossRef]
14. Trelease, R.B. Diffusion of innovations: Smartphones and wireless anatomy learning resources. *Anat. Sci. Educ.* **2008**, *1*, 233–239. [CrossRef]
15. Ashiru-Oredope, D.; Hopkins, S.; Vasandani, S.; Umoh, E.; Oloyede, O.; Nilsson, A.; Kinsman, J.; Elsert, L.; Monnet, D.L.; The #ECDCAntibioticSurvey Project Advisory Group. Healthcare workers' knowledge, attitudes and behaviours with respect to antibiotics, antibiotic use and antibiotic resistance across 30 EU/EEA countries in 2019. *Eurosurveillance* **2021**, *26*, 1900633. [CrossRef]
16. Dyar, O.J.; Hills, H.; Seitz, L.-T.; Perry, A.; Ashiru-Oredope, D. Assessing the knowledge, attitudes and behaviors of human and animal health students towards antibiotic use and resistance: A pilot cross-sectional study in the UK. *Antibiotics* **2018**, *7*, 10. [CrossRef] [PubMed]
17. Higuita-Gutiérrez, L.F.; Roncancio Villamil, G.E.; Jiménez Quiceno, J.N. Knowledge, attitude, and practice regarding antibiotic use and resistance among medical students in Colombia: A cross-sectional descriptive study. *BMC Public Health* **2020**, *20*, 1861. [CrossRef] [PubMed]
18. Huang, Y.; Gu, J.; Zhang, M.; Ren, Z.; Yang, W.; Chen, Y.; Fu, Y.; Chen, X.; Cals, J.W.; Zhang, F. Knowledge, attitude and practice of antibiotics: A questionnaire study among 2500 Chinese students. *BMC Med. Educ.* **2013**, *13*, 163. [CrossRef] [PubMed]
19. Pulcini, C.; Wencker, F.; Frimodt-Møller, N.; Kern, W.; Nathwani, D.; Rodríguez-Baño, J.; Simonsen, G.S.; Vlahović-Palčevski, V.; Gyssens, I.C.; Jacobs, F.; et al. European survey on principles of prudent antibiotic prescribing teaching in undergraduate students. *Clin. Microbiol. Infect.* **2015**, *21*, 354–361. [CrossRef]
20. Hassali, M.A.A.; Sulaiman, S.A.S. Education on Antibiotic Resistance in Medical and Pharmacy Schools: Findings from Curriculum Survey in Selected Southeast Asian Universities. 2011. Available online: https://www.reactgroup.org/uploads/react/resources/213/Education%20on%20antibiotic%20resistance%20in%20medical%20and%20pharmacy%20schools.en.266.pdf (accessed on 10 March 2022).
21. Singh, K.; Sarkar, S.; Gaur, U.; Gupta, S.; Adams, O.P.; Sa, B.; Majumder, M.A.A. Smartphones and Educational Apps Use Among Medical Students of a Smart University Campus. *Front. Commun.* **2021**, *6*, 649102. [CrossRef]
22. Snashall, E.; Hindocha, S. The use of smartphone applications in medical education. *Open Med. J.* **2016**, *3*, 322–327. [CrossRef]
23. Richardson, W. Educational Studies in the United Kingdom, 1940–2002. *Br. J. Educ. Stud.* **2002**, *50*, 3–56. [CrossRef]
24. Ventola, C.L. Mobile devices and apps for health care professionals: Uses and benefits. *Pharm. Ther.* **2014**, *39*, 356–364.
25. Johnson, S.G.; Titlestad, K.B.; Larun, L.; Ciliska, D.; Olsen, N.R. Experiences with using a mobile application for learning evidence-based practice in health and social care education: An interpretive descriptive study. *PLoS ONE* **2021**, *16*, e0254272. [CrossRef]

26. Babatola, A.O.; Fadare, J.O.; Olatunya, O.S.; Obiako, R.; Enwere, O.; Kalungia, A.; Ojo, T.O.; Sunmonu, T.A.; Desalu, O.; Godman, B. Addressing Antimicrobial Resistance in Nigerian Hospitals: Exploring Physicians Prescribing Behavior, Knowledge, and Perception of Antimicrobial Resistance and Stewardship Programs. *Expert Rev. Anti-Infect. Ther.* **2021**, *19*, 537–546. [CrossRef]
27. Marvasi, M.; Casillas, L.; Vassallo, A.; Purchase, D. Educational Activities for Students and Citizens Supporting the One-Health Approach on Antimicrobial Resistance. *Antibiotics* **2021**, *10*, 1519. [CrossRef] [PubMed]
28. Akande-Sholabi, W.; Ajamu, A.T. Antimicrobial stewardship: Assessment of knowledge, awareness of antimicrobial resistance and appropriate antibiotic use among healthcare students in a Nigerian University. *BMC Med. Educ.* **2021**, *21*, 488. [CrossRef] [PubMed]
29. Alex, I.O. Knowledge of antibiotic use and resistance among students of a medical school in Nigeria. *Malawi Med. J.* **2019**, *31*, 133–137. [CrossRef] [PubMed]
30. Bahia, K.; Suardi, S. *The State of Mobile Internet Connectivity 2019*; Gsma: London, UK, 2019.
31. Hagg, E.; Dahinten, V.S.; Currie, L.M. The emerging use of social media for health-related purposes in low and middle-income countries: A scoping review. *Int. J. Med. Inform.* **2018**, *115*, 92–105. [CrossRef]
32. Franco, B.E.; Martínez, M.A.; Rodríguez, M.A.S.; Wertheimer, A.I. The determinants of the antibiotic resistance process. *Infect. Drug Resist.* **2009**, *2*, 1.

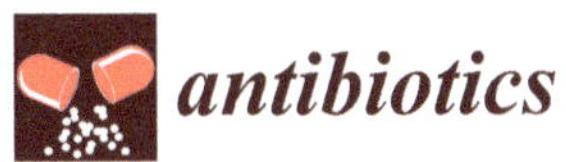

MDPI

Article

Antibiotic Prevalence Study and Factors Influencing Prescription of WHO Watch Category Antibiotic Ceftriaxone in a Tertiary Care Private Not for Profit Hospital in Uganda

Mark Kizito [1,*], Rejani Lalitha [1], Henry Kajumbula [2], Ronald Ssenyonga [3], David Muyanja [4] and Pauline Byakika-Kibwika [1]

1 Department of Medicine, College of Health Sciences, Makerere University, Kampala P.O. Box 7072, Uganda; rejani.lalitha@mak.ac.ug (R.L.); pbyakika@chs.mak.ac.ug (P.B.-K.)
2 Department of Microbiology, College of Health Sciences, Makerere University, Kampala P.O. Box 7072, Uganda; hkajumbula@chs.mak.ac.ug
3 Department of Epidemiology and Biostatistics, College of Health Sciences, Makerere University, Kampala P.O. Box 7072, Uganda; rssenyonga@musph.ac.ug
4 Department of Medicine, Mengo Hospital, Kampala P.O. Box 7161, Uganda; david.muyanja@mengohospital.org
* Correspondence: mkizito2@gmail.com; Tel.: +256-777525087

Abstract: Background: Excessive use of ceftriaxone contributes to the emergence and spread of antimicrobial resistance (AMR). In low and middle-income countries, antibiotics are overused but data on consumption are scarcely available. We aimed to determine the prevalence and factors influencing ceftriaxone prescription in a tertiary care private not-for-profit hospital in Uganda. **Methods:** A cross-sectional study was carried out from October 2019 through May 2020 at Mengo Hospital in Uganda. Patients admitted to the medical ward and who had been prescribed antibiotics were enrolled. Sociodemographic and clinical data were recorded in a structured questionnaire. Bivariate and adjusted logistic regression analyses were performed to determine factors associated with ceftriaxone prescription. **Results:** Study participants were mostly female (54.7%). The mean age was 56.2 years (SD: 21.42). The majority (187, 73.3%) presented with fever. Out of the 255 participants included in this study, 129 (50.6%) participants were prescribed ceftriaxone. Sixty-five (25.5%) and forty-one (16.0%) participants had a prescription of levofloxacin and metronidazole, respectively. Seven participants (2.7%) had a prescription of meropenem. Out of 129 ceftriaxone prescriptions, 31 (24.0%) were in combination with other antibiotics. Overall, broad-spectrum antibiotic prescriptions accounted for 216 (84.7%) of all prescriptions. Ceftriaxone was commonly prescribed for pneumonia (40/129, 31%) and sepsis (38/129, 29.5%). Dysuria [OR = 0.233, 95% CI (0.07–0.77), $p = 0.017$] and prophylactic indication [OR = 7.171, 95% CI (1.36–37.83), $p = 0.020$] were significantly associated with ceftriaxone prescription. **Conclusions:** Overall, we observed a high prevalence of prescriptions of ceftriaxone at the medical ward of Mengo Hospital. We recommend an antibiotic stewardship program (ASP) to monitor antibiotic prescription and sensitivity patterns in a bid to curb AMR.

Keywords: ceftriaxone prescription; prevalence; antibiotic stewardship; Uganda

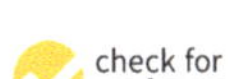

Citation: Kizito, M.; Lalitha, R.; Kajumbula, H.; Ssenyonga, R.; Muyanja, D.; Byakika-Kibwika, P. Antibiotic Prevalence Study and Factors Influencing Prescription of WHO Watch Category Antibiotic Ceftriaxone in a Tertiary Care Private Not for Profit Hospital in Uganda. *Antibiotics* **2021**, *10*, 1167. https://doi.org/10.3390/antibiotics10101167

Academic Editor: Diane Ashiru-Oredope

Received: 20 July 2021
Accepted: 13 September 2021
Published: 26 September 2021

Publisher's Note: MDPI stays neutral with regard to jurisdictional claims in published maps and institutional affiliations.

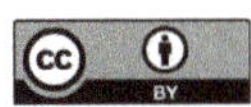

Copyright: © 2021 by the authors. Licensee MDPI, Basel, Switzerland. This article is an open access article distributed under the terms and conditions of the Creative Commons Attribution (CC BY) license (https://creativecommons.org/licenses/by/4.0/).

1. Background

Ceftriaxone is a broad-spectrum, third-generation cephalosporin antibiotic [1]. It is used in the treatment of many community and hospital-acquired infections mainly due to *Streptococcus pneumoniae*, *Streptococcus pyogenes*, *Staphylococcus aureus*, *Escherichia coli*, *Neisseria meningitides*, *Neisseria gonorrhoeae*, *Proteus mirabilis*, and *Enterobacter* spp. [1]. Indications for ceftriaxone use include acute bacterial meningitis, severe pneumonia, complicated intra-abdominal infections, pyelonephritis, severe prostatitis, and sepsis in neonates and children [2].

Ceftriaxone use is high in many low-income countries owing to its broad-spectrum activity, low toxicity, and cheaper cost compared with other antibiotics [3–5]. In Uganda, studies conducted in public healthcare facilities have reported high ceftriaxone prescription rates among hospitalized patients [5–7].

Unfortunately, there are reports of increasing resistance to this commonly prescribed antibiotic, and this is one of the emerging global health issues. For instance, in one review on antimicrobial resistance (AMR) covering Eastern African countries, Gram-negative and Gram-positive resistance to ceftriaxone was very high [8]. In Uganda, a summary of antimicrobial drug resistance patterns from blood cultures collected between June 2013 and October 2014 at Mulago National Referral Hospital showed high resistance of *Enterobacteriaceae* to ceftriaxone [9]. Furthermore, a study done at Uganda Cancer Institute among febrile cancer patients observed that Gram-negative resistance to ceftriaxone was very high [10].

To curb the increasing AMR, the World Health Organization (WHO) recommends continuous monitoring of antibiotic use [11]. Consequently, cephalosporins are frequently identified as a particular target for use evaluation and antibiotic stewardship [12].

In Uganda, similar to many other low-income countries, the private sector is increasingly becoming an important source of health care filling gaps where no or little public health care is available [13]. Half of all Ugandans (49%) utilize the private or private-not-for-profit (PNFP) sector care [14]. Despite this, there is a paucity of data on antibiotic use in private hospitals in Uganda. This study aimed at identifying the prevalence and the factors influencing ceftriaxone prescription at a tertiary care private not-for-profit hospital in Kampala, Uganda.

2. Methods

2.1. Study Setting and Design

A cross-sectional study was carried out from October 2019 through May 2020 at the medical ward of Mengo Hospital in Uganda. Mengo Hospital is a tertiary care private not-for-profit faith-based hospital in Kampala, the capital city of Uganda, with a bed capacity of 300. The medical ward consists of 40 beds and admits an average of 8 patients in 24 h and 240 patients over a month.

2.2. Data Collection

A team of doctors conducted the study at the medical ward of Mengo Hospital. Training and piloting of the study instruments were conducted for the study team before the start of the study. The study was conducted on weekdays. Hospital files for patients admitted to the medical ward of Mengo Hospital were reviewed. Patients with an antibiotic prescription were approached for written informed consent to participate in the study. For participants who could not consent, their next of kin was approached. We administered a structured pretested questionnaire to the study participants or their next of kin to obtain information about their sociodemographic data (age, sex, address), and medical history. Physical examination was performed on all participants. The name of the antibiotic(s) prescribed and the indication(s) for the prescription at the time of admission were extracted from the files.

2.3. Data Handling and Statistical Analysis

We coded and double entered all variables into Epidata version 3.0, and thereafter exported it to STATA® version 14, where the data were cleaned and analyzed. The prevalence of ceftriaxone prescription was defined as a percentage of patients with ceftriaxone prescription among the total number of patients on any systemic antibiotic. Bivariate and adjusted logistic regression analyses were performed to determine factors associated with ceftriaxone prescription. Statistical significance was set at cutoff points of 0.2 and 0.05 for bivariate and adjusted analyses, respectively.

3. Results

Two hundred and seventy-three patients admitted to the medical ward of Mengo Hospital between October 2019 and May 2020 received a prescription of antibiotics. Eighteen patients were excluded; fifteen did not consent while three were below 18 years of age. Out of the 255 enrolled, 129 (50.6%) were prescribed ceftriaxone as shown in Figure 1 below.

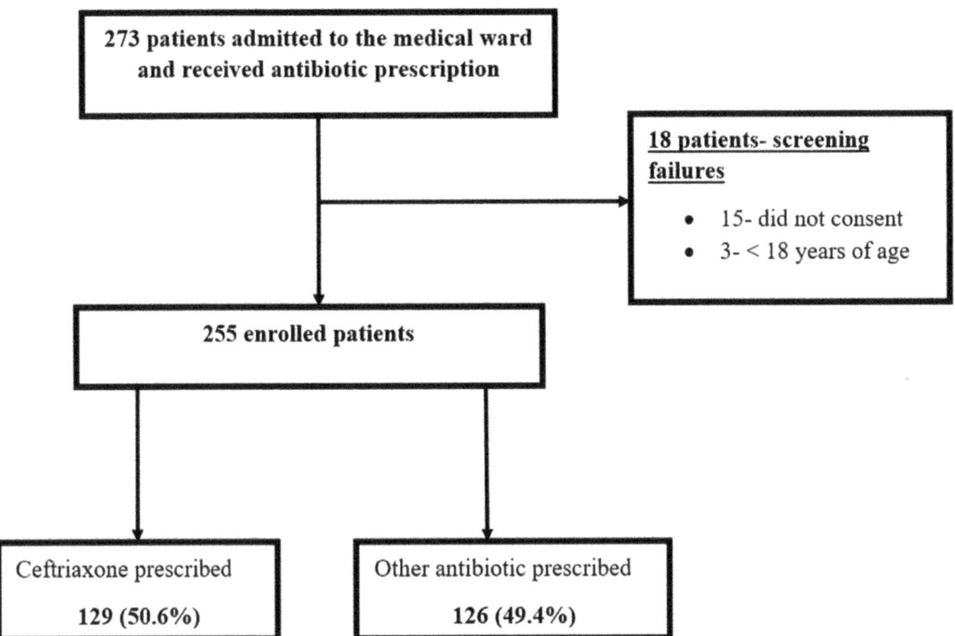

Figure 1. Study profile of hospitalized patients with antibiotic prescription.

3.1. Demographic Characteristics of Study Participants

Among the 255 participants, 54.5% were female. The mean age was 56.2 years (SD: 21.42) with the majority (148, 58%) over 50 years of age. More than half (156, 61.2%) of study participants were Baganda by tribe.

3.2. Clinical Characteristics of Study Participants

The majority of study participants had a fever (see Table 1). The median temperature was 36.5 °C (IQR 36.1–37.0). The median systolic blood pressure was 125 mmHg (IQR 104–147). One hundred and eighteen participants (46.3%) had at least one co-morbidity. Diabetes mellitus was the most prevalent co-morbidity. Nearly a third had crackles on physical examination. More than half of study participants had received antibiotics 5 days before admission (see Table 1).

Table 1. Clinical characteristics of the study participants.

	Frequency (n)	Percentage (%)
Symptoms		
History of fever	187	73.3
History of joint pains	107	42.0
History of cough	103	40.4
History of muscle pains	91	35.7
History of vomiting	90	35.3
History of abdominal pain	86	33.7
History of rapid breathing	78	30.6
History of confusion	77	30.2
History of passing urine frequently	37	14.5
History of wound or ulcer	27	10.6
History of pain on passing urine	20	7.8
History of convulsions	19	7.5
Co-morbidities		
Diabetes mellitus	53	20.8
HIV	39	15.3
Stroke	10	3.9
Chronic lung disease	9	3.5
Malignancy	8	3.1
Heart disease	7	2.7
Chronic liver disease	5	2.0
Chronic kidney disease	3	1.2
Use of antibiotics 5 days prior to admission	145	56.9
Clinical Signs		
Pallor $	101	39.6
Lymphadenopathy	5	2.0
Oral thrush	8	3.1
Skin rash	10	3.9
Wound or ulcer	25	9.8
Bronchial breathing	9	3.5
Crackles	73	28.6
Rhonchi	15	5.9
Temperature ≥ 37.5 °C	54	21.2
Pulse > 100 beats/min	116	45.5
Systolic blood pressure ≤ 100 mmHg	51	20.0
Respiratory rate ≥ 22 breaths/min	70	27.7
Glasgow Coma Scale (GCS)		
>13	204	80.0
≤13	51	20.0
Quick Sequential Organ Failure Assessment (q SOFA) score		
0	127	49.8
1	92	36.1
2–3	36	14.1

$ Pallor (Mild/Moderate 81, Severe 20).

Prevalence of Ceftriaxone Use

Out of 255 study participants, 129 [(50.6%), 95% CI: 44.4–56.7%] were prescribed ceftriaxone. Of these, 40 (31.0%) were prescribed for pneumonia, 38 (29.5%) for sepsis, 14 (10.9%) for gastroenteritis, and 14 (10.9%) for urinary tract infection.

3.3. *Prescribed Antibiotics and Indications*

The most commonly prescribed antibiotics were ceftriaxone and Levofloxacin (see Table 2). Seven patients received meropenem. Of the 255 participants, 71 (27.8%) received a combination of 2 antibiotics. Ceftriaxone and metronidazole, 20 (28.2%), ceftriaxone and azithromycin, 9 (12.7%), and levofloxacin and azithromycin, 6 (8.5%) were the commonest combinations. Two participants received a combination of ceftriaxone, metronidazole, and levofloxacin. Overall, broad-spectrum antibiotic prescriptions accounted for 216 (84.7%) of all prescriptions. Pneumonia and sepsis were the most common indications for antibiotic use (see Table 2).

Table 2. Prescribed antibiotics and indications for antibiotic use.

	Frequency (N = 255) (n)	Percentage (%)
Antibiotics		
Ceftriaxone	129	50.6
Levofloxacin	65	25.5
Metronidazole	41	16.1
Azithromycin	27	10.6
Piperacillin-tazobactam	16	6.3
Amoxicillin/clavulanic acid	16	6.3
Gentamycin	6	2.4
Others *	28	11.0
Indication		
Pneumonia	74	29.0
Sepsis	72	28.3
UTI	37	14.5
Gastroenteritis	33	12.9
Medical prophylaxis **	16	6.3
Others ***	23	9.0

* Cefuroxime (5), Meropenem (5), Flucamox (4) Septrin (3), Ciprofloxacin (2), Imipenem (2) Salbactam (2), Ampiclox (1), Cefazolin (1), Cefixime (1), Cefpodoxime (1) Erythromycin (1). ** Refers to conditions where antibiotics were prescribed without clinical and/or laboratory evidence of infection for example liver cirrhosis complicated by ascites to prevent development of spontaneous bacterial peritonitis. *** CNS infection (5), Cellulitis (5), Sinusitis (2), Tonsillitis (2), PID (1), Abscess (1), Cholecystitis (1), Conjunctivitis (1), Empyema (1), Oral Abscess (1), Pharyngitis (1), Rhino sinusitis (1), and Septic arthritis (1).

3.4. Indications for Commonly Prescribed Antibiotics

Ceftriaxone was commonly prescribed for pneumonia (40/129, 31%) and sepsis (38/129, 29.5%). Levofloxacin was commonly prescribed for sepsis (19/65, 29.2%) and UTI (17/65, 26.2%). Metronidazole was prescribed commonly for gastroenteritis (17/41, 41.5%).

3.5. Factors Associated with Ceftriaxone Prescription

Bivariate and multivariate analyses were performed to identify factors associated with ceftriaxone prescription. Significant factors at bivariate analysis were: sex, dysuria, skin rash, UTI indication, medical prophylactic indication, and HIV disease. Factors significantly associated with ceftriaxone prescription included dysuria and medical prophylactic indication (see Table 3).

Table 3. Multivariate logistic analysis for factors associated with ceftriaxone prescription.

	Adjusted Odds Ratio	(95% Confidence Interval)	*p*-Value
Sex			
Male	1		
Female	0.668	(0.39–1.14)	0.145
History of pain on passing urine			
No	1		
Yes	0.233	(0.07–0.77)	**0.017** *
Indication			
Sepsis	1		
Pneumonia	1.079	(0.55–2.11)	0.825
UTI	0.989	(0.40–2.44)	0.982
GIT Infection	0.670	(0.29–1.61)	0.391
Medical prophylaxis	7.171	(1.36–37.83)	**0.020** *
Others	0.588	(0.22–1.59)	0.296

Table 3. *Cont.*

		Adjusted Odds Ratio	(95% Confidence Interval)	*p*-Value
HIV				
	No	1		
	Yes	1.792	(0.81–3.97)	0.150
Skin Rash				
	No	1		
	Yes	4.671	(0.53–41.22)	0.165

* Statistically significant at 5% level of significance.

4. Discussion

This study was carried out to investigate the prevalence of antibiotic prescription among medical inpatients in a tertiary care private not-for-profit hospital in Kampala, Uganda. The most commonly prescribed antibiotics were ceftriaxone (50.6%), levofloxacin (25.5%), metronidazole (16.1%), azithromycin (10.6%), and piperacillin-tazobactam (6.3%). This is comparable to what has been reported from studies done in public healthcare facilities in Uganda. For instance, a study done at Mulago national referral hospital reported prescription rates of 16% and 6% for metronidazole and azithromycin, respectively [5]. Similar results have also been reported in Tanzania [15], Ethiopia [16], and Egypt [17]. Studies investigating antibiotic prescription patterns in public healthcare facilities in Uganda have reported prescription rates for ciprofloxacin at 10.2% [18] and 19% [5]. A higher levofloxacin prescription rate in this study could likely be attributed to a change in antimicrobial susceptibility patterns. Ceftriaxone, metronidazole, azithromycin, and piperacillin-tazobactam are all listed on the 21st WHO model list of essential medicines 2019 [19] and the ministry of health essential medicines list for Uganda 2016 [20], tools designed to facilitate the appropriate use of antibiotics. Thus, the antibiotic prescription culture at Mengo Hospital is fairly adherent to international and local recommendations. Importantly, levofloxacin, the second most commonly prescribed antibiotic in this study is not listed on these lists. This highlights the need for an antibiotic prescription guideline at this facility in accordance with national and international guidelines to reduce irrational use of levofloxacin, a WHO Watch category antibiotic.

In this study, the indications for antibiotic use were pneumonia (29%), sepsis (28.2%), urinary tract infection (UTI) (14.5%), gastroenteritis (13%), and central nervous system (CNS) infection (2%). Pneumonia was the most common indication for antibiotic use in this study probably because a significant proportion (46.7%) of our study participants were over 60 years and therefore more predisposed to pneumonia [21]. Urinary tract infections are also common in this age group [22]. Our findings are in agreement with what has been reported in other studies [4,16,23,24]. A report by the Uganda National Academy of Sciences on antibiotic resistance in Uganda showed that pneumonia, septicemia, acute diarrhea, and urinary tract infections were the leading bacterial infections among hospitalized patients in Uganda [24]. Another retrospective study investigating the trends of admissions and case fatality rates among medical in-patients at a tertiary hospital in Uganda showed that pneumonia, sepsis, and gastroenteritis were among the leading causes of admissions to the infectious disease wards for a period between January 2011 and December 2014 [23]. Our findings are consistent with findings from studies done in Tanzania [15], Ethiopia [2,16], Eriteria [25], the Netherlands [26], and the US [27,28].

One in every two patients admitted to the medical ward of Mengo Hospital were prescribed ceftriaxone. This is a high prescription rate of ceftriaxone given that it belongs to the watch WHO group of antibiotics that have a high resistance potential and should not be prescribed routinely [29].Ceftriaxone is among the most commonly utilized antibiotics owing to its high potency, a wide spectrum of activity, and a low risk of toxicity [2]. It is used to treat different types of bacterial infections including pneumonia, abdominal, skin and soft tissue, and urinary tract infections [30]. It has the advantage of wide coverage of pathogens, easy administration as it is once-daily dosing–limiting the nursing time needed and a low cost compared with many other antibiotics [31,32]. This probably explains its high prescription rate in this study.

Not surprisingly, studies done in other public healthcare facilities in Uganda have shown a relatively high extent of ceftriaxone prescription; for instance, in a study from a tertiary care hospital in Kampala, the ceftriaxone prescription rate was 43% [7] and 66% [5]. Similar studies done in public healthcare facilities in other parts of Uganda such as Mbarara [33], and Bwindi [6] have reported relatively high ceftriaxone prescription rates of 77.7% and 45%, respectively. Similarly, studies were done in private healthcare facilities in Ethiopia—49% [34], Pakistan—46% [35], and Bangladesh—50% [36]; countries with social and economic indicators of development similar to those of Uganda [37] have also reported a relatively high ceftriaxone prescription rate.

Thus, generally, the observed ceftriaxone use in the present study is irrationally high as this drug should only be used in confirmed severe infections. Overuse of ceftriaxone contributes to antibiotic resistance [38]. To reduce ceftriaxone use and mitigate the rapid development of AMR, hospital antimicrobial stewardship programs should impose and enforce prescription restrictions, set up antibiotic consumption surveillance systems, and deliver appropriate education campaigns to prescribers. Stewardship will increase knowledge on resistance patterns to secure other low-spectrum antibiotics that can still be effectively used. Notably, there is no available published data on resistance rates of bacteria to ceftriaxone at Mengo Hospital. However, studies done in other public healthcare facilities in Uganda have reported resistance rates of 64–66% for *Escherichia coli* [9,10] and 85–100% for Klebsiella pneumoniae [9,10]. It is likely that the resistance rates of bacteria to ceftriaxone at Mengo Hospital are similarly high.

We further investigated factors that may influence ceftriaxone prescription. Factors that were significantly associated with ceftriaxone use included a history of pain on passing urine (dysuria) and medical prophylactic indication. Attending clinicians were 76% less likely to prescribe ceftriaxone to patients with dysuria compared with those with no dysuria. It is not surprising that participants with dysuria were less likely to be prescribed ceftriaxone by the attending clinicians. Dysuria is a well-recognized symptom of urinary tract infections [39]. International [40] and local [41] guidelines recommend nitrofurantoin monohydrate and fluoroquinolones as the first line in the treatment of both uncomplicated and complicated urinary tract infections (acute pyelonephritis), respectively, in adults, and therefore it is likely that clinicians followed these guidelines. Clinicians were seven times more likely to prescribe ceftriaxone for medical prophylaxis compared with sepsis. In our study, medical prophylaxis referred to conditions where antibiotics were prescribed without clinical and/or laboratory evidence of infection for example ceftriaxone prescribed for patients with liver cirrhosis complicated by ascites without evidence of infection to prevent development of spontaneous bacterial peritonitis or antibiotics prescribed for patients with diabetes mellitus and hyperglycemia but no evidence of infection. This implies that whenever clinicians assess patients and find no evidence of infection, they are likely to prescribe ceftriaxone for prophylaxis. This is probably because it is a broad-spectrum antibiotic with activity against a wide range of pathogens. Moreover, qualitative studies done in other healthcare facilities revealed that sometimes clinicians prescribe antibiotics for fear of bad outcomes [42–44]. It is therefore likely that ceftriaxone prescribed for medical prophylaxis was unnecessary. Notably, prophylactic use of antibiotics is a potential driver of antimicrobial resistance [45–48] which is associated with adverse outcomes. This highlights the importance of having a local prescription guideline and whenever appropriate the need to wait for laboratory results before choosing the best antimicrobial therapy.

A strength of this study is that data were collected from a private tertiary care facility, and it could be one of the first studies investigating ceftriaxone prescription in such a setting. This could imply and depict the real practice in many private tertiary hospitals in Uganda. Therefore, our paper presents data from an area and setting of the world with limited available data. We believe it adds valuable information to antibiotic prescribing and stewardship in private healthcare facilities in low-income countries. Results from this study were presented to clinicians and stakeholders at Mengo Hospital and an antimicrobial stewardship committee was set up to promote appropriate antibiotic use at Mengo Hospital.

However, we acknowledge the inherent weaknesses of this study in that first, the prescriptions were strictly based on the physicians' clinical acumen. Second, there are other factors we could not investigate such as influence from pharmaceutical and health insurance companies. It would be important to explore the contribution of these factors toward excessive use of antibiotics in private tertiary healthcare facilities in Uganda. Additionally, this was a single site study and therefore more data may need to be collected from other sites before generalizing the results.

5. Conclusions

Prevalence of ceftriaxone prescription was high in this hospital, mainly for pneumonia and sepsis. We recommend an ASP to monitor antibiotic prescription and sensitivity patterns in a bid to curb AMR.

Author Contributions: The study concept and design were by M.K., H.K., R.L. and P.B.-K., M.K. and D.M. collected the data. M.K. and R.S. analyzed the data. All authors have read and agreed to the published version of the manuscript.

Funding: This study was funded through a grant from Merck KGAA to the Merck-Makerere College of Health Sciences Antimicrobial Research Program.

Institutional Review Board Statement: The study was conducted according to the guidelines of the Declaration of Helsinki, and approved by the Institutional Review Board (or Ethics Committee) of SCHOOL OF MEDICINE RESEARCH AND ETHICS COMMITTEE (protocol code REC REF 2019-081 and date of approval 9 May 2019).

Informed Consent Statement: Informed consent was obtained from all subjects involved in the study.

Data Availability Statement: The datasets used and/or analyzed during the current study are available from the corresponding author on reasonable request.

Acknowledgments: We are indebted to the staff and patients of the medical ward of Mengo Hospital who participated in the study. We thank Moses Grace Kintu for his assistance in data collection.

Conflicts of Interest: The authors declare no conflict of interest.

Abbreviations

AMR	Antimicrobial resistance
ASP	Antibiotic Stewardship Program
BSI	Bloodstream infections
CDC	Centers for Disease Control and Prevention
C. difficile	*Clostridium difficile*
ESBL	Extended spectrum beta-lactamase
IV	Intravenous
GIT	Gastrointestinal
MRSA	Methicillin-resistant Staphylococcus aureus
USA	United States of America
UTI	Urinary tract infection
VRE	Vancomycin-resistant Enterococci
WHO	World Health Organization

References

1. Katzung, B.G. *Basic and Clinical Pharmacology*, 14th ed.; McGraw Hill Professional: New York, NY, USA, 2017.
2. Ayele, A.A.; Gebresillassie, B.M.; Erku, D.A.; Gebreyohannes, E.A.; Demssie, D.G.; Mersha, A.G.; Tegegn, H.G. Prospective evaluation of Ceftriaxone use in medical and emergency wards of Gondar university referral hospital, Ethiopia. *Pharmacol. Res. Perspect.* **2018**, *6*, e00383. [CrossRef] [PubMed]
3. Sileshi, A.; Tenna, A.; Feyissa, M.; Shibeshi, W. Evaluation of ceftriaxone utilization in medical and emergency wards of Tikur Anbessa specialized hospital: A prospective cross-sectional study. *BMC Pharmacol. Toxicol.* **2016**, *17*, 7. [CrossRef] [PubMed]
4. Sonda, T.B.; Horumpende, P.G.; Kumburu, H.H.; van Zwetselaar, M.; Mshana, S.E.; Alifrangis, M.; Lund, O.; Aarestrup, F.M.; Chilongola, J.O.; Mmbaga, B.T.; et al. Ceftriaxone use in a tertiary care hospital in Kilimanjaro, Tanzania: A need for a hospital antibiotic stewardship programme. *PLoS ONE* **2019**, *14*, e0220261. [CrossRef] [PubMed]
5. Kiguba, R.; Karamagi, C.; Bird, S.M. Extensive antibiotic prescription rate among hospitalized patients in Uganda: But with frequent missed-dose days. *J. Antimicrob. Chemother.* **2016**, *71*, 1697–1706. [CrossRef]
6. Rudd, K.E.; Tutaryebwa, L.K.; West, T.E. Presentation, management, and outcomes of sepsis in adults and children admitted to a rural Ugandan hospital: A prospective observational cohort study. *PLoS ONE* **2017**, *12*, e0171422. [CrossRef] [PubMed]
7. Kiguba, R.; Karamagi, C.; Bird, S.M. Antibiotic—Associated suspected adverse drug reactions among hospitalized patients in Uganda: A prospective cohort study. *Pharmacol. Res. Perspect.* **2017**, *5*, e00298. [CrossRef]
8. Ampaire, L.; Muhindo, A.; Orikiriza, P.; Mwanga-Amumpaire, J.; Bebell, L.; Boum, Y. A review of antimicrobial resistance in East Africa. *Afr. J. Lab. Med.* **2016**, *5*, 432. [CrossRef]
9. Kajumbula, H.; Fujita, A.W.; Mbabazi, O.; Najjuka, C.; Izale, C.; Akampurira, A.; Aisu, S.; Lamorde, M.; Walwema, R.; Bahr, N.C.; et al. Antimicrobial drug resistance in blood culture isolates at a tertiary hospital, Uganda. *Emerg. Infect. Dis.* **2018**, *24*, 174–175. [CrossRef]
10. Lubwama, M.; Phipps, W.; Najjuka, C.F.; Kajumbula, H.; Ddungu, H.; Kambugu, J.B.; Bwanga, F. Bacteremia in febrile cancer patients in Uganda. *BMC Res. Notes* **2019**, *12*, 464. [CrossRef] [PubMed]
11. World Health Organization. *Antimicrobial Resistance Global Report on Surveillance: 2014 Summary*; World Health Organization: Geneva, Switzerland, 2014.
12. Robertson, M.B.; Dartnell, J.G.; Korman, T.M.; Ioannides-Demos, L.L.; Kirsa, S.W.; Lord, J.A.; Munafo, L.; Byrnes, G.B. Ceftriaxone and cefotaxime use in Victorian hospitals. *Med. J. Aust.* **2002**, *176*, 524–529. [CrossRef]
13. De Costa, A.; Diwan, V. 'Where is the public health sector?': Public and private sector healthcare provision in Madhya Pradesh, India. *Health Policy* **2007**, *84*, 269–276. [CrossRef] [PubMed]
14. Ministry of Health Uganda (Ed.) *Annual Health Sector Performance Report 2015/2016*; Ministry of Health Uganda: Kampala, Uganda, 2016.
15. Lyamuya, F.; Sheng, T.; Mallya, R.; Uronu, T.S.; Minde, R.M.; Anderson, D.J.; Woods, C.W.; Mmbaga, B.T.; Tillekeratne, L.G. 2029. Prevalence of Antibiotic Use and Administration among Hospitalized Adult Patients at a Tertiary Care Hospital in Kilimanjaro, Tanzania. *Open Forum Infect. Dis.* **2019**, *6*, S681–S682. [CrossRef]
16. Gutema, G.; Håkonsen, H.; Engidawork, E.; Toverud, E.-L. Multiple challenges of antibiotic use in a large hospital in Ethiopia–a ward-specific study showing high rates of hospital-acquired infections and ineffective prophylaxis. *BMC Health Serv. Res.* **2018**, *18*, 326. [CrossRef] [PubMed]
17. Talaat, M.; Saied, T.; Kandeel, A.; El-Ata, G.A.A.; El-Kholy, A.; Hafez, S.; Osman, A.; Razik, M.A.; Ismail, G.; El-Masry, S.; et al. A Point Prevalence Survey of Antibiotic Use in 18 Hospitals in Egypt. *Antibiotics* **2014**, *3*, 450–460. [CrossRef]
18. Mukonzo, J.K.; Namuwenge, P.M.; Okure, G.; Mwesige, B.; Namusisi, O.K.; Mukanga, D. Over-the-counter suboptimal dispensing of antibiotics in Uganda. *J. Multidiscip. Healthc.* **2013**, *6*, 303–310. [PubMed]
19. WHO. *World Health Organization Model List of Essential Medicines: 21st List 2019*; World Health Organization: Geneva, Switzerland, 2019.
20. Ministry of Health Uganda. *Essential Medicines and Health Supplies List for Uganda (EMHSLU)*; December 2016 ed.; Pharmacy, Ed.; Ministry of Health Uganda: Kampala, Uganda, 2016.
21. Henig, O.; Kaye, K.S. Bacterial pneumonia in older adults. *Infect. Dis. Clin.* **2017**, *31*, 689–713. [CrossRef]
22. Detweiler, K.; Mayers, D.; Fletcher, S.G. Bacteruria and urinary tract infections in the elderly. *Urol. Clin.* **2015**, *42*, 561–568. [CrossRef] [PubMed]
23. Kalyesubula, R.; Mutyaba, I.; Rabin, T.; Andia-Biraro, I.; Alupo, P.; Kimuli, I.; Nabirye, S.; Kagimu, M.; Mayanja-Kizza, H.; Rastegar, A.; et al. Trends of admissions and case fatality rates among medical in-patients at a tertiary hospital in Uganda; A four-year retrospective study. *PLoS ONE* **2019**, *14*, e0216060. [CrossRef]
24. UNAS. *Antibiotic Resistance in Uganda: Situation Analysis and Recommendations*; Uganda National Academy of Sciences; Center for Disease Dynamics, Economics & Policy: Kampala, Uganda, 2015; p. 107.
25. Berhe, Y.H.; Amaha, N.D.; Ghebrenegus, A.S. Evaluation of ceftriaxone use in the medical ward of Halibet National Referral and teaching hospital in 2017 in Asmara, Eritrea. A cross sectional retrospective study. *BMC Infect. Dis.* **2019**, *19*, 465. [CrossRef]
26. Aabenhus, R.; Hansen, M.P.; Siersma, V.; Bjerrum, L. Clinical indications for antibiotic use in Danish general practice: Results from a nationwide electronic prescription database. *Scand. J. Prim. Health Care* **2017**, *35*, 162–169. [CrossRef]
27. Fridkin, S.; Baggs, J.; Fagan, R.; Magill, S.; Pollack, L.A.; Malpiedi, P.; Slayton, R.; Khader, K.; Rubin, M.A.; Jones, M.; et al. Vital signs: Improving antibiotic use among hospitalized patients. *Morb. Mortal. Wkly. Rep.* **2014**, *63*, 194–200.

28. Kelesidis, T.; Braykov, N.; Uslan, D.Z.; Morgan, D.J.; Gandra, S.; Johannsson, B.; Schweizer, M.L.; Weisenberg, S.A.; Young, H.; Cantey, J.; et al. Indications and types of antibiotic agents used in 6 acute care hospitals, 2009–2010: A pragmatic retrospective observational study. *Infect. Control. Hosp. Epidemiol.* **2016**, *37*, 70–79. [CrossRef] [PubMed]
29. Klein, E.Y.; Milkowska-Shibata, M.; Tseng, K.K.; Sharland, M.; Gandra, S.; Pulcini, C.; Laxminarayan, R. Assessment of WHO antibiotic consumption and access targets in 76 countries, 2000–2015: An analysis of pharmaceutical sales data. *Lancet Infect. Dis.* **2021**, *21*, 107–115. [CrossRef]
30. Lee, H.; Jung, D.; Yeom, J.S.; Son, J.S.; Jung, S.-I.; Kim, Y.-S.; Kim, C.K.; Chang, H.-H.; Kim, S.-W.; Ki, H.K.; et al. Evaluation of ceftriaxone utilization at multicenter study. *Korean J. Intern. Med.* **2009**, *24*, 374. [CrossRef] [PubMed]
31. Lin, H.-A.; Yang, Y.-S.; Wang, J.-X.; Lin, H.-C.; Lin, D.-Y.; Chiu, C.-H.; Yeh, K.-M.; Lin, J.-C.; Chang, F.-Y. Comparison of the effectiveness and antibiotic cost among ceftriaxone, ertapenem, and levofloxacin in treatment of community-acquired complicated urinary tract infections. *J. Microbiol. Immunol. Infect.* **2016**, *49*, 237–242. [CrossRef]
32. Hurst, A.L.; Olson, D.; Somme, S.; Child, J.; Pyle, L.; Ranade, D.; Stamatoiu, A.; Crombleholme, T.; Parker, S.K. Once-daily ceftriaxone plus metronidazole versus ertapenem and/or cefoxitin for pediatric appendicitis. *J. Pediatr. Infect. Dis. Soc.* **2017**, *6*, 57–64. [CrossRef]
33. Kemigisha, E.; Nanjebe, D.; Boum, Y.; Langendorf, C.; Aberrane, S.; Nyehangane, D.; Nackers, F.; Mueller, Y.; Charrel, R.; Murphy, R.A.; et al. Antimicrobial treatment practices among Ugandan children with suspicion of central nervous system infection. *PLoS ONE* **2018**, *13*, e0205316. [CrossRef]
34. Shimels, T.; Bilal, A.I.; Mulugeta, A. Evaluation of ceftriaxone utilization in internal medicine wards of general hospitals in Addis Ababa, Ethiopia: A comparative retrospective study. *J. Pharm. Policy Pract.* **2015**, *8*, 26. [CrossRef]
35. Saleem, Z.; Saeed, H.; Hassali, M.A.; Godman, B.; Asif, U.; Yousaf, M.; Ahmed, Z.; Riaz, H.; Raza, S.A. Pattern of inappropriate antibiotic use among hospitalized patients in Pakistan: A longitudinal surveillance and implications. *Antimicrob. Resist. Infect. Control.* **2019**, *8*, 188. [CrossRef]
36. Rashid, M.M.; Chisti, M.J.; Akter, D.; Sarkar, M.; Chowdhury, F. Antibiotic use for pneumonia among children under-five at a pediatric hospital in Dhaka city, Bangladesh. *Patient Prefer. Adherence* **2017**, *11*, 1335–1342. [CrossRef]
37. Dalevska, N.; Khobta, V.; Kwilinski, A.; Kravchenko, S. A model for estimating social and economic indicators of sustainable development. *Entrep. Sustain. Issues* **2019**, *6*, 1839–1860. [CrossRef]
38. Srinivasan, A. *Antibiotic Stewardship Grows Up*; Elsevier: Amsterdam, The Netherlands, 2018.
39. Cortes-Penfield, N.W.; Trautner, B.W.; Jump, R.L. Urinary tract infection and asymptomatic bacteriuria in older adults. *Infect. Dis. Clin.* **2017**, *31*, 673–688. [CrossRef] [PubMed]
40. Gupta, K.; Hooton, T.M.; Naber, K.G.; Wullt, B.; Colgan, R.; Miller, L.G.; Moran, G.J.; Nicolle, L.E.; Raz, R.; Schaeffer, A.J.; et al. International Clinical Practice Guidelines for the Treatment of Acute Uncomplicated Cystitis and Pyelonephritis in Women: A 2010 Update by the Infectious Diseases Society of America and the European Society for Microbiology and Infectious Diseases. *Clin. Infect. Dis.* **2011**, *52*, e103–e120. [CrossRef]
41. Ministry of Health Uganda. *Uganda Clinical Guidelines 2016*; Ministry of Health Uganda: Kampala, Uganda, 2016.
42. Md Rezal, R.S.; Hassali, M.A.; Alrasheedy, A.A.; Saleem, F.; Md Yusof, F.A.; Godman, B. Physicians' knowledge, perceptions and behaviour towards antibiotic prescribing: A systematic review of the literature. *Expert Rev. Anti-Infect. Ther.* **2015**, *13*, 665–680. [CrossRef] [PubMed]
43. O'Doherty, J.; Leader, L.F.; O'Regan, A.; Dunne, C.; Puthoopparambil, S.J.; O'Connor, R. Over prescribing of antibiotics for acute respiratory tract infections; a qualitative study to explore Irish general practitioners' perspectives. *BMC Fam. Pract.* **2019**, *20*, 27. [CrossRef]
44. Yantzi, R.; van de Walle, G.; Lin, J. 'The disease isn't listening to the drug': The socio-cultural context of antibiotic use for viral respiratory infections in rural Uganda. *Glob. Public Health* **2019**, *14*, 750–763. [CrossRef]
45. Selekman, R.E.; Shapiro, D.J.; Boscardin, J.; Williams, G.; Craig, J.C.; Brandström, P.; Pennesi, M.; Roussey-Kesler, G.; Hari, P.; Copp, H.L. Uropathogen resistance and antibiotic prophylaxis: A meta-analysis. *Pediatrics* **2018**, *142*, e20180119. [CrossRef]
46. Roldan-Masedo, E.; Sainz, T.; Gutierrez-Arroyo, A.; Gomez-Gil, R.M.; Ballesteros, E.; Escosa, L.; Baquero-Artigao, F.; Méndez-Echevarría, A. Risk factors for gentamicin-resistant E. coli in children with community-acquired urinary tract infection. *Eur. J. Clin. Microbiol. Infect. Dis.* **2019**, *38*, 2097–2102. [CrossRef] [PubMed]
47. Nisha, K.V.; Veena, S.A.; Rathika, S.D.; Vijaya, S.M.; Avinash, S.K. Antimicrobial susceptibility, risk factors and prevalence of bla cefotaximase, temoneira, and sulfhydryl variable genes among Escherichia coli in community-acquired pediatric urinary tract infection. *J. Lab. Physicians* **2017**, *9*, 156–162. [CrossRef]
48. Nieminen, O.; Korppi, M.; Helminen, M. Healthcare costs doubled when children had urinary tract infections caused by extended—Spectrumβ—Lactamase—Producing bacteria. *Acta Paediatr.* **2017**, *106*, 327–333. [CrossRef]

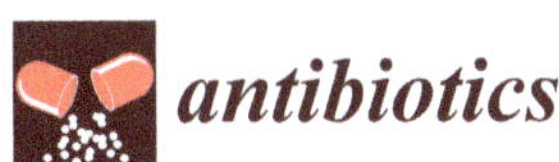

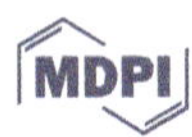

Article

Point Prevalence Survey of Antibiotic Use across 13 Hospitals in Uganda

Reuben Kiggundu [1,*], Rachel Wittenauer [2], JP Waswa [1], Hilma N. Nakambale [3], Freddy Eric Kitutu [4], Marion Murungi [1], Neville Okuna [5], Seru Morries [5], Lynn Lieberman Lawry [6], Mohan P. Joshi [7], Andy Stergachis [2,3] and Niranjan Konduri [7]

1 USAID Medicines, Technologies, and Pharmaceutical Services (MTaPS) Program, Management Sciences for Health (MSH), Kampala P.O. Box 920102, Uganda; jpwaswa@msh.org (J.W.); mmurungi@msh.org (M.M.)
2 School of Pharmacy, University of Washington, Seattle, WA 98105, USA; rwitten1@uw.edu (R.W.); stergach@uw.edu (A.S.)
3 Department of Global Health, University of Washington, Seattle, WA 98105, USA; hilman2@uw.edu
4 Sustainable Pharmaceutical Systems (SPS) Unit, Pharmacy Department, Makerere University School of Health Sciences, Kampala P.O. Box 10217, Uganda; kitutufred@gmail.com
5 Department of Pharmaceuticals and Natural Medicines, Ministry of Health, Kampala P.O. Box 7272, Uganda; nokuna6@gmail.com (N.O.); serumorries@gmail.com (S.M.)
6 Overseas Strategic Consulting, Ltd., Philadelphia, PA 19102, USA; llawry@oscltd.com
7 USAID Medicines, Technologies, and Pharmaceutical Services (MTaPS) Program, Management Sciences for Health (MSH), Arlington, VA 22203, USA; mjoshi@msh.org (M.P.J.); nkonduri@msh.org (N.K.)
* Correspondence: rkiggundu@msh.org

Abstract: Standardized monitoring of antibiotic use underpins the effective implementation of antimicrobial stewardship interventions in combatting antimicrobial resistance (AMR). To date, few studies have assessed antibiotic use in hospitals in Uganda to identify gaps that require intervention. This study applied the World Health Organization's standardized point prevalence survey methodology to assess antibiotic use in 13 public and private not-for-profit hospitals across the country. Data for 1077 patients and 1387 prescriptions were collected between December 2020 and April 2021 and analyzed to understand the characteristics of antibiotic use and the prevalence of the types of antibiotics to assess compliance with Uganda Clinical Guidelines; and classify antibiotics according to the WHO Access, Watch, and Reserve classification. This study found that 74% of patients were on one or more antibiotics. Compliance with Uganda Clinical Guidelines was low (30%); Watch-classified antibiotics were used to a high degree (44% of prescriptions), mainly driven by the wide use of ceftriaxone, which was the most frequently used antibiotic (37% of prescriptions). The results of this study identify key areas for the improvement of antimicrobial stewardship in Uganda and are important benchmarks for future evaluations.

Keywords: point prevalence survey; antimicrobial stewardship; antibiotic use surveillance; antimicrobials; Uganda; hospital; private sector; global health security

check for updates

Citation: Kiggundu, R.; Wittenauer, R.; Waswa, J.; Nakambale, H.N.; Kitutu, F.E.; Murungi, M.; Okuna, N.; Morries, S.; Lawry, L.L.; Joshi, M.P.; et al. Point Prevalence Survey of Antibiotic Use across 13 Hospitals in Uganda. *Antibiotics* **2022**, *11*, 199. https://doi.org/10.3390/antibiotics11020199

Academic Editor: Diane Ashiru-Oredope

Received: 21 December 2021
Accepted: 27 January 2022
Published: 4 February 2022

Publisher's Note: MDPI stays neutral with regard to jurisdictional claims in published maps and institutional affiliations.

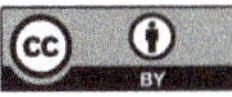

Copyright: © 2022 by the authors. Licensee MDPI, Basel, Switzerland. This article is an open access article distributed under the terms and conditions of the Creative Commons Attribution (CC BY) license (https://creativecommons.org/licenses/by/4.0/).

1. Introduction

Antimicrobial resistance (AMR) is a threat to global health and sustainable development, with adverse health and economic consequences, unless evidence-based efforts are implemented to control its emergence and spread [1,2]. The health and social consequences of AMR include increased morbidity and mortality, increased health care costs, and a projected negative impact on economic growth [3]. More than 700,000 people die annually from AMR, which is estimated to increase to 10 million annually by 2050 if decisive actions are not taken [4]. The potential exacerbating effects of the COVID-19 pandemic on the rise and spread of antimicrobial resistance have increased the urgency to address this problem [5–8]. AMR threatens the effective prevention and treatment of infections and undermines health gains globally as antimicrobials become less effective [9].

Numerous factors contribute to the emergence of AMR [10–12]. Among these factors is the irrational use of antibiotics in health care facilities. A 2015 situational analysis in Uganda showed a high prevalence of AMR to commonly used antibiotics [13]. Recent studies have also demonstrated the high prevalence of multidrug-resistant bacteria in Ugandan hospitals [14]. Further, pharmacokinetic and pharmacodynamic sex-based differences, in addition to gender roles, put females at higher risk of AMR [15]. As part of global efforts to contain AMR, the World Health Organization's (WHO) Global Action Plan on AMR lists five strategic objectives for member countries to adopt and implement. A key aspect of the Global Action Plan is the surveillance of antibiotic use and consumption [16]. Recognizing the importance of antibiotic use surveillance, the Uganda National Action Plan on AMR (2018–2023) includes a strategic objective on surveillance of antibiotic use and consumption [17]. However, a key barrier to implementing this National Action Plan is the lack of current data and surveillance processes to monitor antibiotic use throughout the country, particularly within health facilities. To further strengthen antibiotic use surveillance at health facilities in resource-constrained countries, the WHO developed a standardized point prevalence survey (PPS) template and an associated package of tools which permit uniform collection and comparison of data within and among countries [18].

Recent efforts to measure antibiotic use in sub-Saharan African hospitals have been documented [19–22]. However, there are limited studies that utilize the standardized WHO PPS methodology for resource-limited settings, such as Ugandan hospitals [23–25]. This paper presents data from 13 hospitals in the context of a global health security agenda project for strengthening antimicrobial stewardship programs in low- and middle-income countries. This study was conducted as part of ongoing quality improvement approaches and efforts to build capacity for monitoring antibiotic use in health facilities, with a long-term goal of linkage to each hospital's AMR containment program as well as national efforts to combat AMR [26,27]. These hospitals are depicted in Figure 1.

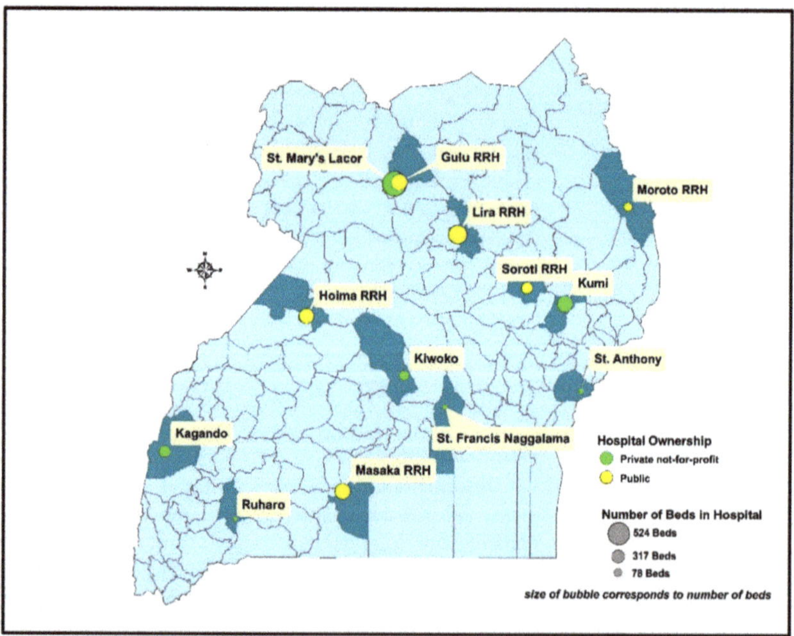

Figure 1. Geographic location of study sites and number of hospital beds.

2. Results

Across the 13 included hospitals, de-identified data for 1077 patients was collected for analysis (Table 1). Of those patients, 609 (56.5%) were female, and the median age was 27 years old (IQR 10–38 years old). Patients were similarly distributed between maternal (28.8%), medical (22.2%), pediatric (22.5%), and surgical (26.3%) wards. Among all patients, at the time of data collection, 97.3% had a peripheral catheter present, 5.6% had a urinary catheter present, 0.5% were intubated, and 0.3% had a central catheter present. In terms of underlying health conditions of the included patients, at the time of data collection, 10.9% had malaria, 4.8% were malnourished, 4.3% were living with HIV, and 1.9% had tuberculosis. Approximately 66% of the included patients were in public hospitals and 34% were in private not-for-profit hospitals. Additional demographic and clinical characteristics of patients are summarized in Table 1 and the hospital characteristics are presented in Figure 1 and Supplementary Table S1.

Table 1. Demographic and clinical characteristics of enrolled patients (n = 1077).

Variable	Number (Proportion) (n = 1077)
Demographics	
Female	609 (56.5%)
Male	468 (43.5%)
Age [a]	27 (10–38)
Hospital ownership	
Public	706 (65.5%)
Private not-for-profit	371 (34.4%)
Hospital	
Gulu RRH	133 (12.3%)
Hoima RRH	103 (9.6%)
Kagando	61 (5.7%)
Kiwoko	43 (4%)
Kumi	47 (4.4%)
Lacor	168 (15.6%)
Lira RRH	119 (11%)
Masaka RRH	127 (11.8%)
Moroto RRH	99 (9.2%)
Ruharo Mission	6 (0.6%)
Soroti RRH	125 (11.6%)
St. Anthony	12 (1.1%)
St. Francis Naggalama	34 (3.2%)
Ward	
Maternal	311 (28.8%)
Medical	239 (22.2%)
Pediatric	243 (22.5%)
Surgical	284 (26.3%)

Table 1. *Cont.*

Variable	Number (Proportion) (n = 1077)
Underlying patient condition	
Central catheter	3 (0.3%)
Peripheral catheter	1049 (97.3%)
Urinary catheter	60 (5.6%)
Intubation	5 (0.5%)
Malaria	118 (10.9%)
Tuberculosis	20 (1.9%)
HIV	46 (4.3%)
COPD	12 (1.1%)
Malnutrition	52 (4.8%)

[a] Age in years expressed as median (interquartile range). Abbreviations: COPD = chronic obstructive pulmonary disease; HIV = human immunodeficiency virus; RRH = regional referral hospital.

2.1. Antibiotic Prevalence

Data were collected on 1387 antibiotics that were prescribed to patients in our study. Of these prescriptions, ceftriaxone was the most prescribed antibiotic (37%), followed by metronidazole (27%), gentamicin (7%), and ampicillin (6%) (Table 2).

Table 2. Prevalence of antibiotic use by indication.

Antibiotic	All Prescriptions (n = 1387)	Community Acquired Infection (n = 577)	Hospital Associated Infection (n = 87)	Medical Prophylaxis (n = 404)	Surgical Prophylaxis (n = 319)
Ceftriaxone	513	183 (35.7%)	21 (4.1%)	177 (34.5%)	132 (25.7%)
Metronidazole	380	121 (31.8%)	26 (6.8%)	98 (25.8%)	135 (35.5%)
Gentamicin	119	70 (58.8%)	12 (10.1%)	22 (18.5%)	15 (12.6%)
Ampicillin	89	55 (61.8%)	5 (5.6%)	27 (30.3%)	2 (2.2%)
Ampicillin-cloxacillin	79	31 (39.2%)	4 (5.1%)	31 (39.2%)	13 (16.5%)
Ciprofloxacin	45	25 (55.6%)	2 (4.4%)	15 (33.3%)	3 (6.7%)
Cloxacillin	27	17 (63%)	1 (3.7%)	5 (18.5%)	4 (14.8%)
Amoxicillin	26	12 (46.2%)	0 (0%)	10 (38.5%)	4 (15.4%)
Azithromycin	19	15 (78.9%)	0 (0%)	3 (15.8%)	1 (5.3%)
Penicillin	16	10 (62.5%)	T0 (0%)	5 (31.3%)	1 (6.3%)
Levofloxacin	15	10 (66.7%)	4 (26.7%)	1 (6.7%)	0 (0%)
Other [a]	59	28 (47.5%)	12 (20.3%)	10 (16.9%)	9 (15.3%)

[a] Other category includes the following antibiotics: nitrofurantoin (n = 10), cefotaxime (n = 7), flucamox (n = 7), cef-sulbactam (n = 5), cefixime (n = 4), meropenem (n = 4), piperacillin-tazobactam (n = 4), sulbactam (n = 4), co-trimoxazole (n = 3), erythromycin (n = 3), ceftazidime (n = 2), amoxyclav (n = 1), doxycycline (n = 1), secnidazole (n = 1), tinidazole (n = 1), clindamycin (n = 1), cefazolin (n = 1).

2.1.1. Prevalence by Indication

Among all the antibiotic prescriptions, the most common indication was for CAI (41.6%), followed by MP (29.1%), SP (23.0%), and HAI (6.3%) (Table 2). For all four indications, ceftriaxone and metronidazole were the two most prescribed antibiotics. For each antibiotic, the most common indication was CAI, except for metronidazole, which was most often prescribed for SP.

2.1.2. Prevalence by Diagnosis

Figure 2 summarizes the most prescribed antibiotic for each of the top five patient diagnoses within indications for CAI and HAI, which are the only two indication categories for which specific diagnosis data were collected. Among CAI indications, the most common diagnoses were clinical sepsis (20%), cellulitis, wound or deep soft tissue infection (19%), pneumonia (18%), gastrointestinal infections (13%), and symptomatic lower urinary tract infections (8%). Among HAI indications, the most common diagnoses were surgical site infections (41%), obstetric or gynecological infections (31%), cellulitis, wound or deep soft tissue infection (7%), intra-abdominal sepsis (7%), and pneumonia (5%). The three most frequently prescribed antibiotics for each of these five most common diagnoses in each indication are also summarized by antibiotic name and the WHO's Access, Watch and Reserve (AWaRE) classification in Figure 2.

Community Acquired Infections		Hospital Acquired Infections	
Diagnosis	**Top Three Prescribed Antibiotics & AWaRe[1]**	**Diagnosis**	**Top Three Prescribed Antibiotics & AWaRe[1]**
Clinical sepsis excluding febrile neutropenia (n=115)[2]	Ceftriaxone (37%)	**Surgical site infection involving skin or soft tissue but not bone** (n=36)	Ceftriaxone (28%)
	Gentamicin (22%)		Metronidazole (25%)
	Ampicillin (20%)		Gentamicin (17%)
Cellulitis, wound, deep soft tissue not involving bone, unrelated to surgery (n=108)[3]	Metronidazole (21%)	**Obstetric or gynaecological infect ions** (n=27)	Metronidazole (44%)
	Ceftriaxone (18%)		Ceftriaxone (22%)
	Ampicillin-cloxacillin (17%)		Gentamicin (7%)
Pneumonia (n=102)[4]	Ceftriaxone (32%)	**Cellulitis, wound, deep soft tissue not involving bone, unrelated to surgery** (n=6)	Gentamicin (33%)
	Gentamicin (22%)		Ampicillin (33%)
	Ampicillin (20%)		Cloxacillin (17%)
Gastrointestinal infections (n=78)[5]	Metronidazole (36%)	**Intraabdominal sepsis, including hepatobiliary** (n=6)	Metronidazole (50%)
	Ceftriaxone (33%)		Ceftriaxone (33%)
	Ciprofloxacin (10%)		Levofloxacin (17%)
Symptomatic lower urinary tract infection (n=44)[6]	Ceftriaxone (48%)	**Pneumonia** (n=4)	Cefixime (25%)
	Ampicillin (7%)		Ceftriaxone (25%)
	Nitrofurantonin (7%)		Gentamicin (25%)
Intraabdominal sepsis, including hepatobiliary (n=33)[7]	Metronidazole (52%)	**Clinical sepsis excluding febrile neutropenia** (n=3)	Gentamicin (33%)
	Ceftriaxone (30%)		Ampicillin (33%)
	Ampicillin-cloxacillin (9%)		Cefotaxime (33%)

Figure 2. Top three antibiotics prescribed for various diagnoses and their AWaRe classification. Notes: [1] WHO AWaRe classification for antibiotics: Access, Watch, Reserve, not classified. [2] First-line treatment recommendation from the Uganda Clinical Guidelines 2016: ampicillin and gentamicin. [3] First-line treatment recommendation: cloxacillin. [4] First-line treatment recommendation: ampicillin and gentamicin (for children < 5yrs) or benzylpenicillin (for older children and adults). [5] First-line treatment recommendation: ceftriaxone and metronidazole, gentamycin (optional). [6] First-line treatment recommendation: nitrofurantoin or ciprofloxacin. [7] First-line treatment recommendation: ampicillin, gentamicin, and metronidazole.

Indications for antibiotics were much more common for CAIs than HAIs. Clinical sepsis, cellulitis, pneumonia, and gastrointestinal infections were the most common CAI diagnoses for antibiotic use. Ceftriaxone and metronidazole are the most prescribed antibiotics at 37% and 27%, respectively.

2.1.3. Prevalence by Hospital

Prescribing patterns, in terms of antibiotic use prevalence, were similar across hospitals (Table 3). Among patients in 13 hospitals in Uganda, antibiotic use was common with 73.7% of patients receiving one or more antibiotics. Among hospitalized patients given an antibiotic, the mean number of antibiotics per patient ranged from 1.6 to 2.0 antibiotics per patient (Table 4). Public hospitals were significantly more likely to be associated with antibiotic use than private hospitals (OR 1.8, $p < 0.01$) (Table 5). Ceftriaxone and metronidazole were the two most prescribed antibiotics in all hospitals, except for Lacor hospital, where gentamicin and ampicillin were prescribed more frequently than ceftriaxone (Table 3). No patients were specifically treated based on antimicrobial susceptibility test laboratory results in any of the hospitals, as no hospitals in this sample regularly conducted sample collection or susceptibility testing as part of their surveillance activities.

Table 3. Prevalence of specific antibiotic use by hospital.

Antibiotic [a]	Total (n = 1387)	Public Hospitals (All Regional Referral Hospitals)						Private Not-for-Profit Hospitals						
		Gulu (n = 144)	Hoima (n = 151)	Lira (n = 170)	Masaka (n = 203)	Moroto (n = 111)	Soroti (n = 157)	Kagando (n = 90)	Kiwoko (n = 44)	Kumi (n = 77)	Lacor (n = 150)	Ruharo Mission (n = 10)	St. Anthony (n = 19)	St. Francis Nag-galama (n = 61)
Ceftriaxone	513	61	66	39	85	62	74	38	12	22	16	4	9	25
Metronidazole	380	43	53	52	62	14	47	28	10	16	33	3	6	13
Gentamicin	119	13	5	22	14	9	2	6	6	8	27	1	2	4
Ampicillin	89	5	2	11	14	6	5	5	5	6	28	0	0	2
Ampicillin-cloxacillin	79	8	7	19	9	11	8	6	0	3	1	0	1	6
Ciprofloxacin	45	6	5	8	4	3	4	1	0	2	11	0	0	1
Cloxacillin	27	0	2	0	0	0	0	0	4	0	20	0	0	1
Amoxicillin	26	6	4	4	1	0	0	4	6	0	1	0	0	0
Azithromycin	19	0	2	3	4	0	1	0	1	1	2	0	0	4
Penicillin	16	0	1	1	0	5	0	0	0	2	7	0	0	0
Levofloxacin	15	0	0	0	2	0	1	1	0	7	1	0	1	2
Other [b]	59	2	4	11	8	1	14	1	0	10	3	2	0	3

[a] Antibiotic AWaRe classification Access, Watch, Reserve, not classified. [b] Other category includes the following antibiotics: Nitrofurantoin (n = 10), cefotaxime (n = 7), flucamox (n = 7), cef-sulbactam (n = 5), cefixime (n = 4), meropenem (n = 4), piperacillin-tazobactam (n = 4), sulbactam (n = 4), co-trimoxazole (n = 3), erythromycin (n = 3), ceftazidime (n = 2), amoxicillin/clavulanic acid (n = 1), doxycycline (n = 1), secnidazole (n = 1), tinidazole (n = 1), clindamycin (n = 1), cefazolin (n = 1).

Table 4. Antibiotic use by hospital.

Care Setting	Mean Antibiotics per Patient (Range)
Hospital ownership	
Public	1.66 (1–4)
Private not-for-profit	1.70 (1–4)
Hospital	
Gulu RRH	1.631 (1–3)
Hoima RRH	1.727 (1–3)
Kagando	1.776 (1–3)
Kiwoko	1.792 (1–4)
Kumi	1.658 (1–3)
Lacor	1.667 (1–3)
Lira RRH	1.953 (1–3)
Masaka RRH	1.685 (1–3)
Moroto RRH	1.325 (1–4)
Ruharo Mission	2.000 (1–3)
Soroti RRH	1.646 (1–3)
St. Anthony	1.727 (1–3)
St. Francis Naggalama	1.625 (1–3)

Table 5. Associations of antibiotic use with characteristics of the study sample.

Variable	Antibiotic Use (*n* [%])	Univariate Model		Multivariate Model [2]	
		Odds Ratio	*p*-Value [1]	Odds Ratio	*p*-Value [1]
Age category					
<2 years	102 (82.9%)	1 (reference)			
2–50 years	569 (71.7%)	0.65	0.01 *	0.63	0.08
>50 years	117 (75.8%)	0.52	0.16	0.70	0.28
Sex					
Female	425 (69.8%)	1 (reference)			
Male	369 (78.8%)	1.15	<0.001 *	1.57	0.003 *
Hospital ownership					
Private not-for-profit	245 (66.0%)	1 (reference)			
Public	549 (77.8%)	1.80	<0.001 *		
Hospital					
Gulu RRH	84 (63.2%)	1 (reference)			
Hoima RRH	88 (85.4%)	3.42	<0.001 *		
Kagando	49 (80.3%)	2.38	0.02 *		
Kiwoko	24 (55.8%)	0.74	0.39		
Kumi	38 (80.9%)	2.46	0.03 *		
Lacor	86 (51.2%)	0.61	0.04 *		
Lira RRH	86 (70.3%)	1.52	0.12		

Table 5. *Cont.*

Variable	Antibiotic Use (*n* [%])	Univariate Model		Multivariate Model [2]	
		Odds Ratio	*p*-Value [1]	Odds Ratio	*p*-Value [1]
Masaka RRH	114 (89.8%)	5.11	<0.001 *		
Moroto RRH	81 (81.8%)	2.62	0.002 *		
Ruharo Mission	5 (83.3%)	2.92	0.33		
Soroti RRH	96 (76.8%)	1.93	0.02 *		
St. Anthony	11 (91.7%)	6.41	0.08		
St. Francis Naggalama	32 (94.1%)	9.33	0.003 *		
Ward					
Maternal	219 (70.4%)	1 (reference)			
Medical	170 (71.1%)	1.04	0.86		
Pediatric	188 (77.4%)	1.44	0.06		
Surgical	217 (76.4%)	1.36	0.10		
Underlying conditions					
HIV (no)	689 (71.7%)	1 (reference)			
HIV (yes)	43 (93.5%)	5.65	0.004 *	5.90	0.003 *
TB (no)	705 (71.9%)	1 (reference)			
TB (yes)	18 (90%)	3.51	0.09		
Malaria (no)	667 (73.2%)	1 (reference)			
Malaria (yes)	85 (72%)	0.94	0.78	0.79	0.31
COPD (no)	752 (73.9%)	1 (reference)			
COPD (yes)	9 (75.0%)	1.06	0.93		
Malnutrition (no)	738 (72.9%)	1 (reference)			
Malnutrition (yes)	49 (94.2%)	6.06	0.002 *	5.78	0.004 *
Hosp in past 90 days (no)	696 (72.8%)	1 (reference)			
Hosp in past 90 days (yes)	65 (80.2%)	1.51	0.15		

[1] Statistical significance is noted by an * for all relationships with $p < 0.05$. [2] Multivariate model includes: age, sex, HIV status, malaria status, and malnutrition status. Abbreviations: RRH = regional referral hospital; COPD = chronic obstructive pulmonary disease; HIV = human immunodeficiency virus; TB = tuberculosis.

2.2. Antibiotic Stewardship Indicators

2.2.1. Guideline Compliance

Among all antibiotics, only 30.1% (*n* = 423) were prescribed in compliance with the Uganda Clinical Guidelines 2016 [28]. Compliance with treatment guidelines was 30.9% of prescriptions in public hospitals and 29.7% in private not-for-profit hospitals (Table 6). In addition to Ruharo (which had 0% compliance but based on a small sample size of 10 total antibiotics), the lowest proportion of prescriptions in alignment with treatment guidelines was recorded at Kumi (15.6%, *n* = 12), and the highest proportion was at Kiwoko (54.5%, *n* = 24). Compliance with prescription guidelines for each antibiotic varied as well. Secnidazole, sulbactam, and tinizadole were always prescribed in accordance with guidelines, and metronidazole was prescribed with a relatively high rate of compliance (63%). All other antibiotics were not prescribed in accordance with guidelines more than half the time. Frequencies of compliance with treatment guidelines by hospital are summarized in Table 6 and compliance by antibiotic is summarized in Supplementary Table S2.

Table 6. Antibiotics prescribed in compliance with Uganda Clinical Guidelines by hospital.

Setting	Guideline Compliance (*n*, %)
Hospital ownership	
Public	289 (30.9%)
Private not-for-profit	134 (29.7%)
Hospital	
Gulu RRH	41 (28.5%)
Hoima RRH	61 (40.4%)
Kagando	17 (18.9%)
Kiwoko	24 (54.5%)
Kumi	12 (15.6%)
Lacor	58 (38.7%)
Lira RRH	61 (35.9%)
Masaka RRH	67 (33%)
Moroto RRH	34 (30.6%)
Ruharo Mission	0 (0%)
Soroti RRH	25 (15.9%)
St. Anthnoy	5 (26.3%)
St. Francis Naggalama	18 (29.5%)

Abbreviations: RRH = regional referral hospital.

Overall, the indication for treatment was documented in patient record notes for 80.1% (n = 1373) of all prescriptions. St. Francis Naggalama recorded the highest proportion of prescriptions with the reason for prescribing antibiotics documented in the notes at 96.8% (n = 61), and Lacor hospital recorded the lowest at 64.3% (n = 153). Among all SP prescriptions, 1% (n = 3) of prescriptions were for 1 dose, 0.7% (n = 2) were multiple doses on day 1, and the remaining was for a longer duration, which was 301 (98.4%) multiple doses on more than 1 day.

2.2.2. WHO AWaRe Classification

Among all 1387 antibiotic prescriptions, 654 (47.2%) were from the Access group, 612 (44.1%) were in the Watch classification, and 9% were unclassified (Figure 3). The most prescribed Watch antibiotics were ceftriaxone (n = 519), ciprofloxacin (n = 45), azithromycin (n = 19), levofloxacin (n = 15), and erythromycin (n = 3). There were no antibiotic prescriptions in the Reserve group. The highest proportion of Access antibiotics was recorded at Lacor hospital (70.5%) and the lowest Access proportion was in Moroto (25.7%). Similarly, the highest proportion of Watch antibiotics was recorded at Moroto hospital (58.4%) and the lowest proportion at Lacor (20.5%).

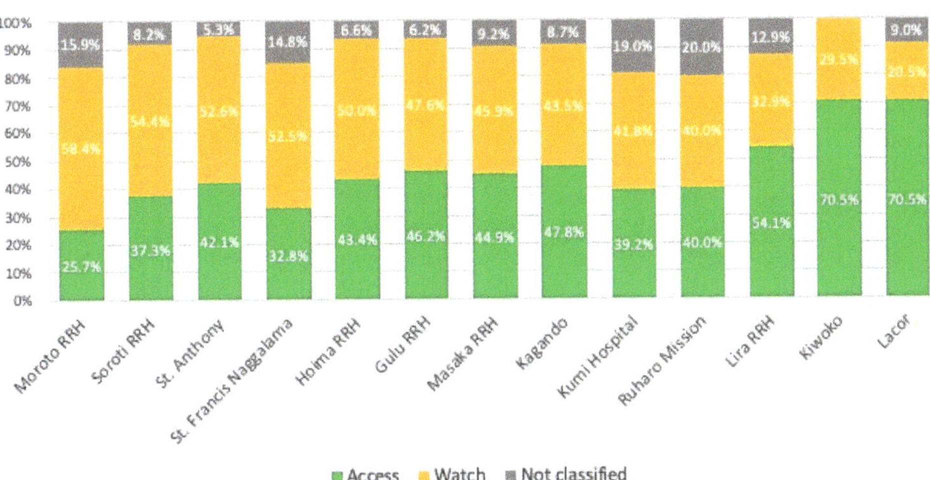

Figure 3. Prescriptions by AWaRe classification per hospital.

2.2.3. Missed Doses

Among all antibiotics with more than 20 prescriptions, ampicillin-cloxacillin (30.4%, n = 24) had the highest proportion of courses that were not administered to patients, followed by metronidazole (15.1%, n = 57). By hospital, Lira hospital and Gulu hospital had the highest percentage of prescriptions that were not administered to patients (25.6%, n = 52; and 16%, n = 31, respectively), and five hospitals had prescriptions that were administered to all patients studied: Hoima, Kagando, Kiwoko, Kumi, and St. Francis Naggalama. The proportion of antibiotic courses that were administered by hospital are summarized in Supplementary Table S3.

2.2.4. Route of Administration

Across all 1387 prescriptions, 11% (n = 157) were administered orally and 88% (n = 1230) were administered parenterally. A switch from parenteral to oral antibiotics was noted for 1.9% (n = 39) among all orally administered antibiotics. Among the antibiotics that were administered parenterally, 925 (75.3%) were administered intermittently, 302 (24.3%) were administered continuously, and 2 (<1%) were administered intramuscularly.

2.3. *Antibiotics per Patient*

Overall, 794 (73.7%) observed patients were on one or more antibiotics. By sex, 425 (69.8%) females and 369 (78.8%) males were on one or more antibiotics. Among patients on antibiotics, 302 (38%) were on one antibiotic, 440 (55%) were on two antibiotics, 44 (6%) were on three antibiotics, and two (<1%) were on four antibiotics. Among patients on any antibiotics, the mean number of antibiotics per patient was 1.55 (range 1–4). The mean number of antibiotics per patient ranged from 1.6 in St. Francis Naggalama Hospital to 2.0 in Ruharo Mission Hospital ($p < 0.001$). In publicly owned hospitals, the mean number of antibiotics per patient was 1.66, and in private not-for-profit hospitals, the mean number of antibiotics was 1.70 ($p = 0.41$) (Table 4).

Several characteristics were associated with significantly increased odds of being on antibiotics based on the univariate analyses (Table 5). These characteristics were being male, public hospital setting, specific hospital, patient HIV status, and patient malnutrition status (Table 5). Males had a 15% increase in the odds of antibiotic use, and public hospital settings had a nearly two-fold increase in antibiotic use than private, not-for-profit hospitals. Among the hospitals surveyed, there were up to nine-fold increases in antibiotic use. Lacor hospital had a 39% decrease in the odds of antibiotic use ($p = 0.04$). HIV and malnutrition patients had a nearly six-fold increase in antibiotic use ($p < 0.001$). Whether a patient was hospitalized in the previous 90 days did not increase the odds of antibiotic use. In the multivariate logistic regression, male sex ($p = 0.003$), HIV status ($p = 0.003$), and malnutrition status ($p = 0.004$) were significantly associated with odds of antibiotic use, while age and malaria status were not (Table 5).

Antibiotics by Sex

Among females, the characteristics associated with increased odds of antibiotic use were attendance at a public hospital (OR 1.60, $p < 0.01$), positive HIV status (OR 4.57, $p = 0.04$), malnourishment status (OR 5.21, $p = 0.03$), and attendance at the following hospitals: Hoima (OR 3.55, $p < 0.01$), Kumi (OR 5.49, $p = 0.03$), Masaka (OR 4.67, $p < 0.01$), and St. Francis Naggalama (OR 5.83, $p = 0.02$). Among males, the characteristics associated with increased odds of antibiotic use were attendance at a public hospital (OR 2.44, $p < 0.01$) and attendance at the following hospitals: Masaka (OR 6.51, $p < 0.01$), Moroto (OR 4.77, $p = 0.01$), and Soroti (OR 3.32, $p = 0.03$) (Supplementary Tables S4 and S5).

3. Discussion

The observed prevalence of antibiotic use of 73.7% is somewhat similar to findings from certain PPS studies conducted in Kenya (67.7%) [29], Botswana (70.6%) [30], Ghana (60.5%) [31] and Jordan (75.6%) [32]. The prevalence of antibiotic use found in this study is high compared to what was found in high-income countries, but similar to findings in other low- and middle-income countries [33]. In contrast, a lower prevalence of antibiotic use was reported in other studies from Kenya (46.7%) [34]; Tanzania (44%) [35]; countries of Ghana, Uganda, Zambia, and Tanzania in the Global PPS (30–57%, with overall prevalence of 50%) [36]; Brazil (52.2%) [37]; Northern Ireland (46.2%) [38]; and Belgium (27.1%) [39]. Cross-national differences may be accounted for by factors such as varying disease burden, antibiotic use guidelines, and policies across countries, including ease of access to antibiotics, differences in patients' characteristics, and types of hospitals.

3.1. *Antibiotic Use and Prevalence by Patient Characteristics*

Both sex (identified by physical or physiological differences) and gender (defined by socially constructed roles) play important roles in AMR, based on sex differences in pharmacokinetics and pharmacodynamics and gender roles [15]. Body weight, blood volume, and fat distribution differences between the sexes have biological effects on how antibiotics are absorbed, distributed, metabolized, and eliminated. This is one of the reasons that females have a greater risk for AMR than males [40]. In this study, males had greater odds of being prescribed an antibiotic compared to females. In many societies where women are considered less valuable than men, gender determines the use of preventative measures and referral for more invasive therapeutic strategies [41]. To understand why, in the study, men were given more antibiotics would require a mixed-methods study to determine if the difference was a population-based difference in the proportion of males versus females, based on clinical indications or standards of care, lack of sex-specific antibiotic guidelines or due to other factors that suggest health inequity at the tertiary care level. Without better data, it is difficult to discern if there are sex differences in diagnosis indications at presentation, standards of care, or health care utilization (e.g., males may present later in the course of the disease) [42]. The WHO PPS does not allow for important data collection and analysis of sex and gender impacts on antibiotic use and AMR. Given WHO's priority to equitably address AMR, the PPS should be updated to include these data in the PPS methodology [43].

3.2. Antibiotic Use Based on Uganda Clinical Guidelines and Hospital Setting

We found that most patients received multiple doses on more than one day, an average of 2.3 antibiotics administered per patient, contrary to WHO recommendations of single antibiotic prophylaxis [44]. In addition to the current practices of antibiotic use driving up the emergence of resistance, it also increases the cost of health care, with an increased risk of adverse drug reactions. There is a lack of guidance on the use of antibiotics in surgery in the Uganda Clinical Guidelines. The lack of guidelines on antibiotic use in surgery is a major concern for AMR emergence and needs to be addressed. Insufficient knowledge, prescriber attitudes, resistance to change, patient expectations exacerbated by scarce resources in countries such as Uganda and several other factors present additional challenges [45].

Use of parenteral antibiotics was very high (88%) compared to oral (12%) in the present study. These values are similar to the use of parenteral antibiotics in Indonesia (85.1%) and Pakistan (91.5%) [46,47]. The overuse of parenteral antibiotics (specifically, using parenteral antibiotics when not indicated or for longer than indicated) often increases costs of care, including costs associated with antibiotics, and nursing time and also increasing the duration of hospital stays; as such, overuse poses a challenge for infection prevention and control, especially in resource-constrained countries, such as Uganda. In this study, reasons for the indication for antibiotic prescription were written in the patient notes somewhat more frequently (80.1% of patients on antibiotics) compared to studies conducted in Indonesia (63.5%) and Pakistan (76.2%).

Our finding of poor adherence to Uganda's Clinical Guidelines (30.1%), along with the high percentage of antibiotics used in the Watch category, further accentuates the need for effective antimicrobial stewardship programs in Uganda, in connection with progress toward universal health coverage [48]. Many factors could contribute to the low adherence to the Uganda Clinical Guidelines, including poor dissemination of the guidelines, lack of proper diagnostic stewardship in hospitals, such as in microbiology and radiology, and long turnaround times for laboratory results. Lastly, in many settings, prescriber preferences and behaviors are a major cause for non-adherence to the guidelines [49]. Similar factors have been described elsewhere as barriers to guideline adherence [50,51]. In contrast, in Tanzania, compliance with national guidelines was high at 84% and South Africa at 90.2% [52,53]. The overall low compliance with Uganda's Clinical Guidelines could be a contributing factor to the observed high prevalence of Watch category antibiotics. In contrast, Lacor hospital, a private-not-for-profit, had a high adherence to the Uganda Clinical Guidelines, 39% less odds of antibiotic use, and hence higher use of the Access category antibiotics, partly attributed to the existence of its hospital antimicrobial stewardship program. The relatively high compliance to national guidelines in Tanzania and South Africa could partly be attributed to the implementation of antibiotic use policies and regulations, along with health care quality improvement initiatives [54,55]. A recent in-depth study of prescribers in Uganda found that stockouts of certain antibiotics, high patient load, prescriber's years of experience, influence of pharmacies and pharmaceutical companies, patient demand, lack of ownership of the dangers of AMR and other factors contributed to poor prescribing practices [56]. Therefore, the Uganda Ministry of Health should strengthen and enforce policies to address the challenge of low compliance to guidelines in health facilities.

Contrary to the general view that inappropriate antibiotic prescribing with respect to indication and quantity is higher in the private sector and based on a situational analysis [13], our findings showed no difference in prevalence of ceftriaxone prescribing, the percentage of guideline compliance, and mean number of antibiotics per patient, which was approximately the same when comparing the public and private-not-for-profit hospitals. Further, public hospitals were associated with 1.8 times higher odds of antibiotic use compared to private hospitals. This could be due to similar disease patterns and common prescriber behavior across both public and private practitioners. Health practitioners (including physicians, nurses, and pharmacists) commonly work in both private and public sectors. So, such working arrangements contribute to prescribing and dispensing behavior across both public and private sectors.

3.3. Proportion of Prescribed Antibiotic Doses Not Administered to Patients

The finding of ampicillin-cloxacillin and metronidazole having a high proportion of doses not administered to patients (coded as "missed doses" in WHO PPS methodology) is not surprising since these drugs are administered at a higher frequency, i.e., every six hours and eight hours, respectively, compared to antibiotics like ceftriaxone, which is administered once a day. Public hospitals have a higher burden of patients and tend to use more higher-frequency dosing drugs. Other possible causes could be essential medicine stockouts, including certain Access group antibiotics, which means the antibiotics were not administered. The latter could also explain the high prevalence and, at times, lack of alignment with clinical guidelines for certain Watch group antibiotics, when the first-line Access group antibiotics ran out of stock [57,58]. These findings have implications for stewardship and may be associated with the emergence of resistance and have been associated with poor treatment outcomes [59,60]. Although causative factors for missed doses may vary between low- and middle-income countries and high-income countries, the use of continuous quality improvement plans has been found to be effective in addressing this challenge [61].

3.4. Route of Administration

The observed high proportion of parenteral antibiotics could point to overall stewardship challenges in health facilities. One possible explanation is the lack of adherence to the Uganda Clinical Guidelines. The observed low compliance with the guidelines (30%) could also explain the high proportion of parenteral antibiotics since most of the first-line drugs for treating common bacterial infections are oral medicines as per the guidelines. Additionally, implementing a hospital-parenteral-to-oral switch program requires regular patient review and availability of microbiology results to guide the switch to determine suitable oral medications. Human resource shortages could hinder regular patient review to switch antibiotics from parenteral to oral. Additionally, the lack of microbiology capacity in most hospitals may negatively affect the clinicians' ability to empirically make decisions for the parenteral-to-oral switch. Lastly, the general belief that parenteral antibiotics work better than oral antibiotics could be a contributing factor [62]. Contributing factors and possible solutions to this challenge have been previously described [63].

3.5. WHO AWaRE Antibiotic Classification

Ampicillin-cloxacillin is listed as "not recommended" in the WHO AWaRe antibiotic classification database. It is considered as an inappropriate fixed-dose combination and is a problem not only in Uganda but in many low- and middle-income countries [64,65]. Ampicillin-cloxacillin was removed from the 2016 Uganda Clinical Guidelines. Reasons for its use could not be elucidated in our study, but it is concerning, given that it is among the top ten most consumed antibiotics nationwide in Uganda [66].

Ceftriaxone, a Watch antibiotic, was the most prescribed antibiotic for patients in these 13 regional hospitals and was used routinely for CAIs, MP, and SP. Ceftriaxone was used empirically as the first-line treatment for CAIs, contrary to Uganda's Clinical Guidelines. Inappropriate use of ceftriaxone, which is a third-generation cephalosporin, can accelerate the emergence of AMR of multidrug-resistant organisms, increase treatment cost, and result in avertable adverse drug effects. In Uganda, one study reported 32% inappropriate use of ceftriaxone in nine health facilities while another study reported a high level of ceftriaxone use at a tertiary care, private not-for-profit hospital [67,68]. A possible explanation for the high prevalence of ceftriaxone could be the ease of use (single daily dose) coupled with its wide spectrum coverage, giving the prescriber a sense of broad-spectrum coverage for most infections encountered in clinical practice.

Not using antimicrobial susceptibility testing when prescribing antibiotics in Uganda is also concerning. This situation is not unique to Uganda as only 2 out of 591 patients that received antibiotics in a PPS study conducted in Tanzania were specifically treated based on antimicrobial susceptibility testing results [52]. Among the challenges in antimicrobial susceptibility testing in sub-Saharan Africa are inadequate resources, weak supply chains for consumables for microbiological laboratory procedures, the timely turn-around of results for clinical decision-making (approximately 22 days in Uganda), and laboratory workforce limitations, such as staffing levels and training [69]. Underuse of culture sensitivity tests in hospitals is pervasive in resource-constrained countries.

This study informs antimicrobial stewardship strategies for Ugandan hospitals by establishing measurable antimicrobial use targets, such as reducing the use of broad-spectrum antibiotics, complying with treatment guidelines and increasing the uptake of antimicrobial susceptibility testing. There is a need to develop and implement feasible strategies for complementing antimicrobial stewardship interventions such as in infection prevention and control and hand hygiene interventions for prevention of health care-associated infection that can reduce the need for antibiotic use. Additionally, the study can serve as a baseline to evaluate future antimicrobial stewardship strategies in Uganda's hospitals. Areas of action could include establishing a funded national system for surveillance of antibiotic use in health facilities to inform antimicrobial stewardship interventions. There is also a need to strengthen implementation and enforcement of policies on the use of antibiotics. This could help reduce the inappropriate use of Watch category antibiotics and increase compliance with the Uganda Clinical Guidelines. For hospitals, survey findings can be used to develop specific continuous quality improvement plans to address the identified gaps. Areas of future research include understanding the potential enablers of implementing antimicrobial stewardship programs in Uganda; behavioral, sex, and gender impacts; and other factors that influence prescribing and consumer behaviors for antibiotics. Comprehensive solutions and multi-pronged approaches to tackle weak laboratory capacity in Uganda and sub-Saharan Africa in general have been extensively described elsewhere. Our study provides further evidence on the need for Uganda to secure appropriate investments to solve this vexing problem, which is an essential component of antimicrobial stewardship [70,71].

3.6. Limitations

Data collection took place over five months, rather than the WHO-recommended three-week window. A major cause of this limitation was the lack of capacity within health facilities to conduct antibiotic use surveys. The longer duration of our study may have resulted in some inconsistencies in antibiotic use patterns based on external factors, such as holidays and changes in disease transmission, including the COVID-19 burden. The PPS study design is restricted to assessing only inpatient antibiotic use. Consequently, antibiotics taken prior to hospitalization or those purchased externally and brought to the hospital are not recorded. The point-in-time nature of the PPS design further limits insight into seasonal patterns in antibiotic use. Even though the study included hospitals from different regions of the country as well as from government and private sectors, there are some limitations in the generalizability of our findings to other hospitals in Uganda and to hospitals in other countries with similar disease burdens and patient demographics.

Our study has numerous strengths. Using the standard WHO PPS methodology allows for comparisons with future studies not only in Uganda but also in other East African settings and sub-Saharan African settings in general. Compared to other PPS studies performed in as few as 1–6 hospitals, the present study included 13 hospitals. Inclusion of public and private not-for-profit hospitals is another strength of the study along with the dispersed geographical coverage of the hospitals in Uganda. Our study built on the existing hospital medicines and therapeutics committee as the mechanism for stewardship interventions. Further, our findings go beyond measuring the use of antibiotics. Several study variables, such as the burden of surgical indications, reasons for antibiotic prescribing, and data on antibiotic use for specific sites, have the potential for additional utility to improve clinical decision making and ensure patient safety. Finally, we are the first to assess sex-disaggregated differences to understand inequities in antibiotic use among males and females by using the PPS methodology.

4. Methods and Materials

All data were collected and analyzed based on the "WHO Methodology for Point Prevalence Survey on Antibiotic Use in Hospitals" version 1.1. The WHO Methodology for Point Prevalence Surveys, published in 2019, is intended to guide the collection of information on prescribing practices of antibiotics and other information relevant to treatment and management of infectious diseases in hospitalized patients [16]. Given challenges associated with data collection and high workload in resource-limited countries such as Uganda, the WHO PPS methodology has been developed with flexibility in mind. The data was collected to inform program activities and not submitted to WHO. Our study used the WHO PPS method over the Global-PPS method given our program's consistent use of standardized WHO tools across countries including Uganda. The WHO-PPS methodology allows for paper-based data entry in hospitals with no access to computer devices.

4.1. Data Collection

4.1.1. Setting

The study was conducted from December 2020 to April 2021 in 13 hospitals in Uganda. Six of the hospitals were public, government owned RRHs and seven were private not-for-profit hospitals. The public hospitals were chosen purposively based on ongoing involvement in related antimicrobial stewardship programs, and the private not-for-profit hospitals were chosen based on geographic location to cover four main regions of the country. Data were collected from all health facilities where our program is working to improve antibiotic use and no sampling of hospitals was done. Uganda has a decentralized health care system, with the lowest level being the Village Health Team and the highest being the National Referral Hospitals. General hospitals provide primary health care, covering the main disciplines of Medicine, Surgery, Pediatrics, and Obstetrics. The RRHs provide all the care provided by the general hospitals and provide specialized care in addition.

4.1.2. Data Collection

Data collection was conducted by staff from each hospital's medicines and therapeutics committee. Training on using the WHO PPS standardized data collection methods, including the paper form, took place one day before the data collection began and included practice sessions. Data were included for all patients admitted to the ward before 8:00 am on the study day as well as all patients discharged on the study day. Data were excluded for patient types listed in the WHO PPS protocol, including all patients who were admitted after 8:00 am, patients in the palliative long-term care wards, patients currently undergoing radiological or surgical procedures, and patients who are still physically present in the ward but who have been officially discharged. Each ward was surveyed completely within one day to minimize impact of patients moving between wards. The variables collected were all core variables in the WHO PPS methodology for hospital, ward, patient, antibiotic, and indication categories of variables.

4.1.3. Study Ethics and Approval

The Uganda Ministry of Health approved this study as part of ongoing technical assistance and implementation of the AMR national action plan [17].

4.2. Data Analysis

After data collection, de-identified data were entered into the WHO PPS Microsoft Excel-based tool by the study team for analysis. Data cleaning checks were performed for all 13 hospitals, and all data entry discrepancies were resolved using the original paper data collection forms. The data cleaning and entry was done as per the WHO methodology/protocol referenced above.

Indication was grouped into four categories: community-acquired infection (CAI), hospital-associated infection (HAI), medical prophylaxis (MP), and surgical prophylaxis (SP). According to the WHO PPS methodology, infection is categorized as HAI if the date of onset is on: Day 3 onwards OR Day 1 or Day 2 AND patient transferred from another hospital OR Day 1 or Day 2 and patient discharged from a hospital (same hospital or another one) in preceding 48 h. Antibiotics were grouped according to 2019 WHO AWaRe classification of antibiotics for evaluation and monitoring of use [72]. Antibiotics in the Access category have a wide range of activity against common pathogens and show low resistance potential; Watch antibiotics have higher resistance potential and are intended to be key targets of stewardship programs and monitoring, and Reserve antibiotics are last-resort options when other alternatives have failed.

Descriptive statistics for the data are presented using mean ± standard deviation or median (IQR) for continuous variables. Results from categorical variables are expressed as proportions and the $\chi 2$ test or Fisher's exact test was used, as appropriate, for comparisons. Univariate logistic regression to assess factors associated with increased odds of antibiotic use was conducted with the following prespecified factors: age (categorized as <2 years, 2–50 years, >50 years), sex, ward, hospital ownership, hospital facility, underlying condition status (HIV, TB, malaria, malnutrition, COPD), hospitalization within previous 90 days, indication category, and whether patient is a referral. This same univariate analysis was then performed disaggregated by sex as well. A multivariate logistic regression was also conducted which included pre-specified variables of interest: age, sex, HIV status, malaria status, and malnutrition status. Significance was evaluated at the alpha = 0.05 level. All analyses were performed using R Studio version 4.0.1 [73].

5. Conclusions

This is the first study in Uganda that was based on the WHO methodology for PPS on antibiotic use in hospitals. These data provide insights into the most common antibiotics used in 13 public and private not-for-profit hospitals throughout the country, including prevalence by patient characteristics, hospital, indication, and diagnosis. Notable findings were the high use of antibiotics among hospitalized patients, the high proportion of patients receiving parenteral antibiotics, the high prevalence of Watch antibiotics (particularly ceftriaxone), antibiotic use for SP nearly always spanning more than one day, low adherence to Uganda Clinical Guidelines, and sex differences in antibiotic use. These findings support the Uganda National Action Plan on AMR in identifying targeted strategies for improving antimicrobial stewardship. The estimates provided herein may also serve as a helpful baseline for the national antimicrobial stewardship technical working committee to promote and facilitate locally appropriate stewardship strategies in hospital settings and catalyze experience sharing and cross-fertilization. Additional research is needed to identify the drivers of inappropriate use in relation to disease burden and operational enablers of effective antimicrobial stewardship programs.

Supplementary Materials: The following are available online at https://www.mdpi.com/article/10.3390/antibiotics11020199/s1, Table S1: Hospital characteristics, Table S2: Associations of antibiotic use with characteristics of females in the study sample, Table S3: Associations of antibiotic use with characteristics of males in the study sample, Table S4: Compliance with Uganda Clinical Treatment Guidelines by antibiotic, Table S5: Adherence by hospital and antibiotic.

Author Contributions: Conceptualization, R.K.; methodology, R.K. and J.W.; training of hospital staff, R.K., J.W. and M.M.; data entry, J.W. and R.K.; formal analysis, R.W. and H.N.N.; writing—original draft preparation, R.K., R.W., J.W., H.N.N., A.S. and N.K.; writing—review and editing, N.O., R.K., R.W., J.W, F.E.K., M.M., L.L.L., S.M., M.P.J., A.S. and N.K.; supervision, R.K., J.W. and N.K.; project administration, R.K., J.W. and N.K.; funding acquisition, R.K. All authors have read and agreed to the published version of the manuscript.

Funding: This study was made possible by the generous support of the American people through the US Agency for International Development (USAID) contract no. 7200AA18C00074.

Institutional Review Board Statement: The Ministry of Health granted permission to the USAID MTaPS program for long-term technical assistance in multisectoral coordination on AMR, infection prevention and control, and antimicrobial stewardship, which includes permission for antibiotic use studies. The conduct of this study is part of the USAID MTaPS program's routine technical assistance to inform priorities for stewardship. The senior administration of all participating hospital sites provided their respective approval and clearance. The study was conducted according to the guidelines of the Declaration of Helsinki.

Informed Consent Statement: Not applicable as there was no direct patient contact and all data were anonymized.

Data Availability Statement: Not applicable.

Acknowledgments: We acknowledge the dedicated efforts of the hospital staff in the 13 participating hospitals in their efforts to collect the data and adhere to the WHO PPS methodology. We thank the senior administration of the 13 participating hospitals in their efforts to facilitate the success of this study as part of the ongoing technical assistance being provided by the USAID MTaPS program. Julius Kisembo is appreciated for his work on Figure 1.

Conflicts of Interest: The authors declare no conflict of interest.

Disclaimer: The contents are the responsibility of the authors and do not necessarily reflect the views of USAID or the US Government.

References

1. Naylor, N.R.; Atun, R.; Zhu, N.; Kulasabanathan, K.; Silva, S.; Chatterjee, A.; Knight, G.M.; Robotham, J.V. Estimating the burden of antimicrobial resistance: A systematic literature review. *Antimicrob. Resist. Infect. Control* **2018**, *7*, 58. [CrossRef] [PubMed]
2. Hay, S.I.; Rao, P.C.; Dolecek, C.; Day, N.P.J.; Stergachis, A.; Lopez, A.D.; Murray, C.J.L. Measuring and mapping the global burden of antimicrobial resistance. *BMC Med.* **2018**, *16*, 78. [CrossRef] [PubMed]
3. Hernando-Amado, S.; Coque, T.M.; Baquero, F.; Martínez, J.L. Defining and combating antibiotic resistance from One Health and Global Health perspectives. *Nat. Microbiol.* **2019**, *4*, 1432–1442. [CrossRef] [PubMed]
4. O'Neill, J. Review on Antimicrobial Resistance Antimicrobial Resistance: Tackling a Crisis for the Health and Wealth of Nations. London: Review on Antimicrobial Resistance. 2014. Available online: https://amr-review.org/Publications.html (accessed on 21 December 2021).
5. Getahun, H.; Smith, I.; Trivedi, K.; Paulin, S.; Balkhy, H.H. Tackling antimicrobial resistance in the COVID-19 pandemic. *Bull. World Health Organ.* **2020**, *98*, 442. [CrossRef]
6. Monnet, D.L.; Harbarth, S. Will coronavirus disease (COVID-19) have an impact on antimicrobial resistance? *Eurosurveillance* **2020**, *25*, 2001886. [CrossRef]
7. Afshinnekoo, E.; Bhattacharya, C.; Burguete-García, A.; Castro-Nallar, E.; Deng, Y.; Desnues, C.; Dias-Neto, E.; Elhaik, E.; Iraola, G.; Jang, S.; et al. COVID-19 drug practices risk antimicrobial resistance evolution. *Lancet Microbe* **2021**, *2*, e135–e136. [CrossRef]
8. Rodríguez-Baño, J.; Rossolini, G.M.; Schultsz, C.; Tacconelli, E.; Murthy, S.; Ohmagari, N.; Holmes, A.; Bachmann, T.; Goossens, H.; Canton, R.; et al. Key considerations on the potential impacts of the COVID-19 pandemic on antimicrobial resistance research and surveillance. *Trans. R. Soc. Trop. Med. Hyg.* **2021**, *115*, 1122–1129. [CrossRef]
9. Bloom, G.; Merrett, G.B.; Wilkinson, A.; Lin, V.; Paulin, S. Antimicrobial resistance and universal health coverage. *BMJ Glob. Health* **2017**, *2*, e000518. [CrossRef]
10. Castro-Sánchez, E.; Moore, L.S.P.; Husson, F.; Holmes, A.H. What are the factors driving antimicrobial resistance? Perspectives from a public event in London, England. *BMC Infect. Dis.* **2016**, *16*, 465. [CrossRef]
11. Vikesland, P.; Garner, E.; Gupta, S.; Kang, S.; Maile-Moskowitz, A.; Zhu, N. Differential Drivers of Antimicrobial Resistance across the World. *Acc. Chem. Res.* **2019**, *52*, 916–924. [CrossRef]
12. Chatterjee, A.; Modarai, M.; Naylor, N.; Boyd, S.E.; Atun, R.; Barlow, J.; Holmes, A.H.; Johnson, A.; Robotham, J. Quantifying drivers of antibiotic resistance in humans: A systematic review. *Lancet Infect. Dis.* **2018**, *18*, e368–e378. [CrossRef]
13. UNAS; CDDEP; GARP-Uganda; Mpairwe, Y.; Wamala, S. *Antibiotic Resistance in Uganda: Situation Analysis and Recommendations*; Uganda National Academy of Sciences: Kampala, Uganda; Center for Disease Dynamics, Economics & Policy: Washington, DC, USA, 2015; p. 107.
14. Kajumbula, H.; Fujita, A.W.; Mbabazi, O.; Najjuka, C.; Izale, C.; Akampurira, A.; Aisu, S.; Lamorde, M.; Walwema, R.; Bahr, N.C.; et al. Antimicrobial Drug Resistance in Blood Culture Isolates at a Tertiary Hospital, Uganda. *Emerg. Infect. Dis.* **2018**, *24*, 174–175. [CrossRef] [PubMed]
15. Soldin, O.P.; Mattison, D. Sex Differences in Pharmacokinetics and Pharmacodynamics. *Clin. Pharmacokinet.* **2009**, *48*, 143–157. [CrossRef] [PubMed]
16. WHO. *Global Action Plan on Antimicrobial Resistance*; The World Health Organization: Geneva, Switzerland, 2015.
17. Antimicrobial Resistance National Action Plan (2018–2023). The Republic of Uganda. 2018. Available online: https://www.heps.or.ug/index.php/publications/antimicrobial-resistance-national-action-plan-uganda-nap (accessed on 21 December 2021).
18. WHO. *World Health Organization Methodology for Point Prevalence Survey on Antibiotic Use in Hospitals*; Version 1.1; World Health Organization: Geneva, Switzerland, 2018.

19. Ogunleye, O.O.; Oyawole, M.R.; Odunuga, P.T.; Kalejaye, F.; Yinka-Ogunleye, A.F.; Olalekan, A.; Ogundele, S.O.; Ebruke, B.E.; Richard, A.K.; Paramadhas, B.D.A.; et al. A multicentre point prevalence study of antibiotics utilization in hospitalised patients in an urban secondary and a tertiary healthcare facilities in Nigeria: Findings and implications. *Expert Rev. Anti-Infect. Ther.* **2022**, *20*, 297–306. [CrossRef] [PubMed]
20. Abubakar, U. Antibiotic use among hospitalized patients in northern Nigeria: A multicenter point-prevalence survey. *BMC Infect. Dis.* **2020**, *20*, 86. [CrossRef]
21. Bediako-Bowan, A.A.A.; Owusu, E.; Labi, A.-K.; Obeng-Nkrumah, N.; Sunkwa-Mills, G.; Bjerrum, S.; Opintan, J.A.; Bannerman, C.; Mølbak, K.; Kurtzhals, J.A.L.; et al. Antibiotic use in surgical units of selected hospitals in Ghana: A multi-center point prevalence survey. *BMC Public Health* **2019**, *19*, 797. [CrossRef]
22. Godman, B.; Momanyi, L.; Opanga, S.; Nyamu, D.; Oluka, M.; Kurdi, A. Antibiotic prescribing patterns at a leading referral hospital in Kenya: A point prevalence survey. *J. Res. Pharm. Pract.* **2019**, *8*, 149–154. [CrossRef]
23. Lanyero, H.; Ocan, M.; Obua, C.; Lundborg, C.S.; Nanzigu, S.; Katureebe, A.; Kalyango, J.N.; Eriksen, J. Antibiotic use among children under five years with diarrhea in rural communities of Gulu, northern Uganda: A cross-sectional study. *BMC Public Health* **2021**, *21*, 1254. [CrossRef]
24. Sekikubo, M.; Hedman, K.; Mirembe, F.; Brauner, A. Antibiotic Overconsumption in Pregnant Women with Urinary Tract Symptoms in Uganda. *Clin. Infect. Dis.* **2017**, *65*, 544–550. [CrossRef]
25. Saito, H.; Inoue, K.; Ditai, J.; Weeks, A.D. Pattern of Peri-Operative Antibiotic Use among Surgical Patients in a Regional Referral and Teaching Hospital in Uganda. *Surg. Infect.* **2020**, *21*, 540–546. [CrossRef]
26. USAID Medicines, Technologies, and Pharmaceutical Services Program. MTaPS Support in Uganda. Available online: https://www.mtapsprogram.org/where-we-work/uganda/ (accessed on 21 December 2021).
27. USAID MTaPS Program. A Technical Guide to Implementing Facility Level Antimicrobial Stewardship Programs in MTaPS Program Countries. Available online: https://www.mtapsprogram.org/wp-content/uploads/2021/03/USAID-MTaPS-Mini-guide-for-facility-AMS-program.pdf (accessed on 21 December 2021).
28. *Uganda Clinical Guidelines. National Guidelines for Management of Common Conditions*; The Republic of Uganda, Ministry of Health: Kampala, Uganda, 2016.
29. Okoth, C.; Opanga, S.; Okalebo, F.; Oluka, M.; Kurdi, A.; Godman, B. Point prevalence survey of antibiotic use and resistance at a referral hospital in Kenya: Findings and implications. *Hosp. Pract.* **2018**, *46*, 128–136. [CrossRef] [PubMed]
30. Paramadhas, B.D.A.; Tiroyakgosi, C.; Mpinda-Joseph, P.; Morokotso, M.; Matome, M.; Sinkala, F.; Gaolebe, M.; Malone, B.; Molosiwa, E.; Shanmugam, M.G.; et al. Point prevalence study of antimicrobial use among hospitals across Botswana: Findings and implications. *Expert Rev. Anti-Infect. Ther.* **2019**, *17*, 535–546. [CrossRef] [PubMed]
31. Amponsah, O.K.O.; Buabeng, K.O.; Owusu-Ofori, A.; Ayisi-Boateng, N.K.; Hämeen-Anttila, K.; Enlund, H. Point prevalence survey of antibiotic consumption across three hospitals in Ghana. *JAC-Antimicrob. Resist.* **2021**, *3*, dlab008. [CrossRef] [PubMed]
32. Abdel-Qader, D.H.; Ismael, N.S.; Albassam, A.; El-Shara', A.; Aljamal, M.S.; Ismail, R.; Abdel-Qader, H.; Hamadi, S.; Al Mazrouei, N.; Ibrahim, O.M. Antibiotics use and appropriateness in two Jordanian children hospitals: A point prevalence study. *J. Pharm. Health Serv. Res.* **2021**, *12*, 166–172. [CrossRef]
33. Pauwels, I.; Versporten, A.; Drapier, N.; Vlieghe, E.; Goossens, H.; Koraqi, A.; Hoxha, I.; Tafaj, S.; Cornistein, W.; Quiros, R.; et al. Hospital antibiotic prescribing patterns in adult patients according to the WHO Access, Watch and Reserve classification (AWaRe): Results from a worldwide point prevalence survey in 69 countries. *J. Antimicrob. Chemother.* **2021**, *76*, 1614–1624. [CrossRef] [PubMed]
34. Maina, M.; Mwaniki, P.; Odira, E.; Kiko, N.; McKnight, J.; Schultsz, C.; English, M.; Tosas-Auguet, O. Antibiotic use in Kenyan public hospitals: Prevalence, appropriateness and link to guideline availability. *Int. J. Infect. Dis.* **2020**, *99*, 10–18. [CrossRef]
35. Horumpende, P.G.; Mshana, S.E.; Mouw, E.F.; Mmbaga, B.T.; Chilongola, J.O.; De Mast, Q. Point prevalence survey of antimicrobial use in three hospitals in North-Eastern Tanzania. *Antimicrob. Resist. Infect. Control* **2020**, *9*, 149. [CrossRef]
36. D'Arcy, N.; Ashiru-Oredope, D.; Olaoye, O.; Afriyie, D.; Akello, Z.; Ankrah, D.; Asima, D.M.; Banda, D.C.; Barrett, S.; Brandish, C.; et al. Antibiotic Prescribing Patterns in Ghana, Uganda, Zambia and Tanzania Hospitals: Results from the Global Point Prevalence Survey (G-PPS) on Antimicrobial Use and Stewardship Interventions Implemented. *Antibiotics* **2021**, *10*, 1122. [CrossRef]
37. Porto, A.; Goossens, H.; Versporten, A.; Costa, S.; Brazilian Global-PPS Working Group. Global point prevalence survey of antimicrobial consumption in Brazilian hospitals. *J. Hosp. Infect.* **2020**, *104*, 165–171. [CrossRef]
38. Elhajji, F.D.; Al-Taani, G.M.; Anani, L.; Al-Masri, S.; Abdalaziz, H.; Qabba'H, S.H.; Al Bawab, A.Q.; Scott, M.; Farren, D.; Gilmore, F.; et al. Comparative point prevalence survey of antimicrobial consumption between a hospital in Northern Ireland and a hospital in Jordan. *BMC Health Serv. Res.* **2018**, *18*, 849. [CrossRef]
39. Vandael, E.; Latour, K.; Goossens, H.; Magerman, K.; Drapier, N.; Catry, B.; Versporten, A.; Belgian Point Prevalence Survey Study Group. Point prevalence survey of antimicrobial use and healthcare-associated infections in Belgian acute care hospitals: Results of the Global-PPS and ECDC-PPS 2017. *Antimicrob. Resist. Infect. Control* **2020**, *9*, 13. [CrossRef] [PubMed]
40. WHO. *Taking Sex and Gender into Account in Emerging Infectious Disease Programmes. An Analytical Framework*; World Health Organization Western Pacific Region: Manilla, Philippines, 2011; ISBN 978 92 9061 532 3.
41. Mauvais-Jarvis, F.; Merz, N.B.; Barnes, P.J.; Brinton, R.D.; Carrero, J.-J.; DeMeo, D.L.; De Vries, G.J.; Epperson, C.N.; Govindan, R.; Klein, S.L.; et al. Sex and gender: Modifiers of health, disease, and medicine. *Lancet* **2020**, *396*, 565–582. [CrossRef]

42. Accorsi, S.; Fabiani, M.; Nattabi, B.; Ferrarese, N.; Corrado, B.; Iriso, R.; Ayella, E.O.; Pido, B.; Yoti, Z.; Corti, D.; et al. Differences in hospital admissions for males and females in northern Uganda in the period 1992–2004: A consideration of gender and sex differences in health care use. *Trans. R. Soc. Trop. Med. Hyg.* **2007**, *101*, 929–938. [CrossRef] [PubMed]
43. WHO. *Tackling Antimicrobial Resistance (AMR) Together: Working Paper 5.0: Enhancing the Focus on Gender and Equity*; World Health Organization: Geneva, Switzerland, 2018.
44. WHO. *Global Guidelines for the Prevention of Surgical Site Infection*, 2nd ed.; World Health Organization: Geneva, Switzerland, 2018.
45. Cooper, L.; Sneddon, J.; Afriyie, D.K.; Sefah, I.A.; Kurdi, A.; Godman, B.; Seaton, R.A. Supporting global antimicrobial stewardship: Antibiotic prophylaxis for the prevention of surgical site infection in low- and middle-income countries (LMICs): A scoping review and meta-analysis. *JAC-Antimicrob. Resist.* **2020**, *2*, dlaa070. [CrossRef] [PubMed]
46. Limato, R.; Nelwan, E.J.; Mudia, M.; de Brabander, J.; Guterres, H.; Enty, E.; Mauleti, I.Y.; Mayasari, M.; Firmansyah, I.; Hizrani, M.; et al. A multicentre point prevalence survey of patterns and quality of antibiotic prescribing in Indonesian hospitals. *JAC-Antimicrob. Resist.* **2021**, *3*, dlab047. [CrossRef]
47. Saleem, Z.; Hassali, M.A.; Versporten, A.; Godman, B.; Hashmi, F.K.; Goossens, H.; Saleem, F. A multicenter point prevalence survey of antibiotic use in Punjab, Pakistan: Findings and implications. *Expert Rev. Anti-Infect. Ther.* **2019**, *17*, 285–293. [CrossRef]
48. WHO. WHO Releases the 2019 AWaRe Classification Antibiotics. 2019. Available online: https://www.who.int/news/item/01-10-2019-who-releases-the-2019-aware-classification-antibiotics (accessed on 21 December 2021).
49. Nambasa, V.; Ndagije, H.; Serwanga, A.; Manirakiza, L.; Atuhaire, J.; Nakitto, D.; Kiguba, R.; Figueras, A. Prescription of Levofloxacin and Moxifloxacin in Select Hospitals in Uganda: A Pilot Study to Assess Guideline Concordance. *Antibiotics* **2020**, *9*, 439. [CrossRef]
50. Maina, M.; McKnight, J.; Tosas-Auguet, O.; Schultsz, C.; English, M. Using treatment guidelines to improve antibiotic use: Insights from an antibiotic point prevalence survey in Kenya. *BMJ Glob. Health* **2021**, *6*, e003836. [CrossRef]
51. Almazrou, S.; Alfaifi, S.; Alfaifi, S.; Hakami, L.; Al-Aqeel, S. Barriers to and Facilitators of Adherence to Clinical Practice Guidelines in the Middle East and North Africa Region: A Systematic Review. *Healthcare* **2020**, *8*, 564. [CrossRef]
52. Seni, J.; Mapunjo, S.G.; Wittenauer, R.; Valimba, R.; Stergachis, A.; Werth, B.J.; Saitoti, S.; Mhadu, N.H.; Lusaya, E.; Konduri, N. Antimicrobial use across six referral hospitals in Tanzania: A point prevalence survey. *BMJ Open* **2020**, *10*, e042819. [CrossRef]
53. Skosana, P.; Schellack, N.; Godman, B.; Kurdi, A.; Bennie, M.; Kruger, D.; Meyer, J. A point prevalence survey of antimicrobial utilisation patterns and quality indices amongst hospitals in South Africa; findings and implications. *Expert Rev. Anti-Infect. Ther.* **2021**, *19*, 1353–1366. [CrossRef] [PubMed]
54. *Policy Guidelines for Implementing Antimicrobial Stewardship*; The United Republic of Tanzania, Ministry of Health, Community Development, Gender, Elderly and Children: Dodoma, Tanzania, 2020.
55. Chetty, S.; Reddy, M.; Ramsamy, Y.; Naidoo, A.; Essack, S. Antimicrobial stewardship in South Africa: A scoping review of the published literature. *JAC-Antimicrob. Resist.* **2019**, *1*, dlz060. [CrossRef] [PubMed]
56. Kagoya, E.K.; Van Royen, K.; Waako, P.; Van Royen, P.; Iramiot, J.S.; Obakiro, S.B.; Kostyanev, T.; Anthierens, S. Experiences and views of healthcare professionals on the prescription of antibiotics in Eastern Uganda: A qualitative study. *J. Glob. Antimicrob. Resist.* **2021**, *25*, 66–71. [CrossRef] [PubMed]
57. Ministry of Health Knowledge Management Portal. Periodic Stock Status Report. Example of One Report Dated 29 April 2021. Available online: http://library.health.go.ug/publications/medicines/ministry-health-stock-status-report-1st-april-2021 (accessed on 21 December 2021).
58. Muyinda, H.; Mugisha, J. Stock-outs, uncertainty and improvisation in access to healthcare in war-torn Northern Uganda. *Soc. Sci. Med.* **2015**, *146*, 316–323. [CrossRef] [PubMed]
59. ReAct Group. Shortages and AMR—Why Should We Care? 4 Consequences of Antibiotic Shortages. 2020. Available online: https://www.reactgroup.org/news-and-views/news-and-opinions/year-2020/shortages-and-amr-why-should-we-care-4-consequences-of-antibiotic-shortages/ (accessed on 21 December 2021).
60. Hwang, B.; Shroufi, A.; Gils, T.; Steele, S.J.; Grimsrud, A.; Boulle, A.; Yawa, A.; Stevenson, S.; Jankelowitz, L.; Versteeg-Mojanaga, M.; et al. Stock-outs of antiretroviral and tuberculosis medicines in South Africa: A national cross-sectional survey. *PLoS ONE* **2019**, *14*, e0212405. [CrossRef]
61. Coleman, J.J.; Hodson, J.; Brooks, H.L.; Rosser, D. Missed medication doses in hospitalised patients: A descriptive account of quality improvement measures and time series analysis. *Int. J. Qual. Health Care* **2013**, *25*, 564–572. [CrossRef]
62. Bonniface, M.; Nambatya, W.; Rajab, K. An Evaluation of Antibiotic Prescribing Practices in a Rural Refugee Settlement District in Uganda. *Antibiotics* **2021**, *10*, 172. [CrossRef]
63. Engel, M.F.; Postma, D.F.; Hulscher, M.E.; van Berkhout, F.T.; Emmelot-Vonk, M.H.; Sankatsing, S.; Gaillard, C.A.; Bruns, A.H.; Hoepelman, A.I.; Oosterheert, J.J. Barriers to an early switch from intravenous to oral antibiotic therapy in hospitalised patients with CAP. *Eur. Respir. J.* **2013**, *41*, 123–130. [CrossRef]
64. Sayer, B.; Bortone, B.; Sharland, M.; Hsia, Y. Fixed-dose combination antibiotics: The search for evidence using the example of ampicillin–cloxacillin. *Br. J. Clin. Pharmacol.* **2021**, *87*, 2996–2999. [CrossRef]
65. Bortone, B.; Jackson, C.; Hsia, Y.; Bielicki, J.; Magrini, N.; Sharland, M. High global consumption of potentially inappropriate fixed dose combination antibiotics: Analysis of data from 75 countries. *PLoS ONE* **2021**, *16*, e0241899. [CrossRef]

66. Namugambe, J.; Delamou, A.; Moses, F.; Ali, E.; Hermans, V.; Takarinda, K.; Thekkur, P.; Nanyonga, S.; Koroma, Z.; Mwoga, J.; et al. National Antimicrobial Consumption: Analysis of Central Warehouses Supplies to in-Patient Care Health Facilities from 2017 to 2019 in Uganda. *Trop. Med. Infect. Dis.* **2021**, *6*, 83. [CrossRef] [PubMed]
67. Kizito, M.; Lalitha, R.; Kajumbula, H.; Ssenyonga, R.; Muyanja, D.; Byakika-Kibwika, P. Antibiotic Prevalence Study and Factors Influencing Prescription of WHO Watch Category Antibiotic Ceftriaxone in a Tertiary Care Private Not for Profit Hospital in Uganda. *Antibiotics* **2021**, *10*, 1167. [CrossRef] [PubMed]
68. Kutyabami, P.; Munanura, E.I.; Kalidi, R.; Balikuna, S.; Ndagire, M.; Kaggwa, B.; Nambatya, W.; Kamba, P.F.; Musiimenta, A.; Kesi, D.N.; et al. Evaluation of the Clinical Use of Ceftriaxone among in-Patients in Selected Health Facilities in Uganda. *Antibiotics* **2021**, *10*, 779. [CrossRef]
69. Barbé, B.; Yansouni, C.; Affolabi, D.; Jacobs, J. Implementation of quality management for clinical bacteriology in low-resource settings. *Clin. Microbiol. Infect.* **2017**, *23*, 426–433. [CrossRef] [PubMed]
70. Jacobs, J.; Hardy, L.; Semret, M.; Lunguya, O.; Phe, T.; Affolabi, D.; Yansouni, C.; Vandenberg, O. Diagnostic Bacteriology in District Hospitals in Sub-Saharan Africa: At the Forefront of the Containment of Antimicrobial Resistance. *Front. Med.* **2019**, *6*, 205. [CrossRef]
71. Lamorde, M.; Mpimbaza, A.; Walwema, R.; Kamya, M.; Kapisi, J.; Kajumbula, H.; Sserwanga, A.; Namuganga, J.F.; Kusemererwa, A.; Tasimwa, H.; et al. A Cross-Cutting Approach to Surveillance and Laboratory Capacity as a Platform to Improve Health Security in Uganda. *Health Secur.* **2018**, *16*, S-76–S-86. [CrossRef]
72. WHO. The 2019 WHO Aware Classification of Antibiotics for Evaluation and Monitoring of Use. 2019. Available online: https://aware.essentialmeds.org/groups (accessed on 21 December 2021).
73. RStudio Team. *RStudio: Integrated Development for R*; RStudio Inc.: Boston, MA, USA, 2020.

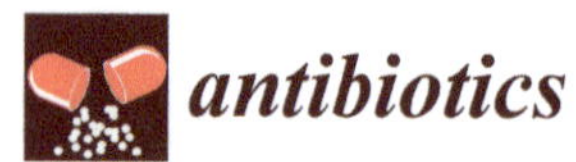
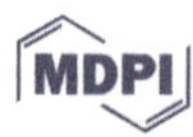

Article

Antibiotic Prescribing Patterns in Ghana, Uganda, Zambia and Tanzania Hospitals: Results from the Global Point Prevalence Survey (G-PPS) on Antimicrobial Use and Stewardship Interventions Implemented

Nikki D'Arcy [1], Diane Ashiru-Oredope [1,*], Omotayo Olaoye [1], Daniel Afriyie [2], Zainab Akello [3], Daniel Ankrah [4], Derrick Mawuena Asima [5], David C. Banda [6], Scott Barrett [7], Claire Brandish [8], Joseph Brayson [7], Peter Benedict [9], Cornelius C. Dodoo [10], Frances Garraghan [11], Josephyn Hoyelah, Sr. [12], Yogini Jani [13], Freddy Eric Kitutu [14], Ismail Musoke Kizito [15], Appiah-Korang Labi [16], Mariyam Mirfenderesky [17], Sudaxshina Murdan [18], Caoimhe Murray [19], Noah Obeng-Nkrumah [20], William J'Pathim Olum [21], Japheth Awuletey Opintan [16], Edwin Panford-Quainoo [22], Ines Pauwels [23], Israel Sefah [24], Jacqueline Sneddon [25], Anja St. Clair Jones [26] and Ann Versporten [23]

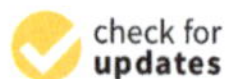

Citation: D'Arcy, N.; Ashiru-Oredope, D.; Olaoye, O.; Afriyie, D.; Akello, Z.; Ankrah, D.; Asima, D.M.; Banda, D.C.; Barrett, S.; Brandish, C.; et al. Antibiotic Prescribing Patterns in Ghana, Uganda, Zambia and Tanzania Hospitals: Results from the Global Point Prevalence Survey (G-PPS) on Antimicrobial Use and Stewardship Interventions Implemented. *Antibiotics* **2021**, *10*, 1122. https://doi.org/10.3390/antibiotics10091122

Academic Editors: Gabriella Orlando and Seok Hoon Jeong

Received: 24 July 2021
Accepted: 13 September 2021
Published: 17 September 2021

Publisher's Note: MDPI stays neutral with regard to jurisdictional claims in published maps and institutional affiliations.

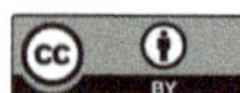

Copyright: © 2021 by the authors. Licensee MDPI, Basel, Switzerland. This article is an open access article distributed under the terms and conditions of the Creative Commons Attribution (CC BY) license (https://creativecommons.org/licenses/by/4.0/).

1 Commonwealth Partnerships Programme on Antimicrobial Stewardship, Commonwealth Pharmacists Association, London E1W 1AW, UK; nikki.darcy@commonwealthpharmacy.org (N.D.); omotayo.olaoye@commonwealthpharmacy.org (O.O.)
2 Pharmacy Department, Ghana Police Hospital, Accra P.O. Box CT104, Ghana; dspdan77@yahoo.com
3 Laro Division, Gulu Regional Referral Hospital, Gulu P.O. Box 166, Uganda; zainake99@gmail.com
4 Korle-Bu Teaching Hospital, Accra P.O. Box 77, Ghana; d.ankrah@kbth.gov.gh
5 LEKMA Hospital, P.M. B Teshie, Nungua, Accra P.O. Box CT104, Ghana; mawuenaasima@gmail.com
6 Department of Pharmacy, University Teaching Hospital, Lusaka P.O. Box 50001, Zambia; banda.chimbi@gmail.com
7 Pharmacy Department, North Tyneside Hospital, Northumbria Healthcare NHS Foundation Trust, Rake Lane, North Shields NE29 8NH, UK; Scott.Barrett@northumbria-healthcare.nhs.uk (S.B.); Joseph.Brayson@northumbria-healthcare.nhs.uk (J.B.)
8 Buckinghamshire Healthcare NHS Trust, Amersham HP7 0JD, UK; claire.brandish@nhs.net
9 Kilimanjaro Christian Medical Centre, Moshi P.O. Box 3010, Tanzania; peterbenedict55@gmail.com
10 School of Pharmacy, University of Health and Allied Sciences, PMB 31, Ho, Ghana; cdodoo@uhas.edu.gh
11 Manchester University NHS Foundation Trust, Oxford Road, Manchester M13 9WL, UK; frances.garraghan@mft.nhs.uk
12 St. Mary's Hospital Lacor, Gulu P.O. Box 180, Uganda; oyella.josephine@lacorhospital.org
13 Centre for Medicines Optimisation Research and Education, University College London Hospitals NHS Foundation Trust, 250 Euston Road, London NW1 2PG, UK; yogini.jani@nhs.net
14 Sustainable Pharmaceutical Systems (SPS) Unit, Pharmacy Department, School of Health Sciences, Makerere University, Kampala P.O. Box 7062, Uganda; freddy.kitutu@mak.ac.ug
15 Entebbe Regional Referral Hospital, Entebbe P.O. Box 29, Uganda; ismailkizito11@gmail.com
16 Medical Microbiology Department, University of Ghana Medical School, Accra P.O. Box GP 4236, Ghana; aklabi@ug.edu.gh (A.-K.L.); jaopintan@ug.edu.gh (J.A.O.)
17 North Middlesex University Hospital NHS Trust, London N18 1QX, UK; mariyam.mirfenderesky@nhs.net
18 UCL School of Pharmacy, University College London, 29-39 Brunswick Square, London WC1N 1AX, UK; s.murdan@ucl.ac.uk
19 St. Francis Hospital, Katete Private Bag 11, Zambia; caoimhe.murray@nhs.net
20 Department of Medical Laboratory Sciences, University of Ghana School of Biomedical and Allied Health Sciences, Accra P.O. Box LG 25, Ghana; nobeng-nkrumah@ug.edu.gh
21 Jinja Regional Referral Hospital, Jinja P.O. Box 43, Uganda; pjathim@gmail.com
22 Liverpool School of Tropical Medicine, Liverpool L3 5QA, UK; 248964@lstmed.ac.uk
23 Laboratory of Medical Microbiology, Vaccine & Infectious Disease Institute (VAXINFECTIO), Faculty of Medicine and Health Sciences, University of Antwerp, Universiteitsplein 1, 2610 Antwerp, Belgium; Ines.Pauwels@uantwerpen.be (I.P.); ann.versporten@uantwerpen.be (A.V.)
24 Department of Pharmacy, Keta Municipal Hospital, Keta-Dzelukope P.O. Box WT82, Ghana; isefah@uhas.edu.gh
25 Scottish Antimicrobial Prescribing Group, Healthcare Improvement Scotland, Delta House, 50 West Nile Street, Glasgow G1 2NP, UK; jacqueline.sneddon@nhs.scot
26 Brighton and Sussex University Hospitals NHS Trust, Brighton BN1 9PX, UK; anja.st.clair-jones@nhs.net
* Correspondence: diane.ashiru-oredope@phe.gov.uk or diane.ashiruoredope@commonwealthpharmacy.org

Abstract: Antimicrobial resistance (AMR) remains an important global public health issue with antimicrobial misuse and overuse being one of the main drivers. The Global Point Prevalence Survey (G-PPS) of Antimicrobial Consumption and Resistance assesses the prevalence and the quality of antimicrobial prescriptions across hospitals globally. G-PPS was carried out at 17 hospitals across Ghana, Uganda, Zambia and Tanzania. The overall prevalence of antimicrobial use was 50% (30–57%), with most antibiotics prescribed belonging to the WHO 'Access' and 'Watch' categories. No 'Reserve' category of antibiotics was prescribed across the study sites while antimicrobials belonging to the 'Not Recommended' group were prescribed infrequently. Antimicrobials were most often prescribed for prophylaxis for obstetric or gynaecological surgery, making up between 12 and 18% of total prescriptions across all countries. The most prescribed therapeutic subgroup of antimicrobials was 'Antibacterials for systemic use'. As a result of the programme, PPS data are now readily available for the first time in the hospitals, strengthening the global commitment to improved antimicrobial surveillance. Antimicrobial stewardship interventions developed included the formation of AMS committees, the provision of training and the preparation of new AMS guidelines. Other common interventions included the presentation of findings to clinicians for increased awareness, and the promotion of a multi-disciplinary approach to successful AMS programmes. Repeat PPS would be necessary to continually monitor the impact of interventions implemented. Broader participation is also encouraged to strengthen the evidence base.

Keywords: antimicrobial resistance; global-pps; antimicrobial surveillance; antibiotics; antimicrobials; antimicrobial stewardship

1. Introduction

Antimicrobial resistance (AMR) is a global, public, and individual health challenge affecting the delivery of safe, effective healthcare in all settings and all countries. The ability of microorganisms to become resistant to the effect of antimicrobials is an inevitable evolutionary process; however, misuse and over-use of antimicrobial agents hastens the development and spread [1,2].

AMR leads to increased mortality rates [3] and duration and cost of patient care [1]. This is of particular concern in low- and middle-income countries (LMICs) due to the reduced availability of appropriate equipment and/or appropriate diagnostic tools, as well as challenges with access to quality antimicrobials [4–7]. The rise in incidence of AMR has led to an increased global focus on antimicrobial stewardship (AMS). Surveillance of antimicrobial use and resistance are core to all AMS activities and understanding how antimicrobials are used allows for a review of current practices and highlights areas for improvement. Point prevalence surveys (PPSs) are a widely recognised surveillance method requiring limited resources to collect information on antimicrobial prescribing practices and other relevant factors in hospitalized patients [8–11].

PPS are a key resource when planning and supporting national and local stewardship interventions in a range of settings, offering a standardised method for comparing data on antimicrobial use across hospitals and countries. The Global Point Prevalence Survey of Antimicrobial Consumption and Resistance (G-PPS; www.global-pps.com/, accessed on 15 May 2021) aims to assess the global prevalence of antimicrobial prescribing and resistance, with an emphasis on countries with low resources, support, and expertise and supports antimicrobial stewardship programs in order to enhance appropriate antimicrobial prescribing [12].

Alongside the evaluation of antimicrobial prescribing practices in hospitals, PPS can identify targets for quality improvement of antimicrobial prescribing and implement and monitor the impact of interventions through repeated surveys. One of the main aims in strengthening global AMS is to reduce the use of antimicrobials that are in the World Health Organization's (WHO) 'Watch' and 'Reserve categories' and 'Not Recommended' group of their AWaRe framework [13,14]. The framework recommends preferred antimicrobial choice for treating common infections—the 'Access' category, based on consideration of benefits versus risks to patients and the potential for resistance. An additional classification—'Not recommended' was added to the framework more recently to include fixed-dose combinations of broad-spectrum antibiotics for which use is not evidence-based [15]. Similarly, the Anatomic Therapeutic Chemical (ATC) classification categorizes drugs active substances into different groups and subgroups according to their therapeutic, pharmacological and chemical properties. WHO endorses the ATC classification as the standard for drug utilization monitoring and research [16].

The Commonwealth Partnerships for Antimicrobial Stewardship programme (CwPAMS), managed by the Commonwealth Pharmacists Association (CPA) and Tropical Health and Education Trust (THET), is a health partnerships programme funded by the UK Official Development Assistance (ODA), through the Department of Health and Social Care's Fleming Fund to address AMR globally [17]. The aim of the programme is to enhance the implementation of protocols and evidenced-based decision making to support antimicrobial prescribing and the capacity for surveillance of antimicrobial consumption and stewardship.

The CwPAMS programme included 12 partnerships between UK health institutions and counterparts in four African Commonwealth countries: Ghana (GH), Uganda (UG), Zambia (ZM), and Tanzania (TZ). The partnerships consisted of volunteer health workers and experts from the five countries who shared skills and knowledge to co-develop strategies to address AMR and AMS. As part of the fulfillment of the aims of the partnership, a Global Point Prevalence Study was used to obtain baseline data and measure the impact of the implementation of AMS programmes across partnership countries.

This paper aims to compare national data on antimicrobial use obtained from 12 hospitals across four countries (Ghana (6), Uganda (4), Zambia (1) and Tanzania (1)) and identify target points for improvement. As part of an additional collaboration, PPS data from a further four hospitals in Ghana and one additional hospital in Zambia (which collected data using the Global PPS platform during the same period as the CwPAMS programme), are also included in the study.

2. Results

2.1. Characteristics of Included Hospitals and Eligible Patients

A total of 4376 patients were included in the survey, with 2169 (50%) treated with antimicrobials across the four countries. From the total number of treated patients, 1366 (63%) were from 10 hospitals in Ghana, 386 (17.8%) from four hospitals in Uganda, 238 (11%) from two hospitals in Zambia, and 179 (8%) from one hospital in Tanzania (Table 1). Of the 17 hospitals included, 3 were identified as primary care, 6 as secondary care and 8 as tertiary care. Additionally, eight hospitals were classed as teaching hospitals, three in both Uganda and Ghana and one in both Zambia and Tanzania.

Table 1 summarises the general characteristics of the patients surveyed across the four countries. More adults were included across all sites than children or neonates. A greater proportion of children were included in Uganda (35%) than the other three countries (Ghana (19%), Tanzania (16%), Zambia (15%). Activities of the wards where patients were surveyed were relatively uniform across the countries, with patients on intensive care wards (IC) making up the smallest proportion of those surveyed (4–20%).

Table 1. Characteristics of wards and patients (treated with at least one antimicrobial) in PPS conducted at 17 hospitals.

Characteristics	Ghana	Uganda	Zambia	Tanzania
Number of Hospitals	10	4	2	1
Number of Treated Patients	1366	386	238	179
Patient Age				
Neonate (≤1 month)	150 (11%)	20 (5%)	32 (13%)	34 (19%)
Child (>1 month–≤17 years)	261 (19%)	136 (35%)	35 (15%)	29 (16%)
Adult (≥18 years)	955 (70%)	214 (56%)	171 (72%)	116 (65%)
Unknown	-	16 (4%)	-	-
Patient Gender				
Male	570 (41.7%)	162 (42%)	96 (40%)	93 (52%)
Female	794 (58.1%)	205 (53%)	142 (60%)	84 (46.9%)
Unknown	2 (0.2%)	19 (5%)	-	2 (1.1%)
Ward Activity				
Medicine	76 (46%)	28 (54%)	9 (45%)	7 (35%)
Surgery	74 (45%)	22 (42%)	7 (35%)	10 (50%)
Intensive Care	15 (9%)	2 (4%)	4 (20%)	3 (15%)

2.2. Prevalence of Antimicrobial Use

The prevalence of antimicrobial use (AMU) was 50% from the 17 sites across the four countries (Table 2). The proportion of patients treated with antimicrobials at the time of the survey was highest in Zambia (57%), followed by Ghana (55%) and Uganda (45%), and was lowest in Tanzania (30%).

Table 2. Prevalence of antimicrobial use in four countries included in PPS.

Country	Admitted Patients	Treated Patients	Prevalence of AMU (%)
Ghana	2502	1366	55
Uganda	862	386	45
Zambia	418	238	57
Tanzania	594	179	30
Total	4376	2169	50

There was a total of 3838 prescriptions recorded in the survey, 2435 (63%) of which were reported from hospitals in Ghana, 710 (18.5%) from Uganda, 402 (10.5%) from Zambia, and 290 (7.5%) from Tanzania.

Of these prescriptions, those in the ATC J01 category (antibacterials for systemic use) were further classified into each of the WHO AWaRe categories (Figure 1). There was no reported use (0%) of the Reserve category of antibiotics in any of the four countries.

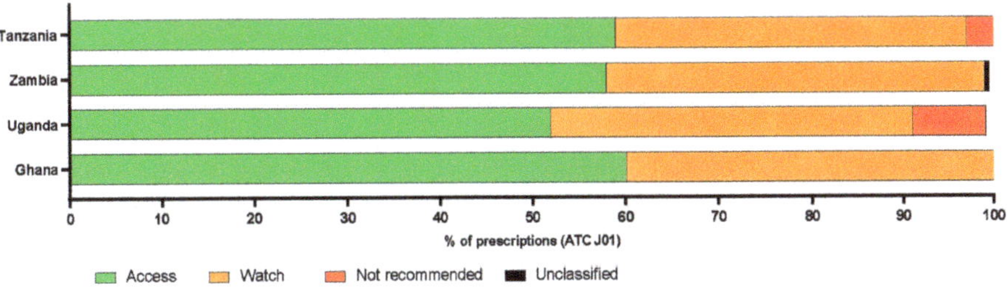

Figure 1. The proportion of antibiotics in the ACT J01 group prescribed in each of four countries.

Antibiotics in the WHO access category were prescribed more frequently than those in other categories across all countries and were prescribed at similar rates, accounting for 60% of the total of ATC J01 antibiotics prescribed in Ghana (1212/2071), 52% in Uganda (309/592), 58% in Zambia (201/347), and 59% in Tanzania (170/288) (Figure 1). Antibiotics in the Watch category were the second most frequently prescribed, again with proportions being similar for all countries (Ghana 42%; *n* = 851, Uganda 39%; *n* = 232, Zambia 41% *n* = 143, Tanzania 38%; *n* = 109). There was no reported use (0%) of the Reserve category antibiotics in any of the four countries.

'Not Recommended' antibiotic combinations were prescribed in Uganda, Tanzania, and Ghana. Ugandan hospitals had the highest prescription rate of these drugs (8%; 48/592) with 47 prescriptions of Ampiclox®® (ampicillin and cloxacillin) (7% of total prescriptions) and one of ciprofloxacin and metronidazole. In Tanzania, Ampiclox®® was prescribed on 9 occasions (3% of total prescriptions). In Ghana, the "Not Recommended" group of antibiotics made up 0.2% of antibiotic prescriptions (4/1212) with ceftriaxone/beta-lactamase inhibitor being prescribed twice, ceftriaxone in combination with another unspecified antibiotic prescribed once and penicillin in combination with another, unspecified antibacterial also prescribed once. Unclassified antibiotics were prescribed very infrequently in all countries.

The proportion of antimicrobials used, as grouped according to the ATC classification level 1, is shown in Table 3. For all countries, antibacterials for systemic use (J01) were the most frequently prescribed, making up 83–99% of prescriptions. Additionally, in Ghana, Uganda, and Zambia, antiprotozoals used as antibacterials (P01AB) made up 4–10% of the prescriptions. Uganda had the highest proportion of prescriptions for antimalarials (P01B) at 4.6% of the total and drugs for treatment of tuberculosis (J04A) at 4.5% of the total. Rates for antibiotics used as intestinal anti-infectives (A07AA), antimycotics and antifungals for systemic use (J02; D01BA) and antivirals for systemic use (J05) were low (0–2%) for all four countries.

Table 3. Proportional antimicrobial use by country grouped by therapeutic subgroup.

Therapeutic Subgroup	Proportional Antimicrobial Use (% of Prescriptions)			
	Ghana	Uganda	Zambia	Tanzania
Antibacterials for systemic use (J01)	85.1	83.4	86.3	99.3
Antimycotics and antifungals for systemic use (J02; D01BA)	0.8	1.3	2.2	0.3
Drugs for treatment of tuberculosis (J04A)	1.2	4.5	0.2	0
Antibiotics used as intestinal anti-infectives (A07AA)	0.5	0.3	0.2	0
Antiprotozoals used as antibacterial agents (P01AB)	8.3	4.2	10.2	0.3
Antivirals for systemic use (J05)	1.4	1.7	0	0
Antimalarials (P01B)	2.8	4.6	0.7	0

The most prescribed antimicrobial across Ghanaian hospitals was metronidazole for systemic use (12% of total prescriptions; 288/2435), compared to ceftriaxone which was prescribed most frequently in the three other countries; Uganda 24% (173/710), Zambia 21% (83/402), and Tanzania 32% (94/290). Full details of the proportions of antimicrobials prescribed in each country can be found in the supplementary data (Tables S1 and S2).

2.3. *Reason for Prescribing Antimicrobials*

The main reasons for prescribing antimicrobials for each country are shown in Figure 2. Across all countries, antimicrobials were most often prescribed for prophylaxis for obstetric or gynaecological surgery, making up between 12 and 18% of total prescriptions (Figure 2). Antimicrobials were next most frequently prescribed for pneumonia or lower respiratory tract infections, in all but Tanzania, where drugs used as medical prophylaxis for new-born risk factors was the second most common reason for prescribing (15% of total).

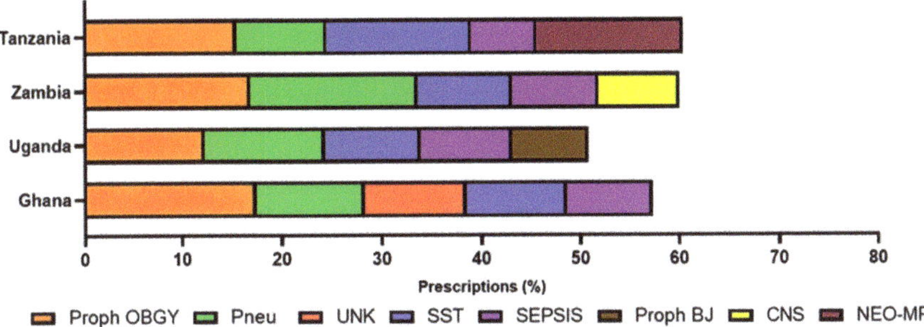

Figure 2. Most common reason for prescribing antimicrobials across 17 hospitals participating in the PPS.

In Ghana, the third most common reason for prescribing was to treat skin and soft tissue infections (equal to prescriptions for completely unknown infections). Uganda had a higher prescription rate for prophylaxis for plastic or orthopaedic surgery than other countries (8%) and prescriptions for infections of the central nervous system were higher in Zambia (8%). Drugs were frequently prescribed for sepsis across all countries (7–9%).

Across all four countries, antimicrobials were frequently prescribed for prophylaxis. This practice was highest in Tanzania, with 48% of all prescribed antimicrobials being for prophylaxis. This was followed by in Ghana (33%), Uganda (27%) and Zambia (27%).

Proph OBGY—prophylaxis for obstetric or gynaecological surgery (caesarean section, no episiotomy, carriage of group B streptococcus); pneu—pneumonia or lower respiratory tract infections; UNK—prescriptions for completely unknown infections; SST—skin and soft tissue infections (cellulitis, wound including surgical site infection, deep soft tissue not involving bone, e.g., infected pressure or diabetic ulcer, abscess); proph BJ—prophylaxis for plastic or orthopaedic surgery (bone or joint); CNS—prescriptions for infections of the central nervous system; NEO-MP—medical prophylaxis for new-born risk factors, e.g., VLBW (very low birth weight) and IUGR (intrauterine growth restriction).

Out of 4376 admitted inpatients, 237 patients (5.4%; range 4.1% in Uganda to 5.1% in Zambia) were treated with antibiotics for systemic use (ATC J01) for at least one healthcare associated infection. Table 4 shows the types of indication for which antimicrobials were prescribed by country. Out of all therapeutic prescribing, community-acquired infections were the most common indication for antimicrobial use. Surgical prophylaxis of >1 day (SP3) was common in all countries, up to 97% of all prescriptions for surgical prophylaxis in Tanzania and Uganda (Table 4). Ghana recorded most antimicrobial prescriptions for which the indication was not known (11%).

Table 4. Type of indication for antimicrobial prescribing.

	Ghana	Tanzania	Uganda	Zambia
Total Number of Prescriptions	2435	290	710	402
Therapeutic use	1344 (55.2%)	134 (46.2%)	477 (67.2%)	288 (71.6%)
Community-Acquired infection; CAI	1074 (79.9%)	89 (66.4%)	416 (87.2%)	257 (89.2%)
Healthcare-Associated Infection; HAI	270 (20.1%)	45 (33.6%)	61 (12.8%)	31 (10.8%)
Prophylactic use	805 (33.1%)	145 (50.7%)	225 (31.7%)	102 (25.4%)
Medical Prophylaxis; MP	172 (7%)	46 (16%)	50 (7%)	17 (4%)
Surgical Prophylaxis; SP	633 (26.0%)	99 (34.1%)	175 (24.6%)	85 (21.1%)
Surgical Prophylaxis One dose; SP1	42 (6.6%)	3 (3.0%)	2 (1.1%)	1 (1.1%)
Surgical Prophylaxis One day; SP2	113 (17.9%)	0 (0%)	3 (1.7%)	2 (2.3%)
Surgical Prophylaxis > 1 day; SP3	478 (75.5%)	96 (97.0%)	170 (97.1%)	83 (96.5%)
Other (OTH)	19 (0.7%)	1 (0.3%)	1 (0.1%)	8 (2%)
Unknown (UNK)	267 (11%)	10 (3%)	7 (1%)	4 (1%)

As mentioned above, one common indication for prescribing antimicrobials in all countries was for prophylaxis for obstetric or gynaecological surgery. The types of antimicrobials prescribed for this indication differed across the four countries. In participating hospitals in Ghana, 16 different drugs were prescribed for OBGY prophylaxis (Table 5), with metronidazole comprising 44% of prescriptions for this indication (186/425). This was split relatively evenly between oral (95/186; 22% of total number of prescriptions) and parenteral administration (91/186; 21.4% of total prescriptions). Of the 186 times metronidazole was prescribed, it was co-administered with another antimicrobial (88%; 164/186). When given orally, it was most commonly prescribed with co-amoxiclav; amoxicillin/clavulanic acid (42/95) and, when given parenterally, it was most commonly prescribed with co-amoxiclav (23/91) or ceftriaxone (22/91).

Table 5. Antimicrobials prescribed for prophylactic OBGY purposes in Ghana (% of total) and AWaRe group.

ATC Code	Drug	% of Prescriptions for Proph-OBGY	AWaRe Classification
P01AB01	Oral Metronidazole	22.4	Access
J01XD01	Parenteral Metronidazole	21.4	Access
J01CF02	Co-amoxiclav/Amoxicillin and enzyme inhibitor	21.6	Access
J01DC02	Cefuroxime	11.8	Watch
J01CA04	Amoxicillin	9.9	Access
J01DD04	Ceftriaxone	6.4	Watch
J01MA02	Ciprofloxacin	1.6	Watch
J01GB03	Gentamicin	1.4	Access
J01FF01	Clindamycin	1	Access
J01FA10	Azithromycin	0.5	Watch
J01AA02	Doxycycline	0.5	Access
J01MA12	Levofloxacin	0.5	Watch
P01AB07	Secnidazole	0.5	Unclassified
J01DD13	Cefpodoxime	0.2	Watch
J01CF05	Flucloxacillin	0.2	Access
J02AC01	Fluconazole	0.2	Unclassified

Again, in Ghana, co-amoxiclav was prescribed as a single agent on 19% of occasions (81/425) and, as described, frequently co-administered with metronidazole (65/186). Cefuroxime was the next most frequently prescribed on 12% of occasions (50/425). The top two drugs that were most prescribed in the participating hospitals in Ghana were in the access category, whereas ceftriaxone is in the Watch category. Whilst the most common reason for prescribing antimicrobials was the same for the other 3 countries, there was less variation in drug type (Figure 3).

In Uganda, metronidazole and ceftriaxone were prescribed together frequently for proph OBGY. Metronidazole was prescribed 47.1% of total prescriptions for proph OBGY (41/87) and ceftriaxone 44% (38/87) (Figure 3). They were co-prescribed on 37 occasions, with ceftriaxone only being prescribed alone once for this indication. All but two prescriptions for metronidazole were parenteral administration.

Metronidazole and ceftriaxone were both prescribed for proph OBGY with the same frequency in Tanzania (49%) but were not co-administered on any occasion to the same patient. Metronidazole was also the most prescribed antimicrobial for prophylactic OBGY purposes in Zambia (44%) and was frequently co-administered with amoxicillin (22%) (Figure 3).

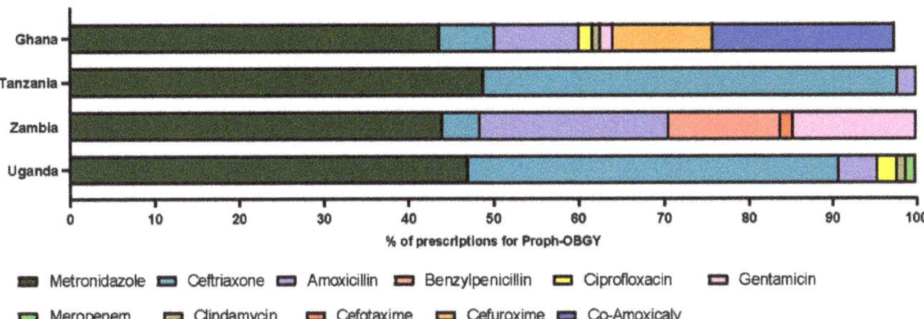

Figure 3. Antimicrobials prescribed for Prophylactic OBGY purposes in four countries (% of total). For Ghana, antimicrobials making up < 1% of prescriptions have been omitted for clarity.

2.4. Antibiotic Prescription by AWaRe Categories and Age, Gender and Countries

Based on a chi-squared test conducted on the general dataset, there was a significant association between antibiotic prescription across the AWaRe categories and countries ($X^2 = 43.80$, $p < 0.001$), gender ($X^2 = 24.81$, $p < 0.001$) and age ($X^2 = 97.74$, $p < 0.001$). From country-specific analysis, there was a significant association between gender and antibiotic prescription across the AWaRe categories in Ghana ($X^2 = 26.67$, $p < 0.001$) and Zambia ($X^2 = 14.12$, $p < 0.001$) while the association was not significant in Uganda ($X^2 = 1.46$, $p = 0.482$) and Tanzania ($X^2 = 0.41$, $p = 0.815$). Furthermore, there was a significant association between age and antibiotic prescription across the AWaRe categories in Ghana ($X^2 = 42.23$, $p < 0.001$), Tanzania ($X^2 = 58.50$, $p < 0.001$) and Uganda ($X^2 = 22.68$, $p < 0.001$). A summary of the statistics is available in Supplementary Tables S3–S5.

2.5. Quality Indicators for Prescribing

Quality indicators for all prescriptions were recorded during each survey and include criteria from the GPPS protocol [18] as shown in Table 6. Stop/review dates (i.e., whether a date of review or stop date of the antimicrobial was recorded in the medical records) were almost always reported in both Uganda (99% of prescriptions) and Tanzania (99%). Indications for prescriptions were well-documented ranging from 66% of all prescriptions in Ghana to 97% in Uganda. The proportion of prescriptions that were guideline-compliant varied widely among the four countries from 55% in Zambia, to 88% in Tanzania (Table 6). Ghana most frequently reported the absence of antimicrobial prescription guidelines (13%). Moreover, in Ghana, in 1096 antimicrobial prescriptions (45%), the information with respect to the guidelines was not assessable because the indication was unknown.

Table 6. Proportion of total prescriptions of all antimicrobials for each of the 4 quality indicators (% of total).

Quality Indicator	Ghana	Uganda	Zambia	Tanzania
Total number of prescriptions	2435	710	402	290
Prescriptions with a documented stop/review date	1579 (67%)	700 (99%)	82 (20%)	289 (99%)
Prescriptions with a documented indication	1601 (66%)	687 (97%)	321 (80%)	248 (86%)
Prescriptions that were guideline-compliant *	858 (84%)	413 (67%)	195 (55%)	237 (88%)
Prescriptions for which no guidelines were available (NA)	313 (13%)	36 (5%)	38 (10%)	1 (0.3%)

* Guideline compliance is calculated as compliance to guidelines (Yes) when guidelines are existing (Yes + No).

2.6. Antimicrobial Stewardship Interventions as a Result of PPS

The key antimicrobial stewardship interventions that were implemented as a result of the PPS data in the CwPAMS programme institutions are summarised in Table 7 with further details in SInfo1: Antimicrobial Stewardship Intervention summaries.

Table 7. AMS interventions at 16 of the 17 hospitals in response to the PPS carried out.

	Hospital															
AMS Intervention	**1**	**2**	**3**	**4**	**5**	**6**	**7**	**8**	**9**	**10**	**11**	**12**	**13**	**14**	**15**	**16**
New guidelines developed	X	X		X	X	X	X	X		X	X			X		
Catalyst for forming AMS committee	X	X	X	X					X	X	X	X	X	X	X	X
Improved access to guidelines through:																
Posters	X	X	X													
Printed copies		X	X								X					X
Promotion of CwPAMS app	X	X		X					X		X			X		
Other: Please state												X				
Training sessions	X	X	X	X	X	X	X	X	X	X	X	X	X	X	X	
Repeat PPS conducted and submitted G-PPS platform	X		X	X										X		
Repeat PPS conducted and analysed internally	X	X	X	X					X		X			X		X
AMS awareness raising	X	X	X	X					X	X	X	X		X		
Data presented to clinicians	X	X	X	X	X	X	X	X	X	X				X		
Data presented to AMS committee or DTC	X	X	X	X					X		X			X	X	
Activities for WAAW	X	X	X	X					X					X		
Antibiogram developed			X													
Drug chart updated or created		X											X			X
Improved laboratory services			X		X	X	X	X			X			X		
Other: Please list below																
Quality improvement project on prescriber's adherence to antibiotics for ambulatory pneumonia management Outpatient A/B prescribing survey		X	X													
Engagement with external stakeholders			X								X					

No details provided by hospital 17.

3. Discussion

The Point Prevalence Surveys presented provide key insights into antibiotic prescribing in selected public or not-for-profit hospitals across Ghana, Tanzania, Uganda, and Zambia. The overall prevalence of antimicrobial use was 50% (30–57%), with most antibiotics prescribed belonging to the WHO 'Access' and 'Watch' groups. No 'Reserve' category antibiotics were prescribed across the study sites; however, there were some prescriptions of 'Not Recommended' antibiotic combinations. While this pattern of antibiotic use may partly be due to the prescriber's consideration of optimality and potential for antimicrobial resistance, in line with WHO's goal of improving antibiotic use through antimicrobial stewardship [19], other authors suggest alternative reasoning [20,21].

Antibiotic prescribing patterns were significantly associated with accessibility and affordability, with broad-spectrum antibiotics in the Access category being more readily available and affordable than antibiotics in the Watch and Reserve categories and the 'Not Recommended' group [20,21]. A recent study on antibiotic availability and use in 20 low- and middle-income countries reported that the median proportion of facilities across countries with availability of Access category antibiotics was 89.5% [22]. Pauwels et al. (2021) reported that low-income countries had the highest percentage of use of Access category antibiotics (63%), the lowest use of Watch category antibiotics (36%) and no Reserve category prescriptions on adult wards across 69 countries [23]. A PPS conducted across six referral hospitals in Tanzania also supports data presented in the current study, reporting 62% of prescriptions for in-patients being from the Access group [24]. In addition to availability and affordability, the similarity in prescription patterns across all four countries in the current study might be associated with the circulating bacterial strains and disease burden across low- and middle-income countries [6,7,25]. The WHO proposes that the AWaRe classification should support monitoring of antibiotic prescribing and inform AMS programmes and has the target that by 2023 at least 60% of national antibiotic consumption should come from the Access category [15]. In data presented here, 60% of the total of ATC J01 antibiotics prescribed in Ghana (1212/2071), 52% in Uganda (309/592), 58% in Zambia (201/347) and 59% in Tanzania (170/288) were in the Access category, demonstrating the hospitals' alignment with the WHO target for national antibiotic consumption.

The antibiotics most commonly prescribed across hospitals in all four countries in the current study were metronidazole and ceftriaxone, with metronidazole being the most prescribed antibiotic across Ghanaian hospitals. These findings are supported by data from the Pauwels et al. study across 69 countries, where ceftriaxone was the most commonly used antibiotic for therapeutic use on adult wards worldwide. In the same study, up to 24% of prescriptions for surgical prophylaxis in sub-Saharan Africa were for metronidazole, followed by ceftriaxone (23%) [23]. A PPS carried at the Korle-Bu Teaching Hospital in Ghana (2018) reported metronidazole as the most frequently prescribed antibiotic, followed by amoxicillin-clavulanic acid, cephalosporins (ceftriaxone, cefuroxime), and cloxacillin [26]. A PPS in Kenya also recorded a higher use of nitroimidazoles compared to beta-lactam antibiotics [27]. Furthermore, a PPS in three hospitals in north-eastern Tanzania reported ceftriaxone, metronidazole, and penicillin as the most prescribed antibiotics [28].

Metronidazole is effective in the treatment of a broad range of anaerobic infections which may be more common in African countries [29]. Metronidazole was used in addition to co-amoxiclav, so this could perhaps be an area to target to reduce use if anaerobic infections are covered by use of other antibiotics. This highlights that it might be useful to increase the awareness and understanding of antibiotic sensitivity. The findings presented here show that metronidazole was primarily prescribed for prophylaxis for obstetrics and gynaecology. Published data demonstrate a similarity between the most commonly prescribed antibiotics in PPSs carried out in other low-income countries. This could be explained by the affordability, availability, and the spectrum of activity of metronidazole and ceftriaxone, as well as their suitability for prophylaxis in certain obstetric and gynaecological procedures [30]. However, the broad-spectrum activity of some antibiotics, particularly cephalosporins, can lead to the over-growth of other bacteria that are resistant to their activity, for example *Clostridiodies difficile*, methicillin-resistant *Staphylococcus aureus* (MRSA), and vancomycin-resistant enterococci (VRE) [31,32]. The use of cephalosporins, in particular, and third-generation drugs such as ceftriaxone, are linked to the rise in incidence of extended-spectrum beta-lactamase (ESBLs)-producing bacteria, leading to a reduction of effective antibiotics [33,34]. Therefore, there remains a need to evaluate prescriber's choices and the frequent prescription of ceftriaxone, which falls within the Watch group of antibiotics in the WHO AWaRe categories.

Reasons for antimicrobial prescribing in other published studies demonstrate a similar pattern to the current study, with lower respiratory tract infections and medical and surgical prophylaxis presented as common reasons for prescribing [24,25]. Prophylaxis for obstetric or gynaecological surgery was the most frequent reason for prescribing in the current study. Although the reasons for antimicrobial prescribing were similar across all four countries, Uganda had the highest prescription rates for antimalarials, drugs for the treatment of tuberculosis (TB). The WHO Global Tuberculosis Report (2020) reported Zambia having the highest incidence of TB (of the four countries included here) in 2019 (300–499 incidences per 100,000 population per year), followed by Tanzania (200–299 incidences per 100,000 population per year) and Ghana and Uganda having similar, lower rates (10–99 incidences per 100,000 population per year) [35]. It is possible that there were localised TB and malaria outbreaks in the regions where the Ugandan hospitals were, but data are not available to confirm or deny this. This data may also be influenced by the time of year the PPS was carried out. If the PPS was conducted in the rainy season, then prescriptions for antimalarials might be higher than if the PPS was done in the dry seasons. The reason for this could also be that TB detection methods may be more robust in Uganda, which may explain the lower prevalence of disease but higher use of drugs. Further analysis and PPS would be required to explain the higher observed rates for unclassified antimicrobials and drugs used in the treatment of TB and malaria seen in Uganda. Antimicrobials were often prescribed when indication was documented (Figure 2). There is a need to improve diagnostic capacity as diagnostic uncertainty might lead to the increase of antimicrobial prescribing [36].

From the 4376 admitted inpatients across the 4 countries, 5.4% were treated with antibiotics for systemic use for at least one healthcare-associated infection (HCAI). Out of all therapeutic prescribing, community acquired infections were the most common reason for antimicrobial use. The rates of HCAI were similar to a large study conducted across acute care facilities in 28 countries in the EU/EAA, where 6.5% of patients had at least one HCAI [37]. Although the European study was conducted over a much larger sample group, the data show a trend towards similar rates of HCAI in the data presented in this study.

The chi-squared test of association revealed significant associations between age, gender, countries, and AWaRe categories. Although the exact nature of the relationship between variables is uncertain, the summary statistics (Supplementary Material: Tables S3–S5) provide more insight into these associations. As observed from descriptive analysis, reasons for antibiotic prescribing differ across populations with some age-specific indications such as 'medical prophylaxis for new-born risk factors' mostly observed in Tanzania and Uganda and gender-specific indications such as 'prophylaxis for obstetric or gynaecological surgery' observed across all countries. While these partly explain significant associations between antibiotic prescribing, gender, and age in specific countries and the general population, our results reflect country-specific trends worthy of further investigation.

Through the Global PPS programme and CwPAMS (for the participating hospitals), all partnerships and additional hospitals in Ghana and Zambia have demonstrated the strengthening of their healthcare workforce knowledge and capacity (Table 7) in the areas of antimicrobial use surveillance and AMS. Prior to the programme, although other hospitals had collated antimicrobial use data through PPS methodology, only one hospital in the four countries had previously conducted data collection to the scale of the Global PPS.

Translating PPS findings into contextualised interventions can be challenging but all CwPAMS health partnerships and hospitals involved have provided information regarding key AMS interventions taken as a result of the Global PPS undertaken at their institutions. These are summarised in Table 7 (for the full text, see Supplementary Data). In an evaluation of the impact of the Global-PPS on local AMS programmes, prolonged surgical antibiotic prophylaxis was the most common target for improvement identified [38]. This study also highlights the need to focus on prolonged surgical antibiotic prophylaxis considering that prescriptions for more than one day for surgical prophylaxis were common. However, antibiotics are only one component that can be used to reduce SSI. The inability to ensure a sterile environment and optimal IPC conditions may result in overuse or antibiotics.

Variations in quality indicators were observed across countries. Consistent with this study, the PPS in 6 reference hospitals in Tanzania observed an 84% adherence of antibiotic prescriptions to the National Standard Treatment Guideline [24]. Similarly, a multi-centre PPS in Ghana also recorded a level of non-compliance to national antimicrobial standard treatment guidelines [39]. The variations observed could be influenced by varying national antimicrobial prescribing policies, hospital protocols and the effectiveness of antimicrobial stewardship intervention programs in study centres across all four countries.

The consistency of data collection via the G-PPS methodology adds rigor and validity to the data presented here. The study demonstrates inclusivity with data obtained from 17 hospitals across four countries in 3 African regions, coupled with a good representation of gender, age groups, and hospital sections. In addition, data were collected by trained health professionals working, for the most part, as part of the Commonwealth Partnerships for Antimicrobial Stewardship.

4. Materials and Methods

Training on the collection of surveillance data for the G-PPS reported in this paper was provided to the CwPAMS health partnerships by the Global PPS team and the CPA, supporting the development of evidence-based standards, guidelines, protocols and the development of a mentorship programme to support sustainability. UK volunteers who had experience of PPS also provided mentorship and in-country support during their visits to Ghana, Uganda, Zambia, and Tanzania. Data collection was carried out by volunteers from individual health partnerships. PPS were conducted between May and December 2019, using the G-PPS methodology as described elsewhere [18]. Data from 17 hospitals across four countries: ten in Ghana, four in Uganda, two in Zambia and one in Tanzania were collected and analysed. Follow-up data were collected in a second PPS for two hospitals but only the data from the first survey are included here.

Age of patients were defined as: adult ($\geq$18 years) Child (>1 month–$\leq$17 years) or neonate ($\leq$1 month). Gender, age, diagnosis (reason for prescribing), indication (therapeutic versus prophylactic prescribing), routes of administration, prescribed antimicrobials dosing regimen, and causative microorganisms were all recorded. Data collection also included a set of prescription-related quality indicators; Prescriptions with a documented stop/review date, prescriptions with a documented indication, prescriptions that were guideline compliant and prescriptions for which no guidelines were available. The G-PPS data collection form is available via: https://www.global-pps.com/documents/ (accessed on 15 September 2021).

Hospitals were classified as primary, secondary, or tertiary care hospitals. All inpatients admitted at 8 a.m. on the day of the PPS were included and data were analysed by country and ward type. The included wards were neonatal medical and intensive-care units, paediatric medical, surgical or haematology-oncology ward and intensive-care units and adult medical, pneumology, surgical, haematology-oncology wards, and intensive-care units.

Prescribed antimicrobials were divided into four main categories using the WHO AWaRe classification [14] and further grouped using the 2021 WHO ATC code classification system [20]. AWaRe groups were Access, Watch, Reserve and Not Recommended. Those that were not included in the classification were recorded as unclassified. Antimicrobials were grouped into therapeutic subgroups (ATC 2 level) following the WHO ATC classification system [20]. The therapeutic subgroups were antibacterials for systemic use (J01), antimycotics and antifungals for systemic use (J02 and D01BA including griseofulvin and terbinafine), drugs for treatment of tuberculosis (J04A), antibiotics used as intestinal anti-infectives (A07AA), antiprotozoals used as antibacterial agents, nitroimidazole derivatives (P01AB), antivirals for systemic use (J05) and antimalarials (P01B).

Antimicrobial stewardship interventions as a result of PPS data: leads of all hospitals were asked to provide a short summary of AMS interventions, detailing the actions taken and any follow up data as a result of the PPS.

Data analysis: The results were analyzed descriptively and analytically using the R software (version 4.1.0) and Microsoft Excel (2016). Antimicrobial use prevalence rates were reported by calculating the number of patients on at least one antimicrobial relative to the number of admitted patients at the time of the PPS using Microsoft Excel (2016). The chi-squared test of association was conducted to compare national data on antimicrobial use and identify associations between dependent and independent variables within the dataset using the R software. The tests investigated the association between countries, gender, age groups, and antibiotic prescription across the AWaRe categories. Age was split into three categories namely: neonates (>1 month), children (1 month–17 years), and adults (18 years and above). Statistical significance was set at $p < 0.05$.

Ethics: Formal ethics approval was not required at any hospital as there was no direct patient contact and all data were anonymized. All sites obtained approval from their respective hospital administration. Ethics review and approval was sought and obtained in Uganda and administrative clearance by the participating hospitals was also given. For the four additional sites in Ghana, formal ethical approval was received.

5. Conclusions

The prevalence of antimicrobial use in the hospitals included in this study was 50% (30–57%), with most antibiotics prescribed belonging to the WHO 'Access' and 'Watch' groups. No 'Reserve' category antibiotics were prescribed across the study sites. Not Recommended antibiotics were prescribed, albeit infrequently. This aligns with previously published data in that the 'Access' and 'Watch' category antibiotics are commonly prescribed in LMICs, although to varying extents across countries.

As a result of the CwPAMS health partnership programme and collaboration with other hospitals, PPS data are available for the most part for the first time, strengthening the global commitment to improved antimicrobial surveillance. AMS interventions as a result of the PPSs conducted include formation of AMS committees, preparation of new AMS guidelines and provision of training. Other common interventions included the presentation of findings to clinicians, thus supporting awareness and the multi-disciplinary approach to successful AMS programmes.

In order to continue to monitor the impact of interventions, repeat PPS should be carried out and to strengthen the quality of data, widening participation is encouraged.

Supplementary Materials: The following are available online at https://www.mdpi.com/article/10.3390/antibiotics10091122/s1, Table S1: Most common reason for antimicrobial prescribing across 17 hospitals participating in the PPS, Table S2: Proportional use of ATC level 5-defined antimicrobials in each of 4 countries, Table S3: Countries and Antibiotic Prescription by AWaRe Categories, Table S4: Gender and Antibiotic Prescription by AWaRe Categories, Table S5: Age and Antibiotic Prescription by AWaRe Categories. SInfo1: Antimicrobial Stewardship Intervention summaries.

Author Contributions: Conceptualization, D.A.-O., A.-K.L., N.O.-N. and J.A.O.; Data curation, D.A. (Daniel Afriye), Z.A., D.A. (Daniel Ankrah), D.M.A., D.C.B., S.B., C.B., J.B., P.B., C.C.D., F.G., J.H.S., Y.J., F.E.K., I.M.K., M.M., S.M., C.M., N.O.-N., W.J.O., E.P.-Q., I.S., J.S. and A.S.C.J.; Formal analysis, N.D., D.A.-O. and O.O.; Methodology, D.A.-O., A.-K.L., N.O.-N., J.A.O. and I.P.; Project administration, N.D.; Supervision, D.A.-O.; Writing—original draft, N.D., O.O., I.P. and A.V.; Writing—review and editing, N.D., D.A.-O., D.A. (Daniel Afriye), Z.A., D.A. (Daniel Ankrah), D.M.A., D.C.B., S.B., C.B., J.B., P.B., C.C.D., F.G., J.H.S., Y.J., F.E.K., I.M.K., A.-K.L., M.M., S.M., C.M., N.O.-N., W.J.O., J.A.O., E.P.-Q., I.P., I.S., J.S., A.S.C.J. and A.V. All authors have read and agreed to the published version of the manuscript.

Funding: This was funded by the Department of Health and Social Care using UK aid funding and is managed by the Fleming Fund. The Fleming Fund is a £265 million UK aid investment to tackle antimicrobial resistance by supporting low- and middle- income countries to generate, use, and share data on AMR. The Fleming Fund programme is managed by the UK Department of Health and Social Care. CwPAMS programme is managed by Commonwealth Pharmacists Association and Tropical Health Education Trust (THET). The views expressed in this publication are those of the author and not necessarily those of the Department of Health and Social Care, the NHS, CPA or THET. The Global Point Prevalence Survey is coordinated at the University of Antwerp, Belgium and supported through an unrestricted grant given to them by bioMérieux and personal Methusalem grant to Herman Goossens from the Flemish government; neither funder had a role with any of the CwPAMS projects. None of the funders had any role in the design of the study; in the collection, analyses, or interpretation of data; in the writing of the manuscript, or in the decision to publish the results.

Institutional Review Board Statement: All sites obtained approval from their respective hospital administration. Ethics review and approval was sought and obtained in Uganda and administrative clearance by the participating hospitals was also given. For the four additional sites in Ghana, formal ethical approval was received.

Informed Consent Statement: Not applicable as there was no direct patient contact and all data were anonymized.

Data Availability Statement: Not applicable.

Acknowledgments: All other members of the 12 CwPAMS partnerships that featured in this article as well CPA and THET teams are acknowledged for their support, contributions, and shared learning throughout the CwPAMS programme: The Commonwealth Pharmacist Association CwPAMS programme Team: Victoria Rutter; Chloe Tuck; Sarah Cavanagh; Khor Wei Ping; Omotayo Olaoye; Ayodeji Matuluko; Tropical Health Education Trust (THET) CwPAMS programme Team: Will Townsend; Richard Skone-James; Beatrice Waddingham.

Conflicts of Interest: The authors declare no conflict of interest.

References

1. WHO Antimicrobial Resistance: Fact Sheets. Available online: https://www.who.int/news-room/fact-sheets/detail/antimicrobial-resistance (accessed on 3 February 2021).
2. McEwen, S.A.; Collignon, P.J. Antimicrobial Resistance: A One Health Perspective. *Microbiol. Spectr.* **2018**, *6*, 6–12. [CrossRef]
3. Cassini, A.; Högberg, L.D.; Plachouras, D.; Quattrocchi, A.; Hoxha, A.; Simonsen, G.S.; Colomb-Cotinat, M.; E Kretzschmar, M.; Devleesschauwer, B.; Cecchini, M.; et al. Attributable deaths and disability-adjusted life-years caused by infections with antibiotic-resistant bacteria in the EU and the European Economic Area in 2015: A population-level modelling analysis. *Lancet Infect. Dis.* **2018**, *19*, 56–66. [CrossRef]
4. Howard, P.; Pulcini, C.; Levy Hara, G.; West, R.M.; Gould, I.M.; Harbarth, S.; Nathwani, D. An international cross-sectional survey of antimicrobial stewardship programmes in hos-pitals. *J. Antimicrob. Chemother.* **2015**, *70*, 1245–1255.
5. Afriyie, D.K.; A Sefah, I.; Sneddon, J.; Malcolm, W.; McKinney, R.; Cooper, L.; Kurdi, A.; Godman, B.; Seaton, R.A. Antimicrobial point prevalence surveys in two Ghanaian hospitals: Opportunities for antimicrobial stewardship. *JAC-Antimicrobial Resist.* **2020**, *2*, dlaa001. [CrossRef]
6. Klein, E.Y.; Van Boeckel, T.P.; Martinez, E.; Pant, S.; Gandra, S.; Levin, S.A.; Goossens, H.; Laxminarayan, R. Global increase and geographic convergence in antibiotic consumption between 2000 and 2015. *Proc. Natl. Acad. Sci. USA* **2018**, *115*, E3463–E3470. [CrossRef]
7. Laxminarayan, R.; Matsoso, P.; Pant, S.; Brower, C.; Røttingen, J.-A.; Klugman, K.; Davies, S. Access to effective antimicrobials: A worldwide challenge. *Lancet* **2015**, *387*, 168–175. [CrossRef]
8. Talaat, M.; Saied, T.; Kandeel, A.; El-Ata, G.A.A.; El-Kholy, A.; Hafez, S.; Osman, A.; Razik, M.A.; Ismail, G.; El-Masry, S.; et al. A Point Prevalence Survey of Antibiotic Use in 18 Hospitals in Egypt. *Antibiotics* **2014**, *3*, 450–460. [CrossRef] [PubMed]
9. Saleem, Z.; Hassali, M.A.; Versporten, A.; Godman, B.; Hashmi, F.K.; Goossens, H.; Saleem, F. A multicenter point prevalence survey of antibiotic use in Punjab, Pakistan: Findings and implications. *Expert Rev. Anti-infective Ther.* **2019**, *17*, 285–293. [CrossRef] [PubMed]
10. Dean, B.; Lawson, W.; Jacklin, A.; Rogers, T.; Azadian, B.; Holmes, A. The use of serial point-prevalence studies to investigate hospital anti-infective prescribing. *Int. J. Pharm. Pr.* **2002**, *10*, 121–125. [CrossRef]
11. Willemsen, I.; Groenhuijzen, A.; Bogaers, D.; Stuurman, A.; van Keulen, P.; Kluytmans, J. Appropriateness of Antimicrobial Therapy Measured by Repeated Prevalence Surveys. *Antimicrob. Agents Chemother.* **2007**, *51*, 864–867. [CrossRef]
12. Goossens, H. Global Point Prevalence Survey of Antimicrobial Consumption and Resistance (2019 GLOBAL PPS). Available online: https://www.global-pps.com/ (accessed on 12 January 2021).
13. Global Action Plan on Antimicrobial Resistance. *Microbe Mag.* **2015**, *10*, 354–355. [CrossRef]
14. WHO. WHO Releases the 2019 AWaRe Classification Antibiotics. Available online: https://www.who.int/medicines/news/2019/WHO_releases2019AWaRe_classification_antibiotics/en (accessed on 12 January 2021).

15. Sharland, M.; Gandra, S.; Huttner, B.; Moja, L.; Pulcini, C.; Zeng, M.; Cappello, B.; Cooke, G.; Magrini, N. Encouraging AWaRe-ness and discouraging inappropriate antibiotic use—The new 2019 Es-sential Medicines List becomes a global antibiotic stewardship tool. *Lancet Infect Dis.* **2019**, *19*, 1278–1280. [CrossRef]
16. World Health Organization. WHOCC-ATC/DDD Index. Available online: https://www.whocc.no/atc_ddd_index/ (accessed on 28 November 2020).
17. Commonwealth Pharmacists Association. Commonwealth Pharmacists Association. Available online: https://commonwealthpharmacy.org/ (accessed on 4 November 2020).
18. Versporten, A.; Zarb, P.; Caniaux, I.; Gros, M.-F.; Drapier, N.; Miller, M.; Jarlier, V.; Nathwani, D.; Goossens, H.; Koraqi, A.; et al. Antimicrobial consumption and resistance in adult hospital inpatients in 53 countries: Results of an internet-based global point prevalence survey. *Lancet Glob. Heal.* **2018**, *6*, e619–e629. [CrossRef]
19. WHO Collaborating Centre for Drug Statistics Methodology. ATC Structure and Principles. Available online: https://www.whocc.no/atc/structure_and_principles/ (accessed on 2 February 2021).
20. Antimicrobial stewardship programmes in health-care facilities in low- and middle-income countries: A WHO practical toolkit. *JAC-Antimicrob. Resist* **2019**, *1*, dlz072. [CrossRef] [PubMed]
21. Sartelli, M.; Hardcastle, T.C.; Catena, F.; Chichom-Mefire, A.; Coccolini, F.; Dhingra, S.; Haque, M.; Hodonou, A.; Iskandar, K.; Labricciosa, F.M.; et al. Antibiotic Use in Low and Middle-Income Countries and the Challenges of Antimicrobial Resistance in Surgery. *Antibiotics* **2020**, *9*, 497. [CrossRef] [PubMed]
22. Knowles, R.; Sharland, M.; Hsia, Y.; Magrini, N.; Moja, L.; Siyam, A.; Tayler, E. Measuring antibiotic availability and use in 20 low- and middle-income countries. *Bull. World Heal. Organ.* **2020**, *98*, 177–187C. [CrossRef]
23. Pauwels, I.; Versporten, A.; Drapier, N.; Vlieghe, E.; Goossens, H.; Koraqi, A.; Hoxha, I.; Tafaj, S.; Cornistein, W.; Quiros, R.; et al. Hospital antibiotic prescribing patterns in adult patients according to the WHO Access, Watch and Reserve classification (AWaRe): Results from a worldwide point prevalence survey in 69 countries. *J. Antimicrob. Chemother.* **2021**, *76*, 1614–1624. [CrossRef]
24. Seni, J.; Mapunjo, S.G.; Wittenauer, R.; Valimba, R.; Stergachis, A.; Werth, B.J.; Saitoti, S.; Mhadu, N.H.; Lusaya, E.; Konduri, N. Antimicrobial use across six referral hospitals in Tanzania: A point prevalence survey. *BMJ Open* **2020**, *10*, e042819. [CrossRef]
25. Hsia, Y.; Lee, B.R.; Versporten, A.; Yang, Y.; Bielicki, J.; Jackson, C.; Newland, J.; Goossens, H.; Magrini, N.; Sharland, M.; et al. Use of the WHO Access, Watch, and Reserve classification to define patterns of hospital antibiotic use (AWaRe): An analysis of paediatric survey data from 56 countries. *Lancet Glob. Heal.* **2019**, *7*, e861–e871. [CrossRef]
26. Labi, A.-K.; Obeng-Nkrumah, N.; Nartey, E.T.; Bjerrum, S.; Adu-Aryee, N.A.; Ofori-Adjei, Y.A.; Yawson, A.E.; Newman, M.J. Antibiotic use in a tertiary healthcare facility in Ghana: A point prevalence survey. *Antimicrob. Resist. Infect. Control.* **2018**, *7*, 1–9. [CrossRef]
27. Maina, M.; Mwaniki, P.; Odira, E.; Kiko, N.; McKnight, J.; Schultsz, C.; English, M.; Tosas-Auguet, O. Antibiotic use in Kenyan public hospitals: Prevalence, appropriateness and link to guideline availability. *Int. J. Infect. Dis.* **2020**, *99*, 10–18. [CrossRef] [PubMed]
28. Horumpende, P.G.; Mshana, S.E.; Mouw, E.F.; Mmbaga, B.T.; Chilongola, J.O.; De Mast, Q. Point prevalence survey of antimicrobial use in three hospitals in North-Eastern Tanzania. *Antimicrob. Resist. Infect. Control.* **2020**, *9*, 1–6. [CrossRef]
29. Löfmark, S.; Edlund, C.; Nord, C.E. Metronidazole Is Still the Drug of Choice for Treatment of Anaerobic Infections. *Clin. Infect. Dis.* **2010**, *50*, S16–S23. [CrossRef] [PubMed]
30. Alekwe, L.O.; Kuti, O.; Orji, E.O.; Ogunniyi, S.O. Comparison of ceftriaxone versus triple drug regimen in the prevention of cesarean section infectious morbidities. *J. Matern. Neonatal Med.* **2008**, *21*, 638–642. [CrossRef]
31. Dancer, S. The problem with cephalosporins. *J. Antimicrob. Chemother.* **2001**, *48*, 463–478. [CrossRef]
32. Byrne, F.; Wilcox, M. MRSA prevention strategies and current guidelines. *Injury* **2011**, *42*, S3–S6. [CrossRef]
33. Lexley, M.; Pereira, P.; Phillips, M.; Ramlal, H. Third generation cephalosporin use in a tertiary hospital in Port of Spain, Trinidad: Need for an antibiotic policy. *BMC Infect Dis.* **2004**, *4*, 1–7.
34. Paterson, D.L. Resistance in Gram-Negative Bacteria: Enterobacteriaceae. *Am. J. Med.* **2006**, *119*, S20–S28. [CrossRef] [PubMed]
35. World Health Organisation. Global Tuberculosis Report 2020. Available online: https://www.who.int/teams/global-tuberculosis-programme/data (accessed on 15 September 2021).
36. Ndhlovu, M.; Nkhama, E.; Miller, J.M.; Hamer, D.H. Antibacterial prescribing practices for patients with fever in the transition from presumptive treatment of malaria to "confirm and treat" in Zambia: A cross sectional study. *Trop. Med. Int. Health* **2015**, *20*, 1696–1706. [CrossRef]
37. Suetens, C.; Latour, K.; Kärki, T.; Ricchizzi, E.; Kinross, P.; Moro, M.L.; Jans, B.; Hopkins, S.; Hansen, S.; Lyytikäinen, O.; et al. Prevalence of healthcare-associated infections, estimated incidence and composite antimicrobial resistance index in acute care hospitals and long-term care facilities: Results from two European point prevalence surveys, 2016 to 2017. *Eurosurveillance* **2018**, *23*, 1800516. [CrossRef]
38. Pauwels, I.; Versporten, A.; Vlieghe, E.; Goosssens, H. *Assessing the Learning Needs and Barriers for Implementation of Anti-Microbial Stewardship in Hospitals That Have Participated in the Global Point Prevalence Survey on Antimicrobial Consumption and Resistance (Global-PPS)*; ICPIC: Geneva, Switzerland, 2019.
39. Bediako-Bowan, A.A.A.; Owusu, E.; Labi, A.-K.; Obeng-Nkrumah, N.; Sunkwa-Mills, G.; Bjerrum, S.; Opintan, J.A.; Bannerman, C.; Mølbak, K.; Kurtzhals, J.A.L.; et al. Antibiotic use in surgical units of selected hospitals in Ghana: A multi-centre point prevalence survey. *BMC Public Health* **2019**, *19*, 1–10. [CrossRef] [PubMed]

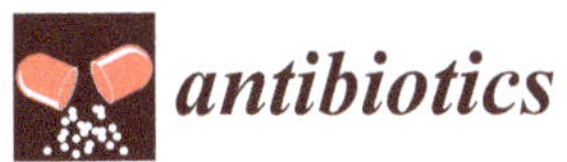

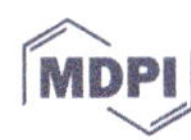

Article

Pharmacist-Driven Antibiotic Stewardship Program in Febrile Neutropenic Patients: A Single Site Prospective Study in Thailand

Kittiya Jantarathaneewat [1,2], Anucha Apisarnthanarak [3], Wasithep Limvorapitak [4], David J. Weber [5] and Preecha Montakantikul [1,*]

1 Department of Pharmacy, Faculty of Pharmacy, Mahidol University, Bangkok 10400, Thailand; kittiyaj@staff.tu.ac.th
2 Department of Pharmaceutical care, Faculty of Pharmacy, Thammasat University, Pathum Thani 12120, Thailand
3 Division of Infectious Diseases, Faculty of Medicine, Thammasat University, Pathum Thani 12120, Thailand; anapisarn@yahoo.com
4 Division of Hematology, Faculty of Medicine, Thammasat University, Pathum Thani 12120, Thailand; Wasithep@tu.ac.th
5 School of Global Public Health, University of North Carolina, Gillings, Chapel Hill, NC 27599-7400, USA; David.Weber@unchealth.unc.edu
* Correspondence: preecha.mon@mahidol.ac.th; Tel.: +66-0-2644-8694

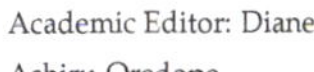

Citation: Jantarathaneewat, K.; Apisarnthanarak, A.; Limvorapitak, W.; Weber, D.J.; Montakantikul, P. Pharmacist-Driven Antibiotic Stewardship Program in Febrile Neutropenic Patients: A Single Site Prospective Study in Thailand. *Antibiotics* **2021**, *10*, 456. https://doi.org/10.3390/antibiotics10040456

Academic Editor: Diane Ashiru-Oredope

Received: 23 March 2021
Accepted: 15 April 2021
Published: 17 April 2021

Publisher's Note: MDPI stays neutral with regard to jurisdictional claims in published maps and institutional affiliations.

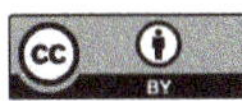

Copyright: © 2021 by the authors. Licensee MDPI, Basel, Switzerland. This article is an open access article distributed under the terms and conditions of the Creative Commons Attribution (CC BY) license (https://creativecommons.org/licenses/by/4.0/).

Abstract: The antibiotic stewardship program (ASP) is a necessary part of febrile neutropenia (FN) treatment. Pharmacist-driven ASP is one of the meaningful approaches to improve the appropriateness of antibiotic usage. Our study aimed to determine role of the pharmacist in ASPs for FN patients. We prospectively studied at Thammasat University Hospital between August 2019 and April 2020. Our primary outcome was to compare the appropriate use of target antibiotics between the pharmacist-driven ASP group and the control group. The results showed 90 FN events in 66 patients. The choice of an appropriate antibiotic was significantly higher in the pharmacist-driven ASP group than the control group (88.9% vs. 51.1%, $p < 0.001$). Furthermore, there was greater appropriateness of the dosage regimen chosen as empirical therapy in the pharmacist-driven ASP group than in the control group (97.8% vs. 88.7%, $p = 0.049$) and proper duration of target antibiotics in documentation therapy (91.1% vs. 75.6%, $p = 0.039$). The multivariate analysis showed a pharmacist-driven ASP and infectious diseases consultation had a favorable impact on 30-day infectious diseases-related mortality in chemotherapy-induced FN patients (OR 0.058, 95%CI:0.005–0.655, $p = 0.021$). Our study demonstrated that pharmacist-driven ASPs could be a great opportunity to improve antibiotic appropriateness in FN patients.

Keywords: antibiotic stewardship; febrile neutropenia; appropriateness; pharmacist-driven; hematology oncologic patient

1. Introduction

Febrile neutropenia (FN) is a life-threatening complication of cancer therapy which can increase morbidity and mortality [1]. Broad spectrum antimicrobial agent administration is an essential part of the treatment of febrile neutropenia to cover hospital-acquired pathogens. Pharmacokinetic alterations of several antibiotics (e.g., piperacillin/tazobactam) were found in febrile neutropenic patients [2,3]. Prescribing antibiotics with common dosage regimens might be inadequate for these patients. Furthermore, incorrect antibiotic dosing was found as the most common non-compliant antibiotic prescription practice in febrile neutropenic patients [4]. Antibiotic optimization would be a challenging method among febrile neutropenic patients. An antibiotic stewardship program (ASP) in immunocompromised patients is suggested by the Infectious Diseases Society of America (IDSA)

2010 guidelines [5]. Recent evidence supports that adherence to an ASP is associated with a lower mortality rate [6]. Although several studies have shown the effectiveness of ASP implementation in febrile neutropenic patients, there is limited evidence of the effectiveness of ASP implementation led by a pharmacist [7–11]. Pharmacist-driven ASPs have been reported to increase antibiotic appropriateness in several studies [12–14]. We believe this is the first study to demonstrate that a pharmacist-driven ASP can be beneficial among febrile neutropenic patients. Our study compared antibiotic appropriateness between a pharmacist-driven ASP and a control group.

2. Results

Ninety febrile neutropenic events occurred in 66 patients. The proportion of men in the control group was higher than the intervention group (57.8% vs. 35.6%, $p = 0.035$). The mean age of all patients was 51.6 $\pm$ 15.6 years. Most patients were diagnosed with cytotoxic chemotherapy-induced febrile neutropenia (74.4%) while twenty patients were identified as a febrile neutropenia during the period of initial hematologic abnormalities diagnosis (22.2%) and only three patients were diagnosed as a febrile neutropenia from other causes such as vitamin B12 deficiency, severe infection, and zidovudine-induced pancytopenia. The majority of our patients had hematologic malignancy (80%) and 8.9% had solid cancer. The Multinational Association for Supportive Care in Cancer (MASCC) risk index median score was 20 (interquartile range (IQR) 17–21). The median absolute neutrophil count was 153.9 cells/mm^3 (IQR 19–520). Fifty-one percent of patients had a history of febrile neutropenia and 55.6% of patients had been exposed to antibiotics within the past 3 months. The median duration of neutropenia was 7 days. The frequency of infectious diseases consultation was similar in both groups. The baseline characteristics are displayed in Table 1.

The major causative organisms were Gram-negative bacteria (43.3%), followed by Gram-positive bacteria (13.3%) and fungi (3.3%). The most common causative Gram-negative bacteria were *Escherichia coli* (33.3%), *Klebsiella pneumoniae* (25.6%), and *Pseudomonas aeruginosa* (10.3%). Most Gram-negative bacteria exhibited multiple-drug resistance (MDR) (69%). More carbapenem-resistant Gram-negative bacteria were often found in the pharmacist-driven ASP group compared to the control group (8.9% vs. 2.2%, $p = 0.167$) while extended spectrum beta-lactamase (ESBL)-producing Gram-negative bacteria were lower than the control group (6.7% vs. 20%, $p = 0.063$). The most common causative Gram-positive bacteria were *Enterococci* spp. (41.7%), *Staphylococcus aureus* (33.3%), and *Corynebacterium* spp. (16.7%). Ampicillin-resistant *Enterococci* spp. was isolated from only in one patient and only one patient had methicillin-resistant *Staphylococcus aureus* (MRSA). Most of the causative organisms were isolated from blood, urine, or sputum (27.8%, 12.2%, and 8.9%, respectively). The most common sources of infection were primary bacteremia, urinary tract infection, and pneumonia (23.3%, 13.3%, and 10%, respectively). However, the causative organisms were not isolated in nearly half of patients.

Overall, antibiotic appropriateness in the pharmacist-driven ASP group was significantly higher than the control group (88.9% vs. 51.1%, $p < 0.001$) (Table 2). In providing empirical therapy, the pharmacist-driven ASP group was more appropriate than the control group (97.8% vs. 77.8%, $p = 0.007$). The appropriate dosage regimen in the pharmacist-driven ASP group was significantly higher than the control group (97.8% vs. 88.7%, $p = 0.049$) as well as appropriate antibiotic coverage (100% vs. 91.1%, $p = 0.041$), while appropriate indications were similar in both groups. When providing therapy for definitive infections, the overall appropriateness was greater in the pharmacist-driven ASP group than in the control group (88.9% vs. 64.4%, $p = 0.004$), as was the duration of therapy (91.1% vs. 75.6%, $p = 0.039$). For therapy if the source of infection was unknown, the overall appropriateness in the pharmacist-driven ASP group also significantly greater than the control group (90% vs. 54.4%, $p = 0.011$). Furthermore, the appropriateness of duration of therapy in the pharmacist-driven group was significantly greater than in the control group (93.2% vs. 75.6%, $p = 0.022$). However, the antibiotic appropriateness in cases of known causative pathogens were not significantly greater than the control group, but there was a trend of improved appropriateness in the pharmacist-driven ASP group. The total antibiotic duration between two groups were similar ($p = 0.948$) (Table 2). The compliance rate to the pharmacist suggestion was 93.8% in the pharmacist-driven ASP group. The most common pharmacist interventions were de-escalation (31.3%), adding additional antimicrobials (18.8%), and avoiding serious drug interaction (18.1%).

Table 1. Baseline characteristics.

Baseline Characteristic	Total (90 FN Episodes), No. (%)	Intervention (45 FN Episodes), No. (%)	Control (45 FN Episodes), No. (%)	*p* Value
Age, mean years ± SD	51.6 ± 15.6	15.6 ± 14.6	52.0 ± 16.7	0.894
Male	42 (46.7)	16 (35.6)	26 (57.8)	0.035
Weight, mean kg ± SD	57.76 ± 1.50	58.94 ± 1.94	60.57 ± 2.30	0.590
Cause of febrile neutropenia				
Cytotoxic chemotherapy	67 (74.4)	34 (75.6)	33 (73.3)	1.000
During period of initial hematologic abnormalities diagnosis	20 (22.2)	10 (22.2)	10 (22.2)	1.000
Other causes [a]	3 (3.33)	1 (2.22)	2 (4.44)	1.000
Active hematologic cancer	72 (80)	34 (75.6)	38 (84.4)	0.496
Active solid cancer	8 (8.9)	4 (8.9)	4 (8.9)	0.496
MASCC score, median (IQR)	20 (17–21)	19 (13–21)	21 (19–21)	0.129
High risk of febrile neutropenia (MASCC < 21)	45 (50)	25 (55.6)	20 (44.4)	0.292
Absolute neutrophil count, median cells/mm^3 (IQR)	153.9 (19–520)	184 (40–645)	77 (13–368)	0.198
Had history of febrile neutropenia	46 (51.1)	20 (44.4)	26 (57.8)	0.206
Recent exposed to antibiotic within past 3 months	50 (55.6)	25 (55.6)	25 (55.6)	1.000
Neutropenia duration, median days (IQR)	7 (4–14)	8 (4–14)	6 (4–10)	0.435
Infectious diseases specialist consultation	50 (55.6)	27 (60)	23 (51.1)	0.396
Time to administer antibiotic, median hours (IQR)	1 (0–4)	1.5 (0–4)	1 (0–4)	0.497
Causative organism identified	49 (54.4)	26 (57.8)	23 (51.1)	0.525
Gram-positive bacteria	12 (13.3)	7 (15.6)	5 (11.1)	0.774
Gram-negative bacteria	39 (43.3)	20 (44.4)	19 (42.2)	0.761
ESBL-producing organisms	12 (13.3)	3 (6.7)	9 (20)	0.118
Carbapenem resistance organisms	5 (5.6)	4 (8.9)	1 (2.2)	0.361

ESBL, extended spectrum beta-lactamase; FN, febrile neutropenia; IQR, interquartile range; MASCC, Multinational Association for Supportive Care in Cancer risk index score; SD, standard deviation. [a] Other causes of febrile neutropenia were from vitamin B12 deficiency, zidovudine-induce pancytopenia and severe infection.

Overall, the antibiotic appropriateness in the pharmacist-driven ASP group was significantly higher than control group (88.9% vs. 51.1%, $p < 0.001$) (Table 2). In providing empirical therapy, the pharmacist-driven ASP group was more appropriate than the control group (97.8% vs. 77.8%, $p = 0.007$). The appropriate dosage regimen in the pharmacist-driven ASP group was significantly higher than the control group (97.8% vs. 88.7%, $p = 0.049$) as well as the appropriate antibiotic coverage (100% vs. 91.1%, $p = 0.041$) while the appropriate indications were similar in both groups. When providing therapy for definitive infections, the overall appropriateness was greater in the pharmacist driven ASP group than in the control group (88.9% vs. 64.4%, $p = 0.004$) as was the duration of therapy (91.1% vs. 75.6%, $p = 0.039$). For therapy if the source of infection was unknown, the overall appropriateness in the pharmacist-driven ASP group was also significantly greater than the control group (90% vs. 54.4%, $p = 0.011$). Furthermore, the appropriateness of duration of therapy in the pharmacist-driven group was significantly greater than in control group (93.2% vs. 75.6%, $p = 0.022$). However, the antibiotic appropriateness in cases of known causative pathogens were not significantly greater than the control group, but there was a trend of improved appropriateness in the pharmacist-driven ASP group. The total antibiotic duration between two groups were similar ($p = 0.948$) (Table 2). The compliance rate to the pharmacist suggestion was 93.8% in the pharmacist-driven ASP group. The most common pharmacist interventions when compared with the control group were de-escalation (22.2% vs. 20%, $p = 0.796$), adding additional antimicrobials (17.8% vs. 8.9%, $p = 0.215$), and avoiding serious drug interaction (6.7% vs. 0%, $p = 0.078$).

Table 2. Study outcomes.

Outcomes	Intervention (45 FN Episodes), No. (%)	Control (45 FN Episodes), No. (%)	*p* Value
Overall appropriateness	40 (88.9)	23 (51.1)	<0.001
Step 1 Empirical therapy	44 (97.8)	35 (77.8)	0.007
Appropriate Indication	45 (100)	45 (100)	-
Appropriate coverage	45 (100)	41 (91.1)	0.041
Appropriate dosage regimen	44 (97.8)	39 (88.7)	0.049
Step 2 Documentation therapy	40 (88.9) [b]	29 (64.4)	0.004
Appropriate indication	43 (95.6)	41 (91.1)	0.361
Appropriate dosage regimen	44 (97.8)	43 (93.3)	0.242
Appropriate duration	41 (91.1)	34 (75.6)	0.039
Length of stay, median days (IQR)	28 (19–42)	23 (16–35)	0.689
30-day infectious diseases related mortality	6 (13.6)	5 (11.1)	1.000
Total antibiotic duration, median days (IQR)	14 (10–23)	15 (10–21)	0.948
antibiotic duration in de-escalation	21 (14–28)	17.5 (15.5–29.5)	0.666
antibiotic duration in escalation	19 (13–34.5)	15 (11–25.5)	0.309

FN, febrile neutropenia; IQR, interquartile range. [b] Total 44 FN episodes since one death occurred before culture was reported.

The 30-day infectious diseases-related mortality and length of stay were similar in both groups (Table 2). In univariate analysis, neither the pharmacist-driven ASP nor ID consultation showed a significant impact on 30-day infectious diseases-related mortality ($p = 0.810$ and 0.267, respectively). However, in multivariate analysis, the pharmacist-driven ASP group and infectious diseases consultation significantly reduced the 30-day infectious diseases mortality in patients with cytotoxic chemotherapy-induced febrile neutropenia (OR 0.058, 95% CI: 0.005–0.655, $p = 0.021$). A history of febrile neutropenia was associated with an increased 30-day infectious diseases mortality, as described in Table 3. The utilization rate of target antibiotics in the pharmacist-driven ASP group tended to be higher than control group (882 Defined Daily Dose (DDD)/1000 patient-day vs. 705.1 DDD/1000 patient-day). The trend of the overall target antibiotic seemed to be higher in both groups (supplementary data, Table S1). The trend of ceftazidime, cefepime, and meropenem utilization was lower in the pharmacist-driven ASP group while piperacillin/tazobactam utilization was higher. In the control group, ceftazidime utilization tended to be decreased, but other target antibiotics' utilization including cefepime, piperacillin/tazobactam, and meropenem were increased. Overall intravenous antibiotic utilization in the pharmacist-driven ASP group declined while amount of utilization in the control group increased.

Table 3. Multivariate analysis of 30-day infectious diseases-related mortality.

Variables	Univariate Analysis			Multivariate Analysis		
	OR	95%CI	*p* Value	OR	95%CI	*p* Value
Pharmacist-driven ASP group and infectious diseases consultation in chemotherapy-induced febrile neutropenic patient	0.184	0.037–0.911	0.038	0.058	0.005–0.655	0.021
Male	0.653	0.176–2.419	0.524	0.744	0.133–4.148	0.736
High risk of febrile neutropenia	5.426	1.098–26.829	0.038	5.155	0.762–34.890	0.093
Had history of febrile neutropenia	5.143	1.040–25.420	0.045	9.380	1.311–67.100	0.026
Carbapenem resistance organisms	8.111	1.015–64.839	0.048	18.771	0.560–628.848	0.102
ESBL producing Gram negative bacteria	2.75	0.614–12.307	0.186	7.417	0.787–69.906	0.080

ASP, antibiotic stewardship program; CI, confidence interval; ESBL, extended spectrum beta-lactamase; MASCC, Multinational Association for Supportive Care in Cancer risk index score; OR, odds ratio.

3. Discussion

The pharmacist-driven ASP group interventions in febrile neutropenic patients showed a favorable effect on antibiotic appropriateness in our study. We found higher antibiotic appropriateness in the pharmacist intervention group than the control group (88.9% vs. 51.1%, $p < 0.001$). When providing empirical therapy, the pharmacist-driven ASP group was more appropriate than the control group, which was different from a previous study [15]. We believe that main reason for this discrepancy was that the previous study evaluated only the prescribed antibiotic appropriateness based on the hospital guidelines and described only the antibiotics indicated for febrile neutropenia, but did not assess the appropriateness of dosage regimens which was included in our assessment of the appropriateness of prescribed antibiotics [15,16]. Moreover, our ASP implementation provided daily review and feedback while the Madran et al. study implemented a hospital guideline and had only a weekly discussion with the ASP team [15]. Likely our study, which provided more frequent feedback, improved the primary physicians' compliance, as noted in a recent study [10]. Furthermore, our results showed that the appropriate dosage regimens were more frequently found in the pharmacist-driven ASP group than the control group (97.8% vs. 88.7%, $p = 0.049$). Our finding was similar to previous studies that the appropriateness was 6.5-fold higher in the pharmacist intervention group then the control group [17]. On the other hand, the appropriateness of antibiotic indication in the pharmacist-driven ASP group resembled the control group, as described in Madran et al. study [15]. However, we also used current standard guidelines and all of our patients had a high risk of febrile neutropenia, similar to the previous study [15].

In documented infection evaluations, the pharmacist-driven ASP group had a greater appropriateness of prescribed antibiotics than the control group (88.9% vs. 64.4%, $p = 0.004$). Our result was similar to previous study in which more appropriateness was found in the intervention group [15]. Moreover, the appropriate duration of therapy was higher in the pharmacist-driven ASP group ($p = 0.039$). Our result was concordant with a previous study that pharmacist-driven ASPs could reduce the duration of antibiotic therapy [18]. However, the appropriateness of antibiotic indication was similar in both groups because our study divided the category of appropriateness into microbial susceptibilities and the penetration of antibiotics to the target site. If pathogens were identified and antibiotics susceptibilities were reported, it could help physicians to choose proper antibiotics. Since most pathogens in the control group were ESBL-producing organisms, this might affect antibiotic appropriateness because carbapenems are drugs of choice for ESBL-producing organisms, and choice of antibiotics was controlled by an infectious diseases physician [19]. In addition, the overall antibiotic appropriateness and proper duration of therapy in the pharmacist-driven ASP group were also greater than the control group when the source of infection was unknown ($p = 0.039$ and 0.066, respectively) (supplementary data, Table S2). However, the total antibiotic duration between two groups did not differ. The reasons for prolonging antibiotic duration in the intervention group were fungal infection (e.g., invasive pulmonary aspergillosis and mucormycosis), superinfection with MDR organisms, and an uncontrolled source of infection. Although the result did not show any difference of antibiotic appropriateness in the case of known causative pathogens and source of infection between the two groups, the pharmacist-driven ASP group tended to use more proper antibiotics than the control group in terms of indication, dose and duration ($p = 0.384$, 0.833, and 0.872, respectively) (supplementary data, Table S3).

Nevertheless, our study did not show a difference in the 30-day infectious diseases-related mortality between the two study groups. Our patients tended to have longer neutropenia durations and higher carbapenem resistance Enterobacteriaceae (CRE) infection rates in the intervention group which differed from a previous study [15]. As a result of rising CRE incidence in Thailand, our patients were more likely to be infected with CRE than reported in a previous study, which might have affected the mortality rate in our study [15,20,21]. However, other ASP studies in febrile neutropenic patients also showed no difference in mortality between two groups as well [10,22–25]. Based on our multivariate analysis, pharmacists should collaborate with other medical personnel such as infectious diseases physicians to improve the 30-day infectious diseases-related mortality in febrile neutropenic patients caused by cytotoxic chemotherapy. This study supports the IDSA Guidelines that ASP team should be made up of a multidisciplinary team to achieve successful ASP implementation [5]. On-site infectious diseases specialists, including an ID physician and pharmacist, can improve the ASP effectiveness in recent study [26]. Hence, a multidisciplinary team would be beneficial for ASP implementation in these specific populations where data are limited, such as febrile neutropenic patients. Notably, although most of the febrile neutropenic patients in our study were caused by cytotoxic chemotherapy, there are some patients caused by hematologic abnormalities during diagnosis in our study which was also mentioned in previous study [27]. Furthermore, our study did not find any difference in the length of stay in both groups, as has been noted in a previous study [10].

Although our target antibiotics utilization in the pharmacist-driven ASP group increased during the study period, which was similar to a previous study, it might have affected inappropriate prescriptions in the control group [10]. For instance, there were some antibiotics improperly used in empirical therapy in the control group such as ceftriaxone, which were not included in our target antibiotics, and antibiotics might have been prescribed at an improper low dose. Therefore, the DDD of target antibiotics in the control group might be lower than expected. Moreover, we implemented a high dose of target antibiotics according to previous pharmacokinetic studies this might have contributed to a higher DDD of target antibiotic in the pharmacist-driven ASP group [2,3]. Besides, the overall intravenous antibiotics in the pharmacist-driven ASP group demonstrated a lower trend than the control group.

Our study had several limitations. First, ward physician rotation could have affected the result. However, the result of this study also showed that the pharmacist intervention group had more appropriateness than the control group. Second, the study was implemented only in medical wards since Thammasat University Hospital did not have a hematology–oncology ward during the study period and we could not fully perform interventions in the other wards such as the emergency department and intensive care unit. Ideally, the ASP implementations in febrile neutropenic patients should be carried out in all wards. Third, we calculated our sample size to demonstrate antibiotic appropriateness rather than 30-day infectious diseases-related mortality. A larger sample size is needed to assess the effect of a pharmacist-driven ASP on 30-day infectious diseases-related mortality. Fourth, we could not evaluate the effect of pharmacist-driven ASPs on antibiotic resistance since the study site did not have an isolation ward for febrile neutropenia patients with multidrug-resistant pathogens. Thus, the acquisition of antibiotic resistance organisms from other patients might have affected our results. Finally, the role of pharmacists in Thailand may be different from western countries. Pharmacists cannot change the antibiotic dosage regimen or discontinue antibiotics by themselves; a physician's signature is needed.

Thus, pharmacist cooperation with a physician was also an important aspect to implement a successful pharmacist-driven ASP in Thailand.

In conclusion, our study showed that a pharmacist-driven ASP in febrile neutropenic patients could improve the antibiotic appropriateness in both empirical and documentation therapy. However, 30-day infectious diseases-related mortality and the length of stay were not different between the groups. Although the target antibiotic utilization in the intervention group increased, we found a reduction in the total antibiotic utilization in the pharmacist-driven ASP group.

4. Materials and Methods

This prospective study was conducted at Thammasat University Hospital in Thailand, a tertiary care and teaching hospital, between 1 August 2019 and 30 April 2020. Two medical wards were pre-designated as the pharmacist-driven ASP group and two other similar medical wards were pre-designated as the control group. Febrile neutropenia in our study was defined as fever (single temperature equivalent to $\geq$38.3 °C orally or equivalent to $\geq$38.0 °C orally over a 1 h period) with neutropenic condition (patient who had $\leq$500 neutrophils per microliter or $\leq$500 neutrophils per microliter and a predicted declined to $\leq$500 neutrophils per microliter over the next 48 h). High risk of febrile neutropenia was identified by the MASCC risk index score less than 21 [28]. Inclusion criteria included adult patients (i.e., age >18 years); patient diagnosed with febrile neutropenia; and patient received antibiotics for treatment of febrile neutropenia. Exclusion criteria included the receipt of antibiotics for febrile neutropenia <24 h, pregnancy, or lactation. This study was approved by the human research ethics committee, Thammasat University (protocol no. MTU-EC-OO-0-078/62).

Our ASP team consisted of an infectious diseases-trained clinical pharmacist, infectious diseases physicians and hematologists. We developed TUH's recommended antibiotic and dosage regimen for empirical therapy in febrile neutropenia, which, adapted from the IDSA 2010 and National Comprehensive Cancer Network (NCCN) 2020 guidelines and distributed to primary physicians prior to the pharmacist-driven ASP, was implemented in two medical wards groups [5,28]. In the intervention group, a clinical pharmacist performed the daily prospective audit and feedback to the primary physician. The pharmacist suggested a suitable antibiotic for each patient, calculated an appropriate dose and recommended the treatment duration for both empirical therapy and documented infection. The antibiotic appropriateness and antibiotic utilization in the intervention group was reported monthly by the clinical pharmacist. Medical personnel practicing in the intervention group were provided education via lectures and posters by the clinical pharmacists during monthly ward conferences. No ASP interventions were performed in the control group. The criteria to evaluate antibiotic appropriateness was adapted from previous studies (supplementary data, Figure S1) [29–31]. In empirical therapy evaluations, a clinical pharmacist evaluated an appropriateness of indications, antibiotic coverage, and dosage regimen of the antibiotics. Therapeutic evaluations for documented infection were divided into 2 groups—unknown source of infection and known causative pathogens and source of infection. Both groups were also evaluated for antibiotic indication, dosage regimen, and duration of antibiotic therapy by pharmacist.

The primary outcome of this study was to compare antibiotic appropriateness between pharmacist-ASP driven group and the control group. Secondary outcomes were to compare antibiotic utilization, patient length of stay, 30-day infectious diseases-related mortality between the intervention and control groups. Target antibiotics in this study were ceftazidime, cefepime, piperacillin/tazobactam, meropenem and imipenem which are recommended as an empirical therapy for febrile neutropenia in current guidelines [28,32,33]. All intravenous antibiotics classes commonly used in these patients were evaluated in this study.

To have an 80% power and 95% confidence interval, the minimum sample size required in each arm, calculated based on a previous study, was 33 subjects [15]. Each outcome was defined as a febrile neutropenic event. All statistical analyses were performed using STATA version 16 (College Station, TX). Chi-square test (two-tailed) was used to compare proportion for categorical variables while t-test was used to compare means for continuous variables. Antibiotic utilization was reported as the defined daily dose per 1000 patient-days. The trend of antibiotic utilization was analyzed by linear regression and reported as the coefficient and p-value. Univariate and multivariate analyses of variables influencing on 30-day infectious diseases-related mortality were performed. All comparisons were 2-sided and a p value < 0.05 was consider statistically significant.

Supplementary Materials: The following are available online at https://www.mdpi.com/article/10.3390/antibiotics10040456/s1, Figure S1: criteria of antibiotic appropriateness evaluation, Table S1: antibiotics utilization, Table S2: antibiotic appropriateness in documentation therapy: unknown source of infection, Table S3: antibiotic appropriateness in documentation therapy: known causative pathogens and source of infection.

Author Contributions: Conceptualization, methodology and formal analysis, P.M., A.A., W.L. and K.J.; investigation, K.J.; writing—original draft preparation, W.L. and D.J.W.; writing—review and editing. All authors have read and agreed to the published version of the manuscript.

Funding: This research received no external funding.

Institutional Review Board Statement: The study was conducted according to the guidelines of the Declaration of Helsinki, and approved by the Institutional Review Board of Thammasat University (protocol no. MTU-EC-OO-0-078/62).

Informed Consent Statement: Informed consent was obtained from all subjects involved in the study.

Data Availability Statement: The data that support the findings of this study are available on request from the corresponding author. The data are not publicly available due to privacy or ethical restrictions.

Acknowledgments: We thank the primary physicians who practiced in the medical wards during the study period at Thammasat University Hospital.

Conflicts of Interest: The authors declare no conflict of interest.

References

1. Talcott, J.A.; Finberg, R.; Mayer, R.J.; Goldman, L. The medical course of cancer patients with fever and neutropenia. Clinical identification of a low-risk subgroup at presentation. *Arch. Intern. Med.* **1988**, *148*, 2561–2568. [CrossRef] [PubMed]
2. Lortholary, O.; Lefort, A.; Tod, M.; Chomat, A.M.; Darras-Joly, C.; Cordonnier, C. Pharmacodynamics and pharmacokinetics of antibacterial drugs in the management of febrile neutropenia. *Lancet Infect. Dis.* **2008**, *8*, 612–620. [CrossRef]
3. Sime, F.B.; Roberts, M.S.; Warner, M.S.; Hahn, U.; Robertson, T.A.; Yeend, S.; Phay, A.; Lehman, S.; Lipman, J.; Peake, S.L.; et al. Altered pharmacokinetics of piperacillin in febrile neutropenic patients with hematological malignancy. *Antimicrob. Agents. Chemother.* **2014**, *58*, 3533–3537. [CrossRef]
4. Naeem, D.; Alshamrani, M.A.; Aseeri, M.A.; Khan, M.A. Prescribing Empiric Antibiotics for Febrile Neutropenia: Compliance with Institutional Febrile Neutropenia Guidelines. *Pharmacy* **2018**, *6*, 83. [CrossRef]
5. Barlam, T.F.; Cosgrove, S.E.; Abbo, L.M.; MacDougall, C.; Schuetz, A.N.; Septimus, E.J.; Srinivasan, A.; Dellit, T.H.; Falck-Ytter, Y.T.; Fishman, N.O.; et al. Implementing an Antibiotic Stewardship Program: Guidelines by the Infectious Diseases Society of America and the Society for Healthcare Epidemiology of America. *Clin. Infect. Dis.* **2016**, *62*, 51–77. [CrossRef] [PubMed]
6. Rosa, R.G.; Goldani, L.Z.; dos Santos, R.P. Association between adherence to an antimicrobial stewardship program and mortality among hospitalised cancer patients with febrile neutropaenia: A prospective cohort study. *BMC Infect. Dis.* **2014**, *14*, 286. [CrossRef] [PubMed]
7. Paskovaty, A.; Pflomm, J.M.; Myke, N.; Seo, S.K. A multidisciplinary approach to antimicrobial stewardship: Evolution into the 21st century. *Int. J. Antimicrob. Agents.* **2005**, *25*, 1–10. [CrossRef]
8. Cheng, V.C.; To, K.K.; Li, I.W.; Tang, B.S.; Chan, J.F.; Kwan, S.; Mak, R.; Tai, J.; Ching, P.; Ho, P.L.; et al. Antimicrobial stewardship program directed at broad-spectrum intravenous antibiotics prescription in a tertiary hospital. *Eur. J. Clin. Microbiol. Infect. Dis.* **2009**, *28*, 1447–1456. [CrossRef]
9. Yeo, C.L.; Chan, D.S.; Earnest, A.; Wu, T.S.; Yeoh, S.F.; Lim, R.; Jureen, R.; Fisher, D.; Hsu, L.Y. Prospective audit and feedback on antibiotic prescription in an adult hematology-oncology unit in Singapore. *Eur. J. Clin. Microbiol. Infect. Dis.* **2012**, *31*, 583–590. [CrossRef]

10. So, M.; Mamdani, M.M.; Morris, A.M.; Lau, T.T.Y.; Broady, R.; Deotare, U.; Grant, J.; Kim, D.; Schimmer, A.D.; Schuh, A.C.; et al. Effect of an antimicrobial stewardship programme on antimicrobial utilisation and costs in patients with leukaemia: A retrospective controlled study. *Clin. Microbiol. Infect.* **2018**, *24*, 882–888. [CrossRef]
11. Ruiz-Ramos, J.; Frasquet, J.; Poveda-Andrés, J.L.; Romá, E.; Salavert-Lleti, M.; Castellanos, Á.; Ramirez, P. Impact of an antimicrobial stewardship program on critical haematological patients. *Farm. Hosp.* **2017**, *41*, 479–487.
12. Storey, D.F.; Pate, P.G.; Nguyen, A.T.; Chang, F. Implementation of an antimicrobial stewardship program on the medical-surgical service of a 100-bed community hospital. *Antimicrob. Resist. Infect. Control* **2012**, *1*, 32. [CrossRef]
13. Rattanaumpawan, P.; Thamlikitkul, V.; Upapan, P. 239A Cluster-Randomized Controlled Trial of Trained Pharmacists and Infectious Disease Clinical Fellows for Approval of Restricted Antibiotics in Hospitalized Medical Patients at Siriraj Hospital. *Open Forum Infect. Dis.* **2014**, *1*, 103. [CrossRef]
14. Apisarnthanarak, A.; Lapcharoen, P.; Vanichkul, P.; Srisaeng-Ngoen, T.; Mundy, L.M. Design and analysis of a pharmacist-enhanced antimicrobial stewardship program in Thailand. *Am. J. Infect. Control* **2015**, *43*, 956–959. [CrossRef]
15. Madran, B.; Keske, Ş.; Tokça, G.; Dönmez, E.; Ferhanoğlu, B.; Çetiner, M.; Mandel, N.M.; Ergönül, Ö. Implementation of an antimicrobial stewardship program for patients with febrile neutropenia. *Am. J. Infect. Control* **2018**, *46*, 420–424. [CrossRef] [PubMed]
16. Van den Bosch, C.M.; Geerlings, S.E.; Natsch, S.; Prins, J.M.; Hulscher, M.E. Quality indicators to measure appropriate antibiotic use in hospitalized adults. *Clin. Infect. Dis.* **2015**, *60*, 281–291. [CrossRef]
17. DeWitt, K.M.; Weiss, S.J.; Rankin, S.; Ernst, A.; Sarangarm, P. Impact of an emergency medicine pharmacist on antibiotic dosing adjustment. *Am. J. Emerg. Med.* **2016**, *34*, 980–984. [CrossRef] [PubMed]
18. Ohashi, K.; Matsuoka, T.; Shinoda, Y.; Mori, T.; Yoshida, S.; Yoshimura, T.; Sugiyama, T. Clinical outcome of pharmacist-led prospective audit with intervention and feedback after expansion from patients using specific antibiotics to those using whole injectable antibiotics. *Eur. J. Clin. Microbiol. Infect. Dis.* **2019**, *38*, 593–600. [CrossRef]
19. Harris, P.N.A.; Tambyah, P.A.; Lye, D.C.; Mo, Y.; Lee, T.H.; Yilmaz, M.; Alenazi, T.H.; Arabi, Y.; Falcone, M.; Bassetti, M.; et al. Effect of Piperacillin-Tazobactam vs Meropenem on 30-Day Mortality for Patients With, E. coli or Klebsiella pneumoniae Bloodstream Infection and Ceftriaxone Resistance: A Randomized Clinical Trial. *JAMA* **2018**, *320*, 984–994. [CrossRef] [PubMed]
20. Chotiprasitsakul, D.; Srichatrapimuk, S.; Kirdlarp, S.; Pyden, A.D.; Santanirand, P. Epidemiology of carbapenem-resistant Enterobacteriaceae: A 5-year experience at a tertiary care hospital. *Infect. Drug Resist.* **2019**, *12*, 461–468. [CrossRef]
21. Righi, E.; Peri, A.M.; Harris, P.N.; Wailan, A.M.; Liborio, M.; Lane, S.W.; Paterson, D.L. Global prevalence of carbapenem resistance in neutropenic patients and association with mortality and carbapenem use: Systematic review and meta-analysis. *J. Antimicrob. Chemother.* **2017**, *72*, 668–677. [CrossRef] [PubMed]
22. Ko, J.H.; Kim, S.H.; Kang, C.I.; Cho, S.Y.; Lee, N.Y.; Chung, D.R.; Peck, K.R.; Song, J.H. Evaluation of a Carbapenem-Saving Strategy Using Empirical Combination Regimen of Piperacillin-Tazobactam and Amikacin in Hemato-Oncology Patients. *J. Korean Med. Sci.* **2019**, *34*, 17. [CrossRef] [PubMed]
23. Kirk, A.; Pierce, J.; Doll, M.; Lee, K.; Pakyz, A.; Kim, J.; Markley, D.; De la Cruz, O.; Bearman, G.; Stevens, M.P. Effect of carbapenem restriction on prescribing trends for immunocompromised wards at an academic medical center. *Am. J. Infect. Control* **2019**, *47*, 1035–1037. [CrossRef] [PubMed]
24. Snyder, M.; Pasikhova, Y.; Baluch, A. Early Antimicrobial De-escalation and Stewardship in Adult Hematopoietic Stem Cell Transplantation Recipients: Retrospective Review. *Open Forum Infect. Dis.* **2017**, *4*, 226. [CrossRef]
25. Paskovaty, A.; Pastores, S.M.; Gedrimaite, Z.; Kostelecky, N.; Riedel, E.R.; Seo, S.K. Antimicrobial de-escalation in septic cancer patients: Is it safe to back down? *Intensive Care Med.* **2015**, *41*, 2022–2023. [CrossRef]
26. Livorsi, D.J.; Nair, R.; Lund, B.C.; Alexander, B.; Beck, B.F.; Goto, M.; Ohl, M.; Vaughan Sarrazin, M.S.; Goetz, M.B.; Perencevich, E.N. Antibiotic stewardship implementation and patient-level antibiotic use at hospitals with and without on-site Infectious Disease specialists. *Clin. Infect. Dis.* **2020**, 388. [CrossRef]
27. Keng, M.K.; Sekeres, M.A. Febrile neutropenia in hematologic malignancies. *Curr. Hematol. Malig. Rep.* **2013**, *8*, 370–378. [CrossRef]
28. NCCN; Clinical Practice Guidelines in Oncology. Clinical Practice Guidelines in Oncology. *Prevention and Treatment of Cancer-Related Infections Version 2.2020 June 5, 2020*. Available online: https://www.nccn.org/professionals/physician_gls/pdf/infections.pdf (accessed on 27 December 2020).
29. Kollef, M.H. Inadequate antimicrobial treatment: An important determinant of outcome for hospitalized patients. *Clin. Infect. Dis.* **2000**, *31*, 131–138. [CrossRef]
30. Kollef, M.H. Rebuttal from Dr Kollef. *Chest* **2017**, *151*, 744–745. [CrossRef]
31. Kollef, M.H. The importance of appropriate initial antibiotic therapy for hospital-acquired infections. *Am. J. Med.* **2003**, *115*, 582–584. [CrossRef]
32. Freifeld, A.G.; Bow, E.J.; Sepkowitz, K.A.; Boeckh, M.J.; Ito, J.I.; Mullen, C.A.; Raad, I.I.; Rolston, K.V.; Young, J.A.; Wingard, J.R. Clinical practice guideline for the use of antimicrobial agents in neutropenic patients with cancer: 2010 Update by the Infectious Diseases Society of America. *Clin. Infect. Dis.* **2011**, *52*, 427–431. [CrossRef] [PubMed]
33. Klastersky, J.; de Naurois, J.; Rolston, K.; Rapoport, B.; Maschmeyer, G.; Aapro, M.; Herrstedt, J. Management of febrile neutropaenia: ESMO Clinical Practice Guidelines. *Ann. Oncol.* **2016**, *27*, 111–118. [CrossRef] [PubMed]

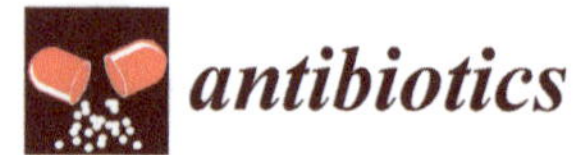

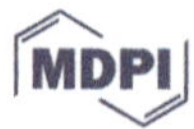

Article

Impact of an Education-Based Antimicrobial Stewardship Program on the Appropriateness of Antibiotic Prescribing: Results of a Multicenter Observational Study

Federica Calò [1], Lorenzo Onorato [1,2], Margherita Macera [1], Giovanni Di Caprio [2], Caterina Monari [1], Antonio Russo [1], Anna Galdieri [3], Antonio Giordano [4], Patrizia Cuccaro [5] and Nicola Coppola [1,*]

1 Department of Mental Health and Public Medicine–Infectious Diseases Unit, University of Campania Luigi Vanvitelli, 80138 Naples, Italy; fede.calo85@gmail.com (F.C.); lorenzoonorato@libero.it (L.O.); macera.margherita@libero.it (M.M.); caterina.monari@gmail.com (C.M.); antoniorusso.ar.ar@gmail.com (A.R.)
2 Infectious Diseases Unit, AORN Sant'Anna and San Sebastiano, 81100 Caserta, Italy; giov.dicaprio@gmail.com
3 Direzione Sanitaria, AOU Vanvitelli, 80138 Naples, Italy; anna.galdieri@policliniconapoli.it
4 Direzione Generale, AOU Vanvitelli, 80138 Naples, Italy; antonio.giordano@policliniconapoli.it
5 Direzione Sanitaria, AORN Sant'Anna and San Sebastiano, 81100 Caserta, Italy; patriziacuccaro@hotmail.com
* Correspondence: nicola.coppola@unicampania.it; Tel.: +39-081-5666223; Fax: +39-081-5666013

Abstract: To evaluate the effect that an education-based Antimicrobial stewardship program (ASP) implemented in two hospitals in southern Italy had on the quality and appropriateness of antibiotic prescription. We conducted a multicenter observational study in two hospitals in the Campania region. Only some departments of both hospitals were already participating in the ASP. We collected data on all patients admitted on the day of evaluation in antibiotic therapy or prophylaxis through a case report form. The primary outcome was to investigate the difference in the appropriateness of the antibiotic prescriptive practice in the departments that had joined the ASP and in those that had not participated in the project (non-ASP). The total number of patients assessed was 486. Of these, 78 (16.05%) were in antibiotic prophylaxis and 130 (26.7%) in antibiotic therapy. The prescriptive appropriateness was better in the units that had joined ASP than in those that had not, with respectively 65.8% versus 22.7% ($p < 0.01$). Patients in the non-ASP units more frequently received unnecessary antibiotics (44.9% versus 0%, $p = 0.03$) and, as surgical prophylaxis, the use of antibiotics not recommended by the guidelines (44.2% versus 0%, $p = 0.036$). Multivariable analysis of the factors associated with prescriptive appropriateness identified ASP units ($p = 0.02$) and bloodstream or cardiovascular infections ($p = 0.03$) as independent predictors of better prescriptive appropriateness. The findings of the present study reinforce the importance of adopting an educational ASP to improve the quality of antimicrobial prescription in clinical practice.

Keywords: antibiotics; antimicrobial stewardship; quality of prescription; prescriptive appropriateness; surgical prophylaxis

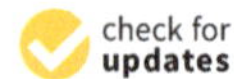

Citation: Calò, F.; Onorato, L.; Macera, M.; Di Caprio, G.; Monari, C.; Russo, A.; Galdieri, A.; Giordano, A.; Cuccaro, P.; Coppola, N. Impact of an Education-Based Antimicrobial Stewardship Program on the Appropriateness of Antibiotic Prescribing: Results of a Multicenter Observational Study. *Antibiotics* **2021**, *10*, 314. https://doi.org/10.3390/antibiotics10030314

Academic Editor: Akke Vellinga

Received: 1 February 2021
Accepted: 16 March 2021
Published: 17 March 2021

Publisher's Note: MDPI stays neutral with regard to jurisdictional claims in published maps and institutional affiliations.

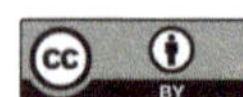

Copyright: © 2021 by the authors. Licensee MDPI, Basel, Switzerland. This article is an open access article distributed under the terms and conditions of the Creative Commons Attribution (CC BY) license (https://creativecommons.org/licenses/by/4.0/).

1. Introduction

Antimicrobial resistance is one of the greatest threats to global health today, leading to increased mortality, higher medical costs and prolonged hospital stays [1]. The number of estimated cases of infections with selected antibiotic-resistant bacteria occurring in 2015 in the EU and European Economic Area (EEA) was 671,689, accounting for about 33,110 attributable deaths and 874,541 disability-adjusted life-years (DALYs) [2]. In particular, among European countries Italy and Greece have the greatest burden of infections due to antibiotic-resistant bacteria [2].

Although antimicrobial agents used to treat infections are lifesaving, their overuse is one of the main drivers of antimicrobial resistance, resulting in the increased emergence and spread of multidrug-resistant bacteria. In hospitals the proportion of broad-spectrum antimicrobials used varied from 16% to 62% across Europe [3]. These drugs are not always necessary, and when their use is required, the selection, dose, route of administration and duration of treatment may be inappropriate [4–7].

To improve antibiotic prescriptions in the hospital setting is of utmost importance to avoid heading into a post-antibiotic era, where common infections and minor injuries can once again kill [1]. Thus, the implementation of programs for optimizing the use of antibiotics in hospitals is a public health priority. Antibiotic stewardship interventions are effective in increasing compliance with antibiotic policy and reducing consumption and duration of antibiotic treatment without, however, leading to an increase in mortality [8,9].

The objectives of the present study were to provide a snapshot analysis of antibiotic use and to investigate the impact of an educational antimicrobial stewardship program (ASP) on the appropriateness of antibiotic prescribing in two hospitals in southern Italy, in order to identify priority areas of intervention and implement measures aimed at optimizing antibiotic prescribing.

2. Materials and Methods

2.1. Study Design and Setting

This study was carried out in two hospitals in Naples and Caserta, in the Campania region of southern Italy. The 268-bed teaching hospital located in Naples serves adults and pediatrics in 30 units; the community hospital in Caserta has about 486 active beds in 23 units. Only the latter is equipped with an emergency department.

A persuasive-educational ASP, based on audit and feedback conducted by a team of infectious disease consultants [8], was started in January 2017 in Naples, and April 2018 in Caserta. The departments included in the ASP were those with the highest consumption of broad-spectrum antibiotics (in terms of defined daily dose) and/or those who had greater interest and willingness to join the project. In particular, five medical units (nephrology, neurology, endocrinology, geriatrics and infectious diseases), six surgical units (thoracic surgery, orthopedics, general surgery, gynecology and otolaryngology) and four intensive care units (ICUs) (of which one was a cardiac surgery ICU) were involved in the ASP. Briefly, we identified a multidisciplinary team, including infectious disease consultants, clinical microbiologists, pharmacists and a statistician. During the audits all patients on antibiotic treatment were evaluated, and recommendations on the indication, choice of antibiotics, route of administration and duration of therapies were given to the physicians in care. For each unit involved in the ASP one or more reference physicians were identified to carry out the audits with the infectious disease consultants. During the audits, carried out once or twice a week at regular intervals depending on the complexity of the unit, the adherence to these indications was evaluated. Furthermore, the infectious disease consultants were responsible for writing and sharing diagnostic and therapeutic protocols, based on the local epidemiology, for the management of the most common infectious syndromes. Moreover, all units of both hospitals had been involved since March 2019 in the "bacteremia program": for five days a week, in the case of bloodstream infections, the microbiology unit informed the infectious disease specialists of positivity to allow better management of the patient.

The present study was prospectively planned by the infectious disease consultants of the ASPs and by the healthcare administration of the two hospitals that approved and institutionalized the ASP. They prepared the study protocol in September 2019 and a pre-formed case report form. The team of infectious disease consultants at both hospitals received the same training and education on local and international infectious guidelines to follow. They also were trained with the same methodology in conducting the ASP.

Thus, the snapshot analysis of antibiotic use and the evaluations of appropriateness of antibiotic prescribing were performed by audit in the two hospitals, respectively, in the week 10–14 of February 2020 in Naples, and 14–23 of November 2019 in Caserta. The audits in Naples were performed by infectious disease consultants operating in Caserta, and the audits in Caserta by those operating in Naples; the consultants were unaware if the units were participating in the ASP or not.

2.2. Data Collection

The pre-formed case report form was filled-in on the days of evaluation by the infectious disease consultants to assess antibiotic prescriptive appropriateness, both in the units that had joined the ASP and in those that had not participated in the project.

The data collected included the following: type of unit, number of patients admitted to the ward in empiric or targeted antibiotic therapy and/or antibiotic prophylaxis (type of antimicrobial, dosage, way of administration, indication and duration). For each antibiotic prescription the appropriateness in relation to the patient's clinical state and guidelines was evaluated. We included all types of antimicrobials in the evaluation: antibacterials and antifungals for systemic use, antituberculosis, antiprotozoal and antimalarials and antivirals for systemic use. We did not include topical antibiotics.

For each patient in antibiotic therapy additional data were collected. They included the type of acquisition of infection (nosocomial, according to US CDC criteria [10], healthcare-associated or community-acquired), presentation with sepsis or septic shock [11], the site of infection and whether the therapy was empirical or targeted.

2.3. Assessment of Appropriateness

The appropriateness of antimicrobial treatment was defined a priori in the phase of planning of the present study (in September 2019). Precisely, treatment was defined adequate if it was active towards the pathogen responsible for infection and if it was correct in dosage, duration and way of administration [12,13]. A therapy was defined empirical prior to the identification of the germ with relative antibiogram or targeted otherwise. Empirical therapy was considered adequate when at least one antimicrobial with activity against the most frequent germs involved in relation to the presumed site of infection was administered [14].

For every antibiotic prescription deemed inappropriate, the reason for inappropriateness was recorded. Only one reason for inadequacy was enough to consider the treatment as inadequate, and it could be considered inadequate for several reasons at the same time. The antibiotic was considered unnecessary when the patient's clinical state did not show evidence of infection. Antimicrobial therapy was considered inadequate when not indicated by the guidelines or when the antibiotic had no activity on the etiology involved [12].

Antimicrobial therapy was considered not recommended when, in the targeted treatment, the antibiotic was active but had an excessively wide range of action for the expected etiologies or, in the case of empirical treatment, it was not recommended by the guidelines. The duration of antimicrobial therapy was considered excessive when it exceeded the recommended limits of the international guidelines.

2.4. Outcomes

The primary outcome was to assess the appropriateness of antibiotic prescribing in the two hospitals; in particular, to assess whether there was a difference in the adequacy of prescriptive practice in the departments that had joined the ASP and in those that had not participated in the project.

The secondary outcome was to identify the main reasons for prescriptive inappropriateness in order to identify priority areas of intervention and put in place measures to optimize antibiotic prescribing.

2.5. Ethics

All methods used in the study were in accordance with the international guidelines, with the standards on human experimentation of the Ethics Committee of the Azienda Ospedaliera Universitaria, University of Campania, and with the Helsinki Declaration of 1975, revised in 2013. Since the leadership of the University of Campania and AORN Caserta formally approved the study, and the data were collected in the aggregate manner during routine clinical activities, no approval was required by the local Ethics Committee.

2.6. Statistical Analysis

Continuous variables were summarized as mean and standard deviation, and categorical variables as absolute and relative frequencies. For continuous variables, the differences were evaluated by the Student *t*-test; categorical variables were compared by the chi-square test, using exact procedures if needed.

Variables with a univariate p value < 0.1 were chosen for inclusion in an exploratory multivariable analysis, which was performed using logistic regression.

3. Results

3.1. Characteristics of Units Participating in the Study

A total of 53 units, between the two hospitals, were assessed; in particular, 19 medical, 25 surgical and 9 ICUs were evaluated. Of the total number of units evaluated 15 had joined the ASP and 38 had not. The total number of patients assessed was 486. Of these, 208 (42.8%) were being treated with antibiotics, specifically 78 (16.1%) were in antibiotic prophylaxis and 130 (26.7%) in antibiotic therapy.

3.2. Appropriateness in ASP and Non-ASP Units

The global adequacy of antimicrobial prescription and a comparative analysis between the wards that had joined the ASP units and those that had not (non-ASP units) are summarized in Table 1.

Table 1. Characteristics and global adequacy of antimicrobial prescription between ASP and non-ASP units.

Variables	ASP	Non-ASP	*p* Value
	Characteristics of Units		
Units N	15	38	–
Beds available N	184	426	–
Patients admitted/ Available beds n/N (%)	117/184 (63.6)	369/426 (86.6)	–
Medical Units n/N (%)	5/15 (33.3)	14/38 (36.8)	0.81
Surgical Units n/N (%)	6/15 (40)	19/38 (50)	0.51
Intensive Care Units n/N (%)	4/15 (26.7)	5/38 (13.2)	0.24
	Characteristics of antibiotic prescriptions		
Antibiotic prophylaxis n/N (%)	14/117 (12)	64/426 (17.3)	0.17
Antimicrobial therapy n/N (%)	27/117 (23.1)	103/426 (27.9)	0.30
	Prescriptive appropriateness		
Appropriate antimicrobial prescription n/N (%)	27/41 (65.8)	38/167 (22.7)	<0.001
Inappropriate antimicrobial prescriptions n/N (%)	14/41 (34.2)	129/167 (77.2)	
	Reason for inappropriate antimicrobial prescription		
Antimicrobial unnecessary n/N (%)	3/14 (21.4)	50/129 (38.7)	0.14
Antimicrobial inadequate n/N (%)	3/14 (21.4)	14/129 (10.8)	0.30
Antimicrobial not recommended n/N (%)	4/14 (28.6)	46/129 (35.6)	0.46
Excessive duration n/N (%)	3/14 (21.4)	40/129 (31)	0.36
Inadequate dose n/N (%)	4/14 (28.6)	19/129 (14.7)	0.24
Inadequate way of administration n/N (%)	0/14 (0)	2/129 (1.5)	0.62
2 reasons for inappropriate antimicrobial prescription n/N (%)	3/14 (21.4)	35/129 (27.1)	0.53
≥3 reasons for inappropriate antimicrobial prescription, n/N (%)	0/14 (0)	3/129 (2.3)	0.55

The prescriptive appropriateness was better in the ASP units than in the non-ASP units (65.8% versus 22.7%, $p < 0.01$). The inappropriateness was more frequently due to unnecessary (38.7%) or not recommended prescriptions (35.6%) or excessive duration (31%) in non-ASP units, while inadequate antibiotic prescription (21.4%) or dosing (28.6%) was more frequent in the ASP group, although the difference was not statistically significant. Patients in the non-ASP units were more frequently treated with third-generation cephalosporins (20.9% versus 7.3%, $p = 0.01$) and quinolones (17.4% versus 2.4%, $p < 0.01$) (Table S1). On the contrary, first-generation cephalosporins were more frequently prescribed for patients in the ASP units (53.6%) than for those in the non-ASP units (10.2%, $p < 0.01$) (Table S1). Only 10 patients were taking other antimicrobials such as antifungals and anti-tuberculosis agents.

3.3. *Factors Associated with Appropriate and Inappropriate Antimicrobial Prescription*

As shown in Table 2, a comparison between appropriate and inappropriate prescriptions showed that antimicrobial therapy was more frequently appropriate in ASP units (41.5% versus 9.8%, $p < 0.01$), especially in medical units (50.8% versus 28.7%, $p < 0.01$) and ICUs (15.4% versus 5.6%, $p = 0.02$).

Table 2. Factors associated with appropriate or inappropriate prescription.

Variables	Appropriate Prescription	Inappropriate Prescription	*p* Value
N° of Antimicrobial prescriptions	65	143	–
Antibiotic prophylaxis, N (%)	16 (24.6)	62 (43.4)	0.01
Antibiotic therapy, N (%)	49 (75.4)	81 (56.6)	0.01
Prescriptions in non-ASP units, N (%)	38 (58.5)	129 (90.2)	<0.01
Prescriptions in ASP units N (%)	27 (41.5)	14 (9.8)	<0.01
	Characteristics of Units		
Medical units, N (%)	33 (50.8)	41 (28.7)	<0.01
Surgical units, N (%)	22 (33.8)	94 (65.7)	<0.01
Intensive care units, N (%)	10 (15.4)	8 (5.6)	0.02
	Appropriateness of antibiotic therapy prescription		
Empiric therapy, n/N (%)	25/49 (51.0)	72/81 (88.9)	<0.01
Prescriptions in non-ASP units, n/N (%)	30/49 (61.2)	73/81 (90.1)	<0.01
Prescriptions in ASP units, n/N (%)	19/49 (38.8)	8/81 (9.9)	<0.01
	Acquisition of infection		
Community-acquired infection, n/N (%)	30/49 (61.2)	44/81 (54.3)	0.44
Healthcare-associated infection, n/N (%)	5/49 (10.2)	5/81 (6.2)	0.40
Nosocomial infection, n/N (%)	11/49 (22.4)	20/81 (28.9)	0.04
Unknown, n/N (%)	3/49 (6.2)	12/81 (14.8)	0.13
	Severity of infection		
Sepsis, n/N (%)	6/49 (12.2)	5/81 (6.2)	0.23
Septic shock, n/N (%)	1/49 (2)	1/81 (1.2)	0.72
	Source of infection		
Unknown source, n/N (%)	1/49 (2)	9/81 (11.1)	0.06
Pneumonia, n/N (%)	9/49 (18.4)	20/81 (24.7)	0.40
Endocarditis/Cardiovascular, n/N (%)	5/49 (10.2)	0/81 (0)	<0.01
Abdominal, n/N (%)	1/49 (2)	15/81 (18.5)	<0.01
Genito-urinary, n/N (%)	6/49 (12.2)	13/81 (16)	0.55
Osteoarticular, n/N (%)	3/49 (6.1)	1/81 (1.2)	0.12
Skin and soft tissues, n/N (%)	5/49 (10.2)	4/81 (4.9)	0.25
Central Nervous System, n/N (%)	1/49 (2)	1/81 (1.2)	0.72
Bloodstream, n/N (%)	9/49 (18.4)	2/81 (2.5)	<0.01
Other, n/N (%)	7/49 (14.3)	7/81 (8.6)	0.31
Missing data, n/N (%)	4/49 (36.4)	7/81 (63.6)	0.92
Collection of microbiology specimen, n/N (%)	37/49 (75.5)	36/81 (44.4)	<0.01

On the contrary, inappropriate prescriptions were more frequently reported in surgical units (65.7% versus 33.8%, $p < 0.01$) due to the inappropriate prescription of antibiotic prophylaxis (43.4% versus 24.6%, $p = 0.01$) (Table 2). Moreover, appropriateness was more frequently reported in the 11 patients with bloodstream infections ($p < 0.01$) and in the 5 patients with bacterial endocarditis ($p < 0.01$); instead, the 16 patients with abdominal infections were more frequently treated with inappropriate antimicrobial therapy ($p < 0.01$). Another factor associated with appropriate prescription was the collection of microbiology specimens ($p < 0.01$), while a factor associated with inappropriate prescription was the presence of nosocomial infections ($p = 0.04$) (Table 2).

Multivariable analysis of the factors associated with prescriptive appropriateness identified ASP units ($p = 0.02$), and bloodstream or cardiovascular ($p = 0.03$) as a source of infections, as independent predictors of better prescriptive appropriateness (Table 3).

Table 3. Logistic regression analysis for independent factors related to prescriptive appropriateness.

Factor	OR	95% CI		*p* Value
		Lower Limit	Upper Limit	
Medical units (ref.)				
Surgical units	0.50	0.12	2.04	0.33
Intensive care units	1.70	0.37	7.79	0.49
ASP (ref.)				
Non-ASP	0.21	0.05	0.85	0.03
Community-acquired infection (ref.)				
Healthcare-associated infection	0.68	0.11	4.13	0.674
Nosocomial infection	0.42	0.12	1.53	0.19
N° sepsis (ref.)				
Sepsis	1.89	0.28	12.88	0.52
Septic shock	0.12	0.00	4.34	0.24
Other sources of infection (ref.)				
Bloodstream or Cardiovascular infections/	7.16	1.19	43.05	0.03
Abdominal	0.39	0.04	3.73	0.41
Collection of microbiology specimen (ref)				
No collection of microbiology specimen	0.42	0.12	1.49	0.18

3.4. Analysis of Antimicrobial Therapy and of Antibiotic Prophylaxis

Considering only antimicrobial therapy, no differences in acquisition, source and severity of infection were observed between the ASP and non-ASP units (Table 4).

Table 4. Adequacy of antimicrobial therapy between ASP and non-ASP units.

Variables	ASP, N (%)	Non-ASP, N (%)	*p* Value
N of antimicrobial therapy prescriptions	27	103	–
	Antibiotic therapy		
Empiric therapy, N (%)	10 (37)	87 (84.5)	<0.01
Target therapy, N (%)	17 (63)	16 (15.5)	<0.01
	Acquisition of infection		
Community-acquired infection, N (%)	16 (59.2)	58 (56.3)	0.78
Healthcare-associated infection, N (%)	4 (14.8)	6 (5.8)	0.11
Nosocomial infection, N (%)	4 (14.8)	27 (26.2)	0.21
Unknown, N (%)	3 (11.1)	12 (13.1)	0.94
	Severity of infection		
Sepsis, N (%)	2 (7.4)	9 (8.7)	0.82
Septic shock, N (%)	2 (7.4)	0 (0)	<0.01
	Source of infection		
Unknown source, N (%)	0 (0)	10 (9.7)	0.09
Pneumonia, N (%)	6 (22.2)	23 (22.3)	0.99
Endocarditis/Cardiovascular	4 (14.8)	1 (1)	<0.01
Abdominal, N (%)	2 (7.4)	14 (13.6)	0.38
Genito-urinary, N (%)	5 (18.5)	14 (13.6)	0.51
Osteoarticular, N (%)	2 (7.4)	2 (1.9)	0.14
Skin and soft tissues, N (%)	3 (11.1)	6 (5.8)	0.33
Central Nervous System, N (%)	0 (0)	2 (1.9)	0.46
Bloodstream, N (%)	3 (11.1)	8 (7.8)	0.57
Other, N (%)	1 (3.7)	13 (12.6)	0.18
Missing data, N (%)	1 (3.7)	10 (9.7)	0.31
Collection of microbiology specimen, N (%)	23 (85.2)	50 (48.5)	<0.01

Table 4. *Cont.*

Variables	ASP, N (%)	Non-ASP, N (%)	*p* Value
	Prescriptive appropriateness		
Appropriate antimicrobial therapy prescription, N (%)	21 (77.7)	34 (33)	<0.01
Inappropriate antimicrobial therapy prescription, N (%)	6 (22.3)	69 (67)	
	Reason for inappropriate antimicrobial therapy prescription		
Antimicrobial unnecessary, n/N (%)	0/6 (0)	31/69 (44.9)	0.03
Antimicrobial inadequate, n/N (%)	1/6 (16.6)	8/69 (11.6)	0.71
Antimicrobial not recommended, n/N (%)	4/6 (66.6)	21/69 (30.4)	0.07
Excessive duration, n/N (%)	0/6 (0)	15/69 (21.7)	0.20
Inadequate dose, n/N (%)	2/6 (33.3)	14/69 (20.3)	0.45
Inadequate way of administration, n/N (%)	0/6 (0)	1/69 (1.4)	0.77
2 reasons for inappropriate antimicrobial therapy prescription, n/N (%)	1/6 (16.6)	17/69 (24.6)	0.66
≥3 reasons for inappropriate antimicrobial therapy prescription, n/N (%)	0/6 (0)	2/69 (2.9)	0.67

In the ASP units the patients were less frequently treated with an empirical antimicrobial therapy (37% versus 84.5%, $p < 0.01$), and microbiological samples were more often collected before the start of therapy (85.2% versus 48.5%, $p < 0.01$); moreover, antimicrobial prescriptions were more frequently appropriate (77.7% versus 33%, $p < 0.01$) (Table 4). Non-ASP wards more frequently gave unnecessary antimicrobials (44.9% versus 0%, $p = 0.03$) (Table 4).

Considering only the antibiotic prophylaxis, as reported in Table 5, ASP units showed better prescriptive appropriateness (57.2% versus 18.8%, $p < 0.01$), whereas, in the non-ASP units the use of antibiotics not recommended by the guidelines was more frequently observed (44.2% versus 0%, $p = 0.04$).

Table 5. Adequacy of antibiotic prophylaxis between ASP and non-ASP units.

Variables	ASP, N (%)	Non-ASP, N (%)	*p* Value
N° of antimicrobial prophylaxis prescriptions	14	64	–
	Units		
General Surgery, n/N (%)	0/6 (0)	7/19 (36.8)	0.19
Urogenital Surgery, n/N (%)	1/6 (16.6)	3/19 (15.8)	0.70
Emergency Surgery, n/N (%)	0/6 (0)	2/19 (10.5)	0.50
Orthopedics, n/N (%)	1/6 (16.6)	1/19 (5.3)	0.23
Head and neck Surgery, n/N (%)	0/6 (0)	4/19 (21.1)	0.33
Thoracic Surgery, n/N (%)	1/6 (16.6)	0/19 (0)	0.03
Abdominal Surgery, n/N (%)	3/6 (50)	2/19 (10.5)	0.01
	Prescriptive appropriateness		
Appropriate antibiotic prophylaxis prescription, N (%)	8 (57.2)	12 (18.8)	<0.01
Inappropriate antibiotic prescription, N (%)	6 (42.8)	54 (81.2)	
	Reason for inappropriate antibiotic prophylaxis prescription		
Antibiotic unnecessary, n/N (%)	2/6 (33.3)	14/54 (26.9)	0.74
Antibiotic inadequate, n/N (%)	2/6 (33.3)	4/54 (7.7)	0.05
Antibiotic not recommended, n/N (%)	0/6 (0)	23/54 (44.2)	0.04
Excessive duration, n/N (%)	3/6 (50)	23/54 (44.2)	0.79
Inadequate dose, n/N (%)	1/6 (16.6)	5/54 (9.6)	0.59
Inadequate way of administration, n/N (%)	0/6 (0)	1/54 (1.9)	0.73
2 reasons for inappropriate antibiotic prophylaxis prescription, n/N (%)	2/6 (33.3)	15/54 (28.8)	0.81
≥3 reasons for inappropriate antibiotic prophylaxis prescription, n/N (%)	0/6 (0)	1/54 (1.9)	0.73

4. Discussion

Antibiotic resistance is rising to dangerously high levels all over the world. Overuse and misuse of antibiotics contribute to the acquisition and spread of infections due to antibiotic-resistant bacteria. In the present study, we report the effects that an education-based ASP implemented in some units of two hospitals in the Campania region of southern Italy had on the appropriateness of antimicrobial prescription. Specifically, we observed a higher antimicrobial prescription appropriateness for both antibiotic therapy and prophylaxis in the units that joined the ASP; moreover, a significant decrease in the use of antibiotics with a high environmental impact, such as third-generation cephalosporins and quinolones, was observed in ASP units. Programs and interventions that aim at optimizing antimicrobial use, i.e., antimicrobial stewardship programs, have grown exponentially in recent years [15], proving effective and important in hospital settings. The introduction of ASP in hospitals involves a series of structured interventions. They first include the institutionalization of the program so that it is recognized and progressively accepted by all the professionals of the hospital. Secondly, it is important to assess the local data on prevalence of antibiotic resistance and the consumption of antibiotics in order to implement tailor-made interventions.

ASPs in hospitals have shown a positive impact, with reduced length of stay, shorter treatment duration without an increase in mortality and a reduction in colonization and infection with resistant bacteria [9,16]. In our previous work [8], we observed a significant decrease in antimicrobial consumption, and in the incidence of bloodstream infections due to multidrug-resistant Gram-negative organisms, in two intensive care units after the implementation of a persuasive educational ASP. Educational interventions, although less immediate than restrictive methods, have a more sustained impact in influencing prescriptive behavior and can yield even better long-term results [17]. Antimicrobial stewardship includes not only limiting inappropriate use, but also optimizing antimicrobial selection, dosing, route and duration of therapy to maximize the clinical cure [18]. Thus, the present study confirms the effects of an ASP on the appropriateness of antimicrobial prescription since the participation in an ASP was an independent factor associated with appropriate antimicrobial prescription.

When analyzing the reason for inappropriate prescriptions, we found a higher frequency of unnecessary (38.7%) or not recommended prescriptions (35.6%) in non-ASP units as compared to ASP units (21.4% and 28.6%, respectively), while inadequate antibiotic prescriptions (21.4%) or dosing (28.6%) was more frequent in ASP groups, although none of these differences reached statistical significance. A commonly feared consequence of narrowing the spectrum of empirical therapy is the prescription of antibiotics that are ineffective against the clinical isolates. However, we should consider that in our study the definition of inadequate empirical therapy does not imply a lack of effectiveness against the isolated strain, but only against the totality of the potentially expected etiologies. Furthermore, we should point out that if we consider the total number of prescriptions, the rate of inadequacy is similar in non-ASP units (14 of 167, 8.4%) and in ASP units (3 out of 41, 7.3%).

Making accurate diagnoses is one of the main goals of the ASP. Overall, the results of the analysis of the antimicrobial therapy in ASP and non-ASP units reinforce the recommendations in pursuing the collection of culture samples before the start of therapy. In addition, we found that non-ASP units make greater use of empirical therapy at the same severity of the patient's clinical state and more often resorted to the use of antibiotics when not necessary, i.e., the patient's clinical state was not suggestive of infection. Indeed, we found a rate of about 50% of unnecessary antimicrobial prescription in non-ASP units.

Similar data come from a study conducted in the United States in 2010–2011 that found at least 30% of antibiotics prescribed in doctors' offices, emergency departments and hospital clinics were unnecessary [19].

In the present study, another factor independently associated with appropriateness in antimicrobial prescription was the presence of bloodstream infections or bacterial endocarditis. These data may be associated with the infectious disease management of bacterial endocarditis and to the structured bacteremia program conducted by infectious disease specialists in ASP and non-ASP units of both hospitals. The infectious disease consultations that were provided to all patients with bloodstream infections have most probably increased the appropriateness of antibiotic prescriptions in this setting and improved the adequacy of patients' management. In fact, some studies showed that advice from infectious disease specialists reduced inappropriate treatment and resulted in better clinical outcomes in the management of sepsis [20,21] and *Staphylococcus aureus* bacteremia [22–24].

Finally, a better prescriptive appropriateness in ASP units was registered even in surgical prophylaxis. One of the strategies of ASP was to optimize surgical antibiotic prophylaxis, ensuring that timely and appropriate antibiotics are administered as recommended before surgery and limiting prolonged use of antibiotic prophylaxis once surgery is over [25]. We found how, not following the guidelines, surgical non-ASP units more frequently used broad-spectrum antibiotics as a first choice for surgical prophylaxis. These findings underline the importance of using a persuasive educational approach that, through audits and drafting of locally adapted guidelines, allows an improvement in the prescribers' knowledge.

This study has several limitations: even using a study setup that minimized bias inherent in subjective parameter estimation (e.g., the use of standardized treatment guidelines), the experts of infectious diseases may have had motivational biases that influenced their clinical judgment. Moreover, baseline data on the antimicrobial appropriates in wards before the beginning of ASP were not available, making it difficult to compare the outcomes before and after the intervention. Finally, the analysis on the relationship between appropriateness and experience of the physicians was not done. The strengths of our study include its multicenter design and the use of structured intervention that can easily be replicated and incorporated into clinical practice to evaluate the appropriateness of antimicrobial prescription.

5. Conclusions

The findings of this study reinforce the importance of adopting an educational ASP in order to improve the quality of antimicrobial prescription in clinical practice and possibly to contribute to a reduction in the global phenomenon of antibiotic resistance. Structured and persuasive interventions aimed at improving prescriber knowledge and compliance, and at optimizing the management of complicated infections such as bacteremia, are of fundamental importance for the success of ASP programs. The efforts of future research should focus on identifying the best strategies to implement an effective stewardship program in hospital settings in order to reduce the misuse of antibiotics.

Supplementary Materials: The following are available online at https://www.mdpi.com/2079-6382/10/3/314/s1, Table S1: Main classes of antimicrobials used in ASP and non-ASP and way of administration.

Author Contributions: N.C., F.C. and L.O. were responsible for the conception and design of the study, interpreted the data, and wrote the paper; M.M., F.C., C.M., G.D.C., L.O. and A.R. conducted the audits as Infectious Disease Consultants and contributed to collecting and analyzing the data; A.G. (Anna Galdieri), A.G. (Antonio Giordano) and P.C. approved and supported the program; L.O. performed the statistical analysis. All authors have read and agreed to the published version of the manuscript.

Funding: No funding has been received for this study.

Institutional Review Board Statement: The study was conducted according to the guidelines of the Declaration of Helsinki. Ethical review and approval were waived for this study since the leadership of the University of Campania and AORN Caserta formally approved the study, and the data were collected in the aggregate manner during routine clinical activities.

Informed Consent Statement: Patient consent was waived due to observational nature of the study.

Data Availability Statement: The datasets used and/or analyzed during the current study are available from the corresponding author.

Acknowledgments: We thank Maria Di Vico, Ilaria De Luca and Roberta Palladino for their invaluable help in the study.

Conflicts of Interest: The authors declare that they have no conflict of interest.

References

1. World Health Organization. Antibiotic Resistance. Available online: https://www.who.int/news-room/fact-sheets/detail/antibiotic-resistance (accessed on 17 March 2021).
2. Cassini, A.; Högberg, L.D.; Plachouras, D.; Quattrocchi, A.; Hoxha, A.; Simonsen, G.S.; Colomb-Cotinat, M.; Kretzschmar, M.E.; Devleesschauwer, B.; Cecchini, M.; et al. Attributable deaths and disability-adjusted life-years caused by infections with antibiotic-resistant bacteria in the EU and the European Economic Area in 2015: A population-level modelling analysis. *Lancet Infect. Dis.* **2019**, *19*, 56–66. [CrossRef]
3. European Centre for Disease Prevention and Control. ECDC Calls for Continued Action to Address Antimicrobial Resistance in Healthcare Settings. Available online: https://www.ecdc.europa.eu/en/news-events/ecdc-calls-continued-action-address-antimicrobial-resistance-healthcare-settings (accessed on 17 March 2021).
4. Plachouras, D.; Kärki, T.; Hansen, S.; Hopkins, S.; Lyytikäinen, O.; Moro, M.L.; Reilly, J.; Zarb, P.; Zingg, W.; Kinross, P.; et al. Antimicrobial use in European acute care hospitals: Results from the second point prevalence survey (PPS) of healthcare-associated infections and antimicrobial use, 2016 to 2017. *Euro Surveill.* **2018**, *23*, 800393. [CrossRef] [PubMed]
5. Zarb, P.; Amadeo, B.; Muller, A.; Draiper, N.; Vankerckhoven, V.; Davey, P.; Goossens, H.; Markova, B.; Jansen, H.; Metz-Gercek, S.; et al. ESAC-3 Hospital Care Subproject Group. Identification of targets for quality improvement in antimicrobial prescribing: The web-based ESAC Point Prevalence Survey 2009. *J. Antimicrob. Chemother.* **2011**, *66*, 443–449. [CrossRef]
6. Hecker, M.T.; Aron, D.C.; Patel, N.P.; Lehmann, M.K.; Donskey, C.J. Unnecessary use of antimicrobials in hospitalized patients: Current patterns of misuse with an emphasis on the antianaerobic spectrum of activity. *Arch. Intern. Med.* **2003**, *163*, 972–978. [CrossRef] [PubMed]
7. Pelullo, C.P.; Pepe, A.; Napolitano, F.; Giuseppe, D.G.; Coppola, N. Perioperative Antibiotic Prophylaxis: Knowledge and Attitudes among Resident Physicians in Italy. *Antibiotics* **2020**, *9*, 357. [CrossRef]
8. Onorato, L.; Macera, M.; Calò, F.; Monari, C.; Russo, F.; Lovene, M.R.; Signoriello, G.; Annibale, R.; Pace, M.C.; Autilio, C.; et al. The effect of an antimicrobial stewardship programme in two intensive care units of a teaching hospital: An interrupted time series analysis. *Clin. Microbiol. Infect.* **2020**, *26*, 782.e1–782.e6. [CrossRef]
9. Davey, P.; Marwick, C.A.; Scott, C.L.; Charani, E.; McNeil, K.; Brown, E.; Gould, I.M.; Ramsay, C.R.; Michie, S. Interventions to improve antibiotic prescribing practices for hospital inpatients. *Cochrane Database Syst. Rev.* **2017**, *2*, CD003543. [CrossRef] [PubMed]
10. Garner, J.S.; Jarvis, W.R.; Emori, T.G.; Horan, T.C.; Hughes, J.M. CDC definitions for nosocomial infections, 1988. *Am. J. Infect. Control.* **1988**, *16*, 128–140. [CrossRef]
11. Singer, M.; Deutschman, C.S.; Seymour, C.W.; Shankar-Hari, M.; Annane, D.; Bauer, M.; Chiche, J.D.; Bellomo, R.; Bernard, G.R.; Coopersmith, C.M.; et al. The Third International Consensus Definitions for Sepsis and Septic Shock (Sepsis-3). *J. Am. Med. Assoc.* **2016**, *315*, 801–810. [CrossRef]
12. American Thoracic Society; Infectious Diseases Society of America. Guidelines for the management of adults with hospital-acquired, ventilator-associated, and healthcare-associated pneumonia. *Am. J. Respir. Crit. Care Med.* **2005**, *171*, 388–416. [CrossRef]
13. Siempos, I.I.; Ioannidou, E.; Falagas, M.E. The Difference between Adequate and Appropriate Antimicrobial Treatment. *Clin. Infect. Dis.* **2008**, *46*, 642–644. [CrossRef] [PubMed]
14. Retamar, P.; Portillo, M.M.; López-Prieto, M.D.; de Cueto, M.; Garcia, M.V.; Gomez, M.J.; Del Arco, A.; Munoz, A.; Sanchez-Porto, A.; Torses-Tortosa, M.; et al. Impact of inadequate empirical therapy on the mortality of patients with bloodstream infections: A propensity score-based analysis. *Antimicrob. Agents Chemother.* **2012**, *56*, 472–478. [CrossRef] [PubMed]
15. Dyar, O.J.; Huttner, B.; Schouten, J.; Pulcini, C.; ESGAP (ESCMID Study Group for Antimicrobial stewardshiP). What is antimicrobial stewardship? *Clin. Microbiol. Infect.* **2017**, *23*, 793–798. [CrossRef] [PubMed]
16. Cox, J.A.; Vlieghe, E.; Mendelson, M.; Wertheim, H.; Ndegwa, L.; Villegas, M.V.; Gould, I.; Levy Hara, G. Antibiotic stewardship in low-and middle-income countries: The same but different? *Clin. Microbiol. Infect.* **2017**, *23*, 812–818. [CrossRef] [PubMed]
17. Tamma, P.D.; Avdic, E.; Keenan, J.F.; Zhao, Y.; Anand, G.; Cooper, J.; Dezube, R.; Hsu, S.; Cosgrove, S.E. What Is the More Effective Antibiotic Stewardship Intervention: Preprescription Authorization or Postprescription Review with Feedback? *Clin. Infect. Dis.* **2017**, *64*, 537–543.
18. Dellit, T.H.; Owens, R.C.; McGowan, J.E., Jr.; Gerding, D.N.; Weinstein, R.A.; Burke, J.P.; Huskins, W.C.; Paterson, D.L.; Fishman, N.O.; Carpenter, C.F.; et al. Infectious Diseases Society of America and the Society for Healthcare Epidemiology of America Guidelines for Developing an Institutional Program to Enhance Antimicrobial Stewardship. *Clin. Infect. Dis.* **2007**, *44*, 159–177. [CrossRef] [PubMed]

19. Fleming-Dutra, K.E.; Hersh, A.L.; Shapiro, D.J.; Bartoces, M.; Enns, A.E.; File, T.M., Jr.; Finkelstein, J.A.; Gerber, J.S.; Hyun, D.Y.; Linder, J.A.; et al. Prevalence of inappropriate antibiotic prescriptions among us ambulatory care visits, 2010–2011. *JAMA—J. Am. Med. Assoc.* **2016**, *315*, 1864–1873. [CrossRef] [PubMed]
20. López-Cortés, L.E.; Del Toro, M.D.; Gálvez-Acebal, J.; Bereciartua-Bastarrica, E.; Fariñas, M.C.; Sanz-Franco, M.; Natera, C.; Corzo, J.E.; Lomas, J.M.; Pasquau, J.; et al. Impact of an Evidence-Based Bundle Intervention in the Quality-of-Care Management and Outcome of Staphylococcus aureus Bacteremia. *Clin. Infect. Dis.* **2013**, *57*, 1225–1233. [CrossRef]
21. Minton, J.; Clayton, J.; Sandoe, J.; Mc Gan, H.; Wilcox, M. Improving early management of bloodstream infection: A quality improvement project. *BMJ* **2008**, *336*, 440–443. [CrossRef]
22. Pérez-Rodríguez, M.T.; Sousa, A.; López-Cortés, L.E.; Martinez-Lames, L.; Val, N.; Baroja, A.; Nodar, A.; Vasallo, F.; Alvarez-Fernandez, M.; Crespo, M.; et al. Moving beyond unsolicited consultation: Additional impact of a structured intervention on mortality in Staphylococcus aureus bacteraemia. *J. Antimicrob. Chemother.* **2019**, *74*, 1101–1107. [CrossRef]
23. Martin, L.; Harris, M.T.; Brooks, A.; Main, C.; Mertz, D. Management and outcomes in patients with Staphylococcus aureus bacteremia after implementation of mandatory infectious diseases consult: A before/after study. *BMC Infect. Dis.* **2015**, *15*, 568. [CrossRef] [PubMed]
24. Lahey, T.; Shah, R.; Gittzus, J.; Schwartzman, J.; Kirkland, K. Infectious diseases consultation lowers mortality from Staphylococcus aureus bacteremia. *Medicine* **2009**, *88*, 263–267. [CrossRef] [PubMed]
25. Tarchini, G.; Liau, K.H.; Solomkin, J.S. Antimicrobial Stewardship in Surgery: Challenges and Opportunities. *Clin. Infect. Dis.* **2017**, *64* (Suppl. 2), S112–S114. [CrossRef] [PubMed]

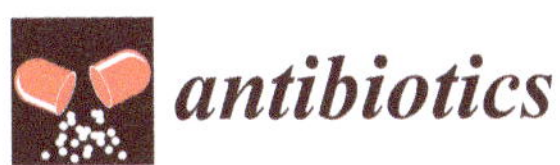 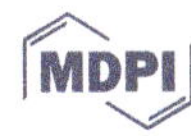

Article

Antimicrobial Stewardship Program Implementation in a Saudi Medical City: An Exploratory Case Study

Saleh Alghamdi [1], Ilhem Berrou [2,*], Eshtyag Bajnaid [3], Zoe Aslanpour [4], Abdul Haseeb [5], Mohamed Anwar Hammad [1] and Nada Shebl [4]

1 Department of Clinical Pharmacy, Faculty of Clinical Pharmacy, Albaha University, Albaha 65779-77388, Saudi Arabia; saleh.alghamdi@bu.edu.sa (S.A.); m.anwar@bu.edu.sa (M.A.H.)
2 Faculty of Health & Applied Sciences, University of the West of England, Staple Hill, Bristol BS16 1DD, UK
3 Department of Clinical Pharmacy, Pharmaceutical Services Administration, King Abdullah Medical City, Makkah 11176, Saudi Arabia; bajnaid.e@kamc.med.sa
4 Department of Clinical and Pharmaceutical Sciences, School of Life and Medical Sciences, University of Hertfordshire, Hatfield AL10 9AB, UK; z.aslanpour@herts.ac.uk (Z.A.); n.a.shebl@herts.ac.uk (N.S.)
5 Department of Clinical Pharmacy, College of Pharmacy, Umm Al Qura University, Makkah 77207, Saudi Arabia; amhaseeb@uqu.edu.sa
* Correspondence: Ilhem.berrou@uwe.ac.uk; Tel.: +44-11-732-84053

Abstract: Antimicrobial stewardship programs (ASPs) in hospitals have long been shown to improve antimicrobials' use and reduce the rates of antimicrobial resistance. However, their implementation in hospitals, especially in developing countries such as Saudi Arabia, remains low. One of the main barriers to implementation is the lack of knowledge of how to implement them. This study aims to explore how an antimicrobial stewardship programme was implemented in a Saudi hospital, the challenges faced and how they were overcome, and the program outcomes. A key stakeholder case study design was used, involving in-depth semi-structured interviews with the core members of the ASP team and analysis of 35 ASP hospital documents. ASP implementation followed a top-down approach and involved an initial preparatory phase and an implementation phase, requiring substantial infectious diseases and clinical pharmacy input throughout. Top management support was key to the successful implementation. ASP implementation reduced rates of multi-drug resistance and prescription of broad-spectrum antimicrobials. The implementation of ASPs in hospital is administrator rather than clinician driven. Outsourcing expertise and resources may help hospitals address the initial implementation challenges.

Keywords: antimicrobial stewardship programs; hospitals; multi-drug resistance

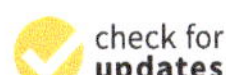

Citation: Alghamdi, S.; Berrou, I.; Bajnaid, E.; Aslanpour, Z.; Haseeb, A.; Hammad, M.A.; Shebl, N. Antimicrobial Stewardship Program Implementation in a Saudi Medical City: An Exploratory Case Study. *Antibiotics* **2021**, *10*, 280. https://doi.org/10.3390/antibiotics10030280

Academic Editor: Seok Hoon Jeong

Received: 7 February 2021
Accepted: 8 March 2021
Published: 9 March 2021

Publisher's Note: MDPI stays neutral with regard to jurisdictional claims in published maps and institutional affiliations.

Copyright: © 2021 by the authors. Licensee MDPI, Basel, Switzerland. This article is an open access article distributed under the terms and conditions of the Creative Commons Attribution (CC BY) license (https://creativecommons.org/licenses/by/4.0/).

1. Introduction

Antimicrobial stewardship programs (ASP) in hospital are interventions to reduce risks of antimicrobial treatment failures, adverse events, hospital acquired infections, rates of antimicrobial resistance and costs associated with antimicrobial prescriptions and prolonged length of stay in hospital [1]. These programs focus on optimizing the choice, dosing and route of administration of antimicrobials, monitoring their prescription and resistance patterns, and continuous provision of education and feedback to prescribers.

The programs were first implemented in the USA in the late 1990s, and started to gain popularity in Europe soon after that [2]. In an international survey carried out in 2015 by the ESCMID Study Group for Antimicrobial Policies (ESGAP) and ISC Group on Antimicrobial Stewardship, 52% of the countries had a national antimicrobial stewardship plan, 58% had ASPs in hospitals and 4% of the countries were planning antimicrobial stewardship strategies [3]. The Netherlands, France [4] and England [5] reported high rates of ASP implementation in hospitals. In the USA, a recent study suggests that 51% of the leading hospitals in the country have an active ASP. Around 59% of these hospitals had

ASP for more than 5 years [6]. However, the status of ASP implementation in hospitals in developing countries is less clear. Various reports point to low levels of implementation [7–9] for various reasons including: a lack of diagnostic testing and antimicrobials, sub-optimal infection prevention and control practices and the prevalent inappropriate prescribing practices [10,11]. Resistant microorganisms may spread from one person to another, one health care facility to another and one country to another [12]. Tackling antimicrobial resistance in developing countries is critical to reduce its burden in those countries, and to strengthen the global effort to contain this threat.

Like in many other developing countries, Saudi hospitals report low levels of ASP implementation, mainly in tertiary hospitals, despite having a national antimicrobial stewardship plan to implement ASPs in hospitals [13]. This is in contrast to reports of high prevalence of antimicrobial resistance and the emergence of new and rare multi-drug resistant strains [14]. Worryingly, these pathogens can spread globally given that Saudi Arabia is a popular destination for millions of international travelers annually for pilgrimage (Hajj).

We recently reported that one of the factors behind the lagging implementation of ASPs in Saudi hospitals is the lack of "know how" to implement them [13]. ASPs are novel to Saudi hospitals, and their implementation would require a significant change to routine practice, where antimicrobials are heavily prescribed, often inappropriately [15,16]. A recent guide by Mendelson et al. details a generic protocol for the implementation and/ or optimization of ASP in hospitals in both developing and developed countries' contexts [17]. However, three issues may be considered. First, the protocol may provide a useful outline of the resources needed and what the programs usually entail, but it may not be sufficiently practical, and may not highlight how implementation challenges can be practically overcome. Second, although the protocol recognises the resource limitations in developing countries, it does not differentiate between implementation in developing vs. developed contexts. Third, the protocol is clinician-oriented; however, in various developing countries, such as Saudi Arabia, it is hospital administrators, not clinicians, who often make decisions about policy implementation [15]. This study aims to explore how an antimicrobial stewardship programme was implemented in a Saudi hospital, the challenges faced and how they were overcome, and the program outcomes. Findings would improve the current knowledge of ASP implementation in developing countries, and provide hospitals in the region with a practical guide to implement these programs.

2. Results

A number of areas emerged as key themes from the interviews: motives for ASP adoption, development and implementation of ASP, implementation challenges, and outcomes. Where useful, we included quotes from the participants to illustrate key points.

2.1. Motives for ASP Adoption in the Medical City

The decision to adopt and implement an antimicrobial stewardship programme was initially made by the chief executive officer (CEO) of the medical city in 2015.

"Leadership support is the biggest thing we have here (at the hospital). It was all from the leadership to begin with. After 2–3 weeks from my appointment, the CEO came to me and said I want to start this (antimicrobial stewardship) programme, and it has to be up and running . . . "

Various factors (stated in no particular order of importance) seem to have influenced this decision. First, the CEO's surgical background heightened the need to improve infection prevention and control, and reduce the prevalence of multi-drug resistant strains in the facility. The CEO's training in an international hospital with a longstanding experience of ASPs influenced their conviction of the benefits of ASPs in the organisation. Second, the CEO perceived the medical city, one of the largest and most highly specialist tertiary centres in the country, to be a pioneer, and an exemplary model for other hospitals in the region to follow suite in relation to implementing ASPs. Third, the special context of the medical city, being a referral facility from other hospitals in the region, means that they often admit patients with complex care needs, who would have spent months in the referring hospitals. These patients tend to be colonized with multi–drug resistant strains, which are then transferred to the medical city. Fourth, the medical city is home to advanced neurosurgery and oncology centres, whose patients are immunocompromised and vulnerable to severe outcomes of multi-drug resistant infections. This context necessitated the adoption and implementation of interventions, such as ASPs, that can reduce the prevalence of multi–drug resistance and optimise the use of antimicrobials.

From the infectious diseases' consultant, clinical microbiologist, the lead antimicrobial pharmacist and infection control consultant's perspectives, the strongest motive to adopt and implement ASPs was the high prevalence of multi-drug resistant (MDR) microorganisms, particularly among Gram–negative bacteria. This was fueled by the high and inappropriate use of antimicrobials. The high prevalence of MDR organisms may have contributed to increased mortality rates, failure of surgical procedures, and may have compromised the safety of immunocompromised patients receiving specialist oncology, cardiac and neurosurgery services. The hospital was also planning to set up a transplant centre and was desperate to reduce the rates of multi-drug resistance.

"They were prescribing very expensive and inappropriate antibiotics and antifungals ... ICU patients were mostly on 3, 4, or 5 antibiotics. It was not justifiable at all ... We needed to start a strong antimicrobial stewardship programme for the patient's sake, and also to educate prescribers".

"We were having outbreaks of multi-drug resistant organisms and there was overuse of antibiotics. We had a major issue with drug resistant *Acinetobacter baumannii* which was sensitive to colistin, and then it became resistant to colistin. So, it became pan-drug resistant *Acinetobacter baumannii*. The infection control experts (in the hospital) said that this was because of the overuse of carbapenems in the ICU, and then the overuse of even colistin in the ICU".

"We have the oncology centre and we wanted to start the transplant centre, and of course the immunocompromised patients needed to have much fewer resistant microorganisms".

It is noteworthy that the MOH antimicrobial stewardship plan does not appear to be a motive for ASP adoption and implementation despite the medical city being a "flagship" MOH organisation.

2.2. *Development and Implementation of the Antimicrobial Stewardship Programme*

Phases of ASP Implementation

The ASP is part of the hospital's patient safety portfolio (PSP) of 10 strategic patient safety programs to address patient safety issues within the hospital and to improve the quality and safety of care. These are shown in Figure 1.

There were two phases of ASP implementation in the medical city.

Phase 1

The ASP aims to improve antimicrobial prescribing practices, reduce the high prevalence of multi–drug resistance in the hospital and the high costs associated with antimicrobials' prescribing.

Initially, the ASP programme was suggested to be part of the medication safety program, but the CEO insisted that the ASP programme should be an independent, standalone programme with its own key performance indicators.

"When we started discussing antimicrobial stewardship, the idea was that it should be part of the medications (safety) programme, but I said no, it needs to be done independently, it needs to stand out, to be very obvious and very evident"

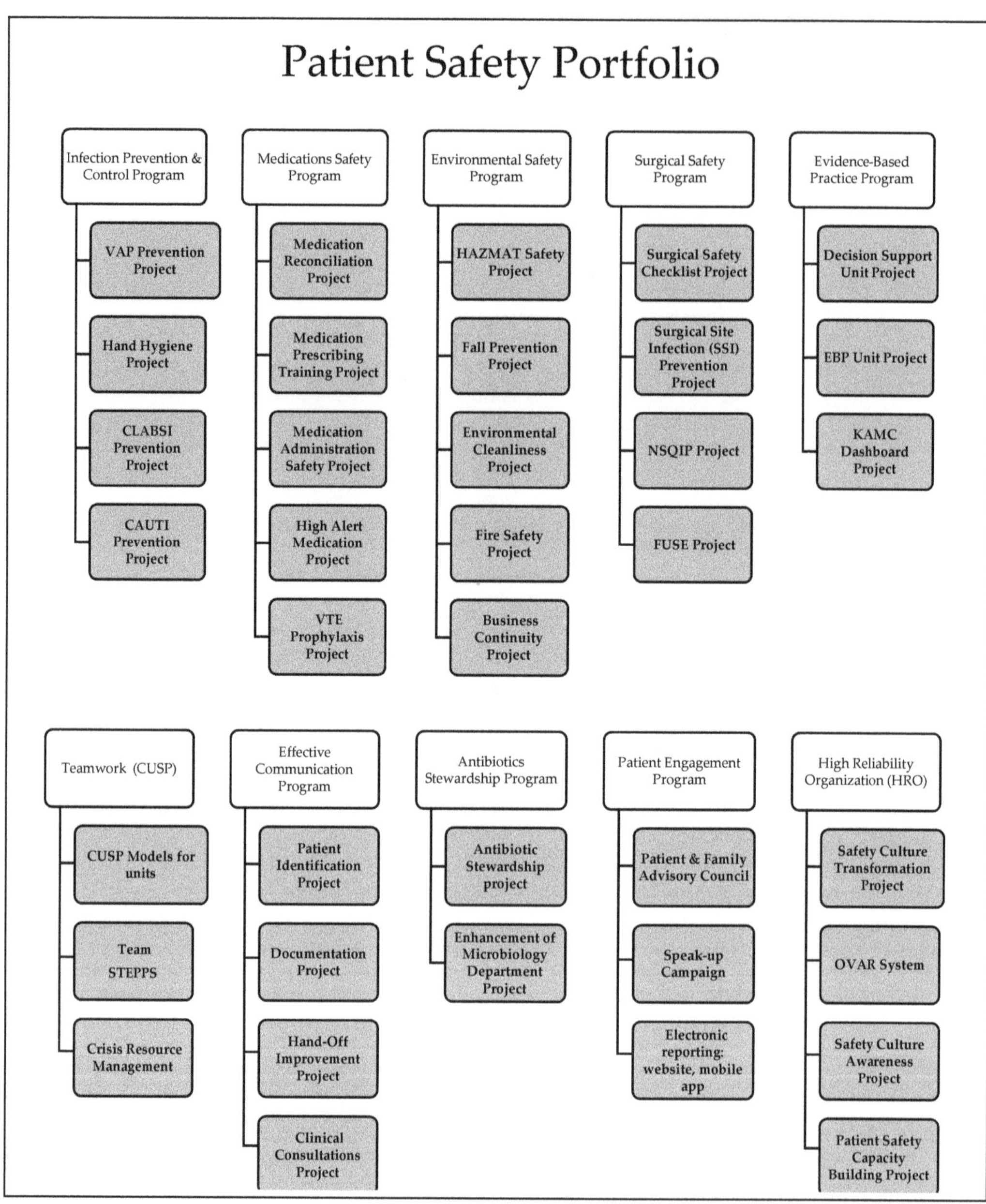

Figure 1. Patient safety portfolio of programs.

The hospital had no expert staff "in house" to set up and implement the ASP, so it outsourced a locum infectious disease pharmacist, who trained in a hospital in the USA. The locum ID pharmacist reviewed current practices and the potential implementation barriers, and provided practical guidelines on how these could be overcome. The hospital then appointed an antimicrobial lead pharmacist, who worked with the locum ID pharmacist, and the ID consultant to draft the hospital ASP policy (based on the Infectious Diseases

Society of America (IDSA) ASP guidelines) [1,18], the formulary restriction list (based on local antibiogram and MDROs surveillance reports), and set up the ASP team.

"we started with first thing formulary restriction based on the MDR (multi-drug resistance) pattern at the hospital. What are the medicines that we need to restrict firstWe started with broad spectrum antibiotics ... carbapenems, meropenem, imipenem, colistin ... and then with the antifungals voriconazole, posaconazole ... then we included caspofungin, micafungin and anidulafungin since they have a high cost ... "

The core members of the ASP team at the medical city were:

- The ID consultant as the director of the ASP program and their ID team;
- The antimicrobial lead pharmacist as the manager of the ASP program and the clinical pharmacists' team;
- Clinical pharmacists;
- Consultant clinical microbiologist and their team;
- The infection control consultant and their team.

The roles and responsibilities of each team member are presented in Figure 2. The ASP team maintained direct (and frequent) communication with key stakeholders such as the heads of ICU, hematology and oncology departments (where antimicrobials' use and resistance were high), and the head nurse (whose team is directly affected by the change in how antimicrobials will be obtained and administered). Those key stakeholders were often invited to take part in ASP team meetings, and become members of the bigger ASP team.

ID consultant- Director of the ASP

Chairs monthly ASP team meetings to discuss progress and feedback

invite key stakeholders to ASP team meetings to increase collaboration with hospital departments (particularly those resistant to ASP recommendations

ID Team

Review DOTs data, quality indicators and ASP forms

Facilitate antimicrobials' prescribing discussions and updates

Deliver the daily ASP tasks (reviewing restriction forms with clinical pharmacists, providing feedback to prescribers)

Maintain 24/7 ID cover for review and approval of restricted antimicrobials

Microbiology Team

Report information on antimicrobial susceptibility

Maintain constant communication (via a daily email) with ID team, clinical pharmacists is sent to team, and infection control consultant regarding antimicrobial resistance rates and selective reporting of antibiotic susceptibility testing

Prepare annual antibiogram

Lead antimicrobial pharmacist- Manager of the ASP

Oversees the day to day delivery of ASP tasks

Coordinates the input from the clinical pharmacists, communication with the ID Team , microbiology and the infection control consultant, and collect DOT data

Clinical pharmacists

Identify patients being prescribed restricted antimicrobials

Ensure appropriate restriction forms are submitted and approved

Review if the antimicrobial is still indicated and if the treatment duration is within the ID recommendation

Discuss with ID team alternative antimicrobials and appropriateness of dosing, and treatment duration

Optimise dosing of antimicrobials based on changes in kidney function and microbiology lab results

Coordinate with clinical pharmacists when patients are transferred to their wards

Infection control Team

Monitor the rate of healthcare acquired infection and incidence rates of multi-drug resistant infections

Share and discuss infection rates data with ASP team members and key stakeholders on a monthly basis

Match infection rates data with rates of antimicrobial consumption and discuss potential solutions with ASP team

Figure 2. Roles and responsibilities of core members of the ASP team. ASP (antimicrobial stewardship programme); ID (Infectious Diseases); DOT (Days of Therapy).

The team developed an antimicrobial restriction form and discussed it with hospital physicians, and clinical and hospital pharmacists. The form was introduced on a trial basis, to get physicians used to filling in the form and discussing prescription decisions with the ID consultant. It was then updated based on prescribers' and pharmacists' feedback, before approval by the medical records committee. A copy of the antimicrobial restriction form and the associated workflow is included in Supplementary File S1.

The remaining steps of the implementation plan were then agreed; these included:

Raising awareness of antimicrobial resistance and the outcomes of inappropriate antimicrobials' use through a hospital-wide health promotion event lasting for a week and coinciding with the World Antimicrobial Awareness Week (18–24 November 2015).

"everyday was targeted to specific people or specific departments. We published a newsletter about antimicrobial stewardship and we had small antimicrobial stewardship contests".

Antimicrobials prescribing training sessions for physicians:

"We let people get used to filling the forms, and know which antibiotics are restricted. Before there was resistance, and now everyone knew that it is just a matter of telling, understanding, and providing feedback ... it will be applied and implemented as restricted antibiotics will not be approved unless it is necessary. If it (restricted antibiotic) is prescribed, it will not be approved by the ID team (unless the form is filled in)"

Training members of the ID team and the clinical pharmacists on how to carry out the daily ASP tasks once the programme goes live at beginning of January 2016.

Phase 2

The two core strategies (restriction and preauthorization, and prospective audit with intervention and feedback) of ASPs were implemented. In January 2016, the plan was to introduce the restriction form into hospital departments with the least prescriptions of broad-spectrum antimicrobials (neuroscience and surgery) to identify potential implementation issues, and manage the workload of the small ID team at the time. However, the hospital decided to roll out the form into all the remaining departments including ICU, hematology and oncology because of the recruitment of more ID clinicians, which expanded the capacity of the ID team to review and authorize physicians' requests of restricted antimicrobials. Furthermore, the ID team provided 24 h, 7 days a week "on call" cover dedicated to reviewing and authorising (or not) restriction forms.

"Each unit is covered by ID (Infectious disease team) for these forms. They meet every morning. They meet with the clinical pharmacist in that unit. They will also review all the (restriction) forms, and if it is justified they will approve it. If they are not satisfied, they look into the patient's file, and then discuss with the prescribers. The discussion with the prescriber is mainly because we want the education to play a role (in the programme)".

In addition to antimicrobials' restriction, the ASP team conducted regular auditing of antimicrobials' prescribing, communicated rates of antimicrobials' prescribing to relevant heads of departments, and provided feedback to prescribers. Prospective audit and feedback were also carried out by the pharmacy team to ensure adherence to antimicrobials' guidelines and optimise antimicrobials' dosing before input from the ID team; the infectious disease physicians and the clinical pharmacists maintained regular contact with the medical team regarding patients on antibiotics. The clinical pharmacists were responsible for documenting the daily follow ups or recommendations on the patients' files. They would document their input under the title "ASP Pharmacy Assessment".

The microbiology team started selective reporting of antibiotic susceptibility testing to reduce physicians' prescribing of restricted antimicrobials such as meropenem and imipenem:

"We follow cascade reporting ... microbiology (started) to minimise the disclosure of all susceptibility reporting".

The ASP team continued to meet monthly to review rates of antimicrobial resistance, DOT (days of therapy) data and the list of restricted antimicrobials. Feedback from physicians and heads of department regarding antimicrobials' prescribing needs was discussed and addressed. Examples include drafting guidelines on the prescribing of oral fosfomycin for UTIs, surgical prophylaxis, granulocytopenia and vancomycin dosing.

"Most of our physicians do not use Fosfomycin because they do not believe that oral medication can be used against multi-drug resistant organisms like ESPL (Extended-Spectrum Beta-Lactamases) or CRB (Chlorine-Resistant Bacteria) ... we have a lot of patients now deescalating to fosfomycin"

Education efforts were ongoing throughout the second phase of implementation. Prescribers' education has been a fundamental component for ASP success at the medical city. Figure 3 shows the timeline for implementing the ASP in the medical city.

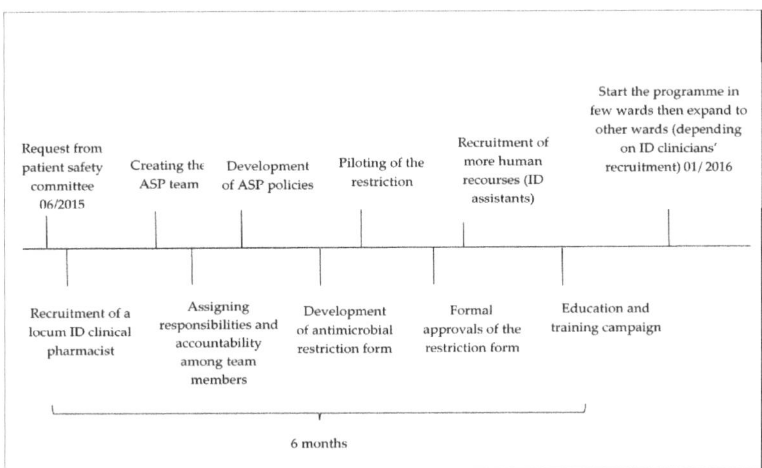

Figure 3. The timeline for implementing the ASP in the medical city.

2.3. *ASP Implementation Challenges*

Various factors affected the implementation of ASP in the medical city.

2.3.1. Shortage of ASP Staff

During the initial phase, the availability of only one ID consultant, and no other clinician with ID expertise forced the ASP team to optimise ID input, and resulted in an initial "short" list of restricted antimicrobials requiring approval from the ID consultant.

"We started with one ID consultant, we did not have anyone else. That's why we needed as much concise shortlist as we can".

During phase 2, the hospital recruited more ID clinicians, resulting in rolling out the ASP across all hospital departments. The shortage of ID physicians has been attributed to the lack of infectious diseases training programs for physicians in the Middle East and most Asian countries.

Shortage of microbiology personnel and facilities at the medical city also challenged the implementation of the programme. The medical city had only one consultant clinical microbiologist, heading a team of microbiology technicians. Supply issues of laboratory consumables and equipment, due to financial pressures, placed constraints on how quickly susceptibility tests were reported:

"we do not have items coming regularly. Sometimes we even run out of gram stain reagents and we need to borrow them from other hospitals ... we would like to have some key equipment like MALDI/TOF (matrix-assisted laser desorption ionization time-of-flight mass spectrometry)... we all know there are financial constraints ... so we have supply issues, space issues and financial issues".

2.3.2. Incompatible IT Systems

One of the biggest challenges to ASP implementation at the medical city, as reported by the participants, was the incompatibility of the electronic medical system in the hospital with the requirements of the ASP, so several data had to be generated manually (antimicrobials' costs data, DOT data and data for the hospital antibiogram). Furthermore, the restriction forms could not be submitted electronically, they had to be filled in manually, and hard copies had to be collected by pharmacists, and reviewed and authorised by ID physicians:

"we have some constraints in our hospital information system … we are trying to work around that";

"The health information system at the hospital is not supportive enough, to get accurate data, as we collect data manually (in all departments), which consumes time and manpower".

Physicians' resistance to ASP formulary restrictions and policies

The physicians were initially resistant to formulary restrictions and the need to obtain ID approval for the prescription of restricted antimicrobials for numerous reasons:

1. Physicians' worry about complications given that their patients tend to be complex, immunocomprosied and systemically unwell.

"At the beginning we faced resistance, especially in the critical areas in haematology and oncology because they (physicians) say our patients are sick".

2. During phase 1, the resistance appears to be mainly towards ID clinicians' involvement. The physicians at the hospital were routinely making antimicrobial prescription decisions without seeking input from the only ID consultant; who would not have been able to provide input to all departments. During phase 2, after the ID consultant, and later the ID team, became more involved in decisions about antimicrobial prescriptions, the physicians started to seek more consultations and input from the ID team:

"Now the doctors trust more the ID (infectious diseases) team with their consultations. I think also since the ID team started to be more involved with the restriction and talking to convince the doctors that this needs de-escalation … ".

3. Resistance to change: Before the implementation of the ASP, the physicians routinely prescribed antimicrobials empirically and prescribed more than one broad-spectrum antimicrobial, without much reliance on susceptibility reporting. The restriction of prescribing options, and the need to rely on susceptibility reporting and ID approval, was a significant change to their routine practice.

"People tend to treat empirically instead of trying to diagnose".

2.4. *Critical Factors for the Sucessful Implementaion of ASP in the Medical City*

A number of factors have been identified as key to the implementation of the ASP in the hospital.

2.4.1. Top Management Support

The decision to adopt and implement ASP in the medical city was made by the CEO. Top management support ensured dedicated financial resources for ID clinicians' and locum ASP pharmacist recruitment. Furthermore, senior managers instructed the hospital departments to engage with the ASP team's educational events and process changes. This support was provided throughout the implementation phases, and was perceived by the participants to be a key determinant of the successful implementation of the ASP:

"There is a lot of commitment from the administration and the leadership";

"Leadership support is the biggest thing we have here".

2.4.2. Project Management Training

When the PSP programmes and projects were outlined, the hospital administration provided project management training (outsourced) to clinicians involved in these projects including the ASP project. This entailed training on how to write policies and project proposals, identify project outcomes, carrying out relevant data analysis, and strategies to influence behavior change.

2.4.3. A Dedicated ASP Team

A key facilitator to ASP implementation was setting up a dedicated ASP team. This meant that there was a specific person (or group) that maintained open, constant communication with the hospital staff regarding ASP, and was always available for assistance with the implementation of the program. The group members had clear roles and responsibilities and communicated frequently to track the progress of the implementation plan and evaluate its outcomes.

2.4.4. Increased ID Clinicians' Involvement in the Prescribing and Monitoring of Antimicrobials

The implementation of ASP in the hospital aimed to change physicians' antimicrobial prescription behaviors, through the restriction of certain antimicrobials, the prescribing of which would require the input of an ID clinician. The ID team ensured that an ID clinician was available over 24 h, 7 days a week to review restriction forms, authorise requests if appropriate and suggest alternative antimicrobials if needed. This increased provision facilitated physicians' cooperation and reduced their resistance to the process changes:

"even weekends they (ID team) come to just sign and review the forms, and there is always an ID on call for antimicrobial stewardship beside the ID on call".

The ID team also delegated antimicrobials' dose optimisation to the pharmacy team in recognition of clinical pharmacists' skills and expertise, and to manage the workload associated with the increased cover:

"The ID consultant sent a memo to the whole hospital that the ID consultant, ID doctors and hospital physicians will recommend the regimen, and the dosing will be the responsibility of the pharmacist. That was a huge thing, and everyone was following this recommendation".

Figure 4 summarizes the nine essential steps for ASP implementation in hospital, fostered by strong senior management support and governed by key implementation strategies. Hospitals in the region should first start by setting up the ASP program as a stand-alone program with defined aims and outcome measures. Then, an ASP team needs to be set up with clear roles and responsibilities, especially in relation to the day-to-day management of the implementation and oversight of the program. The ASP team would need to be trained on how to manage the project, carry out the implementation steps, evaluate interventions and modify the implementation plans based on feedback from users. Relevant ASP interventions would then have to be designed and refined based on clinicians and administrators' feedback, followed by education campaigns and training sessions with the clinicians to improve their engagement and reduce their resistance. Throughout the constant engagement with clinicians and hospital administrators, barriers to implementation need to be identified and addressed prior to implementation. The ASP program can be piloted in departments with the least antimicrobial prescribing and resistance issues, before launching it throughout the remaining departments. This is a cyclical process, and sustaining successful outcomes and good practice may require refining the ASP aims and outcomes, adding more members to the ASP team, further education and training and ongoing exploration and identification of barriers to adherence to ASP policies and procedures. Senior management support is paramount throughout the implementation process. The ASP team should have autonomy in managing and refining the ASP, should focus on achieving the defined ASP outcomes, and employ an education approach to help clinicians adhere to the restrictive requirements of the program.

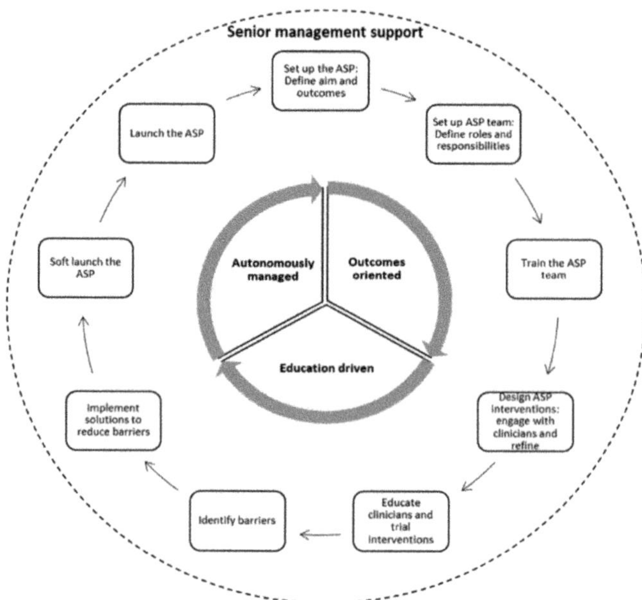

Figure 4. ASP implementation process model.

2.5. Outcomes of ASP implementation

The ASP implementation outcomes set out by the ASP team were: reduction of antimicrobial resistance rates, rates of multi-drug resistant microorganisms, antimicrobials' usage (DOTs) and costs (we were not able to obtain data for all the outcomess). These were used as key performance indicators (KPIs) and were regularly monitored by the ASP committee.

Following the implementation of the ASP in 2016, the hospital achieved a reduction in resistance rates (Table 1) and antimicrobials' usage (Table 2). The hospital either sustained or slightly increased levels of the susceptibility of microorganisms to antimicrobials throughout 2017–2019. However, antimicrobial usage seems to have increased over the years. DOT data of 2019 shows a particularly marked increase compared to data from 2018 (data shown in Tables S1 and S2 of Supplementary File S2) This increase has been attributed to a number of reasons (suggested through personal communication) including: setting up a solid organ transplant center in 2018 and the associated increase in patient numbers and prescribing antimicrobials, an incremental 20% increase in patients' numbers annually and increased numbers of extended-spectrum β-lactamase (ESBL) isolates due to the restriction of prescribing board spectrum antimicrobials, which led to increased use of piperacillin/tazobactam, cefepime and quinolones. Furthermore, Meropenem's use doubled, and micafungin's use tripled from 2018 to 2019. In 2019, the hospital decided to reduce the use of imipenem and limit its use to resistant *Enterococcus facium*, due to cost. The alternative, Meropenen, was more cost-effective, and was being prescribed instead. Similarly, Micafungin was being prescribed as an alternative to the more expensive antifungals caspofungin and anidulafungin in late 2018. Later in 2019, anidulafungin was re-added to the formulary for limited patients with liver impairment.

Table 1. Hospital antibiogram data (2015–2016) showing the percentage of sensitive susceptibilities between specific microorganisms (columns) and antibiotics (rows).

		Microorganisms					
Antibiotics	**Year**	*E. coli*	*A. baumannii*	*Enterobacter spp.*	*S. epidermidis*	*S. aureus*	*MRSA*
Amoxicillin/Clavulanic acid	2015	37	-	-	-	28	-
	2016	49	-	-	-	-	-
Cefepime	2015	45	28	39	-	-	-
	2016	48	22	66	-	-	-
Ciprofloxacin	2015	33	20	60	20	62	47
	2016	36	22	75	20	75	69
Clindamycin	2015	-	-	-		45	-
	2016	-	-	-	28	76	71
Colistin	2015	-	69	-	-	-	-
	2016	-	97	-	-	-	-
Gentamicin	2015	71	24	56	46	75	55
	2016	65	34	79	53	86	71
Piperacillin/Tazobactam	2015	47	-	48	-	-	-
	2016	77	-	64	-	-	-

Table 2. Hospital DOT data for July–Dec 2015 (before ASP implementation) and January–June 2016 (after).

Antibiotics	Total DOT (07–12/2015)	Total DOT (01–06/2016)
Tigecycline	1039.8	624.5
Colistin	2080.9	1417.2
Meropenem	2287.2	2597.3
Imipenem	2365.6	1666.1
TOTAL	7773.5	6305.1 (−18.9%)

In late 2020, we sought updates on the status and outcomes of the ASP in the hospital. Supplementary File S3 includes a summary of personal communications with the hospital' s ASP team.

3. Discussion

Top management initiation and support of ASP implementation in the hospital, combined with a team approach to planning, implementing and monitoring of the ASP has led to the successful implementation of the program in the hospital. The implementation challenges reported in this study have been reported nationally in Saudi Arabia [13], but this hospital demonstrates that implementation remains possible if key players (top management and ASP team members) work together, effectively, to address those challenges.

In this case study, we demonstrate how managerial and clinical interests can be aligned to reduce antimicrobial resistance rates, and pioneer the implementation of ASPs to enhance the hospital's reputation. Alignment of managerial and clinical interests has been shown to be a key determinant of the success of quality improvement interventions [19]. Furthermore, in contrast to a typical top-down order delegation approach, the CEO empowered the members of the ASP team to take over the responsibility of ASP, monitor its key performance indicators, and make autonomous decisions. This empowering leadership strategy was key to the successful implementation of ASP in our study, and was also reported in Steinmann et al. study [20].

The initial lack of "know how" to implement ASPs and the national shortage of ASP team members have widely been reported to hinder ASP implementation [15,21]. However, top management support ensured the allocation of the necessary funds and resources, and outsourcing expert staff to help hospital staff implement ASPs. Other reported examples also include outsourcing laboratory services [22] or pharmacy services [23]. ASP implementation in the hospital could only occur once more ID clinicians were recruited. Other hospitals may not be able follow example given the national shortage of these specialists. To overcome the shortage of ID clinicians, hospitals in South Africa implemented an alternative pharmacist-led ASP [24], highlighting the need to adapt ASP programs and interventions to maximise the use of scarce resources. We also suggested in [13] that regional/local ASP hubs can be set up so that ID and clinical pharmacists' resources are shared to improve ASP implementation in hospitals.

The lack of and/or incompatibility of information technology (IT) systems with antimicrobial stewardship interventions hinders ASP implementation [15,25]. Innovation and integration of compatible IT systems improves the processes and outcomes of ASPs in hospitals [26]. Moreover, physicians' resistance to ASP restrictions on prescribing antimicrobials also affects ASP implementation. In their study, Perozziello et al. [27] suggests that ASP education interventions, instead of restrictive ones, can improve physicians' engagement with ASP implementation. In our study, education, early engagement with physicians, and trialing interventions prior to full implementation increased physicians' engagement despite the initial resistance. This was also shown by Alawi et al. 2016 [28].

ASP implementation in the hospital reduced antimicrobial consumption and rates of some resistant strains, which further strengthens the evidence base for their effectiveness [28–30]. However, restricting antimicrobials may reduce resistance of some strains but increase the resistance of other strains, also known as the "'squeeze the balloon effect" [31]. Resistance rates are also affected by the duration of antimicrobial treatment [32]. These should be considered when evaluating ASP outcomes. It is also important that hospitals monitor resistant rates, especially those of MDR, to target efforts to curb it [33]. Interesting perspectives are emerging, calling for a radical rethinking of what antimicrobial stewardship programs should entail, such as Vickers et al. calling for innovative commercial models to stimulate novel antimicrobial development, and integrating rapid diagnostics and infection control practices within the program [34]. Furthermore, given the enormity of the antimicrobial resistance threat, all possible strategies to identify novel or repurpose old agents to confer antimicrobial properties should be considered, including exploring the antimicrobial properties of essential oils [35].

The findings of our study can help Saudi hospitals develop and implement ASPs. We identified a number of challenges and the strategies to overcome them. Our findings, however, need to be interpreted with caution. First, our case study involves a single hospital. Although there are various lessons to be learnt on ASP implementation, there is no "one size fits all" approach, and other hospitals need to adapt the recommendations of our study before adopting this implementation model. Future research could use a comparative case study approach to analyze the similarities, differences and patterns across different hospitals. Second, we have not explored the effectiveness of ASP post implementation. Although we demonstrate that the ASP led to reduced antimicrobial consumption and a reduction in rates of resistance, an analysis of long-term effects is needed, through a longitudinal study, to understand if ASP processes and outcomes can be sustained. Third, our key informants included ASP team members and the hospital's CEO. Exploring input from other ASP key players, such as hospital information technologists and middle managers could provide further insights on how interventions can be successfully implemented.

4. Methods

This study used a key stakeholder case study design [36], focusing on a tertiary care center (medical city) that implemented an antimicrobial stewardship program in 2016. The hospital has a 1500 bed capacity, consists of a coronary care unit (CCU), cardiac surgery intensive care unit (CSICU) and provides cardiac, hematology, oncology, neuroscience, medical and specialized surgery services. Qualitative methods were used, focusing on in-depth semi-structured interviews and analysis of relevant documents. The core members of the ASP team, including an ID consultant (Director of the ASP), a clinical pharmacist (Manager of the ASP), a consultant clinical microbiologist, an infection control consultant, and the CEO of the medical city were interviewed in July 2017, for 29–45 min. The interviews were conducted face-to-face in the participants' main language (Arabic or

English), audio recorded and transcribed verbatim. Additional data were collected through content analysis of 35 ASP hospital documents.

The interview schedule was developed following a review of the literature and discussions with three ASP pharmacists (two from Saudi Arabia and one from the UK) and two ID consultants (from Saudi Arabia). Questions in the schedule were all open-ended to obtain in-depth views and perspectives of the study participants. The interview schedule has two main sections. The first is a section on background information (three questions), such as the position of healthcare professionals, gender and years of experience. In the second section, 12 open-ended questions were used to explore the components of the ASP in the medical city, members of the ASP team and their responsibilities, the adoption and implementation process of the ASP, and the factors influencing the adoption and implementation process of the ASP in the medical city. Probing questions were also asked based on the responses of the participants to obtain further details.

5. Conclusions

Successful ASP implementation in Saudi hospitals is administrator-driven and requires a hospital leadership that empowers clinicians to take responsibility for implementing the program. Outsourcing expertise and resources could help hospitals address some of the implementation challenges. However, a compatible IT infrastructure that integrates ASP interventions is key to improving implementation and monitoring outcomes.

Supplementary Materials: The following are available online at https://www.mdpi.com/2079-6382/10/3/280/s1, Supplementary File S1: A copy of the hospital's antimicrobial restriction form and the associated workflow is included; Supplementary File S2: Hospital antibiogram data (2015–2019) and DOT data (2018–2019) are included under Tables S1 and S2, respectively. Supplementary File S3: Hospital ASP updates.

Author Contributions: Conceptualization, S.A., I.B. and N.S.; methodology, S.A., I.B. and N.S.; software, S.A. and M.A.H.; validation, S.A., I.B. and N.S.; formal analysis, S.A. and I.B.; investigation, S.A. and E.B.; resources, S.A.; data curation, S.A., E.B., A.H.; writing—original draft preparation, S.A., I.B. and N.S.; writing—review and editing, S.A., I.B., N.S., Z.A.; visualization, S.A., N.S., I.B.; supervision, I.B., N.S., Z.A.; project administration, S.A.; funding acquisition, S.A. All authors have read and agreed to the published version of the manuscript.

Funding: This research is part of S.A. PhD studentship. The PhD studentship of S.A. is funded by Albaha University (Albaha, Saudi Arabia).

Institutional Review Board Statement: This study was approved by the Health and Human Sciences Ethics Committee of the University of Hertfordshire (Hatfield, UK) (protocol no. LMS/PGR/UH/02344). Official permissions to conduct this research was granted by the hospital taking part in this study.

Informed Consent Statement: Informed consent was obtained from all subjects involved in the study.

Data Availability Statement: Data are contained within the article or Supplementary Material (Appendices 1 and 2).

Acknowledgments: We would like to thank all the participants for taking part in this study.

Conflicts of Interest: The authors declare no conflict of interest. The funders had no role in the design of the study; in the collection, analyses, or interpretation of data; in the writing of the manuscript, or in the decision to publish the results.

References

1. Centers for Disease Control and Prevention Core Elements of Hospital Antibiotic Stewardship Programs. Available online: https://www.cdc.gov/antibiotic-use/core-elements/hospital.html (accessed on 28 January 2021).
2. Dyar, O.J.; Huttner, B.; Schouten, J.; Pulcini, C. What is antimicrobial stewardship? *Clin. Microbiol. Infect.* **2017**, *23*, 793–798. [CrossRef] [PubMed]
3. Howard, P.; Pulcini, C.; Hara, G.L.; West, R.M.; Gould, I.M.; Harbarth, S.; Nathwani, D. An international cross-sectional survey of antimicrobial stewardship programmes in hospitals. *J. Antimicrob. Chemother.* **2015**, *70*, 1245–1255. [CrossRef] [PubMed]

4. Kallen, M.C.; Binda, F.; Oever, J.T.; Tebano, G.; Pulcini, C.; Murri, R.; Beovic, B.; Saje, A.; Prins, J.M.; Hulscher, M.E.J.L.; et al. Comparison of antimicrobial stewardship programmes in acute-care hospitals in four European countries: A cross-sectional survey. *Int. J. Antimicrob. Agents* **2019**, *54*, 338–345. [CrossRef]
5. Scobie, A.; Budd, E.L.; Harris, R.J.; Hopkins, S.; Shetty, N. Antimicrobial stewardship: An evaluation of structure and process and their association with antimicrobial prescribing in NHS hospitals in England. *J. Antimicrob. Chemother.* **2019**, *74*, 1143–1152. [CrossRef] [PubMed]
6. Nhan, D.; Lentz, E.J.M.; Steinberg, M.; Bell, C.M.; Morris, A.M. Structure of antimicrobial stewardship programs in leading US hospitals: Findings of a nationwide survey. *Open Forum Infect. Dis.* **2019**, *6*, 1–7. [CrossRef] [PubMed]
7. Wilkinson, A.; Ebata, A.; Macgregor, H. Interventions to reduce antibiotic prescribing in LMICs: A scoping review of evidence from human and animal health systems. *Antibiotics* **2018**, *8*, 2. [CrossRef]
8. Alghamdi, S.; Shebl, N.A.; Aslanpour, Z.; Shibl, A.; Berrou, I. Hospital Adoption of Antimicrobial Stewardship Programmes in Gulf Cooperation Council Countries: A Review of Existing Evidence. *J. Glob. Antimicrob. Resist.* **2018**, *15*, 196–209. [CrossRef] [PubMed]
9. Akpan, M.R.; Isemin, N.U.; Udoh, A.E.; Ashiru-Oredope, D. Implementation of antimicrobial stewardship programmes in African countries: A systematic literature review. *J. Glob. Antimicrob. Resist.* **2020**, *22*, 317–324. [CrossRef]
10. Cox, J.A.; Vlieghe, E.; Mendelson, M.; Wertheim, H.; Ndegwa, L.; Villegas, M.V.; Gould, I.; Hara, G.L. Antibiotic stewardship in low- and middle-income countries: The same but different? *Clin. Microbiol. Infect.* **2017**, *23*, 812–818. [CrossRef]
11. van Dijck, C.; Vlieghe, E.; Cox, J.A. Antibiotic stewardship interventions in hospitals in low-and middle-income countries: A systematic review. *Bull. World Health Organ.* **2018**, *96*, 266–280. [CrossRef]
12. World Intellectual Property Organization Antimicrobial Resistance—A Global Epidemic. Available online: https://www.wipo.int/meetings/en/doc_details.jsp?doc_id=350357 (accessed on 25 January 2021).
13. Alghamdi, S.; Berrou, I.; Aslanpour, Z.; Mutlaq, A.; Haseeb, A.; Albanghali, M.; Hammad, M.A.; Shebl, N. Antimicrobial Stewardship Programmes in Saudi Hospitals: Evidence from a National Survey. *Antibiotics* **2021**, *10*, 193. [CrossRef]
14. Zaman, T.U.; Alrodayyan, M.; Albladi, M.; Aldrees, M.; Siddique, M.I.; Aljohani, S.; Balkhy, H.H. Clonal diversity and genetic profiling of antibiotic resistance among multidrug/carbapenem-resistant Klebsiella pneumoniae isolates from a tertiary care hospital in Saudi Arabia. *BMC Infect. Dis.* **2018**, *18*, 1–11. [CrossRef]
15. Alghamdi, S.; Atef-Shebl, N.; Aslanpour, Z.; Berrou, I. Barriers to implementing antimicrobial stewardship programmes in three Saudi hospitals: Evidence from a qualitative study. *J. Glob. Antimicrob. Resist.* **2019**, *18*, 284–290. [CrossRef]
16. Alsaleh, N.A.; Al-Omar, H.A.; Mayet, A.Y.; Mullen, A.B. Evaluating the appropriateness of carbapenem and piperacillin-tazobactam prescribing in a tertiary care hospital in Saudi Arabia. *Saudi Pharm. J.* **2020**, *28*, 1492–1498. [CrossRef] [PubMed]
17. Mendelson, M.; Morris, A.M.; Thursky, K.; Pulcini, C. How to start an antimicrobial stewardship programme in a hospital. *Clin. Microbiol. Infect.* **2020**, *26*, 447–453. [CrossRef] [PubMed]
18. Dellit, T.H.; Owens, R.C.; Mcgowan, J.E.; Gerding, D.N.; Weinstein, R.A.; Burke, J.P.; Huskins, W.C.; Paterson, D.L.; Fishman, N.O.; Carpenter, C.F.; et al. Infectious Diseases Society of America and the Society for Healthcare Epidemiology of America Guidelines for Developing an Institutional Program to Enhance Antimicrobial Stewardship. *Clin. Infect. Dis.* **2007**, *44*, 159–177. [CrossRef] [PubMed]
19. Pannick, S.; Sevdalis, N.; Athanasiou, T. Beyond clinical engagement: A pragmatic model for quality improvement interventions, aligning clinical and managerial priorities. *BMJ Qual. Saf.* **2016**, *25*, 716–725. [CrossRef] [PubMed]
20. Steinmann, K.E.; Lehnick, D.; Buettcher, M.; Schwendener-Scholl, K.; Daetwyler, K.; Fontana, M.; Morgillo, D.; Ganassi, K.; O'Neill, K.; Genet, P.; et al. Impact of empowering leadership on antimicrobial stewardship: A single center study in a neonatal and pediatric intensive care unit and a literature review. *Front. Pediatr.* **2018**, *6*, 1–12. [CrossRef]
21. Rzewuska, M.; Duncan, E.M.; Francis, J.J.; Morris, A.M.; Suh, K.N.; Davey, P.G.; Grimshaw, J.M.; Ramsay, C.R. Barriers and Facilitators to Implementation of Antibiotic Stewardship Programmes in Hospitals in Developed Countries: Insights From Transnational Studies. *Front. Sociol.* **2020**, *5*, 1–13. [CrossRef]
22. Pan American Health Organization Recommendations for Implementing Antimicrobial Stewardship Programs in Latin America and the Caribbean: Manual for Public Health Decision-Makers. 2018. Available online: https://www.paho.org/en/documents/recommendations-implementing-antimicrobial-stewardship-programs-latin-america-and (accessed on 22 January 2021).
23. Nachtigall, I.; Tafelski, S.; Heucke, E.; Witzke, O.; Staack, A.; Recknagel-Friese, S.; Geffers, C.; Bonsignore, M. Time and personnel requirements for antimicrobial stewardship in small hospitals in a rural area in Germany. *J. Infect. Public Health* **2020**, *13*, 1946–1950. [CrossRef] [PubMed]
24. Brink, A.J.; Messina, A.P.; Feldman, C.; Richards, G.A.; Becker, P.J.; Goff, D.A.; Bauer, K.A.; Nathwani, D.; Van den Bergh, D. Antimicrobial stewardship across 47 South African hospitals: An implementation study. *Lancet Infect. Dis.* **2016**, *16*, 1017–1025. [CrossRef]
25. Kapadia, S.N.; Abramson, E.L.; Carter, E.J.; Loo, A.S.; Kaushal, R.; Calfee, D.P.; Simon, M.S. The Expanding Role of Antimicrobial Stewardship Programs in Hospitals in the United States: Lessons Learned from a Multisite Qualitative Study. *Jt. Comm. J. Qual. Patient Saf.* **2018**, *44*, 68–74. [CrossRef] [PubMed]
26. King, A.; Cresswell, K.M.; Coleman, J.J.; Pontefract, S.K.; Slee, A.; Williams, R.; Sheikh, A. Investigating the ways in which health information technology can promote antimicrobial stewardship: A conceptual overview. *J. R. Soc. Med.* **2017**, *110*, 320–329. [CrossRef]

27. Perozziello, A.; Lescure, F.X.; Truel, A.; Routelous, C.; Vaillant, L.; Yazdanpanah, Y.; Lucet, J.C. Prescribers' experience and opinions on antimicrobial stewardship programmes in hospitals: A French nationwide survey. *J. Antimicrob. Chemother.* **2019**, *74*, 2451–2458. [CrossRef] [PubMed]
28. Alawi, M.M.; Darwesh, B.M. A stepwise introduction of a successful antimicrobial stewardship program: Experience from a tertiary care university hospital in Western, Saudi Arabia. *Saudi Med. J.* **2016**, *37*, 1350–1358. [CrossRef] [PubMed]
29. Nathwani, D.; Varghese, D.; Stephens, J.; Ansari, W.; Martin, S.; Charbonneau, C. Value of hospital antimicrobial stewardship programs [ASPs]: A systematic review. *Antimicrob. Resist. Infect. Control* **2019**, *8*, 1–13. [CrossRef] [PubMed]
30. Rodriguez-Bano, J.; Perez-Moreno, M.A.; Penalva, G.; Garnacho-Montero, J.; Pinto, C.; Salcedo, I.; Fernandez-Urrusuno, R.; Neth, O.; Gil-Navarro, M.V.; Perez-Milena, A.; et al. Outcomes of the PIRASOA programme, an antimicrobial stewardship programme implemented in hospitals of the Public Health System of Andalusia, Spain: An ecologic study of time-trend analysis. *Clin. Microbiol. Infect.* **2019**, *26*, 358–365. [CrossRef]
31. Burke, J.P. Antibiotic Resistance—Squeezing the Balloon? *JAMA* **1998**, *280*, 1270–1271. [CrossRef]
32. De Waele, J.J.; Schouten, J.; Beovic, B.; Tabah, A.; Leone, M. Antimicrobial de-escalation as part of antimicrobial stewardship in intensive care: No simple answers to simple questions—a viewpoint of experts. *Intensive Care Med.* **2020**, *46*, 236–244. [CrossRef]
33. Moglad, E.H. Antibiotics profile, prevalence of extended-spectrum beta-lactamase (ESBL), and multidrug-resistant Enterobacteriaceae from different clinical samples in Khartoum State, Sudan. *Int. J. Microbiol.* **2020**, *2020*, 1–6. [CrossRef] [PubMed]
34. Vickers, R.J.; Bassetti, M.; Clancy, C.J.; Garey, K.W.; Greenberg, D.E.; Nguyen, M.-H.; Roblin, D.; Tillotson, G.S.; Wilcox, M.H. Combating resistance while maintaining innovation: The future of antimicrobial stewardship. *Futur. Microbiol* **2019**, *14*, 1331–1341. [CrossRef] [PubMed]
35. Donadu, M.G.; Le, N.T.; Ho, D.V.; Doan, T.Q.; Le, A.T.; Raal, A.; Usai, M.; Marchetti, M.; Sanna, G.; Madeddu, S.; et al. Phytochemical compositions and biological activities of essential oils from the leaves, rhizomes and whole plant of hornstedtia bella Škorničk. *Antibiotics* **2020**, *9*, 334. [CrossRef] [PubMed]
36. Yin, R.K. *Case Study Research: Design and Methods (Applied Social Research Methods)*, 5th ed.; SAGE Publications: London, UK, 2013; ISBN 1452242569.

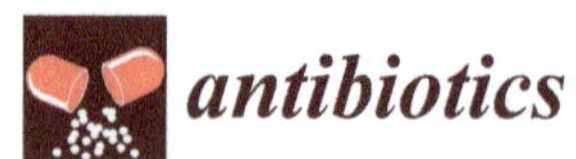

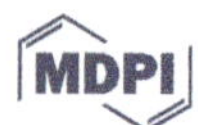

Article

Development of and User Feedback on a Board and Online Game to Educate on Antimicrobial Resistance and Stewardship

Diane Ashiru-Oredope [1,*], Maxencia Nabiryo [1], Andy Yeoman [2], Melvin Bell [2], Sarah Cavanagh [1], Nikki D'Arcy [1], William Townsend [3], Dalius Demenciukas [2], Sara Yadav [1], Frances Garraghan [1], Vanessa Carter [1], Victoria Rutter [1] and Richard Skone-James [3]

1 Commonwealth Pharmacists Association, London E1W 1AW, UK; maxencia.nabiryo@commonwealthpharmacy.org (M.N.); sarah.cavanagh6@nhs.net (S.C.); nikki.darcy@commonwealthpharmacy.org (N.D.); sara.yadav@commonwealthpharmacy.org (S.Y.); frances.garraghan@commonwealthpharmacy.org (F.G.); vanessa.carter@commonwealthpharmacy.org (V.C.); victoria.rutter@commonwealthpharmacy.org (V.R.)

2 Focus Games Ltd., Glasgow G40 1DA, UK; Andy@focusgames.com (A.Y.); melvin@focusgames.com (M.B.); dalius@focusgames.com (D.D.)

3 Health and Education Trust, London NW1 4LE, UK; william.townsend@thet.org (W.T.); Richard.Skone-James@thet.org (R.S.-J.)

* Correspondence: diane.ashiru-oredope@commonwealthpharmacy.org

Abstract: Antimicrobial resistance (AMR), particularly antibiotic resistance, is one of the most challenging global health threats of our time. Tackling AMR requires a multidisciplinary approach. Whether a clinical team member is a cleaner, nurse, doctor, pharmacist, or other type of health worker, their contribution towards keeping patients safe from infection is crucial to saving lives. Existing literature portrays that games can be a good way to engage communities in joint learning. This manuscript describes an educational antimicrobial stewardship (AMS) game that was co-created by a multidisciplinary team of health professionals spanning across high- and low- to middle-income countries. The online AMS game was promoted and over 100 players across 23 countries registered to participate on 2 occasions. The players were asked to share feedback on the game through a short online form. Their experiences revealed that the game is relevant for creation of awareness and understanding on antimicrobial stewardship in both high- and low-to-middle income settings worldwide.

Keywords: antimicrobial resistance (AMR); antimicrobial stewardship (AMS); AMS Game; board game; online game; Commonwealth Partnerships for Antimicrobial Stewardship; CwPAMS; gaming; game-based learning; gamification

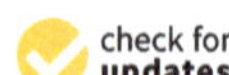

Citation: Ashiru-Oredope, D.; Nabiryo, M.; Yeoman, A.; Bell, M.; Cavanagh, S.; D'Arcy, N.; Townsend, W.; Demenciukas, D.; Yadav, S.; Garraghan, F.; et al. Development of and User Feedback on a Board and Online Game to Educate on Antimicrobial Resistance and Stewardship. *Antibiotics* **2022**, *11*, 611. https://doi.org/10.3390/antibiotics11050611

Academic Editor: Albert Figueras

Received: 12 March 2022
Accepted: 24 April 2022
Published: 1 May 2022

Publisher's Note: MDPI stays neutral with regard to jurisdictional claims in published maps and institutional affiliations.

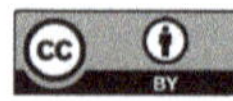

Copyright: © 2022 by the authors. Licensee MDPI, Basel, Switzerland. This article is an open access article distributed under the terms and conditions of the Creative Commons Attribution (CC BY) license (https://creativecommons.org/licenses/by/4.0/).

1. Introduction

Antimicrobial resistance (AMR), particularly antibiotic resistance, is one of the most challenging global health threats of our time [1]. Even under the shadow of COVID-19, AMR posed a substantial threat to patients who developed secondary bacterial infections [2]. AMR causes challenges to the treatment of infections and infectious diseases, including HIV/AIDS, typhoid, cholera, tuberculosis, gonorrhoea, hospital-associated infections, and malaria, which disproportionately affect low- and middle-income countries (LMICs) [1]. AMR is also particularly prevalent and problematic in LMICs where health systems and medical resources, including access to water, sanitation, and hygiene (WASH), are limited, as well as where socioeconomic drivers, such as extreme poverty, increase the risk of communicable diseases exponentially [3]. The Fleming Fund was created in response to this need, and has funded many programmes of work, including the Commonwealth Partnerships for Antimicrobial Stewardship Programme (CwPAMS). CwPAMS addresses AMR through antimicrobial stewardship interventions in eight African Fleming Fund priority countries, using a health partnership approach.

Tackling AMR requires a multidisciplinary approach. Whether a clinical or healthcare team member is a nurse, doctor, pharmacist, cleaner, or other type of health worker, their contribution towards keeping patients safe from infection and the spread of resistant organisms is crucial to saving lives.

Existing literature portrays that games can be a good way to engage communities in joint learning [4,5]. Evidence shows that games have been used to promote health and wellbeing in regard to both infectious and non-infectious diseases [6]. As a health education tool, games have proven to be an enjoyable method that enhances learning through stimulating players' interests and motivation [6,7]. While existing studies largely point to games as an impactful educational tool for children and students, some studies have demonstrated that games can be used as a capacity-building intervention for health professionals [8]. Games can be used for improving health professionals' knowledge and skills, changing their attitudes and performance, and improving how they care for their patients [8]. Despite the strong indication that games can improve knowledge, several studies including those conducted among health professionals do not show sufficient evidence that games can improve performance or change behaviour [7,9–11]. To this end, there is a need for more research with a focus on outcomes that go beyond knowledge assessment, to include outcomes such as skills, behaviour, and patient outcomes [10].

Few existing studies highlight that AMS games can be an innovative way of spreading awareness on AMR. A study conducted in Saudi Arabia among students concluded that gamification using an AMS board game can significantly improve AMR knowledge, with better retention than a conventional lecture [12]. In another study conducted in the UK among children aged 7–15 years, it was reported that antibiotic games improved knowledge on the use of antibiotics for bacterial versus viral infections and ensured that the course of antibiotics was completed [13]. The antimicrobial stewardship (AMS) game described in this manuscript was developed to encourage players (healthcare teams including students, doctors, laboratory staff, pharmacists, and nurses) to discuss AMS and learn what they can do personally, and collectively, to improve stewardship in their organisation and their community. The intention was to create a game for groups to play, and in order to make the game more widely accessible, a physical printed tabletop board game was developed with an online version for groups working remotely. Further, it is intended that the game would encourage the player to understand the scale of the AMR problem and that everyone who uses, dispenses or prescribes antimicrobials is part of the solution to reduce the impact of AMR. Effective training and capacity building are vital to the success of stewardship programmes, particularly when staff are new to the concept. The AMS game is intended to make stewardship training engaging and inclusive, generating fun and enthusiasm with a serious purpose and clear outcomes.

Focus Games Ltd. was the game development partner for this project. Focus Games Ltd. has been a leading developer of 'serious' educational games/game-based learning and simulations since 2004. They have developed over 100 different games for staff, patients, and the public that address a wide range of clinical, health, and wellbeing issues.

Independent evaluations of these games demonstrate that they can improve knowledge and encourage beneficial changes in thinking and behaviour [14].

Subject matter expertise, technical competency, and decision-making are diluted when individuals cannot communicate effectively with the people around them. These interpersonal skills can be learned and developed in the same way that subject matter expertise is developed. However, because these interpersonal 'soft' skills are largely intangible, we need to find appropriate ways of teaching.

Although there is not a definitive theoretical framework for the development of serious games, key elements of good practice have previously been summarised [15]. In development of the AMS game several elements of published good practice [15], were considered for incorporation:

- Competition and goals, with players competing against other players both for the physical and online games.

- Clear rules that define how the game is played.
- Choice through the use of multiple-choice questions.
- Challenges—players are provided with problems to solve in this game. We use the case studies as a way to provide additional challenges.
- Coaching, debriefing, and feedback: to reinforce learning.
- Performance assessment, so players know how they did.
- Mechanics: the elements of the game that control gameplay.

The development of the AMS game involved a wide range of stakeholders from across the globe, who represented the target audience for which the game was being developed. To test the usability of the developed AMS game, we used online platforms to invite interested individuals including healthcare teams to play the AMS game and asked them to share their experiences through an online feedback survey form.

2. Materials and Methods

The game was developed by the Commonwealth Partnerships for Antimicrobial Stewardship Programme (CwPAMS), led by the Commonwealth Pharmacists Association (CPA) and Tropical Health and Education Trust (THET) in partnership with Focus Games Ltd. The CPA was the overall technical lead for developing the antimicrobial stewardship concepts (questions and answers) used in the game. Focus Games Ltd. was responsible for programming the AMS concepts into a playable game. THET's coordination expertise was leveraged in bringing together relevant partners to support the development of the game.

2.1. AMS Game Development

The AMS game used the Focus Games Ltd. development process/pathway (Figure 1).

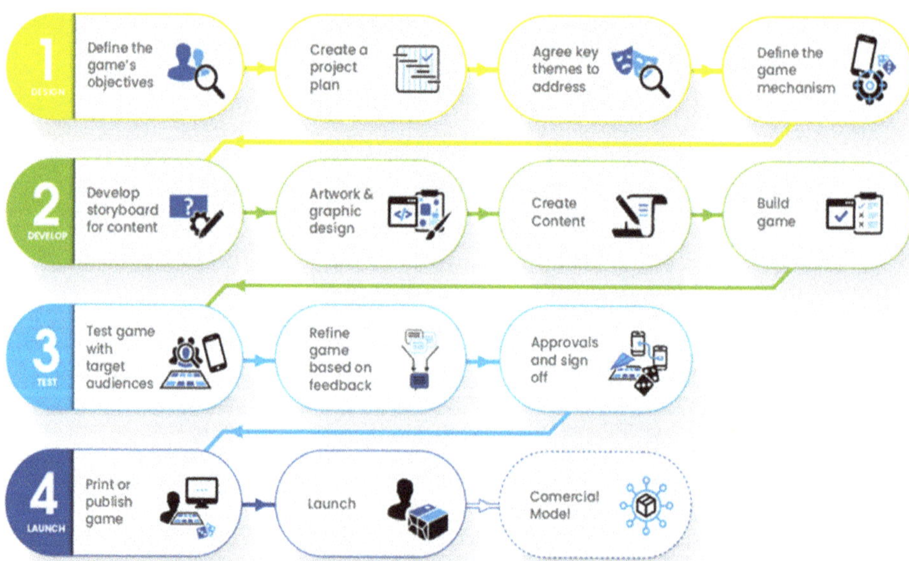

Figure 1. Focus Games Ltd's Game development process/pathway [16].

In order to optimise relationships and collaboration between stakeholders and programme team, Focus Games Ltd. used a range of project management tools to ensure that resources and priorities were managed efficiently and that they were overseen by a programme manager.

At the beginning of the project, a project plan and milestones were agreed upon as well as a specification document which included deliverables pertinent to the project. These deliverables formed the sign-off and approval for the completion of the project.

Focus Games used agile project management processes and tools (Jira). All code development was managed in Bitbucket (GIT repository), ensuring a strong development, test, and live approach. All staff are suitably qualified in their respective disciplines.

The development process for the AMS game included four key phases previously developed by Focus Games Ltd. (Figure 1).

Phase 1—Define Objectives: Requirements for the game outcomes were derived from interviews with and feedback from individual stakeholders, ranging from national to frontline health professionals including pharmacists, doctors, and nurses from eight African countries and the UK. They acted as subject matter experts as well as representatives for the target audience of the game through the development and user testing phases, which included syntax and grammar that was considered acceptable across multiple countries. This identified the learning objectives for the narrative structure of the factual content and how the game design and mechanism will facilitate engagement and learning.

Phase 2—Develop Storyboards: Specific learning objectives and game dynamics were identified based on best practice derived from experience of previous games developed by Focus Games Ltd. This involved the creation of graphic design mock-ups of the game and a written storyboard outline of the factual content. These were discussed and agreed upon by the project team, which included subject matter experts as well as stakeholders across nine countries (Ghana, Kenya, Malawi, Nigeria, Sierra Leone, Tanzania, Uganda, United Kingdom, and Zambia) that were all part of the countries of focus for the CwPAMS programme.

Phase 3—Prototype and Testing: A rapid prototyping approach was used, incorporating data from the pilot scenario and interviews with subject matter experts (SMEs). The game mechanism and design were finalised. The written content was drafted and loaded into the game mechanism. The game was subsequently tested in workshops with SMEs whose feedback informed design iterations.

Phase 4—Refine, Rework, and Launch: production of the final design and implementation of the distribution and commercialisation strategy.

The model and process used are based on practical experience of developing 100 educational games that are being actively used by healthcare professionals around the world. Focus Games have previously evaluated third-party frameworks and models and have found many of them impractical for the purpose of developing game-based learning for the healthcare setting.

2.2. *Target Audience for the AMS Game*

The AMS game is intended to support education on antimicrobial stewardship among current and future healthcare team members, including doctors, nurses, pharmacy teams, laboratory staff, and students.

2.3. *Stakeholder Engagement*

The game was co-created between partners in the UK and eight African countries that were part of the CwPAMS programme to ensure that the game is relevant, effective, and was designed to be used in either a high-income or low- to middle-income setting. The four broad areas addressed in the game are introduction to antimicrobial resistance and stewardship, appropriate use of antimicrobial agents, infection prevention and control, and stewardship and surveillance.

Partners and their network of health professionals were asked to share insights on the game. Twenty-seven stakeholders ranging from national to frontline health professionals, including pharmacists, doctors, and nurses across nine countries (Ghana, Kenya, Malawi, Nigeria, Sierra Leone, Tanzania, Uganda, United Kingdom, and Zambia), were consulted on the type of the game—snakes and ladders, the question cards for the AMS game, and case studies to include in the AMS game. Stakeholders were asked to share broad comments about content and accuracy of the answers to the questions in the game within their context and also asked to suggest any additional questions. To guide the feedback process, a structured feedback form (available as Supplementary File S1) was developed in Microsoft Word and shared with the stakeholders via email. The feedback form covered the following sections: demographics of the respondent (name, title, country, profession, job title, and email address), relevancy of the questions to the country, responsiveness of the questions to the key aspects of AMS, and also provided space for them to suggest other potential topics for inclusion in the game.

Demonstration of the board and online games (Figure 2) are available via https://commonwealthpharmacy.org/press-release-launch-of-the-antimicrobial-stewardship-ams-game/ accessed on 27 April 2022.

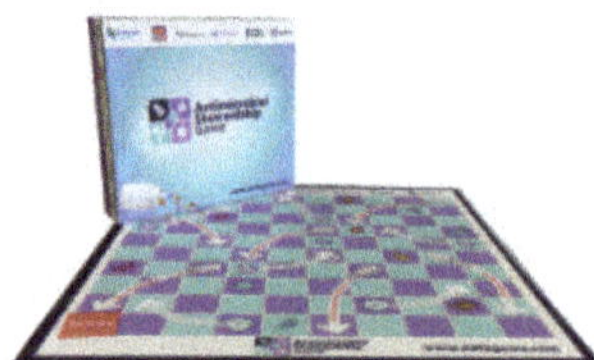
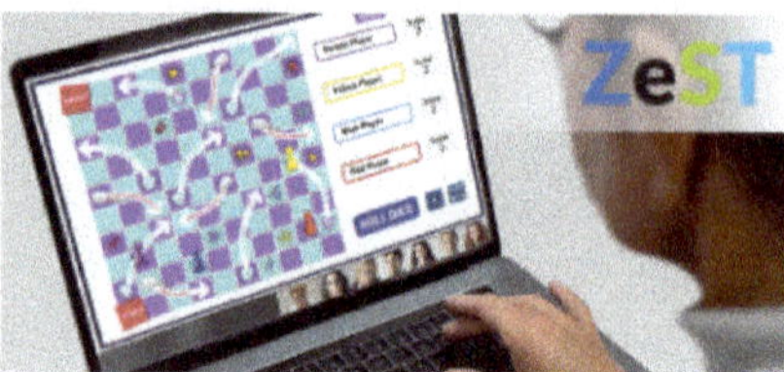

Figure 2. Board and online AMS games [17].

A guide was developed for the facilitators to provide direction on how to host the game (available in Supplementary File S2). Sample questions and answers are available in Supplementary File S3. A prize was planned for the participants of the game. The participants who completed the evaluation form of the game were entered into a draw to win access to the online AMS game for a period of one year

2.4. Recruitment of Participants and Playing the Game

The AMS game was first launched and played in August 2021, and then played again during the World Antimicrobial Awareness Week in November 2021 as part of a global tournament (Supplementary File S4). On both occasions, the game was promoted globally through online channels including email, websites, and social media to encourage people across the globe to register as players or facilitators. The facilitators had a technical background in antimicrobial resistance and stewardship and the project team provided a short briefing session on how to steer the session between the playing teams.

The game was hosted on Zoom, where participants received a Zoom link upon registration and used it to join the game session. Players were allocated to different breakout rooms with facilitators. In each breakout room, players were divided into two teams. Teams took turns to answer and discuss a series of questions and case studies about AMR and AMS that were being shown after the facilitators rolled the dice. The game lasted for 45 min. The facilitators were responsible for organizing players into teams, and moderating the game by displaying questions, encouraging players to discuss the questions and agree on the response, and displaying the correct answer after the players' responses. The facilitator guide is available as Supplementary File S2.

2.5. Feedback from Players of the Game

We collected feedback from individuals who played the AMS game on 24 November 2021. The feedback was collected using an online questionnaire with quantitative and open/free response text-based options hosted on Survey Monkey. This was a short questionnaire with 13 questions that: collected the players' demographic information, examined their experience in antimicrobial stewardship, assessed their knowledge gain and confidence in antimicrobial stewardship after playing the game, and assessed their perceptions on the game in terms of enjoyment and whether they would share lessons from the game and also recommend it to others.

2.6. Data Management

Data were collected anonymously, although survey respondents could voluntarily provide their name and email address should they wish to be contacted afterwards, e.g., for information about game prize winners and future relevant AMR events. All data were anonymised prior to data analysis. The data were held securely by the project team and in line with the General Data Protection Regulation 2016/679 [18].

2.7. Data Analysis

Descriptive statistics on the frequency distributions and percentages were used to analyse the responses. Data were analysed using Stata 14.

3. Results

3.1. Developing the Game: Feedback on Relevance

3.1.1. Demographics of Respondents

Twenty-six stakeholders ranging from national to frontline health professionals, including pharmacists [18], doctors [4], nurses [3], and an epidemiologist [1], across nine countries (Kenya 3, Malawi 3, Nigeria 3, Sierra Leone 3, Tanzania 2, United Kingdom 4, Uganda 3, and Zambia 6), provided responses on the relevance of the game (Table 1).

Table 1. Respondents' feedback on relevance of questions.

	Number of Respondents	Percentage (%)
Questions broadly relevant to your country	$n = 25$	
Yes	25	100
No	0	0
Some questions not at all relevant or inaccurate for your country	$n = 25$	
Yes	10	40
No	15	60
Questions and case studies address key aspects of AMS	$n = 24$	
Yes	24	100
No	0	0

3.1.2. Feedback on Relevance of Questions of the Game

When asked whether the questions were broadly relevant to their countries, all 25 respondents who answered this question said "yes". However, 40% of the 25 respondents mentioned that some questions were not at all relevant or were inaccurate to their countries (Table 1). To this end, respondents shared some of the following suggestions, including questions that could be added to the game:

"What is antibiotic resistance? The response needs to be modified to include inappropriate antibiotic use as a driver of antibiotic resistance not optimal use of the same. The response should also include that antibiotics are not effective against parasites."

"Perhaps consider adding some more questions on the role of IPC and the MTC in AMS."

"I would suggest to add the following topics on hospital-associated infections. Diagnostics on how to identify the presence of a microbe in a patient specimen."

On the other hand, the questions and case studies were found to address the key aspects of AMS, as indicated by all 24 respondents that answered the question.

3.2. Players' Feedback on the AMS Game

3.2.1. Demographics of Respondents

In total, 328 individuals from 23 countries registered to join the online game sessions at the launch of the game in August 2021, and during World Antimicrobial Awareness Week in November 2021. More than 120 attended the two live sessions and 74 participants responded to the AMS game evaluation form. The respondents represented 13 countries across 4 regions: Africa [7], Europe [2], South-East Asia [2], and the Western Pacific region [1] (Table 2). More than half (62.2%) of the respondents were pharmacists. The majority of respondents had experience in AMS, with 20.3% recorded as AMS specialists. However, 10.8% of the respondents were new to AMS.

Table 2. Demographics of respondents (players' feedback).

Country	Number of Respondents (n = 74)	Percentage (%)
European Region	39	52.8
United Kingdom	38	51.4
Hungary	1	1.4
South-East Asia Region	2	2.7
India	1	1.4
Sri Lanka	1	1.4
African region	32	43.2
Uganda	15	20.3
Kenya	7	9.5
Ghana	2	2.7
Nigeria	3	4.1
Sierra Leone	3	4.1
Eswatini	1	1.4
Malawi	1	1.4
Western Pacific Region	1	1.4
Fiji	1	1.4
	Number of respondents (n = 74)	**Percentage (%)**
Role/Profession		
Pharmacist	46	62.2
Student	7	9.5
Doctor	6	8.1
Other (Academic, Environmental Health)	5	6.8
Support staff	4	5.4
Other clinical staff	3	4.05
Laboratory staff	2	2.7
Nurse	1	1.4

Table 2. *Cont.*

Country	Number of Respondents (n = 74)	Percentage (%)
Level of Experience in AMS		
Some knowledge of AMS	30	40.5
Experienced in AMS	21	28.4
Specialist in AMS	15	20.3
New to AMS	8	10.8

3.2.2. Player Enjoyment of the AMS Game

When asked whether they enjoyed playing the AMS game, almost all (91.9%) of the respondents agreed that they enjoyed it (Table 3). The reasons for enjoyment were mainly attributed to: the simplicity of the design of the game, making it easy to play, and the game was viewed as a novel, unique, interactive, and fun approach for empowering participants to tackle AMR. Comments included:

> *"The game was highly entertaining and enriching. You get to learn more of the AMS or rather, fine-tune your knowledge via the game. Will really love to partake again. Kindly keep me posted. Thanks."*

> *"The game was very interesting, straight forward and all-round included the One Health aspect which I am really interested in that I think is the way to go if mitigation of antimicrobial resistance is to be achieved."*

> *"The game is a good way of bringing the awareness to health workers. It should be rolled out across and include students in medicine, nursing, pharmacy, and laboratory."*

> *"What I loved most was that the answers provided by the game were simple, understandable and straightforward to the point and also there was more valuable information attached to the answer thus giving more understanding and meaning."*

Table 3. Enjoyment playing the AMS game.

Enjoyed Playing the AMS Game	Number of Respondents (n = 74)	Percentage (%)
Strongly disagree	2	2.7
Disagree	0	0
Neither disagree nor agree	4	5.4
Agree	26	35.1
Strongly agree	42	56.8

On the other hand, time was a common reason stated as a limitation to enjoyment of the game. The reason for this was attributed towards the short time allocated for the demonstration and not the game itself, whereby players would usually enjoy the game at their own pace. In this perspective, respondents felt that if given more time, the game would be a valuable tool for learning.

> *"The demonstration was a bit rushed so difficult to get a real feel for the game. I can see it could be a useful tool to facilitate discussion around AMS with more junior/inexperienced staff. The game needs to be seen in this light because I feel if the focus becomes on playing the game, answering questions as quickly as possible, etc., then it's true value will be lost."*

> *"A good fun, learned few things for a very short time."*

> *"Cross talking among participants making it difficult to respond … time constraints … facilitators should not talk much."*

3.2.3. Knowledge Gain after Playing the Game

The majority (75.7%) of respondents agreed that they got to know more about AMS after playing the game (Table 4). In this regard, respondents from the African Region agreed more than respondents from the European Region by a difference of 12.1% (Table 5). Qualitatively, respondents mentioned to mainly have gained knowledge on the relevance of One Health in AMS and others perceived the game as an opportunity to refresh the principles and strengthen their knowledge on AMS.

Table 4. Knowledge and confidence gain after playing the game.

	Number of Respondents	Percentage (%)
Know more about AMS after playing the game	$n = 74$	
Strongly disagree	6	8.1
Disagree	3	4.1
Neither disagree nor agree	9	12.2
Agree	35	47.3
Strongly agree	21	28.4
More confident about AMS	$n = 73$	
Strongly disagree	4	5.5
Disagree	3	4.1
Neither disagree nor agree	8	11
Agree	41	56.2
Strongly agree	17	23.3

Table 5. Knowledge gain according to geographic region.

Knowledge Gain	Region			
	African	Europe	South-East Asia	Western Pacific
Strongly disagree	3 (9.3%)	3 (7.7%)	0 (0%)	0 (0%)
Disagree	1 (3.1%)	2 (5.1%)	0 (0%)	0 (0%)
Neither disagree nor agree	2 (6.3%)	7 (17.9%)	0 (0%)	0 (0%)
Agree	14 (43.8%)	19 (48.7%)	1 (50%)	1 (100%)
Strongly agree	12 (37.5%)	8 (20.5%)	1 (50%)	0 (0%)
Total	32 (100%)	39 (100%)	2 (100%)	1 (100%)

> *"I understood that not only human health must be emphasised so as to end antimicrobial resistance but also animal and environmental health. Interacting with more informed players was more informing."*
>
> *"The game was a quick mind check for the principles on AMR."*

Further, when asked to highlight the most important things they learned from the game, respondents commonly stated aspects related to improved understanding of One Health and handwashing as key aspects in AMS. Additionally, respondents acknowledged the gain of understanding of key AMS terminologies, such as "biosecurity" and "watchful waiting". Overall, there were expressions of increase in knowledge on the causes and preventive measures of AMR. It was also realised that there is a need to create more awareness on AMR and AMS and it was commonly stated that games can be a fun and interactive approach for empowering health professionals and other team members to improve AMS.

> *"Actually, it's funny to say but today I learnt that there is a difference between antibiotics and antimicrobials. At first, I thought there was no difference. And I have also learnt about antimicrobial and antibiotic resistance."*
>
> *"I learned that simple practices such as handwashing play a big role in fighting AMR."*
>
> *"Learning is fun when made simple in such innovative ways. I also think it can stick to the brain and allows easy replication in actual practice settings."*

Relatedly, more than three quarters (79.5%) of respondents expressed having more confidence about AMS after playing the game. Respondents associated gaining confidence with acquiring knowledge from the game, thus making them better positioned to create awareness on AMS, as explained by the participants' comments below:

> *"I can now educate my colleagues, the nation and the entire world about the goodness of antimicrobial stewardship."*
>
> *"I think the game is great, since am just an undergraduate student but I have been able to reason out different things with people already in the profession. This has boosted my confidence."*

3.2.4. Sharing Lessons Gained from Playing the Game

The majority (93.3%) (Table 6) of participants responded in agreement about sharing lessons from the game with colleagues. Some voiced reasons as to why they would share lessons and others mentioned platforms they would use for sharing, such as those highlighted below:

Table 6. Sharing lessons gained after playing the game.

	Number of Respondents	Percentage (%)
Sharing lessons with colleagues	$n = 74$	
Strongly disagree	2	2.7
Disagree	0	0
Neither disagree nor agree	3	4.1
Agree	38	51.4
Strongly agree	31	41.9
Sharing lessons with patients	$n = 73$	
Strongly disagree	3	4.1
Disagree	0	0
Neither disagree nor agree	17	23.3
Agree	34	46.6
Strongly agree	19	26
Recommending game to colleagues		
No	2	2.7
Yes	71	97.3

> *"I have to share what I have learnt with others so as to facilitate continuation of learning and flow of information."*
>
> *"I will share during our grants meetings and AMS meeting."*
>
> *"I will promote for use in WAAW (World Antimicrobial Awareness Week)."*
>
> *"It was such an engaging experience and will be helpful for bonding in our hospital teams."*

Concerning sharing lessons from the game with patients, more than half (72.6%) (Table 6) of the respondents expressed willingness to do so for some of the following reasons:

"Completing one's dosage as prescribed by a trained health personnel helps minimise antimicrobial resistance."

"The patients can use the game to learn more about AMS."

Further, almost all (97.3%) of the respondents mentioned that they would recommend the game to their colleagues (Table 6).

4. Discussion

This paper has documented the process of developing the AMS game, and reflections by players. Overall, the healthcare teams who played the game found it enjoyable and reported that it can impart knowledge and confidence in AMS and facilitate shared learning with colleagues and patients.

4.1. AMS Game Development

The AMS game was developed to attract a multidisciplinary team of players to discuss AMS and learn what they can do personally, and collectively, to improve stewardship in their organisation and community. A multi-country and multidisciplinary approach was used in the development of the game. This supported incorporation of the contextual educational needs of both high- and low- to middle-income countries as shared by diverse health professionals, including pharmacists, nurses, and doctors from Africa and Europe. With this, we addressed the gap reported in a scoping review on serious health education games targeting healthcare providers, patients, and public health users, where it was reported that LMICs have rarely been considered in the development of games [18]. Consequently, the AMS game described in this manuscript attracted diverse participants, players, and facilitators across 23 countries. Further, it is recommended that for effectiveness, games should be designed according to the requirements of specific groups of people [19]. The AMS game was designed for teams of healthcare staff at all levels. To cater for the needs of diverse staff members, the game was designed with different levels of complexity so the organiser can select questions to match the learning requirements of each group.

4.2. Players' Feedback on the Game

The results showed that the game was enjoyable, as indicated by almost all (91.9%) participants who shared feedback. As in other studies, the enjoyment of the game was attributed to its simplicity in design, making it easy to understand and play [13,19]. The AMS game was also found to be interactive and thus a component that participants enjoyed. The component of playing the game in teams encouraged discussion and learning among players, which also made it more engaging. A systematic review that explored user engagement features in digital games documented more engaging features that can be considered in digital games: the game should have an attractive storyline, be adaptable to gender and age, high-end realistic graphics, well-defined instructions, in combination with clear feedback and a balance of educational and fun content [20]. Whilst the AMS game described in this manuscript covered all these features in its design and appearance, the gender and age components were not considered and neither did the evaluation of the game cater for these variables. It would be important to explore such in future.

It was evidenced that the game can translate knowledge and create awareness on AMS among the players. Higher knowledge gain was recorded among participants from the African countries compared to those from the European countries by a difference of 12.1%. This could imply that the game is more beneficial to the African countries where there are lower levels of awareness on AMR and AMS, as indicated in several studies [12–23]. It was clear from the study findings that the role of One Health in AMS was one of the most common key lessons gained by players, and this is likely because many of the respondents focused on human health in healthcare settings and likely had less exposure to One Health principles. To this end, the AMS game was relevant in accelerating knowledge on the One Health approach, which is recommended by the WHO as a strategy for health workers to responsibly use antimicrobials [24].

The feedback on the game did not only further expose the inadequacy in knowledge on key terminologies in AMS among health professionals, but instantly created awareness and knowledge on terms such as 'antimicrobial stewardship', 'biosecurity', and 'watchful waiting'. Therefore, the AMS game could be a solution to challenges discovered in studies such as that of Higuita-Gutiérrez et al. [25], where 81.8% of 532 medical students had never heard of the term 'antimicrobial stewardship'. Generally, this AMS game may have the potential to increase awareness among health students and professionals across the globe. It can be considered as part of a wider AMR education programme within universities and health institutions. The online version provides an opportunity for use across multiple institutions.

Following the AMS game tournaments, a substantial portion (75.9%) of players who provided feedback indicated that they gained confidence in AMS and thus would participate in creation of awareness on AMS thereafter. This was further demonstrated when over 90% of the study respondents indicated that they would share lessons from the game with colleagues and patients.

4.3. Strengths and Limitations

Our AMS game was developed with consideration of perspectives from a multidisciplinary team of professionals across the UK and African countries. Hence, this game does not only promote One Health in antimicrobial stewardship but is also among the few games that cater for the antimicrobial stewardship awareness needs of both high- and low- to middle-income countries. Whilst the study results indicated that our AMS game is very likely to improve awareness and understanding of AMS, as a limitation, it should be noted that this was a small study designed to collect initial feedback on the new board and online AMS game. Further, only subjective measurements were used to collect feedback on the educational potential of this AMS game, and the small number of players (respondents) makes statistical analysis infeasible. As such, the results of the current study need to be strengthened by studies employing stronger methodologies. We recommend that future studies consider a randomized controlled trial utilizing objective measurement to evaluate the AMS game among a higher number of respondents sampled from a group of individuals who played the game. It would be important that future studies consider: a greater representation of other types of health professionals as the current study had much higher representation ofpharmacists, evaluate the impact of the players' discussions in the breakout rooms (which was not evaluated in this study), and study the effectiveness of the AMS game in comparison to other AMS education interventions.

Despite these limitations, this study generated more evidence and demonstrated that a board and online AMS game is likely to improve knowledge of antimicrobial stewardship. The AMS board game continues to be promoted, made accessible, and used as an education tool among health professionals [26].

5. Conclusions

We provide a documentation of the process of developing a board and online game on antimicrobial resistance and stewardship; and its potential to educate diverse health care teams in high or low-to-middle- income countries. The game was co-created with a diverse group of stakeholders including national and frontline health professionals from high- and low-income countries. The feedback from the initial players (health professionals) of the game highlighted that the game is enjoyable. Also, that it provides an innovative and engaging opportunity for the players to discuss topics in AMR and AMS; whilst improving and strengthening their knowledge of key topics. Further studies will be useful in evaluating the impact of the AMS game as an educational tool for antimicrobial resistance and stewardship.

Supplementary Materials: The following supporting information can be downloaded at: https://www.mdpi.com/article/10.3390/antibiotics11050611/s1. Supplementary File S1: Questions and comments review: Antimicrobial Stewardship Game. Supplementary File S2: A facilitator's guide was developed to guide the facilitator's on how to run the game. Supplementary File S3: Sample questions and answers from the game cards. Supplementary File S4: Poster for the global tournament.

Author Contributions: Conceptualisation, D.A.-O., and W.T.; data curation, D.A.-O., M.N., A.Y., D.D., S.Y., M.B. and R.S.-J.; formal analysis, D.A.-O. and M.N.; funding acquisition, D.A.-O., V.R. and R.S.-J.; methodology, D.A.-O., M.N. and F.G.; project administration, D.A.-O., M.N., D.D., M.B., N.D. and S.Y.; supervision, D.A.-O.; validation, D.A.-O.; writing—original draft, D.A.-O. and M.N.; writing—review and editing, D.A.-O., M.N., A.Y., M.B., S.C., F.G., R.S.-J. and V.C. All authors have read and agreed to the published version of the manuscript.

Funding: This project and partnership were part of the Commonwealth Partnerships for Antimicrobial Stewardship (CwPAMS) managed by the Tropical Health and Education Trust (THET) and Commonwealth Pharmacists Association (CPA). CwPAMS is a global health partnership programme funded by the Department of Health and Social Care (DHSC) using UK aid funding, managed by the Fleming Fund. The Fleming Fund is a £265 million UK aid investment to tackle AMR by supporting low- and middle-income countries to generate, use, and share data on AMR and is managed by the UK Department of Health and Social Care. The views expressed in this publication are those of the author(s) and not necessarily those of the Department of Health and Social Care, the UK National Health Service, the Tropical Health and Education Trust, or The Commonwealth Pharmacists Association.

Institutional Review Board Statement: Ethical approval was not required as per NHS Health Research Authority guidance and the NHS health research decision tool because this was a service evaluation of CPA's programme of activities to develop and implement the AMS game as part of the CwPAMS programme [27]. All respondents participated strictly in their professional capacity, no identifiable data were collected, and their participation in the survey was in all cases on the basis of informed consent.

Informed Consent Statement: Informed consent was obtained from all participants involved in the study.

Data Availability Statement: Data are contained within the article or Supplementary Material.

Acknowledgments: The authors acknowledge: The Commonwealth Partnerships for Antimicrobial Stewardship (CwPAMS) led by the Commonwealth Pharmacists Association and the Tropical Health and Education Trust (THET) who collaborated with the Focus Games Ltd. to co-develop the AMS Game. Stakeholders and partners from Nigeria: Mashood Lawal, Oluchi Maryann Ezeajughi, Grace Olatunde Olakunri, Jelili AdewaleKilani. Tanzania: Eva Muro and Rajabu Hamidu. Zambia: Derick Munkombwe, Andrew Bambala, Aubrey Kalungia, Brian Muyunda, Webrod Mufwambi, and Chabota Simweemba.Uganda: Winnie Nambatya, Komata Ronald, Vivian Twemanye, Florence Nakakembo, and Oscar Obiga. Kenya: Eric Muringu, Immaculate Kerubo, and Leon Ogoti. Ghana: Mohammed Kudus Moro, Emmanuel Amankrah, Dinah Aryeh-Do, and Afua Akuffo. Sierra Leone: Shuwary Barlatt. Jennet Buck, and Brima Lahai. UK: Abigail Scott, Amber Cavanagh, Amy Hai Yan Chan, Eleanor Bull, Esmita Charani, Elizabeth Beech, Hayley Wickens, Jacqui Sneddon, Lesley Cooper, Manjula Halai, Raymond Anderson, Tatiana Hardy.

Conflicts of Interest: The authors declare no conflict of interest. The funders had no role in the design of the study; in the collection, analyses, or interpretation of data; in the writing of the manuscript, or in the decision to publish the results.

References

1. WHO. Antimicrobial Resistance: Fact Sheets. Available online: https://www.who.int/news-room/fact-sheets/detail/antimicrobial-resistance (accessed on 4 March 2022).
2. Ghosh, S.; Bornman, C.; Zafer, M.M. Antimicrobial Resistance threats in the emerging COVID-19 pandemic: Where do we stand? *J. Infect. Public Health* **2021**, *14*, 555–560. [CrossRef] [PubMed]
3. Pokharel, S.; Raut, S.; Adhikari, B. Tackling antimicrobial resistance in low-income and middle-income countries. *BMJ Glob. Health* **2019**, *4*, e002104. [CrossRef] [PubMed]
4. Shi, J.; Renwick, R.; Turner, N.E.; Kirsh, B. Understanding the lives of problem gamers: The meaning, purpose, and influences of video gaming. *Comput. Hum. Behav.* **2019**, *97*, 291–303. [CrossRef]

5. Looyestyn, J.; Kernot, J.; Boshoff, K.; Ryan, J.; Edney, S.; Maher, C. Does gamification increase engagement with online programs? A systematic review. *PLoS ONE* **2017**, *12*, e0173403. [CrossRef] [PubMed]
6. Nakao, M. Special series on "effects of board games on health education and promotion" board games as a promising tool for health promotion: A review of recent literature. *BioPsychoSocial Med.* **2019**, *13*, 5. [CrossRef] [PubMed]
7. Guest, E.; Jarman, H.; Sharratt, N.; Williamson, H.; White, P.; Harcourt, D.; Slater, A. 'Everybody's Different: The Appearance Game'. A randomised controlled trial evaluating an appearance-related board game intervention with children aged 9–11 years. *Body Image* **2021**, *36*, 34–44. [CrossRef] [PubMed]
8. Akl, E.A.; Sackett, K.M.; Pretorius, R.; Bhoopathi, P.S.S.; Mustafa, R.; Schünemann, H.; Erdley, W.S. Educational games for health professionals. *Cochrane Database Syst. Rev.* **2013**, *2013*, Cd006411.
9. Ijaz, A.; Khan, M.Y.; Ali, S.M.; Qadir, J.; Boulos, M.N.K. Serious games for healthcare professional training: A systematic review. *Eur. J. Biomed. Inform.* **2019**, *15*, 30.
10. Tudor Car, L.; Soong, A.; Kyaw, B.M.; Chua, K.L.; Low-Beer, N.; Majeed, A. Health professions digital education on clinical practice guidelines: A systematic review by Digital Health Education collaboration. *BMC Med.* **2019**, *17*, 139. [CrossRef] [PubMed]
11. Mitchell, G.; Leonard, L.; Carter, G.; Santin, O.; Brown Wilson, C. Evaluation of a 'serious game'on nursing student knowledge and uptake of influenza vaccination. *PLoS ONE* **2021**, *16*, e0245389. [CrossRef] [PubMed]
12. Aboalshamat, K.; Khayat, A.; Halwani, R.; Bitan, A.; Alansari, R. The effects of gamification on antimicrobial resistance knowledge and its relationship to dentistry in Saudi Arabia: A randomized controlled trial. *BMC Public Health* **2020**, *20*, 680. [CrossRef] [PubMed]
13. Hale, A.R.; Young, V.L.; Grand, A.; McNulty, C.A.M. Can gaming increase antibiotic awareness in children? A mixed-methods approach. *JMIR Serious Games* **2017**, *5*, e6420. [CrossRef] [PubMed]
14. Focus Games. Case Studies [Online]. 2021. Available online: https://focusgames.com/case_studies.html (accessed on 20 April 2022).
15. Lameras, P.; Arnab, S.; Dunwell, I.; Stewart, C.; Clarke, S.; Petridis, P. Essential features of serious games design in higher education: Linking learning attributes to game mechanics. *Br. J. Educ. Technol.* **2017**, *48*, 972–994. [CrossRef]
16. Focus Games. Develop a Game [Online]. 2021. Available online: https://focusgames.com/develop_a_game.html (accessed on 17 March 2022).
17. Focus Games. Antimicrobial Stewardship Game. 2021. Available online: https://www.amsgame.com/ (accessed on 17 March 2022).
18. Sharifzadeh, N.; Kharrazi, H.; Nazari, E.; Tabesh, H.; Khodabandeh, M.E.; Heidari, S.; Tara, M. Health education serious games targeting health care providers, patients, and public health users: Scoping review. *JMIR Serious Games* **2020**, *8*, e13459. [CrossRef] [PubMed]
19. Brox, E.; Fernandez-Luque, L.; Tøllefsen, T. Healthy gaming–video game design to promote health. *Appl. Clin. Inform.* **2011**, *2*, 128–142. [PubMed]
20. Schwarz, A.F.; Huertas-Delgado, F.J.; Cardon, G.; DeSmet, A. Design features associated with user engagement in digital games for healthy lifestyle promotion in youth: A systematic review of qualitative and quantitative studies. *Games Health J.* **2020**, *9*, 150–163. [CrossRef] [PubMed]
21. Sharma, A.; Singh, A.; Dar, M.A.; Kaur, R.J.; Charan, J.; Iskandar, K.; Haque, M.; Murti, K.; Ravichandiran, V.; Dhingra, S. Menace of antimicrobial resistance in LMICs: Current surveillance practices and control measures to tackle hostility. *J. Infect. Public Health* **2021**, *15*, 172–181. [CrossRef] [PubMed]
22. Fasina, F.O.; LeRoux-Pullen, L.; Smith, P.; Debusho, L.K.; Shittu, A.; Jajere, S.M.; Adebowale, O.; Odetokun, I.; Agbaje, M.; Fasina, M.M.; et al. Knowledge, attitudes, and perceptions associated with antimicrobial stewardship among veterinary students: A multi-country survey from Nigeria, South Africa, and Sudan. *Front. Public Health* **2020**, *8*, 630. [CrossRef] [PubMed]
23. Chukwu, E.E.; Oladele, D.A.; Awoderu, O.B.; Afocha, E.E.; Lawal, R.G.; Abdus-Salam, I.; Ogunsola, F.T.; Audu, R.A. A national survey of public awareness of antimicrobial resistance in Nigeria. *Antimicrob. Resist. Infect. Control.* **2020**, *9*, 72. [CrossRef] [PubMed]
24. WHO. *Health Workers' Education and Training on Antimicrobial Resistance: Curricula Guide*; WHO: Geneva, Switzerland, 2019.
25. Higuita-Gutiérrez, L.F.; Roncancio Villamil, G.E.; Jiménez Quiceno, J.N. Knowledge, attitude, and practice regarding antibiotic use and resistance among medical students in Colombia: A cross-sectional descriptive study. *BMC Public Health* **2020**, *20*, 1861. [CrossRef] [PubMed]
26. Commonwealth Pharmacists Association. Tweets of the #AMSGame in Use. Available online: https://twitter.com/hashtag/AMSGame?src=hashtag_click&f=live (accessed on 11 March 2022).
27. NHS. Is My Study Research? Available online: http://www.hra-decisiontools.org.uk/research/result7.html (accessed on 9 January 2022).

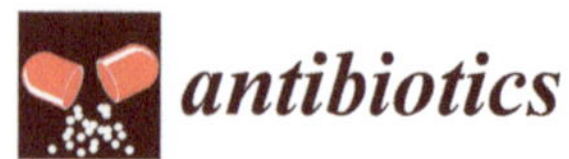

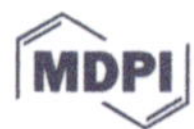

Protocol

Canadian Collaboration to Identify a Minimum Dataset for Antimicrobial Use Surveillance for Policy and Intervention Development across Food Animal Sectors

David F. Léger [1,†], Maureen E. C. Anderson [2,†], François D. Bédard [3], Theresa Burns [4], Carolee A. Carson [1], Anne E. Deckert [1], Sheryl P. Gow [5], Cheryl James [6], Xian-Zhi Li [7], Michael Ott [8] and Agnes Agunos [1,*]

1 Center for Foodborne, Environmental and Zoonotic Infectious Diseases, Public Health Agency of Canada, Guelph, ON N1H 7M7, Canada; david.leger@phac-aspc.gc.ca (D.F.L.); carolee.carson@phac-aspc.gc.ca (C.A.C.); anne.deckert@phac-aspc.gc.ca (A.E.D.)
2 Veterinary Science Unit, Ontario Ministry of Agriculture, Food and Rural Affairs, Guelph, ON N1G 4Y2, Canada; Maureen.E.C.Anderson@ontario.ca
3 Animal Industry Division, Agriculture and Agri-Food Canada, Ottawa, ON K1A 0C5, Canada; francois.bedard@agr.gc.ca
4 Canadian Animal Health Surveillance System, Animal Health Canada, Elora, ON N0B 1S0, Canada; tburns@ahwcouncil.ca
5 Center for Foodborne, Environmental and Zoonotic Infectious Diseases, Public Health Agency of Canada, Saskatoon, SK S7N 5B4, Canada; sheryl.gow@phac-aspc.gc.ca
6 Animal Industry Division, Canadian Food Inspection Agency, Ottawa, ON K1A 0Y9, Canada; cheryl.james@inspection.gc.ca
7 Veterinary Drugs Directorate, Health Canada, Ottawa, ON K1A 0K9, Canada; Xianzhi.li@hc-sc.gc.ca
8 Aquatic Ecosystems Sector, Fisheries and Oceans Canada, Ottawa, ON K1A 0E6, Canada; michael.ott@dfo-mpo.gc.ca
* Correspondence: agnes.agunos@phac-aspc.gc.ca; Tel.: +1-519-400-7895
† Shared first authorship.

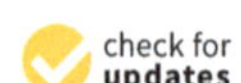

Citation: Léger, D.F.; Anderson, M.E.C.; Bédard, F.D.; Burns, T.; Carson, C.A.; Deckert, A.E.; Gow, S.P.; James, C.; Li, X.-Z.; Ott, M.; et al. Canadian Collaboration to Identify a Minimum Dataset for Antimicrobial Use Surveillance for Policy and Intervention Development across Food Animal Sectors. *Antibiotics* **2022**, *11*, 226. https://doi.org/10.3390/antibiotics11020226

Academic Editor: Diane Ashiru-Oredope

Received: 8 January 2022
Accepted: 8 February 2022
Published: 10 February 2022

Publisher's Note: MDPI stays neutral with regard to jurisdictional claims in published maps and institutional affiliations.

Copyright: © 2022 by the authors. Licensee MDPI, Basel, Switzerland. This article is an open access article distributed under the terms and conditions of the Creative Commons Attribution (CC BY) license (https://creativecommons.org/licenses/by/4.0/).

Abstract: Surveillance of antimicrobial use (AMU) and antimicrobial resistance (AMR) is a core component of the 2017 Pan-Canadian Framework for Action. There are existing AMU and AMR surveillance systems in Canada, but some stakeholders are interested in developing their own AMU monitoring/surveillance systems. It was recognized that the establishment of core (minimum) AMU data elements, as is necessary for policy or intervention development, would inform the development of practical and sustainable AMU surveillance capacity across food animal sectors in Canada. The Canadian Animal Health Surveillance System (CAHSS) AMU Network was established as a multi-sectoral working group to explore the possibility of harmonizing data inputs and outputs. There was a consensus that a minimum AMU dataset for AMU surveillance (MDS-AMU-surv) should be developed to guide interested parties in initiating AMU data collection. This multisectoral collaboration is an example of how consultative consensus building across relevant sectors can contribute to the development of harmonized approaches to AMU data collection and reporting and ultimately improve AMU stewardship. The MDS-AMU-surv could be used as a starting point for the progressive development or strengthening of AMU surveillance programs, and the collaborative work could serve as a model for addressing AMR and other shared threats at the human–animal–environment interface.

Keywords: antimicrobials; multisectoral; stewardship; surveillance; collaboration; antimicrobial use; antimicrobial resistance; food animals

1. Introduction

Surveillance is a vital component of the Global Action Plan for antimicrobial resistance (AMR) published by the World Health Organization (WHO) [1], the Food and Agriculture Organization of the United Nations' (FAO) action plan for AMR 2021-2025 [2] and its predecessor [3], and the World Organisation for Animal Health's (OIE) strategy for AMR and the prudent use of antimicrobials [4]. The FAO-OIE-WHO tripartite collaboration is one example of how resources and expertise can be optimized to implement actions toward mitigating AMR. Surveillance of antimicrobial use (AMU) and AMR is a component of the Canadian plan for "*Tackling Antimicrobial Resistance and Antimicrobial Use: A Pan-Canadian Framework for Action*" [5]. Surveillance data on AMU and AMR are essential for informed decision making to direct other components of the action plan being developed based on this framework, including infection prevention and control, stewardship, and research and innovation. In Canada, AMU/AMR data directly target AMU interventions and have utility in monitoring the impact of regulatory or voluntary changes in AMU practices.

Currently, there are two official data sources that provide information on the types and quantities of antimicrobials intended for use in animals in Canada. The first is the Veterinary Antimicrobial Sales Reporting (VASR) system, in which manufacturers, importers, and compounders are required to submit their annual sales data for medically important antimicrobials to the Veterinary Drugs Directorate at Health Canada [6]. Reporting the sale of medically important antimicrobials [7] is in compliance with the Regulations Amending the Food and Drug Regulations (Veterinary Drugs–Antimicrobial Resistance) [8]. The data providers are also required to include estimates of sales by animal species. The VASR data collection came into effect in 2018, and the data are incorporated in the Canadian Integrated Program for Antimicrobial Resistance Surveillance (CIPARS), otherwise known as the CIPARS VASR component (i.e., pertains to the CIPARS's surveillance component, which conducts the data analysis output, reporting, and communication of the antimicrobial sales data collected). Previously, between 2006 and 2018, the annual national antimicrobial sales data were provided to the CIPARS of the Public Health Agency of Canada by the Canadian Animal Health Institute (CAHI) [9–11], which did not include estimates of sales by animal species but was rather stratified by companion and production animals (production animals included horses) [11]. The second source of data is the CIPARS Farm AMU/AMR Surveillance program, a voluntary initiative that collects data from a network of sentinel veterinarians and producers in specific livestock sectors (pigs, broiler chickens, turkeys, feedlot beef and currently piloting data collection in dairy cattle and layer chickens) across the country [10]. The two AMU data components of CIPARS described above (1. CIPARS VASR sales data, and 2. CIPARS Farm AMU data) are complementary sources of information that contribute to the general landscape of AMU in animals in Canada. These AMU data are useful to understand the AMR trends and patterns across the food supply chain. In addition to the farm program, beginning in 2017, Fisheries and Ocean Canada (DFO) provided open data on the quantities of antimicrobials used in marine and freshwater finfish aquaculture [10]. These data are part of the reporting requirements by aquaculture industry operators under the Aquaculture Activities Regulations authorized under the Fisheries Act [12].

In 2016, the Canadian Animal Health Surveillance System (CAHSS), now an initiative of Animal Health Canada, formerly the National Farmed Animal Health and Welfare Council (https://animalhealthcanada.ca/, accessed on 1 February 2022), brought together individuals representing various government agencies and private industry organizations to discuss AMU and AMR across animal production sectors in Canada. In this inaugural meeting of the CAHSS AMU/AMR Working Group, it was recognized that protecting the effectiveness of antimicrobials while caring for the health and welfare of Canadian animal populations was a key component of national antimicrobial stewardship. There was also a recognition that policy makers, at various levels, lacked a clear understanding around the data necessary to evaluate AMU and to advance stewardship interventions. To address AMU information gaps and assist interested parties in developing their own AMU surveillance programs, the group determined that the elucidation of a "*minimum data set for AMU surveillance*" (MDS-AMU-surv) was a necessary first step. This core list of AMU variables would contribute to the harmonization of data collection at relevant points in the antimicrobial distribution pathway.

At the time of the initial meeting in 2016, there was no existing formal One Health governance mechanism for addressing AMR in Canada. However, the CAHSS AMU/AMR Working Group, combined with joint leadership from the Public Health Agency of Canada (CIPARS) and the Canadian Food Inspection Agency, facilitated the discussions to address activities related to the Pan-Canadian Framework for Action on AMR/AMU. Multisectoral collaboration, described as "more than one sector working together (on a joint program or response to an event)" was identified as the key to addressing zoonoses and other shared threats such as AMR in the human–animal–environment interface [13]. This paper aims to describe the AMU distribution pathway for antimicrobials intended for use in animals in Canada, identify points in the distribution chain where data could be collected to describe the multisectoral collaboration that facilitated the development of the MDS-AMU-surv, and to provide examples of the utility of the MDS-AMU-surv for AMU monitoring and research.

2. Results

The organizations represented by the CAHSS AMU/AMR are listed in the Supplementary Materials.

2.1. Contextual Review of Existing AMU Surveillance Infrastructures and the Antimicrobial Supply Distribution Pathway in Canada

The key players in the Canadian antimicrobial supply distribution pathway are depicted in Figure 1. The distribution is organized into three levels, which also represent existing and potential AMU data collection points:

(1) Manufacturers, importers, and distributors of veterinary drugs (finished products), importers, manufacturers, and compounders of active pharmaceutical ingredients (APIs) (i.e., those who obtain antimicrobials from pharmacies/dispensers of veterinary drugs and human drugs for animal use (blue line in Figure 1). Reporting to VASR is required by regulation;

(2) Prescription and dispensing facilities, including veterinary clinics, feed mills, agri-food companies who employ veterinarians (i.e., corporate veterinarians who prescribe antimicrobials for use in relevant production phases as part of the coordinated supply chain within their network including hatcheries, breeders, commercial growing farms-various commodities, and feedmills), and pharmacies/dispensers of veterinary drugs and human drugs for animal use). Data from this level are not yet available or targeted for a future data collection point;

(3) End users of antimicrobials including pet owners and producers of terrestrial and aquatic food animals. Information on specific terrestrial food animal species is captured through the CIPARS Farm AMU/AMR Surveillance program (voluntary) and aquatic animals via the DFO (by regulation).

The report from the Council of Chief Veterinary Officers in Canada on non-human AMU surveillance [14] was a useful resource for the working group. It provides an understanding of the national infrastructure for AMU data collection and the need for AMU surveillance in Canada. Recently, the document was modified to reflect regulatory changes implemented in December of 2018 in how antimicrobial drug products are distributed/sold. In Figure 1, data availabilities are depicted by the colour of the boxes: blue (available), light blue (partial or captured by another player in the distribution chain), or white (no data; future data collection points). Since 2018, regulations have required that manufacturers, importers, and compounders submit annual data on the volume of medically important antimicrobials sold for veterinary use, by animal species, to the VASR system [8]. Manufacturers and importers of veterinary drugs that also sell or move nonmedically important antimicrobials such as ionophores to other actors are not required to report the total volume of nonmedically important drugs at this time. Importers and manufacturers of APIs are required to have a drug establishment license and follow good manufacturing practices [15]. As stated earlier, prior to 2018, antimicrobial sales data were obtained from CAHI, which is a trade association that represents the majority of manufacturers and distributors of animal health products [16]. The CAHI data collection and analysis were performed by a third party (Impact Vet) [17]. Collated CAHI sales data were then voluntarily shared with CIPARS and included in CIPARS annual reports [10].

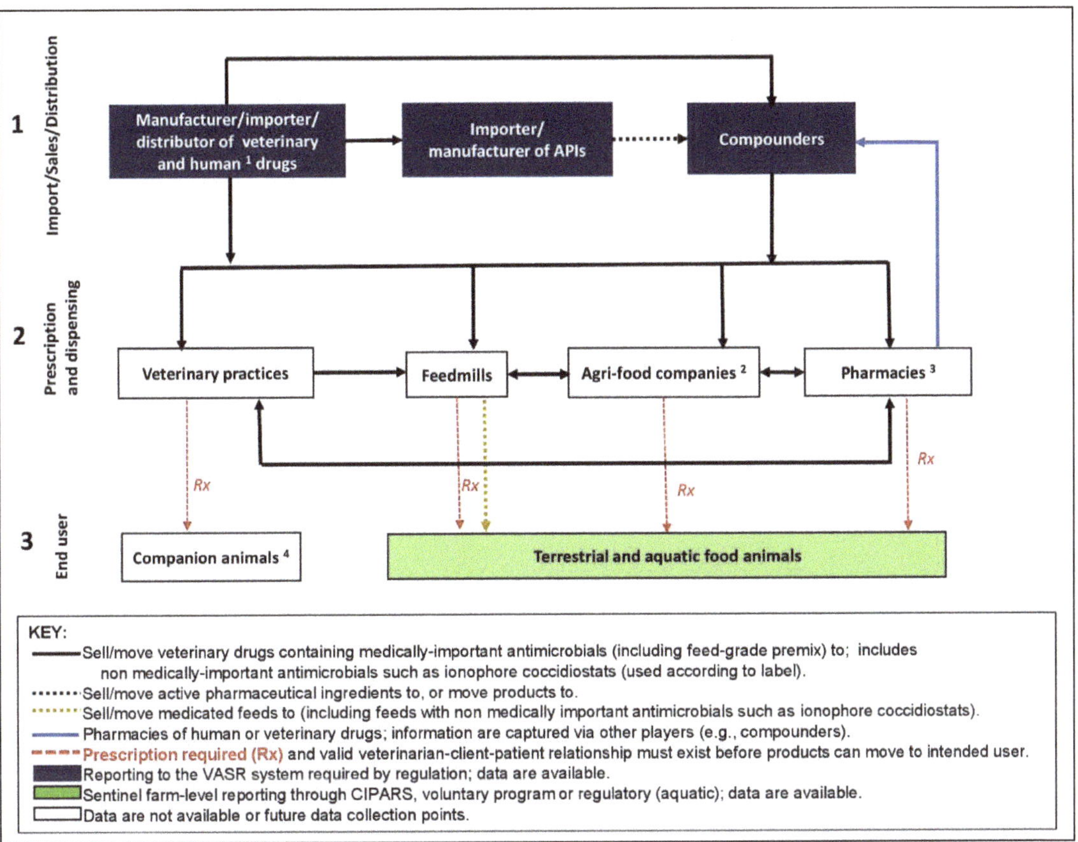

Figure 1. The antimicrobial supply distribution pathway in Canada indicating the existing and future antimicrobial use data collection points. VASR—Veterinary Antimicrobial Sales Reporting system. CIPARS—Canadian Integrated Program for Antimicrobial Resistance Surveillance. [1] Human drugs intended for use animals (largely companion animals). [2] Veterinarians in agrifood companies (corporate veterinarians) prescribe antimicrobials for use in relevant production phases as part of the coordinated supply chain within their network (e.g., hatcheries, breeders, grower farms, and feedmill). [3] Pharmacies of veterinary drugs and human drugs intended for use in animals (i.e., pharmacies of veterinary drugs and human drugs have similar requirements from a regulatory standpoint but differ in where they are dispensing antimicrobials). [4] Companion animals include horses.

With the VASR system, data providers electronically enter information into a secure web-based site under the Canadian Network for Public Health Intelligence at the Public Health Agency of Canada [18]. Information is collected on product characteristics (e.g., Health Canada-assigned drug identification number (DIN), product name, package size, number of packages, ATCvet code, antimicrobial active ingredient, class, and formulation), data provider (manufacturer, importer, and compounder), province, intended animal species of use (high and low estimates of packages sold for 11 different animal species groups), quantities sold, and quantities exported. At the time of writing, there was no system for reporting veterinary prescription and dispensation of antimicrobial products in Canada, but a pilot project in select animal sector/volunteer veterinary practices is underway.

In terms of end user data in terrestrial animals, CIPARS collects farm-level AMU from a network of sentinel veterinarians and producers using species-specific questionnaires or electronic data capture (feedlot beef). The CIPARS program is active in grower–finisher pigs, broiler chickens, turkeys, and feedlot beef with pilot farm-level surveillance in dairy cattle and chicken egg layers, and abattoir-level AMU surveillance (flock sheets) in spent broiler breeder chickens. Farm-level AMU data, animal health, and basic demographics information from the questionnaires are entered into the CIPARS AMU database and exported in Microsoft Excel (Professional Plus 2016) format for further analysis.

A valid veterinarian–client–patient relationship (VCPR) must exist before the finished products containing prescription drugs (including medically important antimicrobials) reach the end user. With the new regulations, veterinary prescriptions and oversight are required for dispensing of medically important antimicrobial products including through feed mills, agrifood companies, and pharmacists. Agrifood companies are similar in structure to vertically integrated systems and have internal veterinary services (i.e., known as corporate veterinarians) who provide oversight of antimicrobial product distribution through company (or partner) feed mills and farms (i.e., as part of the coordinated supply chain, for example in the poultry sector, the hatcheries). The VCPR in the agrifood system is represented in the figure, indicating that a single farmer/producer may interact with different actors in the AMU distribution chain (e.g., corporate veterinary services or independent/private veterinary practice) regarding AMU decisions pertaining to the flock or herd.

2.2. *Stakeholders' Need for AMU Data*

In the initial meeting of the working group, participants were asked for their organization's specific primary objective for AMU surveillance and the utility of the associated data. There were eight food animal sectors and an allied industry (feed mill) that participated in the survey. Responses are shown in Box 1.

Box 1. Participants' responses when asked about their objectives for antimicrobial use surveillance. AMU—antimicrobial use; AMR—antimicrobial resistance.

Primary objectives for antimicrobial use surveillance and the utility of the data collected:

- *"To garner public trust, to demonstrate social responsibility";*
- *"To understand AMU (in my sector)";*
- *"To provide AMU benchmarks (reference or targets) and trends that will inform decision making/policy and demonstrate the impacts of interventions";*
- *"To provide oversight of AMU";*
- *"To reduce reliance on antimicrobials to preserve antimicrobial efficacy";*
- *"To improve/inform/demonstrate antimicrobial stewardship and prudent use";*
- *"To provide international comparisons";*
- *"To guide research priorities";*
- *"To educate the public, veterinarians and producers about AMU/AMR".*

The ability to demonstrate social responsibility was cited by the majority of participants as an overarching objective for the collection of AMU data. However, the ultimate outcome of AMU surveillance indicated was to preserve access to efficacious antimicrobials by strengthening stewardship. Some commodity groups indicated specific AMU surveillance objectives, for example, the need for AMU surveillance data to demonstrate the need for additional licensed antimicrobial options for sheep. Long-term outcomes identified included the ability to address certain AMU practices through the optimization and rationalization of use and to decrease the health burden associated with AMR. Other desired outcomes were related to the sustainability of their commodities, such as economic benefits, impact on production performance parameters, and return on investment. Based on the desired AMU objectives and outcomes, subsequent working group discussions for the inclusion of variables in the MDS-AMU-surv were guided by the AMU/AMR working group vision formed during the first meeting (i.e., in Ottawa, Ontario on 16–19 October 2016). The working group determined that "*AMU surveillance is necessary to inform decision making to objectively address AMU stewardship and to maintain public trust in the sustainable production of safe and affordable food from humanely raised animals*". The working group considered that understanding the need for AMU surveillance could direct the next steps including the development of the MDS-AMU-surv.

2.3. Outputs Desired and Important Considerations When Reporting AMU Data

Several participants emphasized the need for detailed information to better understand AMU in animals. In addition to the ability to quantify AMU, the importance of context was noted (e.g., where—national/regional, who—the population at risk and size, when—time exposed, and why—reason for AMU). Some cautioned that to be successful the surveillance system must not increase the reporting burden on the producer. The group reviewed how existing surveillance platforms such as data from importers/manufacturers/compounders and end-users, as well as future data collection from prescription and dispensation levels, generate the outputs desired by the different sectors (Figure 2).

2.4. The MDS-AMU-Surv Development, Framework for Data Collection, and Data Sources

2.4.1. Core MDS-AMU-Surv Data Elements

A guiding principle for the development of the AMU surveillance capacity considered that there was a "*need for minimum data to tell a coherent story, cognizant of cost and effort*". Exploring existing infrastructure to collect AMU data could optimize resources, again avoiding additional reporting requirements by producers. The working group recognized that national-level organizations (marketing boards or industry sectoral groups) could support existing farm-level data collection (e.g., CIPARS Farm AMU/AMR Surveillance or provincial AMU surveillance initiatives) vs. initiating competing, and possibly redundant, surveillance programs. There was no appetite for regulated use reporting similar to the Yellow Card or Differentiated Yellow Card System in place in other countries such as Denmark [19]. It is important to note that in the aquaculture sector (not yet providing data at the time of MDS-AMU-surv development in 2016–2017), the Aquaculture Reporting Regulations (Fisheries Act, Section 35–36) already required owners and operators of aquaculture establishments to report their annual antimicrobial deposit data [12,20]. There was interest in AMU data capture at the veterinary prescription/dispensing level of the distribution system (white boxes in Figure 1). The core elements of the MDS-AMU-surv are described in Table 1.

2.4.2. Data Source

Several sector representatives indicated that various platforms (i.e., "*what records can you provide?*") could be optimized for data collection that would fulfil the MDS-AMU-surv. Table 1 includes examples of data from existing records that could be used to collect the core MDS-AMU-surv elements and reporting and communications considerations (i.e., different ways to fulfil data requirements for the derivation of AMU metrics and indicators).

2.4.3. AMU Surveillance Framework

As previously described, some sectors were interested in conducting AMU surveillance independent of CIPARS Farm AMU or CIPARS VASR components. Data collected by the industry could thus complement national/published information for the comprehensive assessment of the impact of AMU stewardship actions. These data could also be linked to economic or production variables or indicators not collected through either CIPARS or the VASR system:

- Frequency: An annual frequency of data collection was perceived as being sufficient for tracking AMU over time by the participants in most cases.
- Number of farms: depending on the surveillance objectives and capacity/resources, the sampling frame could be a census of farms across Canada, regional census (e.g., all farms in a given area), random sample (i.e., targets a certain percentage of farms across the area of interest), stratified sample, convenience/voluntary sample, those with electronic records, and those over a certain farm size.
- Who collects the data: existing platforms (government such as CIPARS or other organizations), provincial government, veterinary associations, producer associations, and processor associations were identified as options. These parties have direct access to some data or have a role in the AMU distribution chain (Figure 1).
- Incentives: existing data collection is either voluntary (e.g., CIPARS Farm) or regulatory (e.g., VASR, DFO) in nature. In private sector/industry initiatives, these are industry requirements as part of their on-farm food safety program, but there are no other incentives provided to the producer.

Outputs	*Sales/ Distribution*	*Prescription/ dispensing*	*End-user*
A list of antimicrobial ingredients distributed, sold, purchased or used	Able to provide data	Able to provide data	Able to provide data
Quantitative estimates of non-human [1] *AMU by antimicrobial class*	Able to provide partial data	Ability is dependent on granularity	Able to provide data
Quantitative estimates of non-human AMU by antimicrobial ingredient	Able to provide partial data	Ability is dependent on granularity	Able to provide data
Temporal trends in quantitative estimates of non-human AMU	Able to provide data	Ability is dependent on granularity	Able to provide data
Spatial trends in quantitative estimates of non-human AMU	Able to provide data	Ability is dependent on granularity	Able to provide data
Complete antimicrobial prescribing/dispensing data: dose, frequency, duration and route of administration; identity of animal(s) treated	Unable to provide	Able to provide data	Able to provide data
Provide data by species, commodity/sector	Able to provide partial data	Able to provide data	Able to provide data
Number of animals exposed	Unable to provide	Ability is dependent on granularity	Able to provide data
Trends in quantitative estimates of non-human AMU by reasons for use [2]	Unable to provide	Ability is dependent on granularity	Able to provide data
Trends in quantitative estimates of non-human AMU by clinical impression of the disease [3]	Unable to provide	Ability is dependent on granularity	Able to provide data
Trends in quantitative estimates of extra-label (off-label) drug use for non-human AMU	Able to provide partial data	Ability is dependent on granularity	Able to provide data
Imported product information: Drug Identification Number, imported or compounded AMU	Able to provide data	Ability is dependent on granularity	Able to provide data
Accessed through the Emergency Drug Release by Health Canada	Able to provide data	Able to provide data	Able to provide data
Information on who directed the AMU: producer, feed mill, veterinarian, company	Unable to provide	Able to provide partial data	Able to provide data

Able to provide data [4] — *Ability is dependent on granularity* — *Able to provide partial data* — *Unable to provide*

Figure 2. Antimicrobial use outputs from existing or future data collection points in the antimicrobial supply distribution pathway (figure modified from Reference [14]). [1] Nonhuman antimicrobial use in the table pertains only to animals. [2] Veterinary medical use such as disease treatment, control/metaphylaxis, prevention/prophylaxis, and additionally growth promotion. [3] Clinical impression by the veterinarian with input from producers and postmortem findings with or without laboratory diagnoses. [4] Ability to provide data (green circles) may be different for data collected in certain situations (i.e., confidential business information). AMU—antimicrobial use.

Table 1. Core elements of minimum dataset for antimicrobial use surveillance and considerations for inclusion.

Core Data Elements	Examples of Data That Would Fulfil the Element	Considerations for Surveillance Communication and Reporting
Antimicrobial active ingredient	On-farm treatment records (e.g., flock sheets), Farm purchases, Feed sales, Veterinarian's medical records/prescriptions, Veterinarian's dispensing record, Veterinary purchases, Manufacturer sales	Available in a number of formats, including the product or trade name, or the antimicrobial active ingredient itself. These data can then be easily converted to amount of active ingredient using a glossary of products that provides the concentration of active ingredient (and Anatomical Taxonomic Index codes for veterinary antimicrobials (ATCvet code)). This glossary should be linked to current references (i.e., to be used as a common reference across surveillance programs): Compendium of Medicating Ingredients Brochures [21] and the Drug Products Database [22]; Pharmaceutical products (with DIN) and compounded products (without DIN) as reported in the VASR system; Compendium of Veterinary Products [23]. **Weight of antimicrobials** (i.e., numerator data in some indicator calculations): pertains to the total quantity of AMU across all routes of administration. This is important for analysis of trends and the basis for further quantification of AMU (dose-based indicators).
Biomass unit	On-farm records (e.g., flock sheets), Processor records, Census data (to geographic region), Expert consensus (e.g., proportion of total animals in each production level, multiplier values for biomass calculation (kg) [1])	Required for both numerator (animals treated) and denominator (total animals) estimates. Total population (including mortalities and number of animals introduced to the flock or herd) and weights are important to collect but can come from several different sources, including: • Live pre-slaughter weights; • Slaughter weights; • Actual average treatment weights. In certain sectors, the inclusion of multiple weight and age groups and relevant production class was viewed as useful additional information [2], examples: • Nursery pigs, grow–finisher pigs; • Veal calves, feedlot beef; • Broilers, broiler breeders, layers, layer breeders **Animal biomass** (i.e., denominator data in some indicator estimations composed of the exposed and unexposed groups): pertains to the total number of animals presumably exposed to antimicrobials multiplied by an appropriate multiplier value (kg weight). These data enable comparison of AMU over time and between species.
Reasons for use	Expert consensus (by proportion of total AMU) [3], On-farm records, Veterinary medical records	The ability to capture the main indications for medical AMU, such as for disease prevention/prophylaxis, disease control/metaphylaxis and disease treatment, or growth promotion, was viewed as necessary. More specific reason for using data (e.g., respiratory vs. gastrointestinal vs. other disease treatment) was also desirable but not considered a core necessity. This is additional information for contextualizing AMU and AMR data and the impact of regulatory changes in AMU.
Geographical location	On-farm records, Veterinary records, Processor records, Hatchery delivery receipts	Collecting the province or the region where the animals are raised or antimicrobials sold (for the VASR system) is important to enable geographical comparisons of use.

Table 1. *Cont.*

Core Data Elements	Examples of Data That Would Fulfil the Element	Considerations for Surveillance Communication and Reporting
Time component	Multiple years, Yearly, Monthly, Weekly, Daily, Real-time, Production cycle/s (specify)	Required to compare trends over time and gauge changes in AMU following interventions. There are various time elements that need to be captured for more advanced quantification and analysis [24–27]: • When (age of the animals) animals were likely exposed; • Duration of treatment for each antimicrobial administered (i.e., if available, for one full water treatment course, medicated ration, or total days exposed to all antimicrobials); • Total days at risk (i.e., which is equivalent to the duration of the growing cycle, needed in some AMU indicators such as TI_{1000} or TI_{100} [4]); • Data coverage (e.g., one growing cycle or annually).

[1] Estimates from producers (and producer/farmer associations or marketing boards), researchers, and veterinarians. [2] Studies for identifying the production phase with highest use of antimicrobials, which may be linked to diseases prevalent during that stage. [3] Expert opinion from species-specific veterinarians (derived from their veterinary prescription and animal health records). [4] TI_{1000} or TI_{100}—Treatment Incidence 1000 or 100 (CIPARS used the term) is number of defined daily doses in animals using Canadian standards per 1000 or 100 animal days at risk.

2.5. Application of MDS-AMU-Surv in Analysis and Reporting of Data

As shown in Figure 3, the MSD-AMU-surv core data elements enable the derivation of metrics for the reporting of some commonly used AMU indicators, including those that are count-based, weight-based, and dose-based, which have already been used in existing AMU surveillance systems in Canada [9] and elsewhere [24–29]. Figure 4 shows an example where complementary AMU surveillance components such as the CIPARS VASR and CIPARS Farm AMU Surveillance and other systems utilize the MDS-AMU-surv data elements for informing national AMU stewardship and a more complete picture of the status of AMU in the animal sector in Canada. In any surveillance program, data could be described using a nationally defined categorization system such as Health Canada's Veterinary Drugs Directorate categorization of antimicrobials based on their importance to human medicine [30]. Surveillance data should enable the reporting of AMU aggregated at a national or regional/provincial level. Where possible, reporting by stages of production facilitates the identification of stages deemed to be high users of antimicrobials, and thus opportunities for intervention. The ability to report by primary or main indications for use and disease groups or specific diseases provides value to the collected data. It was recognized that capturing this information for quantitative AMU may be challenging because there are multiple uses for each antimicrobial. In this case, expert opinion may be obtained from participating veterinarians on the most likely reason for AMU. There were suggestions that animal health data such as mortality and occurrences of diseases should be collected to provide context to temporal trends; for example, spikes in total AMU or certain antimicrobials observed during a particular surveillance year may be due to a disease outbreak or emergence.

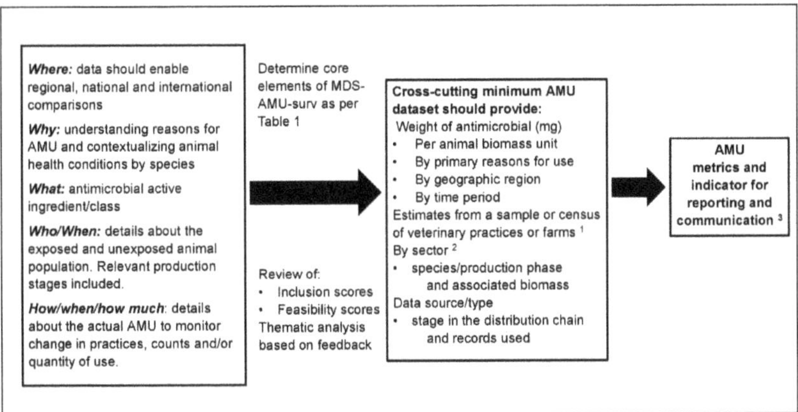

Figure 3. Summary of the considerations for the development of minimum dataset for antimicrobial use surveillance (MDS-AMU-surv), core data elements, outputs, and application. AMU—antimicrobial use. [1] CIPARS program collects information from sentinel farms (pigs, broiler chickens, turkeys, feedlot beef, dairy, and layers). [2] Animal biomass information required for AMU indicator estimations. [3] AMUmetrics and indicators collected are based on the organization/sector's AMU surveillance or study objectives and the stage of the development of the AMU surveillance program (i.e., during the early implementation stages, core elements may be incomplete). In aquaculture (data accessed by CIPARS under open data policy), Aquaculture Activities Regulations (under the Fisheries Act) require all operators/farms to report deposited antimicrobials (i.e., the quantity of antimicrobials prescribed and dispensed for use in aquaculture).

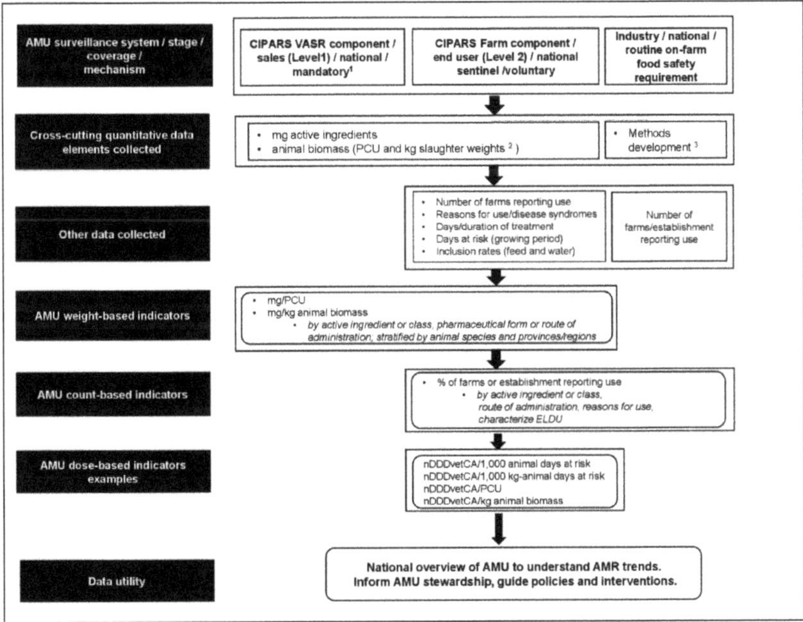

Figure 4. Application of the MDS-AMU-surv in Canadian animal sector. [1] In addition to VASR, CIPARS access open data collected by Fisheries and Oceans Canada under the Aquaculture Activities Regulations of the Fisheries Act. [2] Aquaculture data are not yet reported by biomass unit (i.e., using

the AMU indicators routinely used by CIPARS for AMU reporting in terrestrial animals), but exploration of methodological options for data analysis and future reporting are underway [31]. [3] At the time of writing, the industry (i.e., poultry sector) utilizes count-based indicators to communicate results within their producer networks; as mentioned above, methodology for quantitative AMU indicator analysis and reporting are underway. AMU—antimicrobial use. ELDU—extra-label (off-label) drug use. nDDDvetCA—number of defined daily doses in animals using Canadian standards. PCU—population correction unit. VASR—Veterinary Antimicrobial Sales Reporting system; the data collection platform for national sales data. Levels 1 and 2 pertain to the stage of data collection indicated in Figure 1.

3. Discussion

The development of the MDS-AMU-surv in the Canadian food animal sector demonstrates that different sectors can work together under a voluntary platform. Multisectoral collaboration such as this is useful in addressing components of the Pan-Canadian Framework for action on AMU/AMR in the absence of a formal multisectoral One Health governance mechanism [32]. The authors acknowledge that the working group discussions on MDS-AMU-surv predate the regulatory shifts in AMU; this paper is reflective of the changes including the mandatory reporting requirements to the manufacturers, importers, and compounders, refinements in CIPARS surveillance methodology, and reporting (i.e., metrics and indicators), additional AMU data now provided by the aquaculture industry, and emerging initiatives. AMU monitoring and surveillance programs, whether these are government or industrial sector initiatives [24], are essential components of integrated AMU/AMR surveillance systems [33] and can contribute to national AMU/AMR data reporting and communication [24,34]. For example, food animal sectors in the United Kingdom provide data to the UK Veterinary Antimicrobial Resistance and Sales Surveillance Report [35], the Netherlands Veterinary Medicines Institute [36] program provides data to Monitoring of Antimicrobial Resistance and Antibiotic Usage in Animals in the Netherlands (MARAN) [37], and VetStat is the source of AMU data for the DANMAP of the Danish Programme for the surveillance of antimicrobial consumption and resistance [38]. Competent authorities provide oversight and coordination of AMU/AMR surveillance activities and are also responsible for reporting and communicating the data [24,34]. In various European countries, the livestock industry and other private sector organizations have developed their own AMU monitoring programs, which align with national AMU stewardship goals [24,34]. In addition to monitoring, these programs have set AMU reduction targets and provided benchmarking to promote behaviour change in AMU practices [19,36]. While there is no global consensus on which AMU indicator to use for reporting and for fulfilling various AMU surveillance objectives, existing measurements developed at the national level are used. For example, in Thailand, a set antimicrobial consumption reduction target in animals was based on $mg/PCU_{Thailand}$ [39], and in the Netherlands, a reduction in AMU is measured using species-specific DDDA/animal-year [36].

Membership in CAHSS is voluntary and provides a forum for stakeholder engagement to address specific topic areas in animal health. The AMU/AMR working group membership includes the government, industry, academia, and other interested parties. Representation from various food animal sector is vital in addressing the shared AMR threat in the human–animal–environment interface [13]. In this circumstance, the federal government's participation (Public Health Agency of Canada, Canadian Food Inspection Agency, Agriculture and Agrifood Canada, and Health Canada) provided the expertise regarding AMU surveillance program development, and in return, the government benefited from the information generated to inform policy and action. Industry representation provided practical considerations necessary for a sustainable AMU surveillance framework design. Those from academic institutions could use surveillance initiatives as platforms for research, while veterinary clinics or organizations could apply AMU monitoring principles in their own practice. The MDS-AMU-surv development was specific to AMU surveillance, but it could be used as a model for addressing other components of the global and national

AMR action plans directed at the animal sector or larger stakeholder groups for addressing shared threats in the human–animal–environment interface. Examples of themes that could be discussed by the CAHSS AMU/AMR working group are infection prevention and control (biosecurity, animal health, and transition from AMU-dependent production systems to reduced AMU production systems) and AMU/AMR communication and advocacy. At the time of writing, the CAHSS AMU/AMR working group is exploring the utility of the MDS-AMU-surv for the development of AMU metrics and indicators. Collecting the relevant input parameters through MDS-AMU-surv is essential for describing the AMU information collected and possibly for the alignment of analysis, reporting, and communication with existing AMU surveillance systems.

Detailed data are required for characterizing AMU. The data collected through CIPARS-VASR provide information on total quantity sold for use in all animal species (with total quantities for eleven different animal species groups and aquatic animals) and the diversity and proportion of antimicrobial classes used. This system enables the detection of overall trends in sales and could be used to assess the impacts of regulatory or other changes on AMU at the national or provincial levels. The CIPARS Farm AMU data provide more detailed and specific information regarding AMU in the major food animal species and contextualize sales data such as species-specific AMU and classes used by sector and by disease type. The DFO data provide information on the annual deposit of drugs and pesticides; under the current regulations, each operator is required to report on a yearly basis the amount of drugs deposited, the dates, and the reason for use [12,20]. Farm-level surveillance thus captures other aspects of AMU that are potentially important to the understanding of AMR (e.g., average dose, length of exposure, and production stage). In this regard, the vast majority of countries in Europe also have active AMU monitoring independent of an existing national AMU surveillance program to fulfil other AMU objectives such as benchmarking or targeting AMU quantity reductions within the animal sector (or specific commodity) [24,25].

Recently, in an effort to enhance stewardship of AMU in Canada, additional new AMU monitoring programs have been developed that are independent from the long-standing CIPARS Farm surveillance and the newer CIPARS VASR component. Through a multisectoral collaboration, the province of Québec is developing an AMU surveillance program with the aim of collecting data across the major food animal species raised in the province [40]. The Canadian Veterinary Medical Association is also supporting a veterinary practice AMU data collection system as part of the Stewardship of Antimicrobials by the Veterinarians Initiative (SAVI) [41]. Veterinary prescribing and dispensing data are currently unavailable, which are identified as Level 2 in the Canadian AMU distribution chain (Figure 1). The SAVI pilot project aims to address this AMU data gap. It was recognized that VCPR are complex in some sectors (interactions between multiple actors/players) and that the data may lack the granularity required for understanding the major factors affecting AMU. Methods for data collection at this level should consider potential double reporting (i.e., multiple veterinarians providing oversight to the same establishment or company) when the aim is to quantify AMU, and to contextualize it to the appropriate biomass. Additionally, in recent years, various poultry sectors in Canada have also developed their own AMU data collection as part of their on-farm food safety program and to monitor the progress of their AMU stewardship actions [42,43]. At the industry level, existing platforms in Canada, such as the flock sheets reporting or farm flock health records as part of the poultry on-farm food safety program, are now utilized to collect AMU data. Although the data collected may not be as comprehensive as the CIPARS Farm AMU Surveillance, this generates information (e.g., frequency of use) complementary to the CIPARS Farm AMU Surveillance program. At the time of writing, the methodology for the quantification of the AMU collected is under development. Thus, industry led programs could progressively be built upon to generate quantitative data (i.e., possibly larger coverage such as census vs. sample of farms) enabling much better comparability with existing national or global surveillance programs.

The MDS-AMU-surv proposed in this paper is expected to be sufficient to generate basic AMU metrics and indicators in any livestock sector. CIPARS has advanced its farm-level analysis by developing the defined daily dose in animals using Canadian standards (DDDvetCA) [10,44]. Dose-based indicators were applied to the CIPARS Farm AMU Surveillance data for characterizing AMU trends between species and investigated for their utility for studying AMU–AMR linkages [45]. Additionally, the dose-based indicators were used for monitoring the impact of the changes in voluntary and regulatory AMU practices (i.e., from disease prevention to disease treatment or disease control, progressive elimination of certain classes of antimicrobials) [45,46]. Other sectors intending to develop their capacity for AMU surveillance could progressively improve their data collection and analytic capacity to enable the reporting of indicators relevant to their sector. While there may be different AMU metrics and indicators preferred to inform AMU stewardship in the different sectors, the collection of the MDS-AMU-surv will meet the needs of the government and industry (inform policy, risk assessment, and monitoring of the impact of AMR interventions on the animal–environment–human interface). The MDS-AMU-surv could be progressively improved over time to align with global reporting requirements and the future harmonization of integrated surveillance methods.

4. Materials and Methods

4.1. The CAHSS Working Group

A multistakeholder workshop was held in Ottawa between October 16 and 19, 2016 to gain a better understanding of producer and animal industry needs for AMU surveillance and to define areas where producers and producer associations would find value in collaborating on AMU surveillance. Participants consisted of primarily industry associations, veterinary groups, and government agencies engaged in AMU surveillance in food animals. Following this initial meeting, core CAHSS members (i.e., from the Public Health Agency of Canada, Canadian Food Inspection Agency, Agriculture and Agrifood Canada, and Health) brought together representatives from the government (expertise in public health, veterinary medicine, surveillance, epidemiology, and inspection systems), academia, various livestock animal sectors/marketing boards, and allied industry representatives (e.g., feed mills and pharmaceutical industries) and veterinary associations that had interest in AMU/AMR surveillance, research, and policy development. These representatives ultimately formed the CAHSS AMU/AMR working group. The working group convened in meetings between January 2017 and December 2018 to discuss the development of the minimum AMU dataset. An average of 25 (ranging from 21 to 35) representatives from 24 organizations participated in the quarterly meetings.

4.2. Review of Existing AMU Surveillance Infrastructures and the Antimicrobial Supply Distribution Pathway

In 2017, the government of Canada published the Pan-Canadian Framework for Action on AMU/AMR [5], which aligns with the Global Action Plan on AMR [1]. The MDS-AMU-surv dataset development contributes to the enhancement of the surveillance and stewardship components of the Pan-Canadian Framework. In this regard, several parties, including private sectors, were interested in documenting AMU practices in their sector. The CAHSS AMU/AMR working group recognized the need for a cohesive method for AMU data collection. A report titled "*Non-human antimicrobial use surveillance in Canada: Surveillance Objectives and Options*" was prepared by a Committee under the Council of Chief Veterinary Officers in Canada, which focused on AMU in food-producing animals [14]. Part of this report reviewed earlier versions of Canadian (i.e., CIPARS) and international (e.g., Denmark [38], the Netherlands [37], Sweden [47], and UK VARSS [35]) AMU/AMR surveillance programs and assessed various options in a Canadian context, including potential challenges for data collection (e.g., regulatory vs. voluntary mechanisms for AMU reporting or data collection; availability of resources and industry uptake/interests).

4.3. Survey of CAHSS AMU/AMR WG to Understand the AMU Data Needs

A survey was sent to the working group to better understand the objectives of participating organizations regarding AMU surveillance, desired outputs, and the feasibility of collecting specific data elements. The survey comprised 11 sections (Supplementary Materials I). Responses were collated in Microsoft Excel (Professional Plus 2016), and scores were summarized based on:

- Data inclusion scores: 0—not required, 1—nice to have, and 2—must be included.
- Data collection feasibility scores: 0—not feasible, 1—could start collecting with significant effort, 2—could start collecting with minimal effort, and 3—currently being collected by your organization.

An informal thematic analysis was conducted based on the participating organization's response to the survey when asked about the specific AMU surveillance objectives and the intended utility of the data collected.

4.4. Development of the MDS-AMU-Surv

The intent of the MDS-AMU-surv development was not to create an exhaustive list of variables to be used as a standard by each of the sectors with an interest in collecting AMU data. Instead, the primary consideration was to identify core data elements that could be collected in a number of different ways according to their capacity and capabilities within each commodity/sector and would provide information necessary for development of policies or intervention. Ultimately, the metrics and indicators generated would potentially align with existing national (e.g., CIPARS) and international AMU surveillance programs, for example, the OIE and the European Surveillance for Veterinary Antimicrobial Consumption [28,29], with which industries' or any interested parties' AMU data could be compared.

The list of variables suggested were intended for generating quantitative AMU measurements but could also generate qualitative (count-based) AMU measurements. Obtaining the contextualizing animal demographic data enables the estimation of the most commonly used AMU metrics (e.g., mg/kg animal biomass or mg/population correction unit (PCU)) that could potentially evolve into more advanced measurements (e.g., dose-based indicators) or other relevant indicators for describing AMU.

In aquatic animals, the reporting platform was examined. The owners/licensed operator under the AAR of the Fisheries Act reports antimicrobials deposited to the DFO annually (i.e., prescribed and dispensed for use in aquaculture animals). The reporting platform (Microsoft Excel, Professional Plus 2016) comprises variables largely similar to the MDS-AMU-surv, but animal biomass data have not yet been collected. A link to the current template can be found in Appendix A. At the time of writing, this template is being updated to reflect the changes in the Aquaculture Activities Regulation.

5. Conclusions

The development of the MDS-AMU-surv in the Canadian food animal sector demonstrates that different sectors can work together under a voluntary platform and a collaborative, consensus-building process could be used in future activities related to the Pan-Canadian Framework for Action on AMR.

Supplementary Materials: The following supporting information can be downloaded at: https://www.mdpi.com/article/10.3390/antibiotics11020226/s1, Table S1: Affiliations of the working group involved in the development of the minimum dataset for antimicrobial use surveillance (MDS-AMU-surv) between 2016 and 2017, Table S2: Questionnaire, Inclusion and Feasibility Score.

Author Contributions: Conceptualization: D.F.L. and M.E.C.A.; coordination, recording, and chairing of working group meetings: D.F.L., C.J., F.D.B., T.B. and M.E.C.A.; questionnaire design, survey methodology, and implementation: D.F.L. and M.E.C.A.; formal analysis of survey results, D.F.L. and M.E.C.A.; resources, C.J., T.B. and F.D.B.; writing—original draft preparation, A.A., D.F.L. and A.E.D.; writing—review and editing: D.F.L., M.E.C.A., F.D.B., T.B., C.A.C., A.E.D., S.P.G., X.-Z.L., M.O. and A.A.; project administration: C.J., F.D.B. and T.B.; funding acquisition: C.J., F.D.B. and T.B. All authors have read and agreed to the published version of the manuscript.

Funding: There was no funding received to develop the MDS-AMU-surv. The initial coordination meeting held in Ottawa, Ontario on 16–19 October 2016 was funded by the CFIA, AAFC, and Animal Health Canada, formerly theNational Farmed Animal Health and Welfare Council through the Canadian Animal Health Surveillance System.

Institutional Review Board Statement: Not applicable.

Informed Consent Statement: Not applicable.

Data Availability Statement: Not applicable.

Acknowledgments: The authors acknowledge the representatives from the participating government/associations/organizations in the working group for providing input to the development of the MDS-AMU-surv and for responding to the questionnaires.

Conflicts of Interest: The authors declare no conflict of interest.

Appendix A

Table A1. Template (current at the time of writing of this manuscript) for reporting of pest control products by aquaculture owners and operators to Fisheries and Oceans Canada. The template to be used can also be accessed here: https://view.officeapps.live.com/op/view.aspx?src=https%3A%2F%2Fwww.dfo-mpo.gc.ca%2Faquaculture%2Fmanagement-gestion%2Fdoc%2Fpesticide-deposit-eng.xlsx&wdOrigin=BROWSELINK.

Acronyms or Descriptions:	
AMU	antimicrobial use
AMR	antimicrobial resistance
API	active pharmaceutical ingredient
CAHI	Canadian Animal Health Institute
CAHSS	Canadian Animal Health Surveillance System
CIPARS	Canadian Integrated Program for Antimicrobial Resistance Surveillance: CIPARS VASR component/data from Level 1 in the AMU distribution chain—pertains to the CIPARS surveillance component, which conducts the data analysis and reporting for the antimicrobial sales data collected. CIPARS Farm component/data from Level 3 in the AMU distribution chain (end user)—also known as CIPARS Farm AMU/AMR surveillance program or CIPARS Farm program and pertains to the farm component of CIPARS, which coordinates the voluntary data and sample collection from a network of sentinel veterinary practices and their producers across Canada.
DDDvetCA and nDDDvetCA	defined daily doses in animals using Canadian standards and number of defined daily doses in animals using Canadian standards (milligrams of antimicrobials adjusted by the species-specific DDDvetCA standard for each antimicrobial active ingredient).
MDS-AMU-surv	minimum dataset for antimicrobial use surveillance.
PCU	population correction unit
SAVI	Stewardship of Antimicrobials by Veterinarians Initiative
TI_{100} or TI_{1000}	Treatment Incidence 100 or 1000; CIPARS reports the TI_{1000} antimicrobial use indicator as nDDDvetCA/1000 animal days at risk.

Table A1. *Cont.*

Acronyms or Descriptions:	
VASR	Veterinary Antimicrobial Sales Reporting; the data collection platform for the reporting of sales data (Level 1 of the AMU distribution chain).
VCPR	veterinarian–client–patient relationship

References

1. WHO. Global Action Plan on Antimicrobial Resistance. Available online: https://www.who.int/publications/i/item/9789241509763 (accessed on 18 November 2021).
2. FAO. The FAO Action Plan on Antimicrobial Resistance 2021–2025. Available online: https://www.fao.org/documents/card/en/c/cb5545en (accessed on 19 November 2021).
3. FAO. The FAO Action Plan on Antimicrobial Resistance, 2016–2020. Available online: http://www.fao.org/antimicrobial-resistance/en/ (accessed on 2 July 2018).
4. OIE. The OIE Strategy on Antimicrobial Resistance and the Prudent Use of Antimicrobials. Available online: http://www.oie.int/fileadmin/Home/eng/Media_Center/docs/pdf/PortailAMR/EN_OIE-AMRstrategy.pdf (accessed on 23 September 2018).
5. Government of Canada. Tackling Antimicrobial Resistance and Antimicrobial Use: A Pan-Canadian Framework for Action. Available online: https://www.canada.ca/en/health-canada/services/publications/drugs-health-products/tackling-antimicrobial-resistance-use-pan-canadian-framework-action.html (accessed on 28 September 2018).
6. Government of Canada. Veterinary Antimicrobial Sales Reporting. Available online: https://www.canada.ca/en/public-health/services/antibiotic-antimicrobial-resistance/animals/veterinary-antimicrobial-sales-reporting.html (accessed on 18 November 2021).
7. Government of Canada. List A: List of Certain Antimicrobial Active Pharmaceutical Ingredients. 2020. Available online: https://www.canada.ca/en/public-health/services/antibiotic-antimicrobial-resistance/animals/veterinary-antimicrobial-sales-reporting/list-a.html (accessed on 19 December 2021).
8. Government of Canada. Government of Canada Food and Drugs Act. Regulations Amending the Food and Drug Regulations (Veterinary Drugs—Antimicrobial Resistance). 2017; Volume 151, No. 10. Available online: http://www.gazette.gc.ca/rp-pr/p2/2017/2017-05-17/html/sor-dors76-eng.php (accessed on 25 May 2017).
9. Government of Canada. Canadian Integrated Program for Antimicrobial Resistance Surveillance (CIPARS) 2018: Integrated Findings. Available online: https://www.canada.ca/en/public-health/services/surveillance/canadian-integrated-program-antimicrobial-resistance-surveillance-cipars/cipars-reports/2018-annual-report-integrated-findings.html (accessed on 16 February 2021).
10. Government of Canada. Canadian Integrated Program for Antimicrobial Resistance Surveillance (CIPARS) 2018: Design and Methods. Available online: https://www.canada.ca/en/public-health/services/surveillance/canadian-integrated-program-antimicrobial-resistance-surveillance-cipars/cipars-reports/2018-annual-report-design-methods.html (accessed on 21 December 2021).
11. Government of Canada. Canadian Integrated Program for Antimicrobial Resistance Surveillance. 2016 Annual Report. Available online: http://publications.gc.ca/collections/collection_2018/aspc-phac/HP2-4-2016-eng.pdf (accessed on 16 July 2019).
12. Government of Canada. Aquaculture Activities Regulations. Available online: https://www.dfo-mpo.gc.ca/aquaculture/management-gestion/aar-raa-eng.htm (accessed on 11 December 2021).
13. FAO; OIE; WHO. Tripartite Zoonoses Guide. Available online: https://www.who.int/initiatives/tripartite-zoonosis-guide (accessed on 2 March 2021).
14. CAHSS. Non-Human Antimicrobial Use Surveillance in Canada: Surveillance Objectives and Options. Available online: https://cahss.ca/cahss-tools/document-library/Non-human-antimicrobial-use-surveillance-in-Canada-Surveillance-Objectives-and-Options? (accessed on 18 November 2021).
15. Government of Canada. Oversight on the Quality of Active Pharmaceutical Ingredients for Veterinary Use in Canada. Available online: https://www.canada.ca/en/public-health/services/antibiotic-antimicrobial-resistance/animals/oversight-quality-active-pharmaceutical-ingredients-veterinary-use.html (accessed on 18 November 2021).
16. CAHI. About the Canadian Animal Health Institute. Available online: https://www.cahi-icsa.ca/about-us (accessed on 18 November 2021).
17. Impact Vet. Available online: www.impactvet.com (accessed on 6 January 2022).
18. Government of Canada. Canadian Network for Public Health Intelligence (CNPHI). Available online: https://science.gc.ca/eic/site/063.nsf/eng/98243.html (accessed on 18 November 2021).
19. FAO; The Ministry of Environment and Food, Denmark. Tackling Antimicrobial Use and Resistance in Pig Production Lessons Learned in Denmark. Available online: http://www.fao.org/antimicrobial-resistance/resources/publications-archive/case-studies-series-denmark/en/ (accessed on 16 February 2021).
20. Government of Canada. National Aquaculture Public Reporting Data. Available online: https://open.canada.ca/data/en/dataset/288b6dc4-16dc-43cc-80a4-2a45b1f93383 (accessed on 22 November 2021).
21. Government of Canada. Compendium of Medicating Ingredient Brochure. Available online: https://inspection.canada.ca/animal-health/livestock-feeds/medicating-ingredients/eng/1300212600464/1320602461227 (accessed on 6 January 2022).

22. Government of Canada. The Drug Product Database Online Query. Available online: https://health-products.canada.ca/dpd-bdpp/index-eng.jsp (accessed on 3 January 2022).
23. Animalytix, LLC. Compendium of Veterinary Products, Canada Edition. Available online: https://bam.cvpservice.com/ (accessed on 1 June 2021).
24. Sanders, P.; Vanderhaeghen, W.; Fertner, M.; Fuchs, F.; Obritzhauser, W.; Agunos, A.; Carson, C.; Høg, B.B.; Andersen, V.D.; Chauvin, C.; et al. Monitoring of farm-level antimicrobial use to guide stewardship: Overview of existing systems and analysis of key components and processes. *Front. Vet. Sci.* **2020**, *7*, 540. [CrossRef] [PubMed]
25. AACTING. AACTING Network on Quantification, Benchmarking and Reporting of Veterinary Antimicrobial Usage (AMU) at Farm Level. *Monitoring Systems.* Available online: https://aacting.org/monitoring-systems/ (accessed on 2 June 2018).
26. Collineau, L.; Belloc, C.; Stark, K.D.; Hemonic, A.; Postma, M.; Dewulf, J.; Chauvin, C. Guidance on the selection of appropriate indicators for quantification of antimicrobial usage in humans and animals. *Zoonoses Public Health* **2016**, *64*, 165–184. [CrossRef] [PubMed]
27. Agunos, A.; Gow, S.P.; Deckert, A.E.; Kuiper, G.; Leger, D.F. Informing stewardship measures in Canadian food animal species through integrated reporting of antimicrobial use and antimicrobial resistance surveillance data-part I, methodology development. *Pathogens* **2021**, *10*, 1492. [CrossRef] [PubMed]
28. OIE. Fifth OIE Annual Report on Antimicrobial Agents Intended for Use in Animals. Available online: https://www.oie.int/en/document/fifth-oie-annual-report-on-antimicrobial-agents-intended-for-use-in-animals/ (accessed on 1 June 2021).
29. European Medicines Agency. Sales of Veterinary Antimicrobial Agents in 31 European Countries in 2018. Trends from 2010 to 2018. Tenth ESVAC Report. Available online: https://www.ema.europa.eu/en/veterinary-regulatory/overview/antimicrobial-resistance/european-surveillance-veterinary-antimicrobial-consumption-esvac (accessed on 1 June 2021).
30. Government of Canada. Categorization of Antimicrobial Drugs Based on Importance in Human Medicine. Available online: https://www.canada.ca/en/health-canada/services/drugs-health-products/veterinary-drugs/antimicrobial-resistance/categorization-antimicrobial-drugs-based-importance-human-medicine.html (accessed on 22 November 2021).
31. Narbonne, J.A.; Radke, B.R.; Price, D.; Hanington, P.C.; Babujee, A.; Otto, S.J.G. Antimicrobial use surveillance indicators for finfish aquaculture production: A Review. *Front. Vet. Sci.* **2021**, *8*, 595152. [CrossRef] [PubMed]
32. AMR Network. Available online: https://www.amrnetwork.ca/ (accessed on 22 November 2021).
33. WHO. Integrated Surveillance of Antimicrobial Resistance in Foodborne Bacteria. Application of a One Health Approach. Guidance from the WHO Advisory Group on Integrated Surveillance of Antimicrobial Resistance (AGISAR) In collaboration with Food and Agriculture Organization of the United Nations (FAO), and World Organisation. Available online: https://apps.who.int/iris/bitstream/handle/10665/255747/9789241512411-eng.pdf;jsessionid=C959E32A695A75232D9436A80F69A9D9?sequence=1 (accessed on 3 June 2019).
34. AACTING. Guidelines for Collection, Analysis and Reporting of Farm-Level Antimicrobial Use, in the Scope of Antimicrobial stewardship. Available online: https://aacting.org/aacting-guidelines/ (accessed on 7 January 2022).
35. United Kingdom Veterinary Medicines Directorate. UK-VARSS Veterinary Antimicrobial Resistance and Sales Surveillance 2020. Available online: https://www.gov.uk/government/publications/veterinary-antimicrobial-resistance-and-sales-surveillance-2020 (accessed on 18 November 2021).
36. SDA. General Information about The Netherlands Veterinary Medicines Institute (SDa). Available online: https://www.autoriteitdiergeneesmiddelen.nl/en/about-sda/general (accessed on 16 February 2021).
37. MARAN. MARAN 2019 Monitoring of Antimicrobial Resistance and Antibiotic Usage in Animals in The Netherlands in 2018. Available online: https://rivm.openrepository.com/handle/10029/623134 (accessed on 4 August 2020).
38. DANMAP. DANMAP 2020 Use of Antimicrobial Agents and Occurrence of Antimicrobial Resistance in Bacteria from Food Animals, Food and Humans in Denmark. Available online: https://www.danmap.org/Reports/2020 (accessed on 19 December 2021).
39. Food and Drug Administration Thailand. Thailand's National Strategic Plan on Antimicrobial Resistance 2017–2021 (NSP-AMR)—Goals by the year 2021. Available online: https://amrthailand.net/English (accessed on 1 February 2022).
40. Québec Ministry of Agriculture, Fisheries and Food. Surveillance in Connection with the Use of Antibiotics. Available online: https://www.mapaq.gouv.qc.ca/fr/Productions/santeanimale/maladies/antibio/Pages/Surveillance.aspx (accessed on 19 December 2021).
41. Canadian Veterinary Medical Association. Stewardship of Antimicrobials by Veterinarians Initiative. Available online: https://savi.canadianveterinarians.net/en/about/ (accessed on 18 November 2021).
42. Chicken Farmers of Canada. AMU Strategy, a Prescription for Change. Available online: http://www.chickenfarmers.ca/wp-content/uploads/2018/01/AMU-Magazine_ENG_web-2.pdf (accessed on 7 February 2018).
43. Turkey Farmers of Canada. Guidelines for Antimicrobial Use in the Turkey Industry. Available online: https://www.amstewardship.ca/guidelines-for-antimicrobial-use-in-the-turkey-industry-published-by-the-turkey-farmers-of-canada/ (accessed on 13 April 2020).
44. Bosman, A.L.; Loest, D.; Carson, C.A.; Agunos, A.; Collineau, L.; Leger, D.F. Developing Canadian defined daily doses for animals: A metric to quantify antimicrobial use. *Front. Vet. Sci.* **2019**, *6*, 220. [CrossRef] [PubMed]
45. Agunos, A.; Gow, S.P.; Deckert, A.E.; Leger, D.F. Informing stewardship measures in Canadian food animal species through integrated reporting of antimicrobial use and antimicrobial resistance surveillance data-part II, application. *Pathogens* **2021**, *10*, 1491. [CrossRef] [PubMed]

46. Agunos, A.; Gow, S.P.; Leger, D.F.; Deckert, A.E.; Carson, C.A.; Bosman, A.L.; Kadykalo, S.; Reid-Smith, R.J. Antimicrobial use indices-the value of reporting antimicrobial use in multiple ways using data from Canadian broiler chicken and turkey farms. *Front. Vet. Sci.* **2020**, *7*, 567872. [CrossRef] [PubMed]
47. SWEDRES-SVARM 2019. Sales of Antibiotics and Occurrence of Antibiotic Resistance in Sweden. Available online: https://www.sva.se/en/our-topics/antibiotics/svarm-resistance-monitoring/swedres-svarm-reports/ (accessed on 5 August 2020).

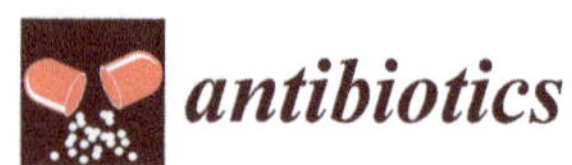 antibiotics

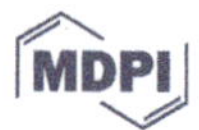

Article

Antibiotic Use in Alpine Dairy Farms and Its Relation to Biosecurity and Animal Welfare

Francesca Menegon, Katia Capello, Jacopo Tarakdjian, Dario Pasqualin, Giovanni Cunial, Sara Andreatta, Debora Dellamaria, Grazia Manca, Giovanni Farina and Guido Di Martino *

Istituto Zooprofilattico Sperimentale delle Venezie, Viale dell'Università 10, 35020 Legnaro, Italy; fmenegon@izsvenezie.it (F.M.); kcapello@izsvenezie.it (K.C.); jtarakdjian@izsvenezie.it (J.T.); dpasqualin@izsvenezie.it (D.P.); gcunial@izsvenezie.it (G.C.); sandreatta@izsvenezie.it (S.A.); ddellamaria@izsvenezie.it (D.D.); gmanca@izsvenezie.it (G.M.); gfarina@izsvenezie.it (G.F.)

* Correspondence: gdimartino@izsvenezie.it

Abstract: The quantification of antimicrobial usage (AMU) in food-producing animals can help identify AMU risk factors, thereby enhancing appropriate stewardship policies and strategies for a more rational use. AMU in a sample of 34 farms in the Province of Trento (north-eastern Italy) from 2018 to 2020 was expressed as defined daily doses for animals per population correction unit according to European Surveillance of Veterinary Antimicrobial Consumption guidelines (DDDvet) and according to Italian guidelines (DDDAit). A retrospective analysis was carried out to test the effects of several husbandry practices on AMU. Overall, the average AMU ranged between 6.5 DDDAit in 2018 and 5.2 DDDAit in 2020 (corresponding to 9 and 7 DDDvet, respectively), showing a significant trend of decrement (−21.3%). Usage of the highest priority critically important antimicrobials (HPCIA) was reduced by 83% from 2018 to 2020. Quarantine management, available space, water supply, animals' cleanliness and somatic cell count had no significant association with AMU. Rather, farms with straw-bedded cubicles had lower AMU levels than those with mattresses and concrete floors ($p < 0.05$). In conclusion, this study evidenced a decrement in AMU, particularly regarding HPCIA, but only a few risk factors due to farm management.

Keywords: AMU; antibiotics; dairy cattle; DDD; biosecurity; animal welfare

check for updates

Citation: Menegon, F.; Capello, K.; Tarakdjian, J.; Pasqualin, D.; Cunial, G.; Andreatta, S.; Dellamaria, D.; Manca, G.; Farina, G.; Di Martino, G. Antibiotic Use in Alpine Dairy Farms and Its Relation to Biosecurity and Animal Welfare. *Antibiotics* **2022**, *11*, 231. https://doi.org/10.3390/antibiotics11020231

Academic Editor: Diane Ashiru-Oredope

Received: 10 January 2022
Accepted: 8 February 2022
Published: 10 February 2022

Publisher's Note: MDPI stays neutral with regard to jurisdictional claims in published maps and institutional affiliations.

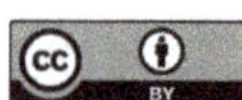

Copyright: © 2022 by the authors. Licensee MDPI, Basel, Switzerland. This article is an open access article distributed under the terms and conditions of the Creative Commons Attribution (CC BY) license (https://creativecommons.org/licenses/by/4.0/).

1. Introduction

The usage of antimicrobials (AMU) to treat large animal populations in intensive livestock production is necessary to avoid animals suffering from bacterial infections and, therefore, to guarantee animal health and welfare [1], but it comes with side effects. In fact, antimicrobial use in both humans and animals leads to antimicrobial resistance (AMR) [2–5].

AMR is a global threat for both human and animal health, as it might compromise the effectiveness of infections' treatment [4,6,7]. In particular, misuse, underdosing and overuse of antimicrobials are the strongest drivers for AMR [8,9]. Hence, action plans on AMR were developed both at a national and international level [9–11]. At the national level, the Italian Ministry of Health promoted a plan against AMR [12], calling for antimicrobial stewardship, with the ultimate goal of providing a coordinated and sustainable strategy to address AMR nationwide. For this purpose, possible benchmarks for farm categorization according to sanitary risk, animal welfare and antimicrobial consumption have been identified [13]. This approach is also endorsed by the EU Farm to Fork strategy [14], which supports a better welfare to improve animal health and food quality and also reduce the need for antimicrobials [15,16]. Within this framework, biosecurity includes all procedures to prevent pathogens from entering a farm and spreading within a farm [17,18]. An improved biosecurity level was proven to positively impact animal health and welfare [17] and to reduce AMU in pigs [19–21] and beef cattle [22]. For dairy cattle, various studies in the literature investigated AMU in cows and calves [23–26]. However, only limited information is available on possible associations between AMU, biosecurity and animal welfare. There are only a few studies available on AMU in the Italian dairy sector, and they do not cover the large variety of livestock systems [27,28]. Therefore, the present study aimed at quantifying AMU in a geographically defined dairy cattle population in Northern Italy (Trentino Alto Adige region) for three years (2018–2020), applying two different dose-based methods. AMU associations with several management factors of biosecurity and animal welfare were also investigated.

2. Results

The average amount of AMU in the inspected 34 dairy farms in 2018, 2019, 2020 was, respectively, 6.48, 6.58 and 5.18 DDDAit/PCU, with a significant decrease ($p < 0.001$) in 2020 compared to both 2018 (−20.1%) and 2019 (−21.3%). Regarding AMU using DDDvet/PCU, the observed average values were 9.03, 8.60, 6.94 for 2018, 2019 and 2020, respectively. Penicillins and first and second generation cephalosporins were the most frequently administered antimicrobial classes, accounting for 34.85% and 13.05% of the overall AMU (Table 1). Antimicrobials classified as highest priority critically important (HPCIA), ranged between 23.52% (in 2018) and 5.32% (in 2020) DDDAit of the total AMU (Table 1). The use of HPCIA was reduced by 83% from 2018 to 2020 (Table 1). HPCIA were more frequently administered via injectable products (Table 2).

Intramammary treatment was the most frequent administration route, representing 53.11% of the total AMU, followed by injectable (45.62%), intrauterine (1.18%) and oral administration routes (0.09%). A significantly lower mean value of DDDAit was observed for all years in lactation compared to dry-off (Table 2), representing, respectively, 37.71% and 62.28% of the intramammary products used.

Table 1. Percentages of defined daily doses for animals per population correction unit (DDDAit/PCU and DDDvet/PCU) administered in 2018–2020 in 34 Alpine dairy cattle farms: Antimicrobials have been grouped and classified according to WHO categorization: HPCIA: highest priority critically important antimicrobials; CIA: critically important antimicrobials; HIA: highly important antimicrobials; IA: important antimicrobials.

	DDDAit %			DDDvet %		
	2018	**2019**	**2020**	**2018**	**2019**	**2020**
HPCIA	23.52	11.03	5.32	27.50	13.26	6.05
Cephalosporins 3rd gen.	10.40	7.05	3.49	14.42	9.14	4.52
Cephalosporins 4th gen.	3.76	0.61	0.00	5.18	0.21	0.00
Fluoroquinolones	6.74	2.09	1.00	5.98	2.19	0.97
Macrolides	2.62	1.29	0.83	1.92	1.72	0.56
Polymyxins	0.00	0.00	0.00	0.01	0.00	0.00
CIA	45.41	47.12	47.55	42.15	46.27	49.91
Aminoglycosides	7.18	7.40	7.32	4.95	5.55	6.06
Ansamycin	5.34	3.55	4.50	6.72	5.38	5.47
Penicillins	32.90	36.16	35.72	30.49	35.35	38.38
HIA	25.01	35.72	36.69	26.55	36.64	37.50
Amphenicols	0.22	0.14	0.12	0.43	0.26	0.22
Cephalosporins 1st and 2nd gen.	11.26	15.81	11.91	14.39	17.65	14.81
Lincosamides	6.09	6.18	10.18	4.13	4.19	7.03
Sulphonamides	3.82	9.74	9.92	3.62	9.94	10.18
Tetracyclines	3.62	3.84	4.56	3.97	4.60	5.26
IA	6.17	6.14	10.44	3.79	3.82	6.54
Aminocyclitols	6.17	6.14	10.44	3.79	3.82	6.54

Table 2. Average Defined daily doses for animals per population correction unit (DDDAit/PCU) administered in 2018–2020 in 34 Alpine dairy cattle farms: Intramammary administered antimicrobials are divided into "dry-off" and "lactation" products, while injectable, intrauterine and oral products are grouped in "not intramammary product" (not IMM). The percentage of highest priority critically important antimicrobials (HPCIA) is also reported.

		2018		2019		2020				
Phase	**n.**	**Mean ± sd**	**% HPCIA**	**Mean ± sd**	**%HPCIA**	**Mean ± sd**	**% HPCIA**	**Year (Y)**	**Phase (P)**	**Y × F**
dry-off	34	2.21 ± 1.21	20.59%	2.45 ± 1.73	5.88%	1.51 ± 1.08	2.94%			
lactation	34	1.42 ± 1.11	35.29%	1.21 ± 0.96	14.71%	1.05 ± 0.80	5.88%	<0.001	<0.001	0.14
not IMM	34	3.10 ± 1.68	94.12%	2.91 ± 1.81	76.47%	2.74 ± 1.96	52.94%			

The analysis of management factors on AMU is shown in Table 3. Five farms performed blanket DCT (dry cow therapy) (3.36 ± 0.22 DDDAit), while 29 farms performed selective DCT using on average 1.44 ± 0.65 DDDAit during the dry-off period. Moreover, in the majority of the farms (i.e., 28 out of 34), microbiological tests for mastitis were routinely performed in symptomatic animals. The presence of a quarantine box, space availability, water quality, animals' cleanliness, presence of ventilation alarm and level of somatic cell count (SCC) did not exhibit any significant association with AMU. Instead, a lower DDDAit was found (p = 0.050) in straw/sawdust bedded cubicles compared to other materials (i.e., mattresses and concrete floor). Overall, the average biosecurity score recorded in farms was 65% (range 37–85%), while the animal welfare average score was 77% (range 63–88%); nonetheless, no significant correlation was found with AMU distribution. On the contrary, the quantity of daily milk produced (mean value 29.7 ± 5.44) was positively correlated with the DDDAit (Spearman's rho = 0.37, p = 0.027).

Table 3. Associations between defined daily doses per animal (DDDAit/PCU) and different management variables in 34 Alpine dairy cattle farms in 2020. Significance for $p < 0.05$.

	n	Mean ± sd	p Value
Quarantine box			
absent	13	5.87 ± 3.25	ns
present	21	4.95 ± 2.19	
Mortality			
<5%	27	5.42 ± 2.76	na
≥5%	7	4.85 ± 2.18	
Sickbay			
present	31	5.14 ± 2.70	na
absent	3	6.98 ± 0.85	
Space available (heifers)			
≥3.5 m^2/animal	20	5.35 ± 2.21	ns
<3.5 m^2/animal	14	5.23 ± 3.24	
Water supply			
≥1 drinker/10 animals	19	5.08 ± 2.06	ns
<1 drinker/10 animals	15	5.57 ± 3.28	
Cleanliness			
<20% of dirty animals	25	5.65 ± 2.72	ns
≥20% of dirty animals	9	4.32 ± 2.23	
Ventilation alarm			
Absent	19	5.43 ± 2.98	ns
present	15	5.13 ± 2.21	
Access to pasture			
No	7	4.62 ± 2.17	na
Yes	26	5.61 ± 2.72	

Table 3. *Cont.*

	n	Mean ± sd	*p* Value
DCT			
Blanket	5	7.85 ± 4.20	na
Selective	29	4.86 ± 2.07	
Somatic cell count			
>150,000 cells/mL	21	5.66 ± 2.84	ns
≤150,000 cells/mL	13	4.72 ± 2.26	
Cubicles material			
Other	10	6.92 ± 3.17	0.05
Straw/sawdust	23	4.74 ± 2.07	
Microbiological tests for mastitis			
Absent	3	4.04 ± 2.15	
Not on a routine basis	3	6.03 ± 0.61	na
For all problematic cows	28	5.36 ± 2.81	

sd: standard deviation; na: not applicable; ns: not significant; DCT: dry cow therapy.

3. Discussion

This study evaluated AMU retrospectively in a sample of holdings, mostly family-run, that we can assume are representative of Alpine dairy farming systems, characterized by small–medium size, usually with access to pasture and without a milking robot. As reported in the European Surveillance of Veterinary Antimicrobial Consumption (ESVAC) in the last decade, Italy was ranked high in Europe in terms of AMU [29]. Compared to other EU studies, this occurrence seems to be confirmed by the present data. For example, an English study [23] reported an average DDDvet of 4.60. However, comparison should be made with caution because these authors did not consider DCT. In terms of DDDAit, the dose-based values in the present study were lower than for DDDvet. DDDAit was defined for each active substance following the summary of Italian products' characteristics: this guaranteed a higher level of precision than DDDvet. Average DDDAit ranged yearly between 6.58 in 2019 and 5.18 in 2020, with a significant variability between farms (2.19–10.34). Considering a three-year timeframe can overcome outlier peak values due to exceptional circumstances and evidenced a significant decreasing trend. A previous Italian study [30] assessed AMU in dairy cattle farms using DDDAit in 2019 in north-western Italy (Lombardy region). These authors observed a similar AMU compared to the present study (4.8 DDDAit per cow/year). However, a different methodology calculation in intramammary products was applied. The number of doses was divided by the Population Correction Unit (PCU) (likewise injectable products) and not by the number of cows, as proposed by the Italian Ministry of Health for this route of administration [31]. The chosen approach can generate an apparently lower consumption estimation compared to the present study. In line with the massive decrease in sales of veterinary antibiotics in European Countries, highlighted in the 10th ESVAC report, the results of the present study show a reduction of 21.3% from 2019 to 2020. This decreasing trend had already been observed from 2007 to 2012 in the Netherlands, where dairy farms registered a −22% reduction of AMU [32]. Conversely, Mazza et al. did not observe a significant decrement in Lombardy. Furthermore, a more prudent AMU was observed during the study period in Alpine farms, with a dramatic reduction in HPCIA (−83%). They were eliminated in intramammary treatments in nearly all the farms. These data are encouraging, considering that in 2015 in Austria, a mean 1.14 DDDvet of HPCIA was used for lactating cows' treatments with intramammary products [33]. In US dairy farms in 2016–2017, 75% of intramammary antimicrobials contained HPCIAs such as ceftiofur and 7% contained cephapirin. These two active principles accounted for almost 82% of the total AMU [34]. The difference between farming system types can also play a major role. Indeed, it has been recently shown [35] that mountain farms with smaller herd sizes, which provide cows with access to pasture and limit concentrates in the diet, use less HPCIA than specialized dairy farms from lowlands. Moreover, it has been widely reported that higher productivity (notably higher milk yield) can be associated with a higher incidence of metabolic disorders, such as mastitis, lameness and other production diseases [36], requiring prompt veterinary intervention. Our results support this evidence, as we traced a positive correlation between milk production and AMU. In line with what is reported in the literature for dairy cattle [27,30,32,34], we found that intramammary medication is the most frequent administration route (53.11%). Previous studies observed a frequency reaching 63% [32] and 78% [34]. In particular, antimicrobial treatments were reported to be more frequent during the dry-off period than during lactation. Dry-off treatments are mainly administered to prevent mastitis in the following lactation [37] but in the present study blanket DCT was performed only in 5 out of 34 farms in 2020. Indeed, most farms (28/34) performed microbiological tests for mastitis in symptomatic animals.

However, no correlation between AMU and SCC was found in the present study. A previous study demonstrated that it is possible to reduce antibiotics in dry-off without increasing somatic cells count (SCC) in the following lactation by implementing management measures to maintain good udder health [38]. For example, some risk factors for *E. coli* mastitis at the herd level include the bedding material and the design of cubicles [39]. The number of cubicles was classified as acceptable in all inspected farms, according to Italian welfare guidelines [13] (ranged between 90–110% of the number of cows) thus this parameter was not an object of analysis. We grouped bedding materials that needed to be frequently replaced, such as straw, sawdust or both, and we compared them to other materials (including mattresses and concrete floor). Therefore, farms that used replaceable materials had lower AMU, which can be attributed to a higher hygiene level guaranteed by a regular replacement of new material. Moreover, in the past, straw also showed a lower incidence of leg injuries in the tarsal joints [40–42], in addition to promoting better animal welfare resulting from higher comfort [42,43] and the presence of manipulable material. On the other hand, other studies observed that sawdust increases the dirtiness of the hindquarters and udder [44] and, compared to straw, it increases the risk of hock skin alterations [45]. Considering these studies, straw can be assumed to be better than sawdust. However, this study does not consider that frequently dry cows are housed separately from lactating cows, and data do not distinguish eventual differences as bedding material between the two phases. Therefore, more detailed studies will be required, including the distinction between dry and lactation period and between straw, sawdust or the use of both of them. No significant correlation between AMU and biosecurity as well as animal welfare scores was observed in the present study. Additionally, no correlation between AMU, biosecurity and animal welfare was found in dairy cattle farms from Lombardy [27], which had similar scores (biosecurity range 21.41–71.56%, animal welfare range 45.32–81.69%). In the beef cattle sector, an improved level of welfare permitted lower usage of antimicrobials, but not a reduction in HPCIA [22]. On the contrary, in 61 Belgian pig farms, AMU was reduced by 52.0%, without impairing the herd production performances, by adopting a series of herd-level interventions concerning biosecurity, vaccination scheme, health care, welfare and zootechnical measures [46]. Similarly, a reduction of 47% of AMU was achieved in pig farms from Belgium, France, Germany and Sweden from birth to slaughter, and farms with bigger compliance achieved a more considerable reduction [19]. However, pig farming is characterized by a general higher AMU than dairy cows (e.g., 16 DDDvet/PCU in 2017 for Tarakdjian et al., 2020 [47]), and this evidence can explain why good management practices are more likely to produce a significant effect in the former than in the latter livestock sector.

4. Materials and Methods

4.1. Data Collection

Thirty-four free-stall farms of mixed-breed dairy cows (i.e., Holstein Friesian, Brown Swiss, Simmental cows) in the Province of Trento (north-eastern Italy) were randomly selected for this study. Farms were located in the area between Garda Lake (south), Stelvio Natural Park (west), Pale di San Martino Natural Park (east) and Bolzano (north), and the altitude ranged from 400 m to 1700 m. Median farm size was 89.5 animals and the mean was 140, representing a small–medium farm in the Italian dairy sector. In 26 of these farms, animals had access to pasture. Farms were visited in 2021; data were collected retrospectively from the farm registry from 2018 to 2020. The biosecurity score was calculated using the Classyfarm protocol, available in Ginestreti et al. [27], and considers 15 items to compute a final score. The final score ranges from 0% to 100%, where 100% is the highest level of biosecurity. Animal welfare was evaluated using Classyfarm protocol, as previously described in Ginestreti et al. [27] and Mazza et al. [30]. The score includes 70 items, 18 of which are animal-based measures (details available in Bertocchi et al. [48]). The final score ranges from 0 to 100%, where 100% corresponds to the maximum level of animal welfare. The most relevant biosecurity and welfare items were also analyzed separately as qualitative variables. These items were the following: average mortality rate (higher or lower than 5%), presence of ventilation alarm and replacement equipment, presence of sick animals' boxes, space available, presence of quarantine boxes, animal cleanliness (less or more than 20% of dirty animals), water (at least one drinker/10 animals), access to pasture, bedding material (straw and/or sawdust/others) and presence of laboratory analyses for mastitis (absent, not on a routine basis, for all problematic cows). Moreover, during the inspection, it was possible to obtain data on average yearly and daily milk production and somatic cell count (SCC) (> or ≤150,000 cells/mL). Based on veterinarians' declarations, it was also possible to distinguish farms applying blanket DCT vs. selective DCT. For each farm, the average number of animals present in the farm for one year was calculated by performing three four-monthly extractions per year from the National data Registry.

4.2. Data Analysis

Overall, AMU per year was quantified using the Defined Daily Dose/Population Cor-rection Unit (DDDAit/PCU) method, proposed by the Italian Ministry of Health [31]. The total amount of mg of an active substance administered for each commercial product was divided by the dosage reported in the summary of products characteristics (SPC), which was reported in the official pharmaceutical handbook [49]. To allow a broader comparison with studies performed in other European countries, AMU was also quantified using DDDvet/PCU [50]. The European Medicines Agency (EMA) provides a standardized daily dosage for each active substance, calculated as the average concentration of various marketed products sold in the European Union (EU) [50]. All intramammary, injectable, intrauterine and oral products were analyzed. Spray AM for external use and ruminal preparations (monensin) were excluded. Oral and injectable antibiotic formulations were calculated per kilogram of animal, while intrauterine and lactating cow intramammary doses (IMM) were calculated per cow. If a range of doses was given, the mean dose was used as the DDDAit [31]. For combination products (e.g., penicillin-streptomycin), the DDDvet was estimated for the main substance, following the guidelines for the DDDvet assignment [50].

Conversely, DDDAit was estimated for both separately, according to the Italian Ministry of Health guidelines [31]. The "PCU" (Population Correction Unit), representing the entire animal biomass "at-risk" present annually in the farm, was calculated by dividing the animals into production categories and multiplying the results by the standard weight attributed to each category. According to the National Reference Centre for Animal Welfare (CreNBA) [31] guidelines, calf, heifer and cow weights were attributed as 100 kg, 300 kg and 600 kg, respectively. Conversely, according to EMA guidelines for DDDvet, the weights attributed were 140 kg, 200 kg, 425 kg for the same previous livestock categories [50]. Antibiotics were grouped according to EMA and WHO classifications, based on their importance to human health [51,52].

4.3. Statistical Analysis

The effects of the phase (dry-off/lactation), year and their interaction on DDDAit distribution were assessed using a linear mixed model; the farm was considered in the model as random effect while the type of phase and year within each farm was included in the repeated effects part of the model, using a compound symmetry covariance structure. The Akaike Information Criterion (AIC) and the residual diagnostics were used to evaluate the model's goodness of fit. Given the model results, the evaluation of the factors collected for each farm in comparison with the DDDAit values was performed considering the year 2020. The Wilcoxon rank-sum test was applied in the case of categorical variables, after having checked the equality of variances using Leven's robust test statistic; regarding continuous variables (i.e., daily milk production, biosecurity and animal welfare scores), the Spearman correlation coefficient was adopted. The HPCIA usage evaluation was performed after dichotomizing the variable (i.e., used at least once or not); given the observed frequencies, only the comparison between 2019 and 2020 for the injectable products was statistically analyzed, using the McNemar test. Given the massive reduction in 2020 of the HPCIAs (only 18 farms used HPCIAs at least once) and the consequent sample size reduction after stratifying by the management variables, HPCIA were not included in the risk factors analysis since the robustness of the statistical analysis would not have been satisfactory. Data analysis was conducted using software SAS v.9.4 (SAS Institute Inc., Cary, NC, USA).

5. Conclusions

This study evidenced a significant decrement in AMU in 34 Alpine dairy farms in 2018–2020, with particular reference to HPCIA. Penicillins and first and second generation cephalosporins were the most frequently administered antimicrobial classes and the most widely used administration route was the intramammary one, specifically during the dry-off period. Replaceable cubicle materials were associated with lower AMU, while quarantine management, available space, water supply, animals' cleanliness and somatic cell count had no significant association with AMU. Furthermore, no association between overall AW and biosecurity score was found. If confirmed by further studies, these results may suggest benchmarks for Alpine dairy farms to promote the reduction of AMU in dairy industry.

Author Contributions: Writing—original draft preparation, F.M.; statistical analysis, K.C.; data collection J.T., D.P., G.C. and S.A.; data analysis, F.M.; supervision, D.D., G.M. and G.F.; project administration, G.D.M. All authors have read and agreed to the published version of the manuscript.

Funding: Data of the present paper originate from the collaboration between IZSVe and Latte Trento s.c.a.

Institutional Review Board Statement: As this was an observational study with commercial animals, specific approval was not needed according to Directive 2010/63/EU.

Informed Consent Statement: Written informed consent was gained from each farmer prior to taking part freely to this research.

Data Availability Statement: The data presented in this study are available on request from the corresponding author. The data are not publicly available due to privacy reason.

Acknowledgments: The authors are thankful to the farmers who collaborated in this project and to Latte Trento s.c.a. for the logistic and financial support.

Conflicts of Interest: The authors declare no conflict of interest.

References

1. Bengtsson, B.; Greko, C. Antibiotic resistance—Onsequences for animal health, welfare, and food production. *Ups. J. Med. Sci.* **2014**, *119*, 96–102. [CrossRef] [PubMed]
2. Roth, N.; Käsbohrer, A.; Mayrhofer, S.; Zitz, U.; Hofacre, C.; Domig, K.J. The application of antibiotics in broiler production and the resulting antibiotic resistance in Escherichia coli: A global overview. *Poult. Sci.* **2019**, *98*, 1791–1804. [CrossRef] [PubMed]
3. EFSA (European Food Safety Authority). The European Union Summary Report on Antimicrobial Resistance in zoonotic and indicator bacteria from humans, animals and food in 2017/2018. *EFSA J.* **2020**, *18*, 6007. [CrossRef]
4. EFSA (European Food Safety Authority). Third joint inter-agency report on integrated analysis of consumption of antimicrobial agents and occurrence of antimicrobial resistance in bacteria from humans and food–Producing animals in the EU/EEA. *EFSA J.* **2021**, *19*, 6712.

5. Chantziaras, I.; Boyen, F.; Callens, B.; Dewulf, J. Correlation between veterinary antimicrobial use and antimicrobial resistance in food-producing animals: A report on seven countries. *J. Antimicrob. Chemother.* **2014**, *69*, 827–834. [CrossRef]
6. Laxminarayan, R.; Matsoso, P.; Pant, S.; Brower, C.; Røttingen, J.A.; Klugman, K.; Davies, S. Access to effective antimicrobials: A worldwide challenge. *Lancet* **2016**, *387*, 168–175. [CrossRef]
7. Gelband, H.; Miller-Petrie, M.; Suraj, P.; Pant, S.; Gandra, S.; Levinson, J.; Barter, D.; White, A.; Laxminarayan, R. The state of the world's antibiotics 2015. *Wound Health S. Afr.* **2015**, *8*, 30–34.
8. Clement, M.; Olabisi, M.; David, E.; Issa, M. Veterinary pharmaceuticals and antimicrobial resistance in developing countries. *IntechOpen* **2019**. [CrossRef]
9. Mendelson, M.; Matsoso, M.P. The World Health Organization global action plan for antimicrobial resistance. *SAMJ S. Afr. Med. J.* **2015**, *105*, 325. [CrossRef]
10. WHO. Global Action Plan on Antimicrobial Resistance. Available online: https://www.who.int/publications/i/item/9789241509763 (accessed on 1 December 2021).
11. Food and Agriculture Organization of the United Nations. *The FAO Action Plan on Antimicrobial Resistance: 2016–2020*; Food and Agriculture Organization of the United Nations: Rome, Italy, 2016. Available online: http://www.fao.org/3/a-i5996e.pdf (accessed on 2 December 2021).
12. Ministero della Salute. *Piano Nazionale di Contrasto dell'Antimicrobico-Resistenza (PNCAR) 2017–2020*; 2017. Available online: https://www.salute.gov.it/imgs/C_17_pubblicazioni_2660_allegato.pdf (accessed on 20 December 2021).
13. Ministero della Salute. Programma Integrato per la Categorizzazione Degli Allevamenti. Guida Interpretativa. Available online: https://www.classyfarm.it/wp-content/uploads/sites/4/2020/02/ba_check_list_bovbuf_2020-1.pdf (accessed on 24 October 2021).
14. European Commission. Farm to Fork Strategy: For a Fair, Healthy and Environmentally-Friendly Food System. Available online: https://ec.europa.eu/food/horizontal-topics/farm-fork-strategy_en (accessed on 14 October 2021).
15. Isomura, R.; Matsuda, M.; Sugiura, K. An epidemiological analysis of the level of biosecurity and animal welfare on pig farms in Japan and their effect on the use of veterinary antimicrobials. *J. Vet. Med. Sci.* **2018**, *80*, 1853–1860. [CrossRef]
16. Stygar, A.H.; Chantziaras, I.; Toppari, I.; Maes, D.; Niemi, J.K. High biosecurity and welfare standards in fattening pig farms are associated with reduced antimicrobial use. *Animal* **2020**, *14*, 2178–2186. [CrossRef]
17. Dewulf, J.; Immerseel, F.V. General principles of biosecurity in animal production and veterinary medicine. In *Biosecurity in Animal Production and Veterinary Medicine: From Principles to Practice*, 1st ed.; Acco Uitgeverij: Leuven, Belgium, 2019; pp. 64–94.
18. Pandolfi, F.; Edwards, S.A.; Maes, D.; Kyriazakis, I. Connecting different data sources to assess the interconnections between biosecurity, health, welfare, and performance in commercial pig farms in Great Britain. *Front. Vet. Sci.* **2018**, *5*, 41. [CrossRef]
19. Collineau, L.; Rojo-Gimeno, C.; Leger, A.; Backhans, A.; Loesken, S.; Okholm Nielsen, E.; Postma, M.; Emanuelson, U.; Beilage, E.; Sjölund, M.; et al. Herd-specific interventions to reduce antimicrobial usage in pig production without jeopardising technical and economic performance. *Prev. Vet. Med.* **2017**, *144*, 167–178. [CrossRef]
20. Laanen, M.; Persoons, D.; Ribbens, S.; de Jong, E.; Callens, B.; Strubbe, M.; Maes, D.; Dewulf, J. Relationship between biosecurity and production/antimicrobial treatment characteristics in pig herds. *Vet. J.* **2013**, *198*, 508–512. [CrossRef]
21. Postma, M.; Backhans, A.; Collineau, L.; Loesken, S.; Sjölund, M.; Belloc, C.; Emanuelson, U.; Beilage, E.; Okholm Nielsen, E.; Stärk, K.D.C.; et al. Evaluation of the relationship between the biosecurity status, production parameters, herd characteristics and antimicrobial usage in farrow-to-finish pig production in four EU countries. *Porc. Health Manag.* **2016**, *2*, 9. [CrossRef]
22. Diana, A.; Lorenzi, V.; Penasa, M.; Magni, E.; Alborali, G.L.; Bertocchi, L.; De Marchi, M. Effect of welfare standards and biosecurity practices on antimicrobial use in beef cattle. *Sci. Rep.* **2020**, *10*, 20939. [CrossRef]
23. Hyde, R.M.; Remnant, J.G.; Bradley, A.J.; Breen, J.E.; Hudson, C.D.; Davies, P.L.; Clarke, T.; Critchell, Y.; Hylands, M.; Linton, E.; et al. Quantitative analysis of antimicrobial use on British dairy farms. *Vet. Rec.* **2017**, *181*, 683. [CrossRef]
24. Obritzhauser, W.; Trauffler, M.; Raith, J.; Kopacka, I.; Fuchs, K.; Köfer, J. Antimicrobial drug use on Austrian dairy farms with special consideration of the use of highest priority critically important antimicrobials. *Berl. Münch. Tierärztl. Wochenschr.* **2016**, *129*, 185–195.
25. Hommerich, K.; Ruddat, I.; Hartmann, M.; Werner, N.; Käsbohrer, A.; Kreienbrock, L. Monitoring antibiotic usage in german dairy and beef cattle farms—A longitudinal analysis. *Front. Vet. Sci.* **2019**, *6*, 244. [CrossRef]
26. Pereyra, V.G.; Pol, M.; Pastorino, F.; Herrero., A. Quantification of antimicrobial usage in dairy cows and preweaned calves in Argentina. *Prev. Vet. Med.* **2015**, *122*, 273–279. [CrossRef]
27. Ginestreti, J.; Lorenzi, V.; Fusi, F.; Ferrara, G.; Scali, F.; Alborali, G.L.; Bolzoni, L.; Bertocchi, L. Antimicrobial usage, animal welfare and biosecurity in 16 dairy farms in Lombardy. *Large Anim. Rev.* **2020**, *26*, 3–11.
28. Ferroni, L.; Lovito, C.; Scoccia, E.; Dalmonte, G.; Sargenti, M.; Pezzotti, G.; Maresca, C.; Forte, C.; Magistrali, C.F. Antibiotic Consumption on Dairy and Beef Cattle Farms of Central Italy Based on Paper Registers. *Antibiotics* **2020**, *9*, 273. [CrossRef]
29. EMA. Sales of Veterinary Antimicrobial Agents in Europe in 31 European Countries in 2018. Available online: https://www.ema.europa.eu/en/documents/report/sales-veterinary-antimicrobial-agents-31-european-countries-2018-trends-2010-2018-tenth-esvac-report_en.pdf (accessed on 10 December 2021).
30. Mazza, F.; Scali, F.; Formenti, N.; Romeo, C.; Tonni, M.; Ventura, V.; Bertocchi, L.; Lorenzi, V.; Fusi, F.; Tolini, C.; et al. The Relationship between Animal Welfare and Antimicrobial Use in Italian Dairy Farms. *Animals* **2021**, *11*, 2575. [CrossRef]

31. Ministero della Salute. Metodologia diCalcolo e di Valutazione del Consumo Degli Antimicrobici nel Settore Veterinario. DDD e DCD Defined Daily Dose Animal for Italy (DDDAit). Available online: https://ddd.veterinariodifiducia.it/MetodologiaDDDConsumoAntimicrobiciV1_2.pdf (accessed on 14 October 2021).
32. Kuipers, A.; Koops, W.J.; Wemmenhove, H. Antibiotic use in dairy herds in the Netherlands from 2005 to 2012. *J. Dairy Sci.* **2016**, *99*, 1632–1648. [CrossRef]
33. Firth, C.L.; Käsbohrer, A.; Schleicher, C.; Fuchs, K.; Egger-Danner, C.; Mayerhofer, M.; Schobersberger, H.; Köfer, J.; Obritzhauser, W. Antimicrobial consumption on Austrian dairy farms: An observational study of udder disease treatments based on veterinary medication records. *Peer J.* **2017**, *5*, e4072.
34. De Campos, J.L.; Kates, A.; Steinberger, A.; Sethi, A.; Suen, G.; Shutske, J.; Safdar, N.; Goldberg, T.; Ruegg, P.L. Quantification of antimicrobial usage in adult cows and preweaned calves on 40 large Wisconsin dairy farms using dose-based and mass-based metrics. *J. Dairy Sci.* **2021**, *104*, 4727–4745. [CrossRef]
35. Zuliani, A.; Lora, I.; Brščić, M.; Rossi, A.; Piasentier, E.; Gottardo, F.; Contiero, B.; Bovolenta, S. Do Dairy Farming Systems Differ in Antimicrobial Use? *Animals* **2021**, *10*, 47. [CrossRef]
36. Oltenacu, P.A.; Broom, D.M. The impact of genetic selection for increased milk yield on the welfare of dairy cows. *Anim. Welf.* **2010**, *19*, 39–49.
37. Green, M.J.; Green, L.E.; Medley, G.F.; Schukken, Y.H.; Bradley, A.J. Influence of dry period bacterial intramammary infection on clinical mastitis in dairy cows. *J. Dairy Sci.* **2002**, *85*, 2589–2599. [CrossRef]
38. Krattley-Roodenburg, B.; Huybens, L.J.; Nielen, M.; van Werven, T. Dry period management and new high somatic cell count during the dry period in Dutch dairy herds under selective dry cow therapy. *J. Dairy Sci.* **2021**, *104*, 6975–6984. [CrossRef]
39. Schukken, Y.H.; Kremer, W.D.; Lohuis, J.A. Escherichia coli mastitis in cattle. I. Clinical diagnosis and epidemiological aspects. *Tijdschr. Diergeneeskd.* **1989**, *114*, 829–838.
40. Fulwider, W.K.; Grandin, T.; Garrick, D.J.; Engle, T.E.; Lamm, W.D.; Dalsted, N.L.; Rollin, B.E. Influence of Free-Stall Base on Tarsal Joint Lesions and Hygiene in Dairy Cows. *J. Dairy Sci.* **2007**, *90*, 3559–3566. [CrossRef] [PubMed]
41. Tucker, C.B.; Weary, D.M.; von Keyserlingk, M.A.G.; Beauchemin, K.A. Cow comfort in tie-stalls: Increased depth of shavings or straw bedding increases lying time. *J. Dairy Sci.* **2009**, *92*, 2684–2690. [CrossRef] [PubMed]
42. Wechsler, B.; Schaub, J.; Friedli, K.; Hauser, R. Behaviour and leg injuries in dairy cows kept in cubicle systems with straw bedding or soft lying mats. *Appl. Anim. Behav. Sci.* **2000**, *69*, 189–197. [CrossRef]
43. Manninen, E.; de Passillé, A.M.; Rushen, J.; Norring, M.; Saloniemi, H. Preferences of dairy cows kept in unheated buildings for different kind of cubicle flooring. *Appl. Anim. Behav. Sci.* **2002**, *75*, 281–292. [CrossRef]
44. Lardy, R.; Des Roches, A.D.B.; Capdeville, J.; Bastien, R.; Mounier, L.; Veissier, I. Refinement of international recommendations for cubicles, based on the identification of associations between cubicle characteristics and dairy cow welfare measures. *J. Dairy Sci.* **2021**, *104*, 2164–2184. [CrossRef]
45. Potterton, S.L.; Green, M.J.; Harris, J.; Millar, K.M.; Whay, H.R.; Huxley, J.N. Risk factors associated with hair loss, ulceration, and swelling at the hock in freestall-housed UK dairy herds. *J. Dairy Sci.* **2011**, *94*, 2952–2963. [CrossRef]
46. Postma, M.; Vanderhaeghen, W.; Sarrazin, S.; Maes, D.; Dewulf, J. Reducing antimicrobial usage in pig production without jeopardizing production parameters. *Zoonoses Public Health* **2017**, *64*, 63–74. [CrossRef]
47. Tarakdjian, J.; Capello, K.; Pasqualin, D.; Santini, A.; Cunial, G.; Scollo, A.; Mannelli, A.; Tomao, P.; Vonesch, N.; Di Martino, G. Antimicrobial use on Italian pig farms and its relationship with husbandry practices. *Animals* **2020**, *10*, 417. [CrossRef]
48. Bertocchi, L.; Fusi, F.; Angelucci, A.; Bolzoni, L.; Pongolini, S.; Strano, R.M.; Ginestreti, J.; Riuzzi, G.; Moroni, P.; Lorenzi, V. Characterization of hazards, welfare promoters and animal-based measures for the welfare assessment of dairy cows: Elicitation of expert opinion. *Prev. Vet. Med.* **2018**, *150*, 8–18. [CrossRef]
49. Ministero della Salute. Sistema Informativo Veterinario. Available online: https://www.vetinfo.it (accessed on 16 November 2021).
50. European Medicines Agency (EMA). Defined Daily Doses for Animals (DDDvet) and Defined Course Doses for Animals (DCDvet): European Surveillance of Veterinary Antimicrobial Consumption (ESVAC). Available online: http://www.ema.europa.eu/docs/en_GB/document_lbrary/Other/2016/04/WC500205410.pdf.45 (accessed on 6 December 2021).
51. European Medicines Agency (EMA). Categorisation of Antibiotics Used in Animals Promotes Responsible Use to Protect Public And Animal Health. Available online: https://www.ema.europa.eu/en/news/categorisation-antibioticsused-animals-promotes-responsible-use-protect-public-animal-health (accessed on 9 November 2021).
52. WHO. *Critically Important Antimicrobials for Human Medicine*, 6th ed.; WHO: Geneva, Switzerland, 2019. Available online: https://apps.who.int/iris/bitstream/handle/10665/312266/9789241515528-eng.pdf (accessed on 6 December 2021).

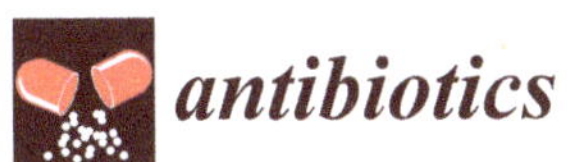

MDPI

Article

Categorisation of Antimicrobial Use in Fijian Livestock Production Systems

Xavier Khan [1,*], Caroline Rymer [1], Partha Ray [1,2] and Rosemary Lim [3]

1 Department of Animal Sciences, School of Agriculture, Policy and Development, University of Reading, P.O. Box 237, Reading RG6 6EU, UK; c.rymer@reading.ac.uk (C.R.); patha.ray@tnc.org (P.R.)
2 The Nature Conservancy, 4245 North Fairfax Drive, Suite 100, Arlington, VA 22203, USA
3 Reading School of Pharmacy, School of Chemistry, Food & Pharmacy, University of Reading, Whiteknights, Reading RG6 6DZ, UK; r.h.m.lim@reading.ac.uk
* Correspondence: x.r.s.khan@pgr.reading.ac.uk

Abstract: Antimicrobial resistance (AMR) is a major global threat to human and animal health. The use of antimicrobials in the livestock sector is considered to contribute to AMR. Therefore, a reduction in and prudent use of antimicrobials in livestock production systems have been advocated. This cross-sectional survey aimed to investigate the extent of imprudent antimicrobial use (AMU) and to determine whether the AMU practice was affected by either the farming system or species of farmed livestock in the largest island (Viti Levu) of Fiji. A total of 276 livestock enterprises were surveyed and antimicrobials were used on 309 occasions over 90 days. Overall, in 298 of 309 (96%) incidents, antimicrobials were used imprudently, comprising antibiotics, 160 of 170 (94%) and anthelmintics, 138 of 139 (99%). Prudent use of antibiotics was associated with commercial farming systems ($X^2 = 13$, $p = 0.001$), but no association was observed with anthelmintic use ($p > 0.05$). Imprudent antibiotic use was associated with dairy (OR = 7.6, CI = 1.41, 41.57, $p = 0.018$) followed by layer and beef ($p > 0.05$) compared to broiler enterprises. Imprudent AMU was more common in the backyard and semi-commercial enterprises compared to commercial broiler enterprises. Policies promoting the prudent use of antimicrobials in Fiji should focus on smaller livestock production systems and enterprises.

Keywords: antibiotics; anthelmintics; prudent use; imprudent use; livestock production systems; Fiji

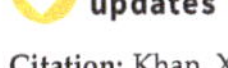

Citation: Khan, X.; Rymer, C.; Ray, P.; Lim, R. Categorisation of Antimicrobial Use in Fijian Livestock Production Systems. *Antibiotics* **2022**, *11*, 294. https://doi.org/10.3390/antibiotics11030294

Academic Editor: Marc Maresca

Received: 4 January 2022
Accepted: 22 February 2022
Published: 23 February 2022

Publisher's Note: MDPI stays neutral with regard to jurisdictional claims in published maps and institutional affiliations.

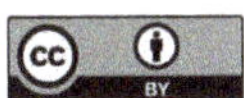

Copyright: © 2022 by the authors. Licensee MDPI, Basel, Switzerland. This article is an open access article distributed under the terms and conditions of the Creative Commons Attribution (CC BY) license (https://creativecommons.org/licenses/by/4.0/).

1. Introduction

Antimicrobial resistance (AMR) is a significant global threat to human and animal health [1]. Antimicrobial use (AMU) in the livestock sector has been considered to contribute to the AMR issue [1,2]. Therefore, a reduction and a prudent use of antimicrobials in livestock production systems have been advocated [1–3]. Food of animal origin is produced using traditional systems in non-commercial farming settings for food and socio-economic security worldwide [4–6]. However, in recent times, increasing demand for foods of animal origin (meat, milk, and eggs) has contributed to the intensification and commercialisation of livestock production systems locally and globally [7–9]. Larger flocks/herds of animals are produced in smaller confinements (sheds, cages, and paddocks) and in a shorter duration than traditional, extensive and free-range systems [6,8,10]. Backyard farming systems continue to produce livestock for domestic consumption, while semi-commercial farmers who are market-orientated produce livestock for domestic consumption and sale [11,12].

Higher flock/herd density with compromised farm biosecurity infrastructure results in higher chances of transmission of diseases amongst flocks/herds; therefore, striking a balance between increasing production and managing farm biosecurity risks has been a challenge faced by livestock farmers [13,14]. As part of a farm-level biosecurity risk management strategy, antimicrobials including antibiotics and anthelmintics (as well as other agents such as vaccines, medicated feed, nutraceuticals, and other herbal preparations) have been used to reduce the risk of microbial infection in the agri-food value chain [15–23].

Antimicrobials have traditionally been used to treat diseases in livestock; however, antimicrobials have also been used prophylactically in flocks/herds of animals and for growth promotion [16,24,25]. The prophylactic use may be predominant in commercial systems due to higher stock density; however, it is presumed that AMU for growth promotion may be more common in systems that have fewer veterinary interventions [22,26,27]. Unnecessary and imprudent use of antimicrobials in livestock production systems is of grave concern due to the risk of emergence and transmission of antimicrobial resistance (AMR) genes via the agri-food value chains to humans [28,29].

The World Organisation for Animal Health (OIE) discourages unnecessary and long-term use of antimicrobials in farmed livestock and advocate the administration of antimicrobials under the supervision of a qualified veterinarian [30,31]. In addition, the use of World Health Organisation (WHO) classified critically important antimicrobials in livestock production systems is prohibited and considered imprudent [32,33]. The imprudent use of antimicrobials has been reported in developing countries, predominantly in the backyard and semi-commercial farming systems, due to lack of access to veterinarians leading to self-prescribing [5,14,16,24]. However, such AMU practices in Fiji are currently unknown. In the United Kingdom (UK), the Veterinary Medicines Directorate (VMD) produced a code of practice on the responsible use of animal medicines in farm animals for livestock keepers, including guidelines for the access, usage and recording of AMU [34]. At a sectoral level, the Responsible Use of Medicines in Agriculture (RUMA) set guidelines for beef, dairy, broiler, layer and other enterprises [35]. Policies on responsible antibiotic use for farm livestock under cascade were also established in the UK, where veterinarians are permitted to prescribe medicines unauthorised for use in livestock [36], but this has not been the case in Fiji. In Fiji, the shortage of veterinary professionals, lack of legislation restricting AMU in livestock and standard therapeutic guidelines have been reported [37]. In addition, Fijian veterinary legislation is outdated since the current one dates to 1956 [38], while the antibiotics and anthelmintics for use in livestock remain unclassified in the current Medicinal Products Act [39]. On the other hand, the existence of a veterinary authority (a standard-setting authority similar to the VMD and BVA) remains unclear, while the legislation targeting antimicrobial residue levels in animal products only outlines standards on milk and milk products, excluding all other animal products [38–40]. Moreover, AMR in the Fijian health sector has also been reported [37].

In the UK, the BVA, in collaboration with VMD, set good practice guidelines for the use of veterinary medicines to assist veterinarians, pharmacists and suitability qualified personnel [41,42]. The VMD guidelines also include off label and cascade use of antibiotics which is only permitted for use under the supervision of veterinarians [36,42]. Hence, deviation from the set regulatory framework and classification on prescribing and dispensing of the antimicrobials is considered imprudent in the UK [43,44]. Antimicrobial legal categories and classification in other South Pacific countries such as Australia and New Zealand are similar to the UK [43–45]. However, the Fijian jurisdiction does not define such specific legal categories and authorisation of veterinary medicines [39]. Our recent study demonstrated moderately high use of antimicrobials which varied by systems and enterprises; however, the quantity of antimicrobials used does not demonstrate whether the antimicrobials were used prudently [46]; therefore, this study aimed to investigate the extent of imprudent AMU in Fiji, and to determine whether this was affected by either farming system or species of farmed livestock.

2. Results

2.1. Characteristics of Antimicrobials Used

The characteristics of AMU in farm enterprises are presented in Table S1. Veterinary antimicrobials were used in 306 of the 309 (99%) incidents, but on three incidents (1%), human antimicrobials were used, which are prohibited for use in food producing livestock. A little over half of the antimicrobials used were antibiotics (n = 170, 55%). Most of the antimicrobials were administered as an oral solution (n = 227, 73%), while a smaller proportion were administered orally as powders ($n = 62$, 20%). All powdered formulations for oral use were reconstituted and administered in drinking water. Most antimicrobials contained a single active pharmaceutical ingredient ($n = 251$, 81%). The majority of administrations were in flocks of poultry or herds of cattle ($n = 253$, 82%) rather than to an individual bird or cow, and 87% (268 of 309) of all administrations were self-prescribed (prescription and administration of antimicrobials to livestock on the farms) by the farmer or farm manager. Antimicrobials were mainly purchased from agricultural or veterinary clinics ($n = 263$, 85%) operated by livestock officers (presumably with tropical agriculture qualifications), referred to as para-veterinarians in the Fijian context.

The most commonly used antimicrobial was anthelmintic of the imidazothiazole derivative class ($n = 72$, 31%) followed by the antibiotic β-lactams ($n = 81$, 26%) and tetracyclines ($n = 58$, 19%) while other antibiotic classes were less frequently used (<10%). A larger proportion of antimicrobials were administered to dairy calves ($n = 82$, 27%) followed by lactating cows ($n = 53$, 17%), bull calves ($n = 42$, 14%) laying hens ($n = 30$, 10%) and broiler breeding birds ($n = 25$, 8%).

2.2. Imprudent Antimicrobial Use Categorisation

The categorisation of AMU practice in livestock enterprises is presented in Table 1. According to the first criterion in the decision-making tree (step 1), all anthelmintics (100%) and almost all antibiotics (98%) passed the step because veterinary antimicrobials were used in 306 of 309 (99%) occasions. The 3 of 309 (1%) uses were imprudent because they were non-veterinary antibiotics. Veterinary anthelmintics were used on 139 of 306 incidents and antibiotics on 167 of 306 incidents (step 2). However, since antibiotics are classified as POM-V and anthelmintics as POM-VPS, antimicrobials were mostly used in an imprudent way, as assessed in step 3 (288 of 306, or 94% of occasions). On this criterion, antibiotics were not prescribed by an authorised prescriber on 156 of 167 (93%) incidents and anthelmintics on 132 of 139 (95%) incidents. In step 4, 18 of 306 (6%) incidents prescribed by the authorised prescriber in step 3 were administered to the target species specified on the label and as per their market authorisation (step 4).

Table 1. Categorisation of 309 incidents where antimicrobials were used in livestock enterprises located in Viti Levu, Fiji.

Steps	AMU Practice	Antimicrobial Type					
		Anthelmintic		Antibiotic		Total	
		n	(%)	*n*	(%)	*n*	(%)
1 * (antimicrobial type)	Prudent	139	(100)	167	(98)	306	(99)
	Imprudent	0	(0)	3	(2)	3	(1)
	Total	139	(100)	170	(100)	309	(100)
3 (prescriber)	Prudent	7	(5)	11	(7)	18	(6)
	Imprudent	132	(95)	156	(93)	288	(94)
	Total	139	(100)	167	(100)	306	(100)
4 (target species)	Prudent	7	(100)	11	(100)	18	(100)
	Imprudent	0	(0)	0	(0)	0	(0)
	Total	7	(100)	11	(100)	18	(100)
5 (purpose of administration)	Prudent	5	(71)	7	(64)	12	(67)
	Imprudent	2	(29)	4	(36)	6	(33)
	Total	7	(100)	11	(100)	18	(100)

Table 1. *Cont.*

Steps	AMU Practice	Antimicrobial Type					
		Anthelmintic		Antibiotic		Total	
		n	(%)	*n*	(%)	*n*	(%)
6+ (cascade)	Prudent	n/a	n/a	11	(100)	11	(100)
	Imprudent	n/a	n/a	0	(0)	0	(0)
	Total	n/a	n/a	11	(100)	11	(100)
7 (AMU records)	Prudent	1	(20)	10	(91)	11	(69)
	Imprudent	4	(80)	1	(9)	5	(31)
	Total	5	(100)	11	(100)	16	(100)
Last step **	Prudent	1	(1)	10	(6)	11	(4)
	Imprudent	138 [a]	(99)	160 [b]	(94)	298 [c]	(96)
	Total	139	(100)	170	(100)	309	(100)

Note: - denotes zero *n* (counts) and % (proportion), * denotes steps as per framework (Table 5) where steps 2a and 2b were verification steps, + denotes step 6, which is only applicable to antibiotics, AMU denotes antimicrobial use, ** last step denotes totals of all steps including human antimicrobials used, [a] denotes anthelmintics imprudent sum = step 1 + step 3 + step 4+ step 5 + step 7, [b] denotes antibiotics imprudent sum = step 1 + step 3 + step 6 + step 7 (steps 4 and 5 are not applicable as antibiotics are prescribed in cascade), [c] denotes antimicrobial imprudent total sum = step 1 + step 3 + step 4 + step 5 + step 6 + step 7, less 4 from step 5 (antibiotics used in cascade).

Based on our evaluation, we found that in 6 of 18 incidents, antimicrobials which we classified as imprudent use were prescribed by an authorised prescriber in step 3 and approved target species in step 4, but we were unaware of the pre-existing condition being treated and therefore classified the use as imprudent in step 5. Since antibiotics should only be used in cascade as per our set framework (Table 5), 11 of 167 (7%) incidents (step 3) antibiotics used were categorised as cascade use in step 6.

On 18 occasions, antimicrobials were administered to authorised target species (step 4); however, only in 5 of 7 incidents were anthelmintics used prudently, and in 7 out of 11 incidents, antibiotics were used prudently. Since antibiotics are prescribed in cascade and all 11 of the 167 incidents were prescribed by the authorised prescriber in step 3, we considered all 11 for cascade use. Maintaining AMU records is essential for antimicrobial stewardship (AMS) programmes. Only 1 out of 5 incidents of anthelmintics were recorded (thus used prudently) whilst 10 out of 11 incidents of antibiotic use were recorded (i.e., prudent) (step 7).

Overall, in 298 of 309 (96%) incidents, antimicrobials were used imprudently. Antibiotics on 160 of 170 (94%) incidents and anthelmintics on 138 of 139 (99%) incidents were used imprudently. The practice of AMU (imprudent, prudent) was associated with the antimicrobial type (anthelmintic, antibiotic), $p = 0.026$, with antibiotic use being marginally more prudent compared to anthelmintics (Table 2).

Table 2. The antimicrobial use practice of 309 occasions when antimicrobials were used on 276 enterprises located in Central and Western divisions of Viti Levu, Fiji.

Antimicrobial Type	Antimicrobial Use Practice			
	Imprudent		Prudent	
	n	% Observed	*n*	% Observed
Anthelmintic	138	99	1	1
Antibiotic	160	94	10	6

n denotes frequency, % denotes percentage observed, Fisher's Exact Test, $p = 0.026$.

2.3. Description of the Types of Antimicrobials Used

OIE classified veterinary critically important antimicrobials (antibiotics only) were used on 55% of 309 incidents, while WHO categorised high priority critically important antimicrobials (macrolides, beta-lactams and third and fourth generation cephalosporins) were used on 3% of occasions (refer Table S1). Antimicrobial agents used as antiparasitic agents (45%) and antimicrobial agents for systemic use (38%) dominated the groups of antimicrobials used. According to the VMP classification, 57% of antimicrobials used were POM-V, and 42% were POM-VPS. Almost half of the administrations (48%) were classified as therapeutic use, while the remaining half was for prophylactic purposes (37%) and growth promotion (15%). Although the prescriber was one of the main prerequisites for categorisation of imprudent use, overall, in 36 incidents (12%), AMU was off label or antimicrobials were used in unauthorised target species, and there were only three incidents (1%) when prohibited antimicrobials were used (Table 3).

Table 3. Classification of antimicrobial formulations used in 309 incidents on 276 livestock enterprises located in Viti Levu, Fiji.

Factor	Sub-Categories	n	(%)
OIE classification	Veterinary critically important	170	(55)
	Unclassified antimicrobials	139	(45)
WHO classification	Highly important	162	(52)
	Unclassified antimicrobials	139	(45)
	High priority critically important	8	(3)
ATC ESVAC classification	Antiparasitic use	139	(45)
	Systemic use	117	(38)
	Intestinal use	26	(8)
	Intramammary use	24	(8)
	Systemic use (humans)	3	(1)
VMD legal distribution category	POM-V	279	(57)
	POM-VPS	131	(42)
	Human antimicrobial	3	(1)
Purpose of administration	Therapeutic	148	(48)
	Prophylactic	115	(37)
	Growth promotion	46	(15)
	Metaphylactic	-	-
Use on target species *	Authorised	270	(87)
	Unauthorised	36	(12)
	Prohibited +	3	(1)

Note: * denotes classification based on National Office of Animal Health (NOAH), - denotes zero n (count) and % (proportion). OIE, World Organization of Animal Health, WHO, World Health Organization, ATC ESVAC, Anatomical therapeutic classification European Surveillance Veterinary Antimicrobial Consumption project, VMD, Veterinary Medicines Directorate, + prohibited use denotes antimicrobials authorised for human use and prohibited for use in livestock raised for food.

In most incidents, farmers self-prescribed anthelmintics (95%) and antibiotics (80%). Para-veterinarians prescribed antibiotics on only 14% of occasions, and veterinarians on only 6% of occasions. There was an association between the type of antimicrobial used and the prescriber, with veterinarians prescribing marginally more antibiotics than anthelmintics ($p < 0.001$) (Figure 1A).

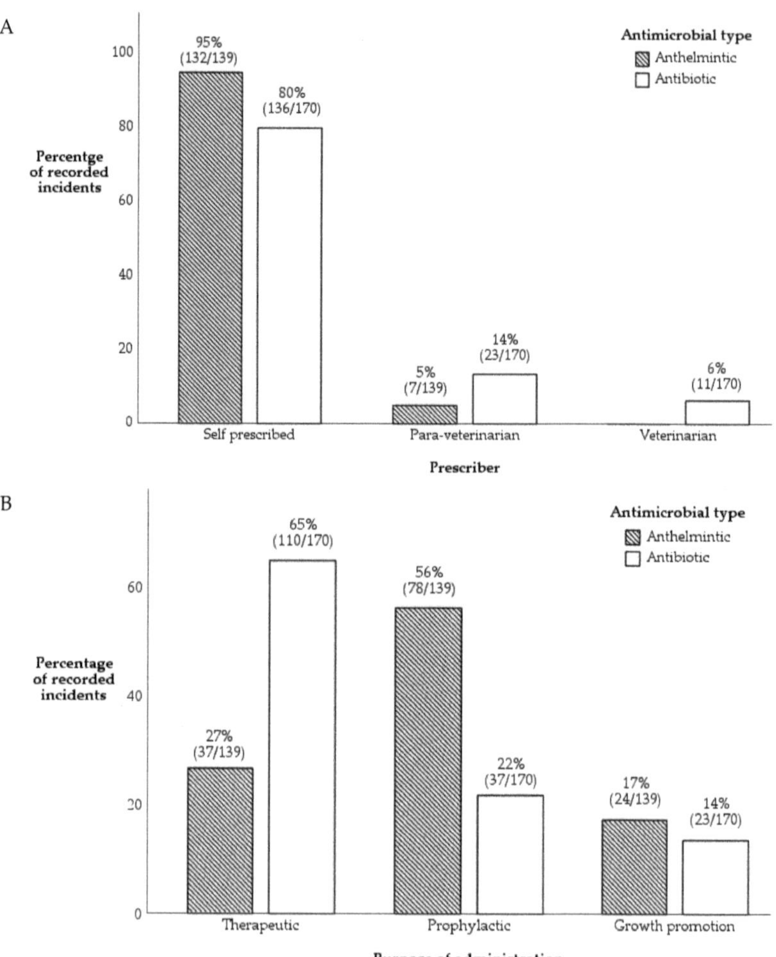

Figure 1. Association of 309 incidents where antimicrobials were used (anthelmintics n = 139, antibiotics n = 170) with (**A**). prescribing pattern (Fisher's exact test, $p < 0.001$), and (**B**). purpose of administration ($X^2 = 48$, $p < 0.001$) in 276 enterprises located in Central and Western division of Viti Levu, Fiji.

Most antibiotics were used therapeutically (65% of occasions), over a fifth (22%) were used prophylactically and 14% as growth promoters. The principal use of anthelmintics was for prophylactic purposes (56%), but on 17% of incidents, anthelmintics were used for growth promotion. There was a significant association between antimicrobial type and purpose of administration type, with greater usage of anthelmintics for prophylaxis ($X^2 = 48$, $p < 0.001$, Figure 1B).

Anthelmintics were used in just over 60% of incidents for parasitic infections, while antibiotics were used in a little over 30% of incidents for growth promotion. Anthelmintic and antibiotics were also used for symptomatic treatment (12% and 26%, respectively). The AMU practice was associated with indications of use, with anthelmintics being mainly used for parasitic infections ($X^2 = 162$, $p < 0.001$, Figure 2).

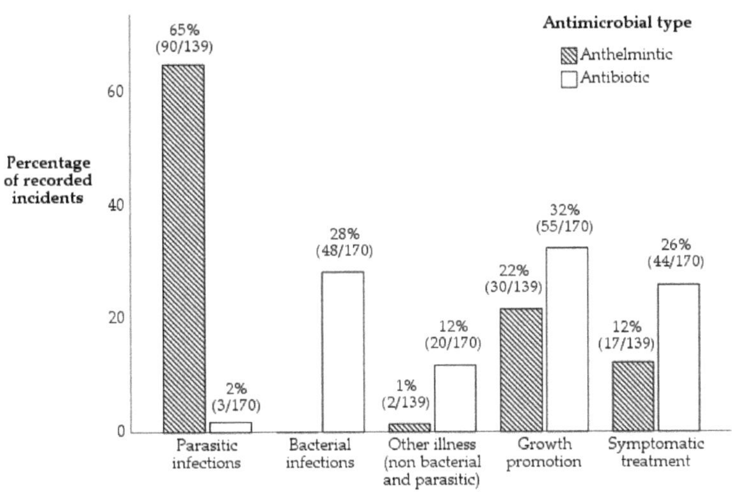

Figure 2. Association between 309 incidents where antimicrobials were used (anthelmintics $n = 139$, antibiotics $n = 170$) and indication of use on 276 enterprises located in the Central and Western division of Viti Levu, Fiji. (Chi-square statistics $X^2 = 162$, $p < 0.001$).

2.4. Prescription of Antimicrobials in Enterprises and Farming Systems

Antimicrobials were not prescribed by veterinarians (Refer Table S1, 298 of 309 incidents) except in broiler enterprises (100%, 11 of 11 incidents). Para-veterinarians were most likely to be used in dairy enterprises (67%, 20 of 30 incidents) and did not prescribe antimicrobials in poultry enterprises ($p = 0.017$, Figure 3A). Farmers self-prescribed antimicrobials in all enterprises, although this was less common in broiler and layer enterprises (10% and 13%, respectively). Farmers self-prescribed antimicrobials most commonly in dairy enterprises (49%, 132 of 268 incidents).

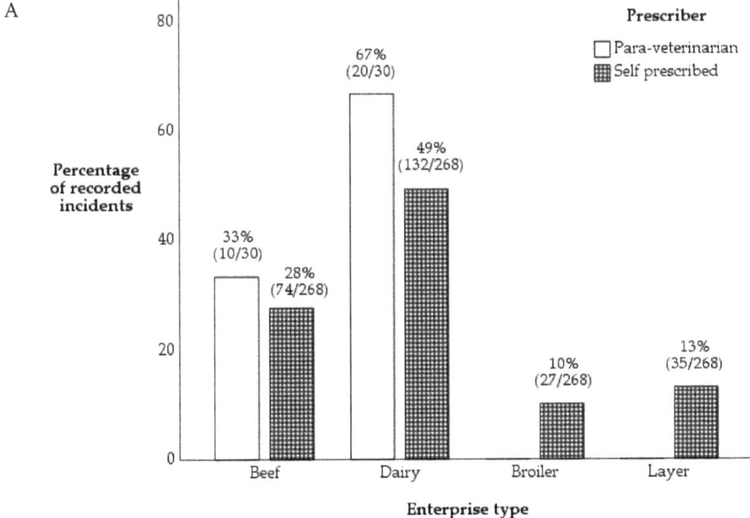

Figure 3. *Cont.*

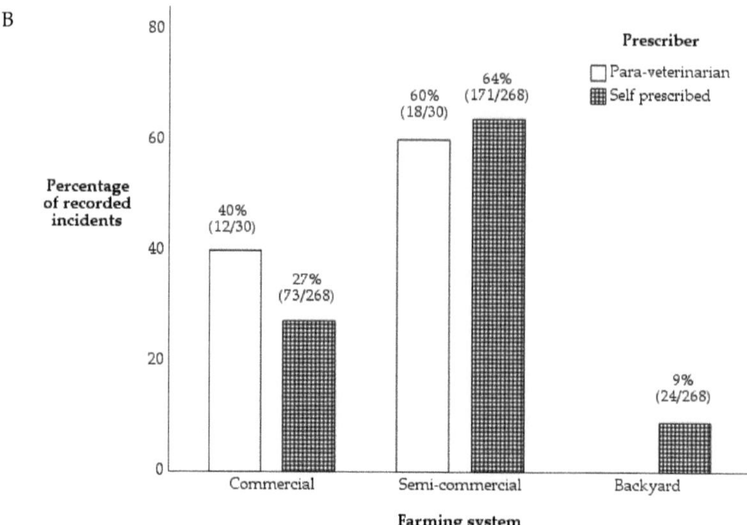

Figure 3. Association between 298 of 309 incidents where antimicrobials were prescribed (para-veterinarians $n = 30$, self-prescribed $n = 268$) and (**A**). different enterprises (Fisherman's exact test, $p = 0.017$) and (**B**). different farming systems (Fisherman's exact test, $p = 0.111$) located in the Central and Western divisions of Viti Levu, Fiji. Veterinarians only prescribed in commercial broiler enterprises ($n = 11$ incidents) and were excluded from the analysis.

Veterinarians only prescribed antimicrobials (refer to Table S1, 298 of 309 incidents) in commercial farming systems (100%, 11 of 11 incidents) while para-veterinarians mostly prescribed in semi-commercial farming systems (60%, 18 of 30 incidents). Self-prescribing was also common in semi-commercial systems (64%) and commercial farming systems (40%). Veterinarians and para-veterinarians did not prescribe any antimicrobials for use in backyard farming systems. However, there was no statistically significant association between prescriber and farming system ($p = 0.111$, Figure 3B).

2.5. Associations and Logistic Regression Modelling of Farming System and Enterprise Type with AMU Practice

Amongst the different farming systems, antibiotics were used imprudently in more incidents in the semi-commercial farming system (98%). The situation was only marginally better in the backyard (92%) and commercial (76%) farming systems. There was an association between farming systems and AMU practice where prudent use mainly was in commercial farming systems ($X^2 = 13$, $p = 0.001$).

The antibiotics were administered imprudently on more incidents in dairy (96%) followed by layer (95%) and beef (94%); however, the situation was better in broiler enterprises (75%). There was an association between AMU practice and enterprise type ($X^2 = 10$, $p = 0.022$), where broiler enterprises were more likely to use antimicrobials prudently.

All anthelmintics administered in the backyard and semi-commercial farming systems were used imprudently. Anthelmintic use was imprudent in beef, dairy and layer enterprises and only slightly better in broiler enterprises. There was no association between anthelmintic use practice and farming systems and enterprise types ($p > 0.05$).

Imprudent use was also more likely to be practiced in dairy enterprises (OR = 7.6, CI = 1.41, 41.57, $p = 0.018$, Table 4) followed by layer enterprises and beef enterprises compared to broiler enterprises; however, our finding was statistically insignificant for layer and beef enterprises ($p > 0.05$).

Table 4. Summary of association and logistic regression modelling of farming systems and enterprise types with antimicrobial use practice on livestock farms located in Central and Western divisions of Viti Levu, Fiji.

Antimicrobial Type +	Factor	Sub-Categories	*n*	(%)	AMU Practice		Chi-Square Tests		Logistic Regression		
					% Imprudent	% Prudent	χ^2	*p*-Value	*p*-Value	OR	95% CI
Antibiotic	Farming system	Backyard	12	(11)	92	8			-	-	-
		Semi commercial	65	(59)	98	2	13	0.001	-	-	-
		Commercial	34	(31)	76	24			-	-	-
	Enterprise type	Beef	18	(16)	94	6			0.125	5.67	0.62, 52.09
		Dairy	48	(43)	96	4	10	0.022	0.018	7.60	1.41, 41.57
		Broiler	24	(22)	75	25				1	
		Layer	21	(19)	95	5			0.093	6.66	0.73, 60.81
Anthelmintic	Farming system	Backyard	8	(9)	100	0			-	-	-
		Semi commercial	61	(65)	100	0	-	0.248	-	-	-
		Commercial	25	(27)	96	4			-	-	-
	Enterprise type	Beef	33	(35)	100	0			-	-	-
		Dairy	51	(54)	98	2	-	0.837	-	-	-
		Broiler	1	(1)	100	0			-	-	-
		Layer	9	(10)	100	0			-	-	-

Note: reference category is commercial for farming systems, broiler for enterprise type, *n* denotes the frequency, % denotes percentage, AMU, antimicrobial use, OR denotes odds ratio, CI denotes confidence interval. - denotes logistic regression modelling was not executed as there was no association (Fisher's exact test, $p > 0.05$) in the anthelmintic model and unbalanced antibiotic model for the farming system, + denotes two models (antibiotic, anthelmintic).

3. Discussion

The present study, to our knowledge, is the first study categorising AMU in livestock production systems in Fiji. The study revealed that in 96% of incidents (298 of 309), antimicrobials were used imprudently on 276 enterprises. The evaluation revealed that 94% (160 of 170 incidents) of antibiotic (POM-V) use and 99% (138 of 139 incidents) of anthelmintic (POM-VPS) use were categorised as imprudent. Although antimicrobials were purchased from veterinary clinics, presumably operated by para-veterinarians, the prescription and administration of antimicrobials to livestock on the farms were done by the farmers (95% self-prescribed). The results also suggest that most POM-V and POM-VPS were sold to farmers without prescription, concurring with the findings of studies in other developing countries [24,47].

The results also suggest that 12% of antimicrobials were administered to unauthorised target species, thus deviating from the market authorisation and the label. Given that 87% of antimicrobials were used in authorised target species, we presume that these antimicrobials were used correctly; used as per indications given in the market authorisation and the labels of the antimicrobials (see Table 3). The indications for which the antimicrobials were used were at the discretion of the farmers. Nonetheless, the actual administration on the farm depends on the farmers' decision-making process where the farmers' intention, attitude and available resources play a fundamental role in deciding the AMU [48], which differs from the UK, where the antibiotics are only prescribed by the veterinarians while anthelmintics by a pharmacist or suitably qualified person or a veterinarian [49].

On the other hand, the unauthorised prescription and administration of antimicrobials are of grave concern. There is a high chance of incorrect dosing, non-compliance to the correct duration of use, and off-label use resulting in imprudent use similarly reported in studies in other countries [47]. Europe and the UK banned the use of antibiotics for growth promotion [50,51]; however, antibiotics continue to be used for growth promotion in the Asian Pacific region [16,52]. The current study's findings confirmed that antimicrobials were used for growth promotion and were also administered prophylactically in livestock farms in Fiji. We presume there may be chances of justified and right intentions for using the antimicrobials in livestock to mitigate farm biosecurity risks [26]. However, using antimicrobials without consulting veterinary professionals poses a greater chance of antimicrobials being used imprudently [48]. We also believe that some imprudent use may be due to a lack of knowledge and understanding of antimicrobials, as participants reported using anthelmintics and antibiotics to treat similar diseases. In was beyond the scope of this study to explain the motivations behind the AMU practice.

Although antimicrobials were used imprudently in the vast majority of incidents (96%), most of them were used on authorised species (Table 1, Step 4). This finding further infers that although there was easy access to antimicrobials, only 12% of antimicrobials were administered to unauthorised species at the farm level (Table 3). However, we could not elucidate if antimicrobials were under or overdosed; therefore, randomised longitudinal quantitative studies that collect the body weights of animals and the ailments treated at the point of treatment with the antimicrobials would be more appropriate. Subsequently, the individual dose and course doses according to the indication for use could be more accurately estimated so that the under or overuse of antimicrobials in the different enterprises could be evaluated.

In the current study, antimicrobials were usually administered to the flock or herd rather than individual animals, which suggested that antimicrobials might have been used on clinically healthy animals. Prophylactic use of antibiotics in animals has been discouraged by OIE [53], but to maintain biosecurity, prophylactic use may be justifiable for economic and welfare reasons. Nevertheless, the prophylactic use of anthelmintics has been found to be beneficial in reducing the number of macroparasite infections reported in other studies [54]. Some studies have reported that one of the motivations for implementing biosecurity was increasing profit through higher farm production [15,55]. Therefore, we suggest further studies to explore and understand the motivations for implementing biosecurity measures such as prophylactic use of antimicrobials in flocks and herds of cattle and poultry. We further suggest exploring the farm biosecurity risk mitigation strategies employed on farms, reducing the incidence and transmission of diseases, thus reducing the need for antimicrobials. This will enable the development and recommendation of more uniform sectoral and enterprise-level risk management strategies. Exposing clinically healthy herds and flocks of animals to antimicrobials may further contribute to the risk of AMR, as demonstrated in other studies [29]. Therefore, in the Fijian jurisdiction, we suggest that care must be taken when administering antimicrobials at the herd and flock level. In addition, all administrations should be executed in consultation and under the supervision of suitably qualified veterinarians following the guidance of the WHO, OIE and FAO [2,3]. We also found that veterinary critically important antibiotics [33] and antibiotics critically important for human medicine [32], such as tetracyclines and β-lactam penicillin, were commonly used and were similarly reported in other developing countries [22,51,52].

Our results also revealed that antibiotics were used under the cascade, and the record-keeping of AMU was inconsistent. We could not establish a general understanding of the importance of maintaining AMU records amongst the livestock farmers and veterinarians. Evaluating and demonstrating an understanding of the decision-making process for cascade use of antibiotics could not be established; however, the cascade use of antibiotics by farmers, without consultation and supervision of veterinarians, is alarming. Contrarily, in the UK, antibiotics can only be used and prescribed by veterinarians under the cascade, adhering to stringent regulatory requirements [36,49]. Therefore, the development and implementation of regulatory frameworks on the cascade use of antibiotics similar to the UK [41,56] would assist the Fijian livestock production sector. In addition, we were also unable to assess the role of the para-veterinarians in veterinary service delivery and AMU decision-making process; therefore, it is crucial to clearly define the roles of para-veterinarians in the legislative frameworks in Fiji so that all POM-VPS (anthelmintics) are appropriately prescribed by para-veterinarians and other professionals as practiced in the

UK and other countries [30,36,41]. Given that we were unable to precisely evaluate the roles of the para-veterinarians and veterinarians at large in veterinary service delivery and livestock production, we suggest further studies exploring and understanding the knowledge, attitude and behaviour of the veterinarian and para-veterinarian towards antimicrobial prescribing, AMU and veterinary practice so that policy recommendations could be made to improve veterinary services and strengthen AMS programmes.

Based on the indications of use, antibiotics were used most frequently for growth promotion followed by treatment for bacterial infections and symptomatic treatment; however, antibiotics being used for the treatment of other illness (non-bacterial and parasitic) is of grave concern since such use is contraindicated in the market authorisation and label of the antibiotics. The use of antibiotics for bacterial infections may be justified due to its compliance to market authorisation and label; however, all other uses (parasitic infections, growth promotion, symptomatic treatment and non-bacterial and parasitic illness) described in Figure 2 are considered as imprudent use and contribute to the growing risks of AMR as reported in another study [29].

Our findings revealed that antibiotics were used therapeutically (65%) and anthelmintics prophylactically (56%) (Figure 1B), but the indications of use (Figure 2) showed that a higher proportion of anthelmintics were used (correctly) for parasitic infections compared to antibiotics which were used for growth promotion. Our study also revealed that antimicrobials were used mainly in the early phase of livestock production (Table S1), probably to prevent animal mortality which is more prevalent when the animal is younger [5,18] and to ensure the sustainability of production, which would serve as an income source to the household [6]. Our results show that the percentage of imprudent AMU was higher in semi-commercial and backyard systems. The high use of antimicrobials may contribute to the development of AMR [29] and higher chances of antimicrobial residues being found in food of animal origins as reported in other studies [25,57], therefore contributing risks to all in the agri-food value chain. Given that most enterprises raised livestock in the backyard and semi-commercial farming systems (Table 4), there is considerable reliance for Fijians on the semi-commercial and backyard farming systems despite the commercial farming system being the primary source of food in the agri-food chain, similarly demonstrated in other studies [6]. Therefore, further studies investigating antimicrobial residue levels in beef, milk, poultry meat and eggs are required, so that antimicrobial residue limits could be established and unnecessary exposure of antimicrobials to Fijians via the agri-food value chain could be minimised. Furthermore, understanding of the drivers for AMU practice in all farming systems over a prolonged duration is required so that necessary policies targeting behavioural interventions could be recommended for incorporation in AMS programmes.

There was a more prudent use of antimicrobials in commercial farming systems, and we presume that the imprudent use of antimicrobials in the backyard and semi-commercial farming system may be due to lack of accessibility to veterinary services, compromised farm biosecurity infrastructure and lack of knowledge and understanding on antimicrobials and AMR, which have also been reported in other studies [8,10,12,14,48]. Our evaluation of prescribing patterns in farming systems and enterprises revealed that veterinarians only prescribed antimicrobials in commercial farming systems and broiler only enterprises. We believe this is due to the easy access of in-house veterinarians in commercial enterprises. In addition, commercial broiler farmers are financially capable of accessing veterinary services considering the financial investments and mitigating financial losses that can result from compromised farm biosecurity [15,58]. Therefore, improving the veterinary services by recruiting more qualified veterinarians and creating training opportunities locally may improve veterinary services to all farmers resulting in POM-V (antibiotics) only being prescribed by veterinarians. This will also enable easy access of veterinarians by semi-commercial and backyard farming systems as well as other specialists and mixed enterprises. We presume improving veterinary services and engaging farmers and veterinarians in AMS programmes may improve and promote prudent use of antimicrobials.

Since the actual disease or ailments for which antimicrobials were administered was unknown, there may be chances of incorrect interpretation and classification of antimicrobials. However, this present study provides the framework for categorising antimicrobials and can be used in developing countries where information on AMU and AMR is scarce. We were unable to execute the logistic modelling for antibiotic use in different farming systems and anthelmintic use in different farming systems and enterprises due to lack of statistical association and unbalanced model due to unequal representation in all categories; therefore, we suggest equal representation to be considered in the inclusion criteria for future studies so that logistic modelling could be executed.

The high prevalence of imprudent use categorisation may also be due to the framework used, which was based on international standards. In the absence of the Fijian national medicine's directorate and legal classification of veterinary antimicrobials, using the UK, EU and OIE regulatory framework on veterinary antimicrobials use as a reference point was the best available choice. Since the UK and EU's food production systems and standards are a robust encompassing regulatory framework targeting every stage of the agri-food value chain, these standards enabled us to best evaluate AMU practice. Additionally, it was not possible to compare imprudent AMU practice in Fiji with other countries due to limited information regarding the categorisation of AMU practice. Nevertheless, despite vast differences in livestock production between developed and developing countries, AMR is a global threat to all countries. Therefore, the applicability of the international standards is well justified as it helped us establish the current situation on the AMU practice in Fiji.

4. Materials and Methods

4.1. Study Design and Data Collection

A cross-sectional survey was conducted between May and August 2019 on 236 livestock farms comprising 276 enterprises in Fiji's largest island's Western and Central divisions (Viti Levu). Livestock farmers and managers were recruited using a purposive and snowball sampling method. This study's design and data collection method was part of the principal survey published earlier [46]. The AMU dataset from the principal survey was used in this present study for the categorisation of AMU practice.

4.2. Data Management and Analysis

In the absence of a Fijian classification system for veterinary antimicrobials, a seven-step framework was developed using the VMD, BVA, ESVAC and OIE guidelines [36,41,56,59,60] to categorise the AMU (antibiotics and anthelmintics) into either prudent or imprudent use (Table 5). We used a similar approach used in the human health sector where imprudent use of antibiotics was defined as either using antibiotics without prescription, incomplete course and non-compliance to instructions of use [51].

All antimicrobials were classified according to their legal distribution category and market authorisation before being categorised into prudent and imprudent use. While antibiotics were classified as Prescription Only Medicine–Veterinarian (POM–V), anthelmintics were considered Prescription Only Medicine–Veterinarian, Pharmacist, Suitably Qualified Person (POM–VPS). In the current study, Suitably Qualified Persons were livestock officers (agriculture veterinary clinics staff and field officers and other non-government livestock officers) since they undertake para-veterinarian duties. The titles (livestock officer and para veterinarian) are used interchangeably in Fiji as there is no prescribed definition and competencies outlined in the current legislative framework.

Table 5. Framework for categorisation of antimicrobial use practice in livestock farms.

Step	Categories	Description	Procedure
1	Antimicrobial type	Verify if veterinary antimicrobial or human antimicrobial was used.	If veterinary antimicrobial was used, proceed to step 2A; if human antimicrobial was used, use was categorised as imprudent.
2	Antimicrobial class	Classify into class: antibiotics or anthelmintics.	Identify the class of the antimicrobial and then proceed to step 2B.
	Legal distribution categories of veterinary antimicrobials	Classify into either: • Authorised Veterinary Medicine–General Sales List (AVM–GSL), • Non-Food Animal Veterinarian, Pharmacist, a Suitably qualified person (NFA-VPS), • Prescription Only Medicine–Veterinarian, Pharmacist, Suitably Qualified Person (POM–VPS), • Prescription Only Medicine–Veterinarian (POM–V).	Identify and classify the veterinary antimicrobial if antibiotics were used and then proceed to step 3. (NOTE: all antibiotics used orally, parenterally and in-feed were classified as POM-V, anthelmintics as POM-VPS, and suitably qualified person (SQP) was a person trained and registered to sell veterinary medicine from agriculture store)
3	Prescriber	Verify the prescriber; • POM–V can only be prescribed by a Veterinarian, • POM–VPS (Veterinarian, Pharmacist, Suitably qualified person), • NFA–VPS (Veterinarian, Pharmacist, Suitably qualified person), • AVM–GSL (General, Self-prescribed, Other farmers).	If prescribed by the authorised prescriber, then proceed to step 4; if not, the use was categorised as imprudent. (NOTE: for steps 4 to 7, if prescribed not in accordance to step 3, then the use was categorised as imprudent at all steps)
4	Target species	Verify the species administered with approved target species according to market authorisation (MA) and label (authorised, unauthorised).	If deviated from the MA, label and prescribed by the veterinarian, or prescribed as per the MA, label and by the authorised prescriber, then proceed to step 5; if not, the use was categorised as imprudent.
5	Purpose of administration	Verify the purpose and establish the administration type: • Therapeutic, • Prophylactic, • Metaphylactic, • Growth promotion.	If prescribed for growth promotion, then the use was categorised as imprudent. If deviated from the MA, label and prescribed by the veterinarian, or prescribed as per the MA, label and by the authorised prescriber, then proceed to step 6; if not, the use was categorised as imprudent.
6	Cascade use	Verify the use of veterinary antimicrobial and prescriber.	If deviated from the MA, label and prescribed by the veterinarian in steps 4 and 5, then the use was categorised as cascade and then proceed to step 7; if not, the use was categorised as imprudent.
7	Farm AMU records	Verify if records were maintained.	If used under the cascade and maintained the antimicrobial use records, then the use was categorised as prudent; if not, the use was categorised as imprudent.

The seven-step framework included classifying veterinary antimicrobial use into 1. Antimicrobial type, 2. Antimicrobial class and legal distribution category of antimicrobial, 3. Prescriber of antimicrobials, 4. Target species (authorised as per label or market authorisation), 5. Purpose of administration (metaphylactic, prophylactic, therapeutic, and growth promotion), 6. Antibiotics used under the cascade and 7. Maintenance of farm AMU records (Table 5). All antimicrobials administered on different incidents were individually evaluated and categorised into prudent/imprudent use. Since only antibiotics can be prescribed in cascade, Step 6 was only applicable to antibiotics [36,49].

All AMU was categorised into prudent and imprudent use based on the intended therapeutic indications (purpose of use) of use reported by the farmer and farm manager (refer to Box 1).

Box 1. Therapeutic Indication Classification.

- All antimicrobials used for deworming were classified as used to treat/prevent parasitic infections.
- All antimicrobials used for mastitis and other infections were classified as used to treat/prevent bacterial infections.
- All antimicrobials used for other illnesses were classified as used to treat/prevent non-bacterial and parasite infections.
- All antimicrobials used for increasing outputs were classified as used for growth promotion.
- All antimicrobials used for gastrointestinal (diarrhoea), respiratory (flu), and viral illness were classified as symptomatic treatment.

All (n = 309 incidents) intended therapeutic indications of use were individually evaluated and categorised using the framework (Table 5) by the first author, a doctoral candidate and pharmacist with experience in agro security, food security and one health (XK), and verified by co-authors, an animal scientist with a doctoral degree and extensive experience in animal sciences (poultry)(CR), academic veterinarian and animal scientist with a doctoral degree with extensive experience in animal sciences (cattle) (PR) and one female academic pharmacist with a doctoral degree in medicine use and safety and extensive experience in qualitative research (RL).

Descriptive statistics were used to summarise the categorical variables; the pharmaceutical, pharmacological, clinical, legal category, therapeutic indications of use, prescribing pattern, source, and purpose of administration (herd/flock vs individual, prophylactic vs therapeutic, growth promotion). Subsequently, AMU practice (prudent/imprudent use) by the farming system and enterprise types were also summarised. The percentage of imprudent antibiotic and anthelmintic uses per enterprise (antibiotic used, n = 111 and anthelmintics used, n = 94) was calculated using the equation below.

$$\text{Percentage of imprudent use} = \frac{\text{Number of times AM used imprudently}}{\text{Total number of times AM used per enterprise}} \times 100 \qquad (1)$$

where AM is antimicrobial, and the number of times is incidents on which antimicrobials were used.

The percentage of imprudent use was binary coded into prudent (0% = prudent, coded 0) and imprudent (>0–100% = imprudent, coded 1) for antibiotics and anthelmintics.

4.3. Statistical Analysis

Data were analysed using IBM SPSS Software V27. The Pearson's chi-square or Fisher's exact test as appropriate was used to investigate the association between the dependent binary-coded variable (prudent = 0 and imprudent = 1) with the antimicrobial types used (antibiotic, anthelmintic), farming system and enterprise type.

To evaluate prescribing patterns, access and use of antimicrobials, the chi-square test or Fisher's exact test as appropriate was also used to investigate the association between antimicrobial types (antibiotic and anthelmintic) and the prescriber of antimicrobials, purpose of administration, and the indication of use (parasitic infections, bacterial infections, other illness, growth promotion, symptomatic treatment). Subsequently, the Fisher's exact test was also used to investigate the association between prescribers of antimicrobials with farming systems and the enterprise type. The veterinarian prescriber category was excluded from the analysis since they only prescribed in commercial broiler enterprises.

The enterprise type (independent variable) was fitted in the binary logistic regression model with the antibiotic use practice (outcome variable). The Hosmer and Lemeshow test was used to evaluate the model fit. From descriptive analysis, the enterprise with the highest percentage of prudent AMU was set as the reference category; thus, broiler enterprises were selected as the reference category in the modelling. The logistic modelling was not executed for antibiotic use practice in different farming systems due to unequal representation of sample, while the anthelmintic use practice modelling was also not performed due to lack of statistical association. For all analyses, $p< 0.05$ was considered statistically significant.

5. Conclusions

This present study suggests that anthelmintics and antibiotics were used imprudently in all enterprises. Imprudent AMU was more common in the backyard and semi-commercial enterprises compared to commercial enterprises. Policies promoting the prudent use of antimicrobials in Fiji should focus on smaller livestock production systems and mixed enterprises. Transformation and improvement of policies on AMU, improving veterinary services and regulating the access, prescribing, and dispensation of antimicrobials is warranted to promote prudent use of antimicrobials at the country level. Concurrently, follow-up studies to understand AMU drivers in Fijian food production systems is essential as information obtained will enable the development of targeted behavioural interventions to promote prudent AMU in livestock production systems.

Supplementary Materials: The following supporting information can be downloaded at: https://www.mdpi.com/article/10.3390/antibiotics11030294/s1, Table S1: Characteristics of 309 antimicrobials used in 236 livestock farms comprising of 276, enterprises located in Viti Levu, Fiji.

Author Contributions: X.K. contributed to conceptualisation, methodology, software, data collection, validation, project administrations, formal analysis, interpretation, writing—original draft preparation, writing—review and editing; C.R., P.R. and R.L. contributed to conceptualisation, methodology, analysis, reviewing and editing, interpretation, and supervision. All authors have read and agreed to the published version of the manuscript.

Funding: This research received no external funding.

Institutional Review Board Statement: Ethical approval for this study was obtained from the University of Reading's School of Agriculture, Policy and Development Ethical Committee (Ref #: 00772P).

Informed Consent Statement: Informed consent was obtained from all subjects involved in the study.

Data Availability Statement: The data presented in this study are available on request from the corresponding author.

Acknowledgments: We would like to thank the Animal Health and Production division team of the Ministry of Agriculture, Fiji, who provided field support, livestock farmers and farm managers who participated in this study.

Conflicts of Interest: The authors declare no conflict of interest.

References

1. WHO. Antimicrobial Resistance. Available online: http://www.who.int/en/news-room/fact-sheets/detail/antimicrobial-resistance (accessed on 1 December 2021).
2. OIE. Antimicrobial Resistance (AMR). Available online: http://www.oie.int/en/for-the-media/amr/ (accessed on 10 December 2021).

3. WHO; FAO; OIE. Taking a Multisectoral, One Health Approach: A Tripartite Guide to Addressing Zoonotic Diseases in Countries. Available online: http://www.fao.org/ag/againfo/resources/en/publications/TZG/TZG.htm (accessed on 1 December 2021).
4. Davidova, S.; Agunos, A.; Fredriksson, L.; Bailey, A. Subsistence and semi-subsistence farming in selected EU new member states. *Agric. Econ.* **2009**, *40*, 733–744. [CrossRef]
5. Sultana, R.; Nahar, N.; Rimi, N.A.; Azad, S.; Islam, M.S.; Gurley, E.S.; Luby, S.P. Backyard poultry raising in Bangladesh: A valued resource for the villagers and a setting for zoonotic transmission of avian influenza. A qualitative study. *Rural. Remote Health* **2012**, *12*, 1927. [CrossRef] [PubMed]
6. Rapsomanikis, G. The Economic Lives of Smallholder Farmers. Available online: http://www.fao.org/3/i5251e/i5251e.pdf (accessed on 1 December 2021).
7. Cao, Y.; Li, D. Impact of increased demand for animal protein products in Asian countries: Implications on global food security. *Anim. Front.* **2013**, *3*, 48–55. [CrossRef]
8. Henriksen, J.; Rota, A. Commercialization of livestock production; towards a profitable and market-oriented smallholder livestock production system. *Livest. Res. Rural. Dev.* **2013**, *26*.
9. Henchion, M.; Hayes, M.; Mullen, A.; Fenelon, M.; Tiwari, B. Future Protein Supply and Demand: Strategies and Factors Influencing a Sustainable Equilibrium. *Foods* **2017**, *6*, 53. [CrossRef]
10. Malusi, N.; Falowo, A.B.; Idamokoro, E.M. Herd dynamics, production and marketing constraints in the commercialization of cattle across Nguni Cattle Project beneficiaries in Eastern Cape, South Africa. *Pastoralism* **2021**, *11*, 1–12. [CrossRef]
11. Kahan, D. Market Oriented Farming. Available online: www.fao.org/3/a-i3227e.pdf (accessed on 1 December 2021).
12. Mariyono, J. Stepping up from subsistence to commercial intensive farming to enhance welfare of farmer households in Indonesia. *Asia Pac. Policy Stud.* **2019**, *6*, 246–265. [CrossRef]
13. Keutchatang, F.D.P.T.; Ntsama, I.S.B.; Nama, G.M.; Kansci, G. Biosecurity Practices and Characteristics of Poultry Farms in Three Regions of Cameroon. *J. World's Poult. Res.* **2021**, *11*, 64–72. [CrossRef]
14. Moya, S.; Chan, K.W.; Hinchliffe, S.; Buller, H.; Espluga, J.; Benavides, B.; Diéguez, F.J.; Yus, E.; Ciaravino, G.; Casal, J. Influence on the implementation of biosecurity measures in dairy cattle farms: Communication between veterinarians and dairy farmers. *Prev. Vet. Med.* **2021**, *190*, 105329. [CrossRef]
15. Adeyonu, A.G.; Otunaiya, A.O.; Oyawoye, E.O.; Okeniyi, F.A. Risk perceptions and risk management strategies among poultry farmers in south-west Nigeria. *Cogent Soc. Sci.* **2021**, *7*, 1891719. [CrossRef]
16. Hosain, M.Z.; Kabir, S.M.L.; Kamal, M.M. Antimicrobial uses for livestock production in developing countries. *Vet. World* **2021**, *14*, 210–221. [CrossRef] [PubMed]
17. Kruse, A.B.; Nielsen, L.R.; Alban, L. Herd typologies based on multivariate analysis of biosecurity, productivity, antimicrobial and vaccine use data from Danish sow herds. *Prev. Vet. Med.* **2018**, *181*, 104487. [CrossRef] [PubMed]
18. Hoelzer, K.; Bielke, L.; Blake, D.P.; Cox, E.; Cutting, S.M.; Devriendt, B.; Erlacher-Vindel, E.; Goossens, E.; Karaca, K.; Lemiere, S.; et al. Vaccines as alternatives to antibiotics for food producing animals. Part 1: Challenges and needs. *Vet. Res.* **2018**, *49*, 64. [CrossRef] [PubMed]
19. Zhanteng, S.; Hongting, Z.; Zhiming, X.; Decheng, S. Residue accumulation, distribution, and withdrawal period of sulfamethazine and N-acetylsulfamethazine in poultry waste from broilers. *Chemosphere* **2021**, *278*, 130420. [CrossRef]
20. Tzamaloukas, O.; Neofytou, M.C.; Simitzis, P.E. Application of Olive By-Products in Livestock with Emphasis on Small Ruminants: Implications on Rumen Function, Growth Performance, Milk and Meat Quality. *Animals* **2021**, *11*, 531. [CrossRef]
21. Abebe, B.A.; Chane Teferi, S. Ethnobotanical Study of Medicinal Plants Used to Treat Human and Livestock Ailments in Hulet Eju Enese Woreda, East Gojjam Zone of Amhara Region, Ethiopia. *Evid. Based Complementary Altern. Med.* **2021**, *2021*, 1–11. [CrossRef]
22. Van Cuong, N.; Nhung, N.T.; Nghia, N.H.; Mai Hoa, N.T.; Trung, N.V.; Thwaites, G.; Carrique-Mas, J. Antimicrobial Consumption in Medicated Feeds in Vietnamese Pig and Poultry Production. *Ecohealth* **2016**, *13*, 490–498. [CrossRef]
23. Edwards, L.E.; Hemsworth, P.H. The impact of management, husbandry and stockperson decisions on the welfare of laying hens in Australia. *Anim. Prod. Sci.* **2021**, *61*, 944–967. [CrossRef]
24. Ayukekbong, J.A.; Ntemgwa, M.; Atabe, A.N. The threat of antimicrobial resistance in developing countries: Causes and control strategies. *Antimicrob. Resist. Infect. Control.* **2017**, *6*, 1–8. [CrossRef]
25. Bamidele Falowo, A.; Festus Akimoladun, O. Veterinary Drug Residues in Meat and Meat Products: Occurrence, Detection and Implications. *Vet. Med. Pharm.* **2019**, *3*, 194. [CrossRef]
26. Raasch, S.; Postma, M.; Dewulf, J.; Stärk, K.D.C.; grosse Beilage, E.J.P.H.M. Association between antimicrobial usage, biosecurity measures as well as farm performance in German farrow-to-finish farms. *Porc. Health Manag.* **2018**, *4*, 30. [CrossRef] [PubMed]
27. Murphy, C.P.; Carson, C.; Smith, B.A.; Chapman, B.; Marrotte, J.; McCann, M.; Primeau, C.; Sharma, P.; Parmley, E.J. Factors potentially linked with the occurrence of antimicrobial resistance in selected bacteria from cattle, chickens and pigs: A scoping review of publications for use in modelling of antimicrobial resistance (IAM.AMR Project). *Zoonoses Public Health* **2018**, *65*, 957–971. [CrossRef] [PubMed]
28. Rega, M.; Carmosino, I.; Bonilauri, P.; Frascolla, V.; Vismarra, A.; Bacci, C. Prevalence of ESβL, AmpC and Colistin-Resistant E. coli in Meat: A Comparison between Pork and Wild Boar. *Microorganisms* **2021**, *9*, 214. [CrossRef] [PubMed]
29. Ström, G.; Boqvist, S.; Albihn, A.; Fernström, L.L.; Andersson Djurfeldt, A.; Sokerya, S.; Sothyra, T.; Magnusson, U. Antimicrobials in small-scale urban pig farming in a lower middle-income country—Arbitrary use and high resistance levels. *Antimicrob. Resist. Infect. Control.* **2018**, *7*, 35. [CrossRef]

30. EU. Guidelines for the Prudent Use of Antimicrobials in Veterinary Medicine. Available online: https://ec.europa.eu/health/sites/health/files/antimicrobial_resistance/docs/2015_prudent_use_guidelines_en.pdf (accessed on 1 August 2021).
31. EMA. *Categorisation of Antibiotics in the European Union. Categorisation of Antibiotics Used in Animals Promotes Responsible Use to Protect Public and Animal Health*; EMA: Amsterdam, The Netherlands, 2019.
32. WHO. *Critically Important Antimicrobials for Human Medicine—6th Revision*; World Health Organization: Geneva, Switzerland, 2019.
33. OIE. *OIE List of Antimicrobials of Veterinary Importance*; OIE: Paris, France, 2007.
34. VMD. *Code of Practice on the Responsible Use of Animal Medicines on the Farm*; VMD: Addlestone, UK, 2014.
35. RUMA. Measuring Antibiotic Use—Dairy, Beef, Poultry. Available online: https://www.ruma.org.uk/measuring-antibiotic-use/ (accessed on 15 November 2021).
36. VMD. *The Cascade: Prescribing Unauthorised Medicines*; VMD: Addlestone, UK, 2015.
37. Loftus, M.; Stewardson, A.J.; Naidu, R.; Coghlan, B.; Jenney, A.; Kepas, J.; Lavu, E.; Munamua, A.; Peel, T.; Sahai, V.; et al. Antimicrobial resistance in the Pacific Island countries and territories. *BMJ Glob. Health* **2020**, *5*, e002418. [CrossRef]
38. Goverment of the Republic Fiji. *Veterinary Surgeons Act 1956*; Goverment of the Republic Fiji: Suva, Fiji, 2012.
39. Goverment of the Republic Fiji. *Medicinal Products Act 2011*; Goverment of the Republic Fiji: Suva, Fiji, 2011.
40. Goverment of the Republic Fiji. *Food Safety Reulations 2009*; Goverment of the Republic Fiji: Suva, Fiji, 2019.
41. BVA. *Good Practice Guide on Veterinary Medicines*; BVA: London, UK, 2007.
42. BVA. *Responsible Use of Antimicrobials in Veterinary Practice: The 7 Point Plan*; BVA: London, UK, 2019.
43. Bennani, H.; Cornelsen, L.; Stärk, K.D.C.; Häsler, B. Characterisation and mapping of the surveillance system for antimicrobial resistance and antimicrobial use in the United Kingdom. *Vet. Rec.* **2021**, *188*. [CrossRef]
44. VMD. *Product Information Database*; VMD: Addlestone, UK, 2020.
45. APVMA. Australian Pesticides and Veterinary Medicines Authority. Available online: https://apvma.gov.au/ (accessed on 1 December 2021).
46. Khan, X.; Rymer, C.; Ray, P.; Lim, R. Quantification of antimicrobial use in Fijian livestock farms. *One Health* **2021**, *13*, 100326. [CrossRef]
47. Phares, C.A.; Danquah, A.; Atiah, K.; Agyei, F.K.; Michael, O.-T. Antibiotics utilization and farmers' knowledge of its effects on soil ecosystem in the coastal drylands of Ghana. *PLoS ONE* **2020**, *15*, e0228777. [CrossRef]
48. Sadiq, M.B.; Syed-Hussain, S.S.; Ramanoon, S.Z.; Saharee, A.A.; Ahmad, N.I.; Mohd Zin, N.; Khalid, S.F.; Naseeha, D.S.; Syahirah, A.A.; Mansor, R. Knowledge, attitude and perception regarding antimicrobial resistance and usage among ruminant farmers in Selangor, Malaysia. *Prev. Vet. Med.* **2018**, *156*, 76–83. [CrossRef]
49. VMD. *Responsible Antibiotic Use under the Cascade*; VMD: Addlestone, UK, 2014.
50. Casewell, M.; Friis, C.; Marco, E.; McMullin, P.; Phillips, I. The European ban on growth-promoting antibiotics and emerging consequences for human and animal health. *J. Antimicrob. Chemoth.* **2003**, *52*, 159–161. [CrossRef]
51. Afari-Asiedu, S.; Oppong, F.B.; Tostmann, A.; Ali Abdulai, M.; Boamah-Kaali, E.; Gyaase, S.; Agyei, O.; Kinsman, J.; Hulscher, M.; Wertheim, H.F.L.; et al. Determinants of Inappropriate Antibiotics Use in Rural Central Ghana Using a Mixed Methods Approach. *Front. Public Health* **2020**, *8*, 90. [CrossRef] [PubMed]
52. Ting, S.; Pereira, A.; Alves, A.d.J.; Fernandes, S.; Soares, C.d.C.; Soares, F.J.; Henrique, O.d.C.; Davis, S.; Yan, J.; Francis, J.R.; et al. Antimicrobial Use in Animals in Timor-Leste Based on Veterinary Antimicrobial Imports between 2016 and 2019. *Antibiotics* **2021**, *10*, 426. [CrossRef] [PubMed]
53. OIE. *Terrestrial Animal Health Code Chapter 6.10*; OIE: Paris, France, 2017.
54. Roesel, K.; Dohoo, I.; Baumann, M.; Dione, M.; Grace, D.; Clausen, P.-H. Prevalence and risk factors for gastrointestinal parasites in small-scale pig enterprises in Central and Eastern Uganda. *Parasitol. Res.* **2017**, *116*, 335–345. [CrossRef] [PubMed]
55. Laanen, M.; Maes, D.; Hendriksen, C.; Gelaude, P.; De Vliegher, S.; Rosseel, Y.; Dewulf, J. Pig, cattle and poultry farmers with a known interest in research have comparable perspectives on disease prevention and on-farm biosecurity. *Prev. Vet. Med.* **2014**, *115*, 1–9. [CrossRef] [PubMed]
56. EMA. Guidance on Collection and Provision of National Data on Antimicrobial Use by Animal Species/Categories 2018. Available online: https://www.ema.europa.eu/en/documents/scientific-guideline/guidance-collection-provision-national-data-antimicrobial-use-animal-species/categories_en.pdf (accessed on 10 November 2021).
57. Adesiyun, A.; Offiah, N.; Lashley, V.; Seepersadsingh, N.; Rodrigo, S.; Georges, K. Prevalence of antimicrobial residues in table eggs in Trinidad. *J. Food Prot.* **2005**, *68*, 1501–1505. [CrossRef]
58. Caudell, M.A.; Dorado-Garcia, A.; Eckford, S.; Creese, C.; Byarugaba, D.K.; Afakye, K.; Chansa-Kabali, T.; Fasina, F.O.; Kabali, E.; Kiambi, S.; et al. Towards a bottom-up understanding of antimicrobial use and resistance on the farm: A knowledge, attitudes, and practices survey across livestock systems in five African countries. *PLoS ONE* **2020**, *15*, e0220274. [CrossRef] [PubMed]
59. Teale, C.; Moulin, G. Prudent use guidelines: A review of existing veterinary guidelines. *Rev. Sci. Tech. OIE* **2012**, *31*, 343. [CrossRef]
60. OIE. OIE Standards, Guidelines and Resolution on Antimicrobial Resistance and the Use of Antimicrobial Agents. Available online: https://web.oie.int/delegateweb/eng/ebook/AF-book-AMR-ANG_FULL.pdf?WAHISPHPSESSID=03152ead00d06990fa9066b7b71fcabc (accessed on 1 December 2021).

MDPI
St. Alban-Anlage 66
4052 Basel
Switzerland
Tel. +41 61 683 77 34
Fax +41 61 302 89 18
www.mdpi.com

Antibiotics Editorial Office
E-mail: antibiotics@mdpi.com
www.mdpi.com/journal/antibiotics

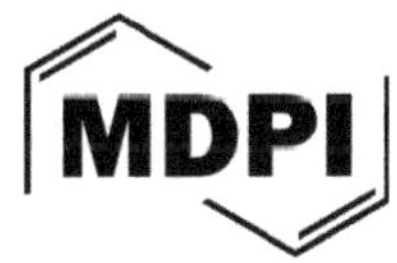

www.ingramcontent.com/pod-product-compliance
Lightning Source LLC
LaVergne TN
LVHW071546170726
843515LV00008B/2222